Second Edition

PHARMACOTHERAPY

Casebook

a patient-focused approach

Second Edition

PHARMACOTHERAPY

Casebook

a patient-focused approach

Edited by
Terry L. Schwinghammer, PharmD, FCCP, FASHP, BCPS
Associate Professor, Department of Pharmaceutical Sciences
School of Pharmacy, University of Pittsburgh
Pittsburgh, Pennsylvania

with

Joseph T. DiPiro, PharmD, FCCP
Panoz Professor, College of Pharmacy, Head, Department of Clinical
and Administrative Sciences,
University of Georgia College of Pharmacy
Clinical Professor of Surgery, Medical College of Georgia
Augusta, Georgia

Robert L. Talbert, PharmD, FCCP, BCPS
Professor and Division Head, College of Pharmacy
University of Texas at Austin
Professor, Departments of Medicine and Pharmacology
University of Texas Health Science Center at San Antonio
San Antonio, Texas

Gary C. Yee, PharmD, FCCP
Professor and Chair, Department of Pharmacy Practice,
College of Pharmacy,
University of Nebraska Medical Center
Omaha, Nebraska

Gary R. Matzke, PharmD, FCP, FCCP
Professor of Pharmaceutical Sciences and Medicine
Schools of Pharmacy and Medicine
Center for Clinical Pharmacology,
University of Pittsburgh
Pittsburgh, Pennsylvania

Barbara G. Wells, PharmD, FASHP, FCCP, BCPP
Professor and Dean, Idaho State University College of Pharmacy
Pocatello, Idaho

L. Michael Posey, RPh
President
Pharmacy Editorial and News Services
Athens, Georgia

APPLETON & LANGE
Stamford, Connecticut

www.appletonlange.com

99 00 01 02 / 10 9 8 7 6 5 4 3 2 1

Executive Editor: Cheryl L. Mehalik
Development Editor: Kathleen McCullough
Senior Production Editor: Jeanmarie Roche
Art Manager: Eve Siegel
Production Service: Rainbow Graphics, LLC
Designer: Mary Skudlarek

PRINTED IN THE UNITED STATES OF AMERICA

Marie A. Abate, PharmD, Professor and Associate Chair of Clinical Pharmacy; Director of the West Virginia Drug Information Center, West Virginia University School of Pharmacy, Morgantown, West Virginia

Cesar Alaniz, PharmD, Clinical Assistant Professor, University of Michigan College of Pharmacy; Clinical Pharmacist, University of Michigan Hospitals, Ann Arbor, Michigan

Peter L. Anderson, PharmD, Fellow in Antiviral Pharmacology, Department of Clinical Pharmacology, College of Pharmacy, University of Minnesota, Minneapolis, Minnesota

Edward P. Armstrong, PharmD, BCPS, FASHP, Associate Professor, Department of Pharmacy Practice and Science, University of Arizona College of Pharmacy, Tucson, Arizona

Tana R. Bagby, PharmD, Adjunct Assistant Clinical Professor, Department of Pharmacy Practice, University of Georgia College of Pharmacy, Athens, Georgia

Laura A. Bartels, PharmD, Assistant Professor of Pharmacy, Department of Pharmacy Practice, Albany College of Pharmacy, Union University, Albany, New York

Leslie L. Barton, MD, Professor of Pediatrics and Pediatric Infectious Diseases; Director, Pediatric Residency Program, Department of Pediatrics, University of Arizona School of Medicine, Tucson, Arizona

Susan D. Bear, BS, PharmD, Clinical Specialist, Department of Pharmacy, University Hospital, Charlotte, North Carolina

Karen Beauchamp, BPharm, RPh, Pharmacy Practice Resident, Southwest Washington Medical Center, Vancouver, Washington

Amy J. Becker, PharmD, Hematology-Oncology Clinical Pharmacy Specialist, University of Iowa Hospitals & Clinics, Iowa City, Iowa

Reina Bendayan, PharmD, Assistant Professor, Faculty of Pharmacy, University of Toronto, Toronto, Ontario, Canada

William H. Benefield, Jr., PharmD, BCPP, FASCP, Clinical Assistant Professor of Pharmacy, University of Texas at Austin; Clinical Assistant Professor of Pharmacology, University of Texas Health Sciences Center at San Antonio; Clinical Pharmacologist, San Antonio State School, San Antonio, Texas

Brian K. Bond, PharmD, was Doctor of Pharmacy Candidate, West Virginia University School of Pharmacy, Morgantown, West Virginia at the time of this writing.

Karim A. Calis, PharmD, MPH, BCPS, BCNSP, FASHP, Coordinator, Drug Information Service and Endocrinology Clinical Pharmacy Specialist, Warren G. Magnuson Clinical Center, National Institutes of Health, Bethesda, Maryland; Associate Clinical Professor, Medical College of Virginia, Virginia Commonwealth University, Richmond, Virginia; Clinical Associate Professor, University of Maryland, Baltimore, Maryland

Bruce R. Canaday, PharmD, BCPS, FASHP, FAPhA, Clinical Professor, University of North Carolina Schools of Pharmacy and Medicine; Pharmacotherapy Director, Coastal Area Health Education Center, Wilmington, North Carolina

Bruce C. Carlstedt, PhD, Professor, Department of Pharmacy Practice, Purdue University School of Pharmacy and Pharmacal Sciences, West Lafayette, Indiana

Daniel T. Casto, PharmD, FCCP, was Associate Professor, College of Pharmacy, University of Texas at Austin and Department of Pediatrics and Pharmacology, University of Texas Health Science Center, San Antonio, Texas at the time of this writing

Marie A. Chisholm, PharmD, Assistant Professor, Department of Pharmacy Practice, University of Georgia College of Pharmacy, Athens, Georgia

Susan Chuck, PharmD, Infectious Diseases Fellow, Department of Pharmacy Practice, University of Illinois at Chicago College of Pharmacy, Chicago, Illinois

Lawrence J. Cohen, PharmD, BCPP, FASHP, FCCP, Professor of Pharmacy, Psychiatry, and Behavioral Sciences, University of Oklahoma Health Sciences Center, Oklahoma City, Oklahoma

Julie A. Cold, PharmD, BCPP, Assistant Professor, Department of Pharmacy Practice, Mercer University Southern School of Pharmacy, Atlanta, Georgia

James D. Coyle, PharmD, Assistant Professor, Department of Pharmacy Practice and Administration, Ohio State University College of Pharmacy, Columbus, Ohio

Brian L. Crabtree, PharmD, BCPP, Associate Professor of Clinical Pharmacy Practice, Department of Clinical Pharmacy Practice, University of Mississippi School of Pharmacy, Jackson, Mississippi

Simon Cronin, PharmD, MS, Clinical Assistant Professor, University of Michigan School of Pharmacy, Ann Arbor, Michigan

Terri G. Davidson, PharmD, Chief Executive Officer, Clinical Pharmacy Associates, Inc.; Senior Medical Writer, Cortex Communications, Inc., Tucker, Georgia

Andrea Eggert, PharmD, BCPP, Was Clinical Assistant Professor of Pharmacy, Department of Pharmacy Practice and Administration, University of Texas at Austin at the time of this writing

Victor A. Elsberry, PharmD, BCNSP, Assistant Professor, Department of Pharmacy Practice and Science, University of Arizona College of Pharmacy, Tucson, Arizona

Brian L. Erstad, PharmD, FASHP, FCCM, Associate Professor, Department of Pharmacy Practice and Science, University of Arizona College of Pharmacy, Tucson, Arizona

Charles W. Fetrow, PharmD, Clinical Pharmacist, Department of Pharmacy Services, St. Francis Medical Center, Pittsburgh, Pennsylvania

John O. Fleming, MD, Associate Professor, Department of Neurology, University of Wisconsin, Madison, Wisconsin

Courtney V. Fletcher, PharmD, Professor, Department of Clinical Pharmacology, College of Pharmacy, University of Minnesota, Minneapolis, Minnesota

Rex W. Force, PharmD, BCPS, Assistant Professor, Departments of Pharmacy Practice and Family Medicine, Idaho State University, Pocatello, Idaho

Carla B. Frye, PharmD, BCPS, Associate Professor, Department of Pharmacy Practice, Butler University College of Pharmacy and Health Sciences, Indianapolis, Indiana

Ashesh J. Gandhi, PharmD, Clinical Cardiology Specialist, Department of Pharmacy, Allegheny University Hospitals—Hahnemann, Philadelphia, Pennsylvania

Marie E. Gardner, PharmD, Clinical Associate Professor, Department of Pharmacy Practice and Science, University of Arizona College of Pharmacy, Tucson, Arizona

Barry E. Gidal, PharmD, Associate Professor, School of Pharmacy and Department of Neurology, University of Wisconsin, Madison, Wisconsin

Patrick P. Gleason, PharmD, BCPS, Assistant Professor, Department of Pharmaceutical Sciences; Assistant Professor of Medicine, Department of General Internal Medicine, University of Pittsburgh Schools of Pharmacy and Medicine, Pittsburgh, Pennsylvania

Barry R. Goldspiel, PharmD, FASHP, Oncology Clinical Pharmacy Specialist, Pharmacy Department, National Institutes of Health Clinical Center, Bethesda, Maryland

Jean-Venable (Kelly) R. Goode, PharmD, BCPS, Assistant Professor, Department of Pharmacy, Virginia Commonwealth University School of Pharmacy, Richmond, Virginia

Elizabeth S. Gray, PharmD, Assistant Professor, Department of Pharmacy, Virginia Commonwealth University School of Pharmacy, Richmond, Virginia

Paige Robbins Gross, RPh, Staff Pharmacist, University of Pittsburgh Medical Center, Pittsburgh, Pennsylvania

Amy J. Guenette, PharmD, BCPS, Clinical Coordinator, Department of Pharmacy, Wausau Hospital, Wausau, Wisconsin

Wayne P. Gulliver, MD, FRCPC, Associate Professor of Medicine (Dermatology), Faculty of Medicine, Memorial University of Newfoundland, St. John's, Newfoundland, Canada

John G. Gums, PharmD, Professor, Department of Pharmacy Practice, Community Health and Family Medicine, University of Florida College of Pharmacy, Gainesville, Florida

R. Donald Harvey III, PharmD, BCPS, Hematology/Oncology Resident, University of North Carolina at Chapel Hill, Chapel Hill, North Carolina

Amy M. Heck, PharmD, Specialized Resident in Drug Information and Pharmacotherapy, Warren G. Magnuson Clinical Center, National Institutes of Health, Bethesda, Maryland

Richard N. Herrier, PharmD, Assistant Professor, Department of Pharmacy Practice and Science, University of Arizona College of Pharmacy, Tucson, Arizona

Mary M. Hess, PharmD, Assistant Professor, Department of Pharmacy and Therapeutics, University of Pittsburgh School of Pharmacy; Critical Care Specialist, Department of Pharmacy, University of Pittsburgh Medical Center, Pittsburgh, Pennsylvania

Kimberly Heying, PharmD, Oncology Pharmacy Resident, Department of Pharmacy Services, University Hospital, Cincinnati, Ohio

Catherine A. Heyneman, PharmD, MS, Assistant Professor, Department of Pharmacy Practice, Idaho State University College of Pharmacy, Pocatello, Idaho

Mark T. Holdsworth, PharmD, BCPS, Associate Professor, University of New Mexico School of Pharmacy, Albuquerque, New Mexico

Jon D. Horton, PharmD, Clinical Pharmacist, Department of Pharmacy, York Health System, York, Pennsylvania

Denise L. Howrie, PharmD, Associate Professor of Pharmacy and Pediatrics, Schools of Pharmacy and Medicine, University of Pittsburgh; Clinical Coordinator, Pharmacy Services, Children's Hospital of Pittsburgh, Pittsburgh, Pennsylvania

Jonathan P. Hubbard, DO, Resident Physician, Department of Family Medicine, Idaho State University, Pocatello, Idaho

Timothy J. Ives, PharmD, MPH, FCCP, BCPS, Associate Professor, Department of Family Medicine, University of North Carolina, Chapel Hill, North Carolina

Linda A. Jaber, PharmD, Associate Professor, Department of Pharmacy Practice, Wayne State University College of Pharmacy, Detroit, Michigan

Mark W. Jackson, MD, FACG, Private Practice in Gastroenterology, Knoxville, Tennessee

Scott Jacober, DO, CDE, Associate Professor of Medicine, Department of Internal Medicine, Division of Endocrinology, Metabolism and Hypertension, Wayne State University School of Medicine, Detroit, Michigan

Michael W. Jann, PharmD, FCP, FCCP, Professor of Pharmacy Practice, Mercer University Southern School of Pharmacy, Atlanta, Georgia

Douglas D. Janson, PharmD, BCNSP, Clinical Pharmacy Specialist in Nutrition Support, University of Pittsburgh Medical Center; Assistant Professor, Department of Pharmacy and Therapeutics, University of Pittsburgh School of Pharmacy, Pittsburgh, Pennsylvania

Donna M. Jermain, PharmD, BCPP, Assistant Professor, Department of Medicine and Psychiatry, Texas A&M University Health Sciences Center; Coordinator of Pharmacy Research and Education, Department of Pharmacy, Scott & White Memorial Hospital, Temple, Texas

Kjel A. Johnson, PharmD, BCPS, Clinical Specialist, Health America of Pennsylvania, Inc.; Assistant Professor, Department of Pharmaceutical Sciences, University of Pittsburgh School of Pharmacy, Pittsburgh, Pennsylvania

Steven V. Johnson, PharmD, BCPS, Clinical Instructor, University of Minnesota College of Pharmacy, Minneapolis; Clinical Pharmacy Specialist/Manager, Regions Hospital, St. Paul, Minnesota

Melanie S. Joy, PharmD, Clinical Instructor and Research Coordinator, School of Medicine, Division of Nephrology and Hypertension, University of North Carolina, Chapel Hill, North Carolina

Barbara L. Kaltenbach, PharmD, Pharmacy Practice Resident, Department of Pharmacy, University of Iowa Hospitals and Clinics, Iowa City, Iowa

Daniel T. Kennedy, PharmD, BCPS, Assistant Professor, Department of Pharmacy, Virginia Commonwealth University School of Pharmacy, Richmond, Virginia

Tien T. Kiat-Winarko, PharmD, BSc, Assistant Professor of Clinical Pharmacy, University of Southern California School of Pharmacy; Director of Pharmacy, USC Pharmacy at the Doheny Eye Institute, Los Angeles, California

Aaron D. Killian, PharmD, BCPS, Assistant Professor, Department of Pharmacy Practice, School of Pharmacy, Texas Tech University Health Sciences Center at Amarillo, Amarillo, Texas

Krista M. King, PharmD, BCOP, Clinical Pharmacy Specialist in Lymphoma, Division of Pharmacy, University of Texas MD Anderson Cancer Center, Houston, Texas

Cynthia K. Kirkwood, PharmD, Assistant Professor, Department of Pharmacy, Virginia Commonwealth University School of Pharmacy, Richmond, Virginia

Daren L. Knoell, PharmD, Assistant Professor, Department of Pharmacy Practice and Administration, Ohio State University College of Pharmacy, Columbus, Ohio

Cynthia P. Koh-Knox, PharmD, Pharmacy Practice Resident, Clarian Health Partners—Methodist Hospital, Indianapolis, Indiana

Robert J. Kuhn, PharmD, Professor and Vice Chair of Ambulatory Services, Division of Pharmacy Practice and Science, University of Kentucky College of Pharmacy, Lexington, Kentucky

Lyle K. Laird, PharmD, BCPP, Assistant Professor, Department of Pharmacy Practice, University of Colorado School of Pharmacy, Denver, Colorado

Nancy P. Lam, PharmD, BCPS, Assistant Professor, Colleges of Pharmacy and Medicine, and Pharmacotherapist, Digestive and Liver Diseases, University of Illinois at Chicago, Chicago, Illinois

Rebecca M. Law, PharmD, Associate Professor, School of Pharmacy, Memorial University of Newfoundland, St. John's, Newfoundland, Canada

Cara Lawless-Liday, PharmD, Assistant Professor, Department of Pharmacy Practice and Administrative Sciences, College of Pharmacy, Idaho State University, Pocatello, Idaho

W. Greg Leader, PharmD, Assistant Professor, Department of Clinical Pharmacy, West Virginia University School of Pharmacy, Morgantown, West Virginia

Mary Lee, PharmD, BCPS, FCCP, Associate Dean and Professor, Department of Pharmacy Practice, Chicago College of Pharmacy, Downer's Grove, Illinois

Christine A. Lesch, PharmD, Infectious Diseases Research Fellow, Department of Pharmacy Practice, University of Illinois at Chicago College of Pharmacy, Chicago, Illinois

James S. Lewis II, PharmD, Pharmacy Practice Resident, Department of Pharmacy, Southwest Washington Medical Center, Vancouver, Washington

Celeste C. Lindley, PharmD, MS, FASHP, FCCP, BCPS, Associate Professor, School of Pharmacy, University of North Carolina at Chapel Hill, Chapel Hill, North Carolina

Sherry Luedtke, PharmD, Assistant Professor, Department of Pharmacy Practice, Texas Tech University Health Sciences Center School of Pharmacy, Amarillo, Texas

Mark S. Luer, PharmD, Assistant Professor, Department of Pharmacy Practice, College of Pharmacy, University of Arkansas for Medical Sciences, Little Rock, Arkansas

Steven J. Martin, PharmD, BCPS, Assistant Professor, Department of Pharmacy Practice, University of Toledo College of Pharmacy, Toledo, Ohio

Barbara J. Mason, PharmD, Professor of Pharmacy, Department of Pharmacy Practice, Idaho State University College of Pharmacy; Ambulatory Care Clinical Pharmacist, Veterans Affairs Medical Center, Boise, Idaho

Rae Ann Maxwell, RPh, PhD, Director of Pharmacy, Western Psychiatric Institute and Clinic; Director of the Investigational Drug Service, University of Pittsburgh Medical Center; Assistant Professor, Department of Pharmacy and Therapeutics, University of Pittsburgh School of Pharmacy, Pittsburgh, Pennsylvania

James W. McAuley, RPh, PhD, Assistant Professor, Departments of Pharmacy Practice and Neurology, Ohio State University, Columbus, Ohio

Alex K. McDonald, PharmD, Specialty Resident in Drug Information, University of North Carolina and Glaxo-Wellcome Inc., Chapel Hill, North Carolina

Elaine McGhee, MD, Clinical Assistant Professor, Department of Pediatrics, University of Pittsburgh School of Medicine, Pittsburgh, Pennsylvania

William McGhee, PharmD, Clinical Pharmacist, Children's Hospital of Pittsburgh; Assistant Professor, Department of Pharmacy and Therapeutics, University of Pittsburgh School of Pharmacy, Pittsburgh, Pennsylvania

Margaret E. McGuinness, PharmD, Assistant Professor of Pharmacy Practice, Oregon State University College of Pharmacy; Clinical Pharmacist—Internal Medicine and Oncology, Portland Veterans Affairs Medical Center, Portland, Oregon

Renee-Claude Mercier, PharmD, Assistant Professor of Pharmacy, University of New Mexico College of Pharmacy, Albuquerque, New Mexico

Joette M. Meyer, PharmD, was Clinical Assistant Professor, Department of Pharmacy Practice, University of Illinois at Chicago College of Pharmacy, Chicago, Illinois at the time of this writing

Laura Boehnke Michaud, PharmD, Clinical Pharmacy Specialist—Breast Oncology, Division of Pharmacy, University of Texas MD Anderson Cancer Center, Houston, Texas

W. Alexander Morton, PharmD, BCPP, Professor of Pharmacy Practice, College of Pharmacy; Associate Professor of Psychiatry and Behavioral Sciences, Department of Psychiatry and Behavioral Sciences, Medical University of South Carolina, Charleston, South Carolina

Laura Mulloy, DO, Acting Chief of Nephrology and Associate Professor of Medicine, Department of Medicine, Medical College of Georgia, Augusta, Georgia

Pamela J. Murray, MD, MPH, Associate Professor of Pediatrics and Obstetrics, Gynecology and Reproductive Sciences, University of Pittsburgh School of Medicine, Pittsburgh, Pennsylvania

James J. Nawarskas, PharmD, Assistant Professor of Pharmacy, University of New Mexico College of Pharmacy, Albuquerque, New Mexico

B. Nhi Nguyen, PharmD, Cardiology Fellow, Department of Clinical Pharmacy, University of Tennessee College of Pharmacy, Memphis, Tennessee

Dannielle C. O'Donnell, PharmD, BCPS, Assistant Professor, University of Texas at Austin College of Pharmacy, Austin, Texas

Michael A. Oszko, PharmD, BCPS, Associate Professor, Department of Pharmacy Practice, University of Kansas School of Pharmacy, Kansas City, Kansas

Linda M. Page, PharmD, Clinical Research Associate, Ventures-Drug Delivery Business, Medtronic Neurological, Minneapolis, Minnesota

Robert B. Parker, PharmD, Associate Professor, Department of Clinical Pharmacy, University of Tennessee College of Pharmacy, Memphis, Tennessee

Beth Bryles Phillips, PharmD, Clinical Pharmacist in Ambulatory Care, Department of Pharmaceutical Care, University of Iowa Hospitals & Clinics, Iowa City, Iowa

Bradley G. Phillips, PharmD, Assistant Professor, Division of Clinical and Administrative Pharmacy, University of Iowa College of Pharmacy, Iowa City, Iowa

Page H. Pigg, PharmD, Pharmacist Account Manager, First Health Services Corporation, Glen Allen, Virginia

Charles D. Ponte, PharmD, BCPS, CDE, FAPhA, FASHP, FCCP, Professor, Department of Clinical Pharmacy and Family Medicine, Schools of Pharmacy and Medicine, Robert C. Byrd Health Sciences Center, West Virginia University, Morgantown, West Virginia

Tara L. Posey, PharmD, Ambulatory Care Clinician, University of Pittsburgh Medical Center; Assistant Professor, Department of Pharmacy and Therapeutics, University of Pittsburgh School of Pharmacy, Pittsburgh, Pennsylvania

Jane M. Pruemer, PharmD, FASHP, Oncology Clinical Pharmacy Specialist, Department of Pharmacy Services, University Hospital, Cincinnati, Ohio

Thomas W. Redford, PharmD, Assistant Professor, Division of Clinical and Administrative Pharmacy, University of Iowa College of Pharmacy, Iowa City, Iowa

Richard S. Rhodes, PharmD, Associate Professor, Department of Pharmacy Practice, Idaho State University College of Pharmacy, Pocatello, Idaho

Denise H. Rhoney, PharmD, Assistant Professor, Department of Pharmacy Practice, Wayne State University College of Pharmacy and Allied Health Professions, Detroit, Michigan

Ted L. Rice, MS, BCPS, Pharmacy Specialist—Trauma, University of Pittsburgh Medical Center; Associate Professor, Department of Pharmacy and Therapeutics, University of Pittsburgh School of Pharmacy, Pittsburgh, Pennsylvania

Milissa A. Rock, RPh, CDE, Community Practice Resident and Clinical Instructor of Pharmacy, Department of Pharmacy, Virginia Commonwealth University School of Pharmacy, Richmond, Virginia

Keith A. Rodvold, PharmD, FCCP, BCPS, Professor of Pharmacy Practice and Associate Professor of Medicine in Pharmacy, Departments of Pharmacy Practice and Infectious Diseases, University of Illinois at Chicago, Chicago, Illinois

Carol J. Rollins, MS, RD, PharmD, BCNSP, Coordinator, Nutrition Support Team and Clinical Pharmacist for Home Infusion Therapy, Arizona Health Sciences Center, Tucson, Arizona

Meredith L. Rose, PharmD, Assistant Professor, Department of Pharmacy and Therapeutics, University of Pittsburgh School of Pharmacy; Clinical Specialist, University of Pittsburgh Medical Center, Pittsburgh, Pennsylvania

Daniel Sageser, PharmD, Oncology Clinical Specialist and Hospice Pharmacy Team Leader, Southwest Washington Medical Center, Vancouver, Washington

Nannette A. Sageser, PharmD, Clinical Pharmacist and Director of the Anticoagulation Service, Southeast Washington Medical Center, Vancouver, Washington

Beata Saletnik, PharmD, Adjunct Clinical Faculty, Idaho State University College of Pharmacy; Veterans Affairs Medical Center, Boise, Idaho

Kristine E. Santus, PharmD, Ambulatory Care Resident, Department of Pharmacy, University of Pittsburgh Medical Center; Clinical Instructor, Department of Pharmacy and Therapeutics, University of Pittsburgh School of Pharmacy, Pittsburgh, Pennsylvania

Jennifer L. Schoelles, PharmD, Pediatric Specialty Resident, University of Kentucky Children's Hospital, Lexington, Kentucky

Rowena N. Schwartz, PharmD, Associate Professor, Department of Pharmacy and Therapeutics, University of Pittsburgh School of Pharmacy; Coordinator of Pharmacy Programs, University of Pittsburgh Cancer Institute, Pittsburgh, Pennsylvania

Terry L. Schwinghammer, PharmD, FCCP, FASHP, BCPS, Associate Professor, Department of Pharmaceutical Sciences, University of Pittsburgh School of Pharmacy, Pittsburgh, Pennsylvania

Mollie Ashe Scott, PharmD, BCPS, Assistant Professor, Department of Pharmacy Practice, Campbell University School of Pharmacy, Buies Creek, North Carolina; Clinical Specialist in Family Medicine, Duke University, Durham, North Carolina

Amy L. Seybert, PharmD, Assistant Professor, Department of Pharmacy and Therapeutics, University of Pittsburgh School of Pharmacy; Clinical Specialist, University of Pittsburgh Medical Center, Pittsburgh, Pennsylvania

Susan Shaffer, PharmD, Specialty Resident in Drug Information, University of North Carolina School of Pharmacy and Glaxo-Wellcome Inc., Chapel Hill, North Carolina

Penny S. Shelton, PharmD, BCPP, FASCP, Assistant Professor, Department of Pharmacy Practice, Campbell University School of Pharmacy, Buies Creek, North Carolina; Clinical Specialist in Geriatrics, Dorothea Dix Hospital, Raleigh, North Carolina

Susan J. Skledar, RPh, MPH, Clinical Instructor, Department of Pharmacy and Therapeutics, University of Pittsburgh School of Pharmacy, Pittsburgh, Pennsylvania

Jill Slimick-Ponzetto, PharmD, BCPS, Clinical Pharmacist, Department of Pharmacy, Veterans Affairs Medical Center; Instructor, Department of Pharmacy and Therapeutics, University of Pittsburgh School of Pharmacy, Pittsburgh, Pennsylvania

Ralph E. Small, PharmD, FCCP, FASHP, FAPhA, Professor of Pharmacy and Medicine, School of Pharmacy, Medical College of Virginia, Virginia Commonwealth University, Richmond, Virginia

Catherine A. Smith, PharmD, Hematology/Oncology Pharmacy Resident, Department of Pharmaceutical Services, Emory University Hospital, Atlanta, Georgia

Jerry D. Smith, PharmD, Manager of Pharmacy Services, Simkin, Inc., and Clinical Assistant Professor, Department of Community Health and Family Medicine, College of Medicine, University of Florida, Gainesville, Florida

Judith A. Smith, PharmD, Oncology Pharmacy Practice Resident, Pharmacy Department, National Institutes of Health Clinical Center, Bethesda, Maryland

Renata Smith, PharmD, Infectious Disease Specialty Resident, Department of Pharmacy Practice, University of Illinois at Chicago College of Pharmacy, Chicago, Illinois

Denise R. Sokos, PharmD, Specialty Pharmacy Resident in Adult Internal Medicine, West Virginia University Hospitals, Morgantown, West Virginia

Christine L. Solberg, PharmD, BCPS, CSPI, Research Associate, Department of Surgery, Regions Hospital, St. Paul, Minnesota

Alka Z. Somani, PharmD, Clinical Pharmacist in Ambulatory Care/Transplantation, Department of Pharmacy, University of Pittsburgh

Medical Center; Assistant Professor, Department of Pharmacy and Therapeutics, University of Pittsburgh School of Pharmacy, Pittsburgh, Pennsylvania

Suellyn J. Sorensen, PharmD, BCPS, Assistant Professor of Pharmacy Practice, Department of Pharmacy Practice, Butler University College of Pharmacy and Health Sciences; Clinical Pharmacist in Infectious Diseases, Clarian Health Partners, Indianapolis, Indiana

William J. Spruill, PharmD, Associate Professor, Department of Clinical and Administrative Sciences, University of Georgia College of Pharmacy, Athens, Georgia

Mary K. Stamatakis, PharmD, Assistant Professor, Department of Clinical Pharmacy, West Virginia University School of Pharmacy, Morgantown, West Virginia

Virginia L. Stauffer, PharmD, BCPS, Clinical Pharmacist, Department of Geriatric Medicine, Methodist Medical Group, Indianapolis, Indiana

Jennifer Stoffel, PharmD, BCPS, Assistant Professor, Department of Pharmacy and Therapeutics, University of Pittsburgh School of Pharmacy; Transplant Clinical Pharmacist, University of Pittsburgh Medical Center, Pittsburgh, Pennsylvania

Jennifer A. Torma, PharmD, Clinical Assistant Professor, Rutgers University College of Pharmacy and Oncology Pharmacy Specialist, Hackensack University Medical Center, Hackensack, New Jersey. At the time of this writing, she was Oncology Specialty Pharmacy Resident, University of Pittsburgh Medical Center, Pittsburgh, Pennsylvania

Sharon M. Tramonte, PharmD, Clinical Assistant Professor, Department of Pharmacy and Pharmacology, University of Texas Health Sciences Center at Austin; Clinical Pharmacologist, Department of Pharmacology, San Antonio State School, San Antonio, Texas

James A. Trovato, PharmD, Assistant Professor, Department of Pharmacy Practice and Science, School of Pharmacy, and Greenebaum Cancer Center, University of Maryland, Baltimore, Maryland

Tate N. Trujillo, PharmD, Critical Care Resident, Cardiopulmonary Care Center, Clarian Health Partners, Indiana University Hospital, Indianapolis, Indiana

Gretchen M. Tush, PharmD, BCPS, Assistant Professor, Department of Pharmacy, Virginia Commonwealth University School of Pharmacy, Richmond, Virginia

J. Edwin Underwood, Jr., PharmD, Associate Professor, Samford University McWhorter School of Pharmacy, Birmingham; Clinical Pharmacist, Lloyd Noland Hospital and Ambulatory Center, Fairfield, Alabama

Chad M. VanDenBerg, PharmD, Clinical Neuroscience Fellow, Department of Pharmacy Practice, Mercer University of Southern School of Pharmacy, Atlanta, Georgia

William E. Wade, PharmD, FASHP, FCCP, Associate Professor, Department of Clinical and Administrative Sciences, University of Georgia College of Pharmacy, Athens, Georgia

Mary Louise Wagner, MS, PharmD, Associate Professor, Department of Pharmacy Practice, Rutgers University College of Pharmacy, Piscataway, New Jersey

Donna S. Wall, PharmD, BCPS, Clinical Pharmacist, Cardiopulmonary Care Center, Clarian Health Partners, Indiana University Hospital, Indianapolis, Indiana

Carla Wallace, PharmD, BCPS, Assistant Professor, Department of Pharmacy Practice, St. Louis College of Pharmacy, St. Louis, Missouri

Amy L. Whitaker, PharmD, Community Pharmacy Practice Resident, Virginia Commonwealth University School of Pharmacy, Richmond, Virginia

Dennis M. Williams, PharmD, FASHP, FCCP, BCPS, Assistant Professor, Department of Pharmacy Practice, University of North Carolina School of Pharmacy, Chapel Hill, North Carolina

Susan R. Winkler, PharmD, BCPS, Clinical Assistant Professor, Department of Pharmacy Practice, University of Illinois at Chicago College of Pharmacy, Chicago, Illinois

Maria Yaramus, PharmD, PharmD Candidate, Duquesne University Mylan School of Pharmacy, Pittsburgh, Pennsylvania

Peggy C. Yarborough, MS, CDE, FAPP, FASHP, NAPP, Associate Professor, Campbell University School of Pharmacy, Buies Creek, North Carolina; Director of Pharmacotherapy—Wilson, Area L Area Health Education Center, Rocky Mount, North Carolina

Winnie M. Yu, PharmD, BCPS, Assistant Professor, Department of Pharmacy and Therapeutics, University of Pittsburgh School of Pharmacy; Clinical Specialist, University of Pittsburgh Medical Center, Pittsburgh, Pennsylvania

Nancy S. Yunker, PharmD, Assistant Professor, Department of Pharmacy, Virginia Commonwealth University School of Pharmacy, Richmond, Virginia

Margaret B. Zak, PharmD, Assistant Professor, Department of Pharmacy and Therapeutics, University of Pittsburgh School of Pharmacy; Clinical Specialist in Infectious Disease, Department of Pharmacy, University of Pittsburgh Medical Center, Pittsburgh, Pennsylvania

William C. Zamboni, PharmD, Assistant Professor, Department of Pharmacy Practice and Science, School of Pharmacy; Department of Developmental Therapeutics, Greenebaum Cancer Center, University of Maryland, Baltimore, Maryland

Basil J. Zitelli, MD, FAAP, Professor of Pediatrics, Department of Pediatrics, Children's Hospital of Pittsburgh, Pittsburgh, Pennsylvania

Contents

PART FIVE
Nutrition and Nutritional Disorders
Gary R. Matzke, PharmD, FCP, FCCP, Section Editor

Note: Additional cases with questions and suggested answers may be found on the Internet at www.pharmacy.pitt.edu/ce/pharmacotherapy.

Preface

The purpose of this second edition of the *Pharmacotherapy Casebook* remains the same as the first edition: to help students in the health professions develop the skills required to identify and resolve drug-related problems through the use of patient case studies. Case studies can actively involve students in the learning process, engender self-confidence, and promote the development of skills in independent self-study, problem analysis, decision making, oral communication, and teamwork. Patient case studies can also be used as the focal point of discussions about pathophysiology, medicinal chemistry, pharmacology, and pharmacotherapeutics of individual diseases. By integrating the biomedical and pharmaceutical sciences with pharmacotherapeutics, case studies can help students appreciate the relevance and importance of a sound scientific foundation in preparation for practice.

The patient cases in this book are intended to complement the scientific information presented in the Fourth Edition of the textbook *Pharmacotherapy: A Pathophysiologic Approach*. The second edition of the casebook contains 131 new cases, 17 more than the first edition. As before, cases are organized into organ system sections that correspond to those of the *Pharmacotherapy* textbook. Students should read the relevant textbook chapter to become thoroughly familiar with the pathophysiology and pharmacotherapy of each disease state before attempting to make "decisions" about the care of patients described in this casebook. By using these realistic cases to practice creating, defending, and implementing pharmaceutical care plans, students can begin to develop the skills and self-confidence that will be necessary to make the real decisions required in professional practice.

In addition to an increase in the *number* of cases in this edition, there is also an increase in case *complexity*. The patient presentations usually contain multiple disease states and drug-related problems, which more closely mirrors actual practice. As a guide for instructors, each case is identified as being one of three complexity levels; this classification system is described in more detail in Chapter 1. This edition also contains an increased *variety* of cases. There are new disease state cases in the Renal, Endocrine, Infectious Disease, and other sections. The casebook also contains cases for which there is no corresponding textbook chapter. These cases are included because of the recent introduction of important new therapies for these medical problems (e.g., cigarette smoking, urinary incontinence, benign prostatic hyperplasia, and erectile dysfunction). This will require students to explore other sources of background reading to prepare answers to these case questions. Users of the first edition will quickly notice that the layout of the patient presentation section has been improved by condensing the information and displaying it in a manner that more closely mimics actual patient records.

The second edition has retained the four introductory chapters, and several have undergone substantial revision.

- Chapter 1 describes the format of case presentations and the means by which students and instructors can maximize the usefulness of the casebook. A systematic approach is consistently applied to each case. The steps involved in this approach include:

  1. Identification of real or potential drug-related problems
  2. Determination of the desired therapeutic outcome
  3. Determination of therapeutic alternatives
  4. Design of an optimal individualized pharmacotherapeutic plan
  5. Identification of methods of evaluate the therapeutic outcome
  6. Provision of patient counseling
  7. Communication and implementation of the pharmacotherapeutic plan

- In Chapter 2, the philosophy and implementation of active learning strategies is presented. This chapter sets the tone for the casebook by describing how these approaches can enhance student learning. The chapter offers a number of useful active learning strategies for instructors and provides advice to students on how to maximize their learning opportunities in active learning environments.
- Chapter 3 presents an efficient method of patient counseling developed by the Indian Health Service. The information can be used as the basis for simulated counseling sessions related to the patient cases.
- Chapter 4 describes two methods for documenting clinical interventions and communicating recommendations to other health care providers. These include the traditional SOAP note and the more pharmacy-specific FARM note. Student preparation of SOAP or FARM notes for the patient cases in this book will be excellent practice for future documentation in actual patient records.

It should be emphasized that the focus of classroom discussions about these cases should be on the *process* of solving patient problems as much as it is on finding the actual answers to the questions themselves. Isolated scientific facts learned today may be obsolete or incorrect tomorrow. Health care providers who can identify patient problems and solve them using a reasoned approach will be able to adapt to the continual evolution in the body of scientific knowledge and contribute in a meaningful way to improving the quality of patients' lives.

We are grateful for the broad acceptance the first edition of the casebook has received. It was adopted by at least 26 schools of pharmacy and 12 nurse practitioner programs. It was also used in institutional staff development efforts and by individual pharmacists wishing to upgrade their pharmaceutical care skills. It is our hope that this second edition will be even more valuable in assisting health care practitioners to meet society's need for safe and effective drug therapy.

Acknowledgments

I would like to thank the 165 case and chapter authors from 84 schools of pharmacy, hospitals, and other institutions who contributed their scholarly efforts to this casebook. I am especially appreciative of their diligence in meeting short deadlines and adhering to the unique format of the casebook. The next generation of pharmacists will benefit from the willingness of these authors to share their expertise.

My sincere appreciation is also extended to the other Section Editors of this casebook, whose careful review and critique of the cases also contributed to the quality of the final product. I am also grateful for the secretarial assistance of Ms. Diane Kenna at the University of Pittsburgh School of Pharmacy.

I am indebted to the following colleagues for their assistance in obtaining and interpreting illustrations to assist in the learning process: Lydia C. Contis, MD, Division of Hematopathology, William Pasculle, MD, Department of Microbiology, and Orlando F. Gabriele, MD, Department of Radiology, University of Pittsburgh Medical Center (UPMC); Terence W. Starz, MD, Department of Medicine, University of Pittsburgh School of Medicine;

Philip J. Nerti, RPh, Health Center Pharmacy Central, Pittsburgh; and Jason Lazar, MD, Winthrop University Hospital, Long Island, New York. The expert photography of Donald Koch and Lisa Dehainaut of the Creative Services/Medical Photography Department at UPMC is also gratefully acknowledged.

I would like to thank Cheryl L. Mehalik, Editor-in-Chief/Health Related Professions, Jeanmarie Roche, Senior Production Editor, Robin Lazrus, Aquisitions Editor, and Jessica Hirshon, Associate Editor/Health Related Professions, at Appleton & Lange. Their cooperation, advice, and commitment were instrumental in bringing this publication from concept to reality. The meticulous production services provided by Bennie Sauls and the staff of Rainbow Graphics, LLC are also appreciated.

My greatest debt of gratitude is owed to my wife, Donna, and children, Amanda and Steven, who shared in large measure in the production of this work by virtue of their sacrifice of hundreds of weekend and evening hours with me. Their understanding, support, and encouragement were vital to the successful completion of this book.

Terry L. Schwinghammer, PharmD, FCCP, BCPS

PART ONE

Principles of Patient-focused Therapy

Terry L. Schwinghammer, PharmD, FCCP, FASHP, BCPS, Section Editor

CHAPTER 1

Introduction: How to Use This Casebook

Terry L. Schwinghammer, PharmD, FCCP, FASHP, BCPS

WHY DO CASE STUDIES ENHANCE LEARNING IN THE CURRICULUM?

The main goals of the case method are to develop the skills of self-learning, critical thinking, and decision making. When case studies are used in the formal curricula of the health care professions or for independent study by health care professionals, the focus of attention should be on learning the *process* of solving drug-related problems, rather than simply finding the scientific answers to the problems themselves. Students do learn scientific facts during the resolution of case study problems, but they usually learn more of them from their own independent study and from discussions with their peers than they do from the instructor. Information recall is reinforced by working on subsequent cases with similar problems. Traditional programs in the health care professions that rely heavily on the lecture format tend to concentrate on scientific content and the rote memorization of facts rather than the development of higher-order thinking skills.

Case studies provide the personal history of an individual patient and information about one or more health problems that must be solved. The learner's job is to work through the facts of the case, analyze the available data, gather more information, develop hypotheses, consider possible solutions, arrive at the optimal solution, and consider the consequences of his or her decisions.[1] The role of the teacher is to serve as coach and facilitator rather than as the source of "the answer." In fact, in many cases there is more than one acceptable answer to a given question. Because instructors do not need to possess the correct answer, they need not be experts in the

field being discussed. Rather, the students become teachers and learn from each other through thoughtful discussion of the case.

FORMAT OF THE CASEBOOK

Background Reading

The patient cases in this casebook are intended to be used as the focal point for independent self-learning by individual students and for in-class problem-solving discussions by student groups and their instructors. If meaningful learning and discussion are to occur, students must come to discussion sessions prepared to discuss the case material rationally, propose reasonable solutions, and defend their pharmacotherapeutic plans. This requires a strong commitment to independent self-study prior to the session. The cases in this book were prepared to correspond with the scientific information contained in the fourth edition of *Pharmacotherapy: A Pathophysiologic Approach.*[2] For this reason, thorough familiarity with the corresponding textbook chapter is recommended as the primary method of student preparation. Other primary and tertiary literature should also be consulted as necessary to supplement the textbook readings. For some of the cases in this second edition of the casebook, there is no corresponding textbook chapter. It therefore becomes mandatory that students explore other reference materials for the necessary background information before completing the answers to these cases.

The cases selected for inclusion in the casebook represent common diseases likely to be encountered by general pharmacy practitioners. As a result, not all of the *Pharmacotherapy* textbook chapters have an associated patient case in the casebook. On the other hand, some of the textbook chapters have several corresponding cases in the casebook.

Levels of Case Complexity

In this second edition, each case is identified at the top of the first page as being one of three levels of complexity. Instructors may use this classification system to select cases for discussion that correspond to the experience level of the student learners. These levels are defined as follows:

Level I. An uncomplicated case; only the single textbook chapter is required to complete the case questions. Little prior knowledge of the disease state or clinical experience is needed.
Level II. An intermediate-level case; several textbook chapters or other reference sources may be required to complete the case. Prior clinical experience may be helpful in resolving all of the issues presented.
Level III. A complicated case; multiple textbook chapters and substantial clinical experience are required to solve all of the patient's drug-related problems.

Developing Ability Outcomes

At the beginning of each case, four to five ability outcomes are included for student reflection. The focus of these outcomes is on achieving competency in the clinical arena, not simply on learning isolated scientific facts. These items indicate some of the functions that the student should be expected to be able to perform in the clinical setting as a result of studying the case, preparing a pharmacotherapeutic plan, and defending his or her recommendations.

The ability outcomes provided are meant to serve as a starting point to stimulate student thinking, but they are not meant to be all inclusive. In fact, students should also generate their own personal ability outcomes and learning objectives for each case. By so doing, students take greater control of their own learning, which serves to improve personal motivation and the desire to learn.

PATIENT PRESENTATION

The format and organization of cases reflect those usually seen in actual clinical settings. The patient's medical history and physical examination findings are provided in the following standard outline format.

Chief Complaint
The chief complaint is a brief statement of the reason why the patient consulted the physician, *stated in the patient's own words*. In order to convey the patient's symptoms accurately, no medical terms or diagnoses are used.

HPI
History of present illness is a more complete description of the patient's symptom(s). General features usually included in the HPI are:

- Date of onset
- Precise location

- Nature of onset, severity, and duration
- Presence of exacerbations and remissions
- Effect of any treatment given
- Relationship to other symptoms, bodily functions, or activities (e.g., activity, meals)
- Degree of interference with daily activities

PMH
The past medical history includes serious illnesses, surgical procedures, and injuries the patient has experienced previously. Minor complaints (e.g., influenza, colds) are generally omitted.

FH
The family history includes the age and health of parents, siblings, and children. For deceased relatives, the age and cause of death are recorded. In particular, heritable diseases and those with a hereditary tendency are noted (e.g., diabetes mellitus, cardiovascular disease, malignancy, rheumatoid arthritis, obesity).

SH
The social history includes not only the social characteristics of the patient, but also the environmental factors and behaviors that may contribute to the development of disease. Items usually included are the patient's marital status, number of children, educational background, occupation, physical activity, hobbies, dietary habits, and use of tobacco, alcohol, or other drugs.

Meds
The medication history should include an accurate record of the patient's current prescription and non-prescription medication use. Because pharmacists possess extensive knowledge of the thousands of prescription and non-prescription products available, they can perform a valuable service to the health care team by obtaining a complete medication history that includes the names, doses, schedules, and duration of therapy for all medications, including herbal therapies and non-traditional remedies.

All
Allergies to drugs, food, pets, and environmental factors (e.g., grass, dust, pollen) are recorded. An accurate description of the reaction that occurred should also be included. Care should be taken to distinguish adverse drug effects ("upset stomach") from true allergy ("hives").

ROS
In the review of systems, the examiner questions the patient about the presence of symptoms related to each body system. In many cases, only the pertinent positive and negative findings are recorded. In a complete ROS, body systems are generally listed starting from the head and working toward the feet and may include the skin, head, eyes, ears, nose, mouth and throat, neck, cardiovascular, respiratory, gastrointestinal, genitourinary, endocrine, musculoskeletal, and neuropsychiatric systems. The purpose of the ROS is to evaluate the status of each body system and to prevent the omission of pertinent information. Information that was included in the HPI is not repeated in the ROS.

PE
The exact procedures performed during the physical examination vary depending upon the chief complaint and the patient's medical history. A suitable physical assessment textbook should be consulted for the specific pro-

cedures that may be conducted for each body system. The general sections for the PE are outlined as follows:

Gen (general appearance)
VS (vital signs)—blood pressure, pulse, respiratory rate, temperature; weight and height are usually included in this casebook, although they are not technically considered to be vital signs)
Skin (integumentary)
HEENT (head, eyes, ears, nose, and throat)
Lungs/Thorax (pulmonary)
Cor or CV (cardiovascular)
Abd (abdomen)
Genit/Rect (genitalia/rectal)
MS/Ext (musculoskeletal and extremities)
Neuro (neurologic)

Labs

The results of laboratory tests are included with almost all cases, and reference ranges for most tests are included in **Appendix A.** Occasionally, another reference text will be needed to identify the usual reference range. It should be noted that reference values differ among laboratories, so the values given in Appendix A should be considered as a general guide only. Institution-specific reference ranges should be used in actual clinical settings.

All of the cases include some physical examination and laboratory findings that are within normal limits. For example, a description of the cardiovascular examination may include a statement that the point of maximal impulse is at the fifth intercostal space; laboratory evaluation may include a serum sodium of 140 mEq/L. The presentation of actual findings (rather than simple statements that the heart examination and the serum sodium were normal) reflects what will be seen in actual clinical practice. More importantly, listing both normal and abnormal findings requires students to carefully assess the complete database and identify the pertinent positive and negative findings for themselves. A valuable portion of the learning process is lost if students are only provided with findings that are abnormal and are known to be associated with the disease being discussed.

The patients described in this casebook have been given fictitious names in order to humanize the situations and encourage students to remember that they will one day be caring for patients, not treating disease states. However, in the actual clinical setting, patient confidentiality is of utmost importance, and patient names should not be used during group discussions in patient care areas unless absolutely necessary. In order to develop student sensitivity to this issue, instructors may wish to avoid using these fictitious patient names during class discussions. In this casebook, patient names are given only in the initial presentation; they are not used in subsequent questions or other portions of the case.

The issues of race, ethnicity, and gender also deserve thoughtful consideration. The traditional format for case presentations usually begins with a description of the patient's age, race, and gender, as in: "The patient is a 65-year-old white male. . . ." Single-word racial labels such as "black" or "white" are actually of limited value in many cases and may actually be misleading in some instances.[3] For this reason, racial descriptors have been excluded from the opening line of each presentation. When ethnicity is pertinent to the case, this information is presented in the social history or physical examination. Finally, patients in this casebook are referred to as men or women, rather than males or females, to promote sensitivity to human dignity.

The patient cases in this casebook include medical abbreviations and drug brand names, just as medical records do in actual practice. Although these customs are sometimes the source of clinical problems, the intent of their inclusion is to make the cases as realistic as possible. A list of abbreviations used in the casebook is included in **Appendix B.** This list is limited to commonly accepted abbreviations; thousands more exist, which makes it difficult for the novice practitioner to efficiently assess patient databases. Most institutions have an approved list of accepted abbreviations; these lists should be consulted in practice to facilitate one's understanding and to avoid using abbreviations in the medical record that are not on the official approved list.

The casebook also contains some photographs of commercial drug products. These illustrations are provided as examples only and are not intended to imply endorsement of those particular products.

Pharmaceutical Care and Drug-related Problems

Modern drug therapy has played a crucial role in improving the health of people by enhancing the quality of life and extending life expectancy. The advent of biotechnology has led to the introduction of unique compounds for the prevention and treatment of disease that were unheard of a decade ago. Each year the Food and Drug Administration approves approximately two dozen new drug products that contain active substances that have never before been marketed in the United States. Although the cost of new therapeutic agents has received intense scrutiny in recent years, drug therapy actually accounts for a relatively small proportion of overall health care expenditures. Appropriate drug therapy is cost effective and may actually serve to reduce total expenditures by decreasing the need for surgery, preventing hospital admissions, and shortening hospital stays.

Improper use of prescription medications is a frequent and serious problem and has been estimated to cause approximately 200,000 deaths, 9 million hospitalizations, and expenditures of $76 billion annually in direct patient care costs. A societal need for better use of medications clearly exists. Widespread implementation of pharmaceutical care has the potential to positively impact this situation by the design, implementation, and monitoring of rational therapeutic plans to produce defined outcomes that improve the quality of patients' lives.[4]

The new mission of the pharmacy profession is to render pharmaceutical care. Schools of pharmacy are implementing new instructional strategies to prepare future pharmacists to provide pharmaceutical care. New entry-level PharmD programs have an increased emphasis on patient-focused care, as evidenced by more experiential training, especially in ambulatory care. Many programs are structured to promote self-directed learning, develop problem-solving and communication skills, and instill the desire for lifelong learning.

In its broadest sense, pharmaceutical care involves the identification, resolution, and prevention of potential drug-related problems. A drug-related problem is an event or circumstance involving drug therapy that actually or potentially interferes with the patient's ability to achieve an optimal medical outcome. Eight major types of drug-related problems have been identified that may potentially lead to an undesirable event that has physiologic, psychological, social, or economic ramifications.[5] These problems include:

1. *Untreated indications.* The patient needs drug therapy for a specific indication but is not receiving it.

2. *Improper drug selection.* The drug currently prescribed is either ineffective or toxic.
3. *Subtherapeutic dosage.* Too little of the correct drug has been prescribed.
4. *Failure to receive drugs.* The patient is not taking or receiving the drug prescribed.
5. *Overdosage.* Too much of the correct drug is being given.
6. *Adverse drug reactions.* The patient has a medical condition resulting from an adverse drug reaction.
7. *Drug interactions.* A medical problem has resulted from a drug–drug, drug–food, or drug–laboratory interaction.
8. *Drug use without indication.* The patient is taking a drug for which there is no valid medical indication.

Because this casebook is intended to be used in conjunction with the *Pharmacotherapy* textbook, one of its purposes is to serve as a tool for learning about the pharmacotherapy of disease states. For this reason, the primary problem to be identified and addressed for most of the patients in the casebook is the need for drug treatment of a specific medical indication (problem #1). Other actual or potential drug-related problems may coexist during the initial presentation or may develop during the clinical course of the disease.

Patient-focused Approach to Case Problems

In this casebook, each patient presentation is followed by a set of patient-focused questions that remain essentially the same for each case. These questions are applied consistently from case to case to demonstrate that a systematic patient care process can be successfully applied regardless of the underlying disease state(s). The questions are designed to enable students to identify and resolve problems related to pharmacotherapy. They help students recognize what they know and what they do not know, thereby guiding them in determining what information must be learned to satisfactorily resolve the patient's problems.[6] A description of each of the steps involved in solving drug-related problems is included in the following paragraphs.

1. Identification of real or potential drug-related problems

The first step in the patient-focused approach is to collect pertinent patient information, interpret it properly, and determine whether drug-related problems exist. Some authors prefer to divide this process into two or more separate steps because of the difficulty that inexperienced students may have performing these complex tasks simultaneously.[4,7] This step is analogous to documenting the subjective and objective patient findings in the SOAP format. It is important to differentiate the process of identifying the patient's drug-related problems from making a disease-related medical diagnosis. In fact, the medical diagnosis is known for the majority of patients seen by pharmacists. However, pharmacists must be capable of assessing the patient's database to determine whether drug-related problems exist that warrant a change in drug therapy. In the case of pre-existing chronic diseases such as asthma or rheumatoid arthritis, one must be able to assess information that may indicate a change in severity of the disease. This process involves reviewing the patient's symptoms, the signs of disease present on physical examination, and the results of laboratory and other diagnostic tests. Some of the cases require the student to develop complete pa-

tient problem lists. Potential sources for this information in actual practice include the patient or his or her advocate, the patient's physician or other health care professionals, and the patient's medical chart or other records.

After the drug-related problems are identified, the clinician should determine which of them are amenable to pharmacotherapy. Alternatively, one must also consider whether any of the problems could have been caused by drug therapy. In some cases (both in the casebook as well as in real life), not all of the information needed to make these decisions will be available. In that situation, providing precise recommendations for obtaining additional information needed to satisfactorily assess the patient's problems can be a valuable contribution to the patient's care.

2. Determination of the desired therapeutic outcome

After pertinent patient-specific information has been gathered and the patient's drug-related problems have been identified, the next step is to define the specific goals of pharmacotherapy. The primary therapeutic outcomes include:

- Cure of disease (e.g., bacterial infection)
- Reduction or elimination of symptoms (e.g., pain from cancer)
- Arresting or slowing of the progression of disease (e.g., rheumatoid arthritis)
- Preventing a disease or symptom (e.g., cardiovascular disease)

Other important outcomes of pharmacotherapy include:

- Not complicating or aggravating other existing disease states
- Avoiding or minimizing adverse effects of treatment
- Providing cost-effective therapy
- Maintaining the patient's quality of life

Sources of information for this step may include the patient or his or her advocate, the patient's physician or other health care professionals, medical records, and the *Pharmacotherapy* textbook or other literature references.

3. Determination of therapeutic alternatives

Once the intended outcome has been defined, attention can be directed toward identifying the kinds of treatments that might be beneficial in achieving that outcome. The clinician should ensure that all feasible pharmacotherapeutic alternatives available for achieving the predefined therapeutic outcome(s) are considered before choosing a single therapeutic regimen. Non-drug therapies (e.g., diet, exercise, psychotherapy) that might be useful should be included in the list of therapeutic alternatives when appropriate. Useful sources of information on therapeutic alternatives include the *Pharmacotherapy* textbook and other references, as well as the clinical experience of the health care provider and other involved health care professionals.

4. Design of an optimal individualized pharmacotherapeutic plan

The purpose of this step is to determine the drug, dosage form, dose, schedule, and duration of therapy that are best suited for a given patient. Individual patient characteristics should be taken into consideration when weighing the risks and benefits of each available therapeutic alternative. For example, an asthma patient who requires new drug therapy for hypertension might better tolerate treatment with a thiazide diuretic rather than a β-blocker. On the other hand, a hypertensive patient with gout may be better served by use of a β-blocker rather than a thiazide diuretic.

The reason for avoiding specific drugs should be stated in the therapeutic plan. Potential reasons for drug avoidance include drug allergy, drug–drug or drug–disease interactions, patient age, renal or hepatic impairment, adverse effects, poor compliance, and high treatment cost.

The specific dose selected may depend upon the indication for the drug. For example, the dose of aspirin used to treat rheumatoid arthritis is much higher than that used to prevent myocardial infarction. The likelihood of compliance with the regimen and patient tolerance come into play in the selection of dosage forms. The economic, psychosocial, and ethical factors that are applicable to the patient should also be given due consideration in design of the pharmacotherapeutic regimen. An alternative plan should also be in place that would be appropriate if the initial therapy fails or cannot be used.

5. Identification of parameters to evaluate the outcome

One must identify the clinical and laboratory parameters necessary to assess the therapy for achievement of the desired therapeutic outcome and for detection and prevention of adverse effects. The outcome parameters selected should be specific, measurable, achievable, directly related to the therapeutic goals, and have a defined end point. As a means of remembering these points, the acronym SMART has been used (Specific, Measurable, Achievable, Related, and Time bound). If the goal was to cure a bacterial pneumonia, one should outline the subjective and objective clinical parameters (e.g., relief of chest discomfort, cough, and fever), laboratory tests (e.g., normalization of white blood cell count and differential), and other procedures (e.g., resolution of infiltrate on chest x-ray) that provide sufficient evidence of bacterial eradication and clinical cure of the disease. The intervals at which data should be collected are dependent upon the outcome parameters selected and should be established prospectively. It should be noted that expensive or invasive procedures may not be repeated after the initial diagnosis is made.

Adverse effect parameters must also be well defined and measurable. For example, it is insufficient to state that one will monitor for potential drug-induced "blood dyscrasias." Rather, one should identify the likely specific hematologic abnormality (e.g., anemia, leukopenia, or thrombocytopenia) and outline a prospective schedule for obtaining the appropriate parameters (e.g., obtain monthly hemoglobin/hematocrit, white blood cell count, or platelet count, respectively).

Monitoring for adverse events should be directed toward preventing or identifying serious adverse effects that have a reasonable likelihood of occurrence. For example, it is not cost effective to obtain periodic liver function tests in all patients taking a drug that causes mild hepatic abnormalities only rarely, such as omeprazole. On the other hand, serious patient harm may be averted by outlining a specific screening schedule for drugs associated more frequently with hepatic abnormalities, such as methotrexate for rheumatoid arthritis or troglitazone for diabetes mellitus.

6. Provision of patient counseling

The concept of pharmaceutical care is based on the existence of a covenantal relationship between the patient and the provider of care. Patients are our partners in health care, and our efforts may be for naught without their informed participation in the process. For chronic diseases such as diabetes mellitus, hypertension, and asthma, patients may have a greater role in managing their diseases than do health care professionals. Self-care is becoming more widespread as increasing numbers of prescription medications receive over-the-counter status. For these reasons, patients must be provided with sufficient information to enhance compliance, ensure successful therapy, and minimize adverse effects. Chapter 3 describes patient interview techniques that can be used efficiently to determine the patient's level of knowledge. Additional information can then be provided as necessary to fill in knowledge gaps. In the questions posed with individual cases, students will be asked to provide the kind of information that should be given to the patient who has limited knowledge of his or her disease. Under the Omnibus Budget Reconciliation Act (OBRA) of 1990, for patients who accept the offer of counseling, pharmacists should consider including the following items:

- Name and description of the medication (which may include the indication)
- Dosage, dosage form, route of administration, and duration of therapy
- Special directions or procedures for preparation, administration, and use
- Common and severe adverse effects, interactions, and contraindications (with the action required should they occur)
- Techniques for self-monitoring
- Proper storage
- Prescription refill information
- Action to be taken in the event of missed doses

Instructors may wish to have simulated patient interviewing sessions for new and refill prescriptions during the case discussions to practice medication counseling skills. Factual information should be provided as concisely as possible to enhance memory retention. An excellent source for information on individual drugs is the *USP-DI Volume II: Advice for the Patient*.[8]

7. Communication and implementation of the pharmacotherapeutic plan

The most well-conceived plan is worthless if it languishes without implementation because of inadequate communication with prescribers or other health care providers. Permanent, written documentation of significant recommendations in the medical record is important to ensure accurate communication among practitioners. Oral communication alone can be misinterpreted or transferred inaccurately to others. This is especially true because there are many drugs that sound alike when spoken but that have different therapeutic uses.

The SOAP format (Subjective, Objective, Assessment, Plan) has been used by clinicians for many years to assess patient problems and communicate findings and plans in the medical record. However, writing SOAP notes may not be the optimal process for learning to solve drug-related problems, because several important steps taken by experienced clinicians are not always apparent and may be overlooked. For example, the precise therapeutic outcome desired is often unstated in SOAP notes, leaving others to presume what the desired treatment goals are. Health care professionals using the SOAP format also commonly move directly from an assessment of the patient (diagnosis) to outlining a diagnostic or therapeutic plan, without necessarily conveying whether careful consideration has been given to all available feasible diagnostic or therapeutic alternatives. The plan itself as outlined in SOAP notes may also give short shrift to the monitoring parameters that are required to ensure successful therapy and to detect and prevent adverse drug effects. Finally, there is often little suggestion provided as to the treatment information that should be conveyed to the most important individual involved: the patient. If SOAP notes are used for documenting drug-related problems, consideration should be given to including each of these components.

In Chapter 4 of this casebook, the FARM note is presented as a useful method of consistently documenting therapeutic recommendations and implementing plans.[9] This method can be used by students as an alternative to the SOAP note to practice communicating pharmacotherapeutic plans to other members of the health care team. Although preparation of written communication notes is not included in written form with each set of case questions, instructors are encouraged to include the composition of a SOAP or FARM note as one of the requirements for successfully completing each case study assignment.

Clinical Course

The process of pharmaceutical care entails an assessment of the patient's progress in order to ensure achievement of the desired therapeutic outcomes. A description of the patient's clinical course is included with many of the cases in this book to reflect this process. Some cases follow the progression of the patient's disease over months to years and include both inpatient and outpatient treatment. Follow-up questions directed toward ongoing evaluation and problem solving are included after presentation of the clinical course.

Self-study Assignments

Each case concludes with several study assignments related to the patient case or the disease state that may be used as independent study projects for students to complete outside class. These assignments generally require students to obtain additional information that is not contained in the corresponding *Pharmacotherapy* textbook chapter.

References

Selected literature references that are specific to the case at hand are included with most cases. These references may be useful to students for answering the questions posed. The *Pharmacotherapy* textbook contains a more comprehensive list of references pertinent to each disease state.

DEVELOPING ANSWERS TO CASE QUESTIONS

The use of case studies for independent learning and in-class discussion may be unfamiliar to many students. For this reason, it may initially be difficult for students to devise complete answers to the case questions. **Appendix C** contains the answers to three cases in order to demonstrate how case responses might be prepared and presented. Additional cases with questions and suggested answers may be found on the Internet at www.pharmacy.pitt.edu/ce/pharmacotherapy. The recommended answers provided in the appendix and on the Website were contributed by the authors of the cases, but they should not necessarily be considered the sole "right" answer. Thoughtful students who have prepared well for the discussion sessions may arrive at additional or alternative answers that are also appropriate.

With diligent self-study, practice, and the guidance of instructors, students will gradually acquire the knowledge, skills, and self-confidence to develop and implement pharmaceutical care plans for their own future patients. The goal of the casebook is to help students progress along this path of lifelong learning.

References

1. Herreid CF. Case studies in science: A novel method of science education. J College Sci Teaching 1994;23:221–229.
2. DiPiro JT, Talbert RL, Yee GC, et al., eds. Pharmacotherapy: A Pathophysiologic Approach, 4th ed. Stamford, CT, Appleton & Lange, 1999.
3. Caldwell SH, Popenoe R. Perceptions and misperceptions of skin color. Ann Intern Med 1995;122:614–617.
4. Hepler CD, Strand LM. Opportunities and responsibilities in pharmaceutical care. Am J Hosp Pharm 1990;47:533–543.
5. Strand LM, Morley PC, Cipolle RJ, et al. Drug-related problems: Their structure and function. Drug Intell Clin Pharm 1990;24:1093–1097.
6. Delafuente JC, Munyer TO, Angaran DM, Doering PL. A problem-solving active-learning course in pharmacotherapy. Am J Pharm Educ 1994;58:61–64.
7. Winslade N. Large-group problem-based learning: A revision from traditional to pharmaceutical care-based therapeutics. Am J Pharm Educ 1994;58:64–73.
8. Micromedex, Inc. USP-DI volume II: Advice for the Patient, 19th ed. Englewood, CO, 1999.
9. Canaday BR, Yarborough PC. Documenting pharmaceutical care: Creating a standard. Ann Pharmacother 1994;28:1292–1296.

CHAPTER 2

Active Learning Strategies

Elizabeth S. Gray, PharmD
Gretchen M. Tush, PharmD, BCPS
Cynthia K. Kirkwood, PharmD

INTRODUCTION

Everyone is faced with situations daily that require use of problem-solving skills. For example, trying to find the quickest route to a gas station in a major city, or determining the most effective method to train your dog not to bark at the neighbors. In the hospital, you may need to identify the etiology of nausea and vomiting in a patient on your internal medicine service. In order to solve problems, we call upon our previous experiences with similar situations, observe, investigate, ask appropriate questions, and finally come to a conclusion or resolution.

Students who graduate from pharmacy school will have the opportunity to pursue many different career paths. They must be prepared to take direct responsibility for patient outcomes by practicing pharmaceutical care. Pharmacists will need to use their skills in communications, problem solving, independent learning, drug information retrieval, and knowledge of disease state management.[1,2] In order to prepare students to practice in this manner, pharmacy educators are moving away from traditional methods of teaching and are using active learning strategies in the classroom. In therapeutics courses, students are given actual written patient cases as the basis for learning. Students may be asked to identify the significant findings, develop a drug-related problem list, create an assessment statement, consider all feasible therapeutic alternatives, make therapeutic recommendations, develop a monitoring plan, formulate a written communication note for other health care providers, and decide how they would educate the patient about new drug therapies. This process actively engages students in problem solving because it requires them to integrate knowledge gained in other areas of the curriculum with specific patient information. As a result, students learn skills that they will use on a daily basis in their future practice sites.

TRADITIONAL TEACHING

In pre-pharmacy course work, and even in some pharmacy school courses, most students are taught using traditional methods. The student comes to class, and the teacher lectures on a predetermined subject that does not require student preparation. Students are passive recipients of information and are usually tested by written examinations that employ a multiple-choice or short answer format. With this method, students are tested primarily on their ability to recall isolated facts and do not learn to apply their knowledge to situations that they will ultimately encounter in pharmacy practice. They are rewarded only by receiving an exam or course grade that may or may not reflect their actual ability to use knowledge to improve patient care. In order to teach students to be lifelong learners, it is essential to stimulate them to be inquisitive and actively involved with the learning that takes place in the classroom. This requires that teachers move away from more comfortable teaching methods and learn new techniques that will help students "learn to learn."

ACTIVE LEARNING STRATEGIES

During the last 15 years, active learning has been defined in many ways, and various methods are described in the educational literature. Simply put, active learning means involving students in the learning process.[3] In classes with active learning formats, students are involved in much more than listening. The transmission of information is de-emphasized and replaced with the development of skills. Most proponents agree that active learning allows students to become engaged in the learning process while developing cognitive skills. Learning is reinforced when students actually apply their knowledge to new situations.[4] In order for active learning to be successful, it requires willing students, innovative teachers, and administrative support within the school.[5] Control of learning must be shifted from the teacher to the students; this provides an opportunity for students to become active participants in their own learning. Although it sounds frightening at first, students *can* take control of their own learning. Knowledge of career and life goals can help students make decisions about how to spend their educational time. Warren[6] identifies several traits that prepare students for future careers:

- Analytical thinking
- Polite assertiveness
- Tolerance
- Communication skills
- Understanding of one's own physical well-being
- The ability to continue to teach oneself after graduation

After going through the active learning process, most students realize that knowledge is easily acquired, but developing critical thinking skills aids in lifelong learning.[5]

Teachers implement active learning exercises into classes in a variety of ways. Some of the active learning strategies give students the opportunity to pause and recall information, cooperate and collaborate in groups, solve problems, and generate questions.[7] More advanced methods include use of simulation, role-playing, debates, peer teaching, problem-based learning, and case studies.[8] Tests and quizzes evaluate student comprehension of material. Each of these strategies allows students to demonstrate their skills.

Didactic lectures can be enhanced by several active learning strategies. The "pause procedure" is designed to enhance student retention and comprehension of material.[9] It involves 15- to 20-minute mini-lectures with 2- to 3-minute pauses for students to rework their notes, discuss the material with their peers for clarification, and develop questions.[10] This strategy can be incorporated into a 50-minute lecture up to three times. Students are able to assess their understanding of the material and formulate opinions. The pause procedure is a useful method for classes that require retention of factual information.[8] With the "think-pair-share" exercise, students are asked to write down the answer to a question and turn to a classmate to compare answers. This method provides immediate feedback to students.[11]

Another active learning technique for classroom sessions is to involve the students in short writing assignments. Writing helps students identify knowledge deficits, clarify understanding of the material, and organize thoughts in a logical manner. Students can be asked to write questions related to the reading assignment and submit them for discussion at the next class session. Alternatively, students can formulate questions and answers before class, and then discuss them in small groups. The "shared paragraph exercise" requires students to write a paragraph at the end of class summarizing the major concepts that were presented. The paragraph is then shared with a partner to clarify the material and receive feedback.[8] Discussions of any misconceptions can be conducted in class or one-on-one with the teacher. Sample test questions may also be used to assess student comprehension of the presentation and facilitate class discussion.

Tests and quizzes are effective tools to help students review the class presentations or reading assignments. Quizzes can be administered several times during class and may or may not be graded. Quizzes given at the beginning of class help stimulate students to review information they did not know and listen for clarification during lecture. Quizzes at the end of the class session allow students to use their problem-solving skills by applying what they have just learned to a patient case or problem.

Problem-solving skills can be developed during a class period by applying knowledge of disease state management to a patient case. Application reinforces the previously learned material and helps students understand the importance of the topic in a real-life situation. Problem-based learning (PBL) is a teaching method in which a problem is used as the stimulus for developing critical thinking and problem-solving skills for acquiring new knowledge. The process of PBL starts with the student identifying the problem in a case. The student spends time either alone or in a group exploring and analyzing the problem and identifying learning resources needed to solve the problem. After acquiring the knowledge, the student applies it to solve the problem.[12] Small or large groups can be established for case discussions to help students develop communication skills, respect for other students' opinions, satisfaction for contributing to the discussion, and the ability to give and accept criticism.[12]

Cooperative or collaborative learning strategies involve students in the generation of knowledge.[8] Students are randomly assigned to groups of 4 to 6 at the beginning of the school term. Several times during the term, each group is given a patient case and a group leader is selected. Each student in the group volunteers to work on a certain portion of the case. The case is discussed in class and each member receives the same grade. After students have finished working in their small groups or during large group sessions, the teacher serves as a facilitator of the discussion rather than as a lecturer. The students actively participate in the identification and resolution of the problem. The integration of this technique helps with development of skills in decision making, conflict management, and communication.[7] Group discussions help students develop concepts from the material presented, clarify ideas, and develop new strategies for clinical problem solving. These skills are essential for lifelong learning and will be used by the students throughout their careers.

CASE STUDIES

Case studies are used by a number of pharmacy schools to teach disease state management.[1,13,14] Case studies are a written description of a real-life problem or situation. Only the facts are provided, usually in chronological sequence similar to what would be encountered in a patient care setting. Many times, as in real life, the information given is incomplete or important details are not available. When working through a case, the student must distinguish between relevant and irrelevant facts and become accustomed to the fact that there is no single "correct" answer. The use of cases actively involves the student in the analysis of facts and details of the case, selection of a solution to the problem, and defense of his or her solution through discussion of the case.[15]

Students enrolled in such courses find that the case study method requires a large amount of preparation time outside of class. In class, active participation is essential for the maximum learning benefit to be achieved. Because of the various backgrounds of the students in class, students learn different perspectives when dealing with patient problems. Some general steps proposed by McDade[15] for students when preparing for class include:

- Skim the text quickly to establish the broad issues of the case and the types of information presented for analysis.
- Reread the case very carefully, underlining key facts as you go.
- Note on scratch paper the key issues and problems. Next, go through the case again and sort out the relevant considerations and decisions for each problem.

- Prioritize problems and alternatives.
- Develop a set of recommendations to address the problems.
- Evaluate your decisions.

EXPECTATIONS OF STUDENTS AND TEACHERS

Active learning provides students with an opportunity to take a dynamic role in the learning process. The students are expected to participate in class discussions and be creative in formulating their own opinions. This method also requires that students listen and be respectful of the thoughts and opinions of their classmates. Assigned readings and homework must be completed before class in order to use class time efficiently for questions that are not answered in other reference material. In order to prepare answers or appropriate therapeutic recommendations, students may have to look beyond the reference materials provided by the teacher; they may have to perform literature searches and use the library to retrieve additional information. It is important for students to justify their recommendations. The active learning strategies outlined previously allow students to comprehend the material presented, participate in peer discussions, and formulate opinions as in real-life situations.

In order to implement active learning strategies in the classroom, teachers must overcome the anxiety that change often creates. Experimenting with active learning methods such as the pause technique and slowly implementing a change in the classroom may work best. Using any of the active learning strategies requires teachers to encourage as much classroom discussion as possible instead of lecturing. Use of a wireless microphone is helpful in encouraging student participation in large classrooms. Teachers should make an effort to learn the names of all students so they can more easily interact with them. In addition, teachers should have a preconceived plan for how the class discussion will go and stick to it. Hutchings recommends envisioning what the chalkboard should look like at the end of the session before beginning.[16]

MAXIMIZING ACTIVE LEARNING OPPORTUNITIES: ADVICE TO STUDENTS

Taking initiative is the key to deriving the benefits of active learning. It is crucial to recognize the three largest squelchers of initiative: laziness, fear of change, and force of habit.[17] You will find that time management is important. Be sure to schedule adequate time for studying, prepare for class by reading ahead, use transition times wisely, identify the times of day that you are most productive, and focus on the results rather than the time to complete an activity.[6]

In active learning, you are expected to talk about what you are learning, write about it, relate it to past experiences, and apply it to your daily life. In a sense, you repeatedly manipulate the information until it becomes a part of you. Some techniques to use when studying are to compare, contrast, and summarize similarities and differences between disease states and pharmacotherapy. In class, take advantage of every opportunity to present your own work. Attempt to relate personal experiences or outside events to topics discussed in class, and always be an active participant in class or group discussions.[18]

When reading assignments, summarize the information and take notes. These will be your notes to study for the course exams and to review for the pharmacy state board examination. While taking notes in class, leave a wide margin on the left to write down questions that you generate later when reviewing the notes.[11] Alternatively, make lists of questions from class or readings to discuss with your colleagues or faculty or try to answer them on your own. When time allows, seek out recent information on subjects that interest you. In class, always try to determine the "big picture."[18]

Some other methods for maximizing active learning are to review corrected assignments and exams for information that you do not understand and seek clarification from faculty. Complete assignments promptly and minimize short-term memorization. Attend class regularly and ask questions when you do not understand something. Give others a chance to contribute and try not to embarrass other students.[18]

In active learning, much of what you learn you will learn on your own. You will probably find that you read more, but you will gain understanding from reading. At the same time, you are developing a critical lifelong learning skill. Your reading will become more "depth processing" in which you focus on:

- The intent of the article
- Actively integrating what you read with previous parts of the text
- Trying to use your own ability to make a logical construction
- Thinking about the functional role of the different parts of an argument

In writing, consider summarizing the major points of each class. Writing about a topic develops critical thinking, communication, and organization skills. In classes that involve active learning, you may write for "think-pair-share" exercises, quizzes, summary paragraphs, and other activities. Stopping to write allows you to reflect on the information you have just heard and reinforces learning. Discussions may occur in large or small groups. Discussing material helps you to apply your knowledge, verbalize the medical and pharmacologic terminology, engage in active listening, think critically, be a leader or a follower, and develop interpersonal skills. When working in groups, all members should participate in problem solving. Teaching others is an excellent way to learn the subject matter.[6]

HOW TO USE THE CASEBOOK

This casebook has been prepared to assist in the development of each student's understanding of a disease and its management as well as problem-solving skills. It is important for students to realize that learning and understanding the material will be guided through problem solving. Students are encouraged to solve each of the problems individually or with others in a study group before discussion of the problem and topic in class. Being prepared for class is essential!

As problems are solved, the student begins to understand that each problem may not have a single solution or answer. The student will begin to appreciate the variety and complexity of diseases that are encountered in different patient populations. In some cases, more detailed information from the patient will play a pivotal role in drug therapy selection and monitoring. In others, most of the diagnoses may be resolved through use of laboratory analysis or specific medical tests. Some cases may require a much more in-depth assessment of the patient's disease state and treatment rendered so far. Other cases may involve initiation of both nonpharmacologic and pharmacologic therapy, ranging from single to multiple drug regimens.

Regardless of disease and/or treatment complexity, students must rely on knowledge previously learned in the areas of anatomy, biochemistry, microbiology, immunology, physiology, pathophysiology, medicinal chemistry, pharmacology, pharmacokinetics, and physical assessment. As a consequence, it will be necessary for the student to review previous notes, handouts, or textbooks. Students can use MEDLINE searches for primary literature, drug reference books, the Internet, and faculty experts as information sources. These resources and the textbook *Pharmacotherapy: A Pathophysiologic Approach* will be essential in supporting each student's ability to solve the problems successfully. Understanding the usefulness and limitations of these resources will be beneficial in the future. Likewise, discussions in study groups and class should lead to a further understanding of disease states and treatment strategies.

SUMMARY

The use of case studies and other active learning strategies will enhance the development of essential skills necessary to practice in any setting, including community pharmacy, health-system pharmacy, long-term care, home care, managed care, and the pharmaceutical industry. The role of the pharmacist will change dramatically in the next century; thus, it is important for students to acquire knowledge and develop the lifetime skills required for continued learning. Teachers who incorporate active learning strategies into the classroom are facilitating the development of lifelong learners who will be able to adapt to any changes that may occur in the profession of pharmacy.

References

1. Winslade N. Large-group problem-based learning: A revision from traditional to pharmaceutical care-based therapeutics. Am J Pharm Educ 1994;58:64–73.
2. Kane MD, Briceland LL, Hamilton RA. Solving problems. US Pharmacist 1995;20:55–74.
3. Tanenbaum BG, Cross DS, Tilson ER, et al. How to make active learning work for you. Radiol Technol 1998;69:374–376.
4. Moffett BS, Hill KB. The transition to active learning: A lived experience. Nurs Educator 1997;22:44–47.
5. Rangachari PK. Active learning: In context. Adv Physiol Educ 1995;13: S75–S80.
6. Warren G. Carpe Diem: A Student Guide to Active Learning. Landover, MD, University Press of America, 1996.
7. Bonwell CC, Eison JA. Active Learning: Creating Excitement in the Classroom. ASHE-ERIC Higher Education Report no. 1. Washington, DC, George Washington University, School of Education and Human Development, 1991.
8. Shakarian DC. Beyond lecture: Active learning strategies that work. JOPERD May–June 1995, 21–24.
9. Ruhl KL, Hughs CA, Schloss PJ. Using the pause procedure to enhance lecture recall. Teacher Educ Spec Educ 1987;10:14–18.
10. Rowe MB. Pausing principles and their effects on reasoning in science. In: Brawer FB, ed. Teaching the Sciences. New Directions for Community Colleges, no. 31. San Francisco, Jossey-Bass, 1980.
11. Elliot DD. Promoting critical thinking in the classroom. Nurs Educator 1996;21:49–52.
12. Walton HJ, Matthews MB. Essentials of problem-based learning. Med Educ 1989;23:542–558.
13. Hartzema AG. Teaching therapeutic reasoning through the case-study approach: Adding the probabilistic dimension. Am J Pharm Educ 1994;58:436–440.
14. Delafuente JC, Munyer TO, Angaran DM, et al. A problem-solving active-learning course in pharmacotherapy. Am J Pharm Educ 1994;58:61–64.
15. McDade SA. An Introduction to the Case Study Method: Preparation, Analysis, and Participation. New York, Teachers College Press, 1988.
16. Hutchings P. Using Cases to Improve College Teaching. Washington, DC, American Association of Higher Education, 1993.
17. Robbins A. Awaken the Giant Within. New York, Simon & Schuster, 1991.
18. Chickering AW, Gamson ZF, Barsi LM. Seven Principles for Good Practice in Undergraduate Education. Racine, WI, The Johnson Foundation, 1989.

CHAPTER 3 ....

Case Studies in Patient Communication

Marie E. Gardner, PharmD
Richard N. Herrier, PharmD

INTRODUCTION

Pharmacy practice has always been founded on both strong technical and people skills. Although all pharmacists are well versed in the technical aspects of the profession, most are not so well prepared regarding interpersonal communication within the clinical context. In contemporary pharmacy practice, good communication skills are critical for achieving optimal patient outcomes and increasing pharmacists' satisfaction with their professional roles. The goal of this chapter is to summarize some of the communication skills required to provide quality care and to provide cases with which to practice these skills. The focus is limited to the essential communication skills needed for symptom assessment and medication consultation and some useful strategies to improve compliance and monitor clinical progress. Readers are encouraged to review aspects of basic communication skills in other sources.[1–5]

BASIC MEDICATION CONSULTATION

Consultation on medication use is one of the most fundamental and important activities of the pharmacist, whether care is provided in a community pharmacy, clinic, or institutional site. Consultation on new medications is mandated by the Omnibus Budget Reconciliation Act of 1990, and most states require counseling for all patients on either new or both new and refill prescriptions.[6,7]

The traditional method of consulting involves providing information: the pharmacist "tells" and the patient "listens." There is little true dialogue or exchange of information. When questioning patients, the pharmacist often asks closed-ended questions such as, "Do you understand?" or, "Do you have any questions?" These closed-ended questions, which can be answered with a yes or no, provide little or no information about what the patient knows about the medication or what concerns the patient may have. When the pharmacist merely provides information and the conversation is essentially one-way, there is no opportunity to ascertain what the patient may know or think about the medication.

The pharmacist–patient consultation techniques developed by the Indian Health Service three decades ago, and further refined in collaboration with colleagues around the country, teach an interactive method of consultation that seeks to verify what the patient knows about the medication and "fill in the gaps" of knowledge only when needed.[2] Research shows that people forget 90% of what is heard within 60 minutes of hearing it.[1] Any counseling technique that is based on the pharmacist speaking most of the time will be ineffective, because patients will almost immediately forget what they heard. By making the patient an active participant in the process, increased learning will occur. Engaging patient participation in the exchange requires the use of specific, open-ended questions that seek to understand what the patient already knows about the medication, followed with new information and a summary at the end of the consultation. The specific techniques will now be discussed in more detail.

Basic Medication Consultation Skills

The interactive technique for consulting on medications uses open-ended questions that start with *who, what, where, when, why,* and *how*. The patient's answers should provide specific information rather than a simple yes or no. In fact, if the patient answers with a yes or no, one should be suspicious of a language barrier or problem with cognition.

Two sets of open-ended questions are used in the consultation. One is for new prescriptions (*Prime Questions*), and the other is for refill prescriptions (*Show-and-Tell Questions*), as shown in Table 1. Using these questions when counseling provides an interactive process that engages the

TABLE 1. Medication Consultation Skills

Prime Questions

1. What did your doctor tell you the medication is for?

   or

   What were you told the medication is for?
   What problem or symptom is it supposed to help?
   What is it supposed to do?
2. How did your doctor tell you to take the medication?

   or

   How were you told to take the medication?
   How often did your doctor say to take it?
   How much are you supposed to take?
   What did your doctor say to do when you miss a dose?
   What does three times a day mean to you?
3. What did your doctor tell you to expect?

   or

   What were you told to expect?
   What good effects are you supposed to expect?
   What bad effects did your doctor tell you to watch for?
   What should you do if a bad reaction occurs?

Show-and-Tell Questions

1. What do you take the medication for?
2. How do you take it?
3. What kind of problems are you having?

patient, thereby making him or her an active participant in the learning process. The questions provide an organized approach to ascertain what the patient already knows about the medication. Utilizing a systematic approach has been associated with improved recall of prescription instructions.[8] The pharmacist can praise the patient for correct information recalled, clarify points misunderstood, and add new information as needed. It spares the pharmacist from repeating information already known by the patient, which is an inefficient use of time. The steps in the consultation process are described next.

1. Open the Consultation

When the prescription is ready and the patient is called for counseling, establish rapport by introducing yourself by name and stating the purpose of the consultation. Then verify the patient's identity, either by asking for identification or at least by asking, "And you are . . . ?" If the patient is non-English speaking, hard of hearing, or otherwise unable to provide his or her name, you have identified a barrier in the consultation that must be overcome before discussing the medication.

If time permits and a private space is available, suggest that the consultation be conducted there and move to that area. This will be important for patients who have hearing problems or those needing extra privacy, such as patients receiving vaginal creams or those with AIDS. Sit facing the patient, and maintain the appropriate interpersonal distance (1½ to 2 feet) during the consultation.

2. Conduct the Counseling Session

Begin by asking the *Prime Questions* if the prescription is a new one, or use the *Show-and-Tell* method for a refill prescription. If the patient is able to tell you what the medication is for, you may choose to probe further or move to the next question. Probing further may be helpful when the patient answers in broad or vague terms. As an example, if a patient receiving a beta blocker tells you that the medication is for "my heart," you may wish to ask in an open-ended fashion, "What is it supposed to do for your heart?" Avoid asking, "Is it for chest pains?" or similar closed-ended questions, because you may alarm the patient by your suggestions, and you might waste time if multiple questions are asked. If the patient does not know what the medication is for or says, "Don't you know?" you should then ask why he or she visited the physician. The patient may describe symptoms of a condition known to be treatable with the medication in question. If so, indicate what symptoms the medication will help. If the patient is totally unaware, a referral back to the physician is indicated, lest the pharmacist judge in error the indication for the medication.

After verifying that the patient knows what the medication is for, ask the second prime question. Often, patients are unaware of the dosage instructions or indicate, "It's on the label, isn't it?" Be aware of the optimal dosing instructions, because the patient may correctly respond "twice a day," but you may need to advise on exact timing, or whether to take the drug with meals. Other questions to include under the second prime question are: (1) how long to take the medication, (2) exactly how much or how often to take it when the medication is prescribed as needed, (3) what to do when a dose is missed, and (4) how to store the medication. Rather than providing facts, consider asking the patient, "What did the doctor say about how long to take this medication?" or, "What will you do if you miss a dose?" Asking a question of the patient prompts his or her attention, whereas "telling" the information is more passive for the patient and the patient may not listen as well. Think of the counseling session as an opportunity to find out what the patient knows, rather than a place to showcase your knowledge. Keep the information you provide brief and to the point.

After verifying patient understanding about how to take the medication, proceed to the third prime question. Often, patients have been told nothing about beneficial or adverse effects. On the other hand, patients may describe anticipated results from the medication. If beneficial effects are mentioned, follow with, "What side effects were you warned about?" to determine the patient's knowledge of potential side effects. Other questions subsumed under this third prime question relate to how the patient will know if the medication is working, what precautions to take while taking the medication, and what to do if the medication does not work.

If the patient is unaware of potential adverse effects from the drug therapy, mention the most common or most serious adverse effects, and describe what to do if they occur. Research shows that patients want information about their medications, especially adverse effects, and that providing such information does not lead to the development of those reactions in most cases.[9-12] Recent work on communicating about the risk of drug reactions suggests a four-quadrant model in which each quadrant requires specific communication skills.[13] The quadrants contain a combination of either high or low probability of occurrence with high or low levels of severity or magnitude. An example of high probability and high magnitude is cancer chemotherapy, which entails frequent and severe toxicities. Empathic communication should be the lead skill in discussing the risk of therapy in this case. The combination of high probability and low magnitude is exemplified by gastric complaints from erythromycin. Pharmacists often encounter patients with common, bothersome side effects. Useful communication skills include providing information about how the medication will work and why it is a good therapy for them, as well as how to manage expected side effects.

When there is low probability but high magnitude (e.g., stroke from an oral contraceptive), careful attention to and assessment of the patient's perceptions about the possible side effects are needed. Be aware of how the patient's perceptions may differ from your own. Because the patient may only hear, "This is unlikely to happen but . . ." and tune out the specifics about the toxicity, it is helpful to ask the patient for feedback on the discussion of toxicity. In the final quadrant, the low probability and low magnitude of risk may be associated with a perception that the medication may have little value to the patient. Heavy-handed tactics to convince, frighten, or otherwise threaten the patient will not be effective. Questioning patients to determine their view of what benefits might be accrued from taking the medication is necessary. Follow with comments to match their assessment. For example, when a patient says, "Well, I could get an allergic reaction to this," the issue of the adverse effect is first and foremost in her mind, whereas the pharmacist may think, "I have never seen anyone allergic to this." Rather than try to convince the patient that no one becomes allergic to it, one might say, "Yes, that is possible. Which do you think is worse—putting up with the pain or taking a chance on the medication?" This brings into the open the discussion of both the risks and benefits of treatment. If the pharmacist can bring the patient along the thought continuum with a discussion of potential benefits, the patient may decide to give it a try. At times, the authors have found it useful to "contract" with the patient. For example, "Sam, we have discussed both the good and bad about taking this medicine, and I know you still have concerns about side effects. I really think this medicine is best for you. Would you be willing to try it for a week, and I will check in with you after a few days to see how things are going?" More often than not, the anticipated adverse effects do not appear.

Using skills described in the sections above for confronting adverse reactions or the fear of them will set the stage for better patient compliance. However, just the act of having to take a medication when one is not used to doing so poses compliance problems. When a patient has a new medication, and after using the prime questions to counsel the patient, it may be helpful to raise compliance concerns. A *universal statement* is a useful opener. It describes the situation for a group, then narrows down to focus on the individual. For example, "Mrs. Green, many patients have trouble fitting medications into their daily schedule. What problems do you foresee in taking this medicine?" It may be necessary to probe into their daily habits and help them find a way to tie medication taking into a particular activity. For instance, if the patient always makes coffee in the morning, having the medication nearby may be sufficient reminder to promote compliance. Be sure to use a partnership approach. Additional compliance-enhancing skills are discussed later in this chapter.

3. Close the Consultation

Most consultations are a combination of the patient knowing some information and the pharmacist providing additional information as the prime questions are reviewed. Because of this, it is important to close the consultation with the *final verification*. Think of the final verification as asking the patient to "play back" everything learned in order to check that the information is complete and accurate. Say to the patient, "Just to make sure I didn't leave anything out, please go over with me how you are going to use the medication." Although the language seems bulky, if the question were phrased, "Just to make sure you've got this . . .," the patient may feel embarrassed if he or she does not recall important facts. At this point, the patient should describe correct use of the medication. Any errors can be corrected and any omissions clarified. Then ask the patient if there is anything else he or she needs and offer assistance as required.

A similar process is used for refill prescriptions. The *Show-and-Tell Questions* verify patient understanding of proper use of chronic medications or medications that the patient has used in the past. The pharmacist begins the process by showing the medication to the patient; that is, by opening the bottle and displaying the contents. Then, the patient tells the pharmacist how he uses the medication by answering the questions shown in Table 1. Note that the doctor is omitted as a reference, since the patient should have been counseled properly by the pharmacist before this and should have all information needed for proper medication usage. The show-and-tell technique allows the pharmacist to detect problems with compliance or unwanted drug effects. If the patient answers incorrectly to the second question, the patient may be non-compliant or the physician may have changed the dosage. The pharmacist will need to further define the reason for the discrepancy. The second show-and-tell question also allows the pharmacist to ask the patient to demonstrate use of an inhaler or injectable medication or how to measure liquid doses to assure proper usage.

Some pharmacists have difficulty asking the third question, fearing that they may arouse suspicion in the patient. However, research discounts this notion, as previously discussed. If potential adverse effects were discussed when the patient was initially counseled, it seems natural, and certainly relevant and important, to query the patient about adverse effects at the refill visit. If new symptomatology is present, explore this further using the *Key Symptom Questions*. Because it is important to evaluate new symptoms critically, we will describe this in detail next.

Exploring Symptoms

At the prescription counter, over the telephone, or at a bedside visit, the patient may mention symptoms that could be related to drug therapy. Knowing how to explore the patient's symptoms and evaluate their relationship to either the disease or its treatment is a key component of the pharmacist's assessment skills. The first step is to get the patient to more fully reveal information about the symptom. An introductory statement such as "Tell me more about it" will encourage the patient to provide more specific details. After this, the *Key Symptom Questions* should be used. These seven focused, open-ended questions, based on medical interviewing techniques, seek specifics that will help define whether the symptom is related to drug therapy.[14,15] They are:

1. *Onset/timing:* When did you notice this, or When did it start?
2. *Duration:* How long have you had this problem?
3. *Context:* Under what circumstances does this symptom appear?
4. *Quality:* What does it feel like?
5. *Quantity:* How much and how often do you notice it?
6. *Treatment:* What makes it better, or What have you done about it?
7. *Associated symptoms:* What other symptoms are you having?

Without proper attention to detail, many pharmacists make assumptions that the symptom expressed is due to a disease state and do not adequately address it. Or they may jump to conclusions about the cause of the symptom and recommend a treatment without knowing the true cause. For example, a patient taking a nonsteroidal anti-inflammatory drug who complains of fatigue might be recommended a vitamin if the pharmacist thinks the patient is tired from inadequate nutrition. Probing the symptom of fatigue with the questions listed above may reveal that the fatigue started after the medication was begun and is accompanied by gastric distress, suggesting anemia from gastrointestinal blood loss as a possible cause for the fatigue.

The *Key Symptom Questions* are also important when there is a tendency to attribute *every* symptom to a medication, as patients are sometimes inclined to do. For instance, a pharmacy student reviewed the chart of a patient with bipolar illness, seizures, and Parkinsonism. The patient was receiving several medications including carbamazepine and carbidopa/levodopa. The patient complained of blurred vision and insomnia, which the student felt were due to the medications. When the patient was interviewed using the questioning technique described, she indicated that she had blurred vision only out of the left eye and that she had insomnia "since the day I was born." Answers to further questions suggested that her symptoms were not likely to be related to her drug therapy.

Knowledge of each drug's side effect profile and the disease state symptomatology is essential to be able to determine whether the symptom resulted from the drug therapy or the disease state. In some cases, it could be either, in which case it is important to ascertain the onset of the symptom. If the symptom began or worsened after starting a new medication, then there is a higher likelihood that the problem is drug related.

Students and new practitioners are often confused about what to do once the symptom has been explored. Determining the seriousness of the problem is sometimes difficult. It is helpful to ask yourself, "What is the worst thing that can happen in this case? If this is an adverse reaction to the medication, what will happen if the medication is continued? What will happen to the patient (and disease process) if the medication is stopped?" Easily discernible side effects, such as dizziness from an antihypertensive, are managed by practical suggestions to the patient without discontinuation of drug therapy. Even so, the patient may elect to stop taking the medication, and the pharmacist must think ahead to those consequences and advise the patient accordingly. More serious toxicities require either calling the patient's physician or advising the patient to discuss the problem with the physician as soon as possible, rather than suggesting stopping the medication.

The most important aspect of addressing symptoms is to obtain enough information to make an informed clinical judgment. This is accomplished by using the *Key Symptom Questions* outlined earlier.

Barriers in the Consultation

The clinical skills described will be easily applied in situations where there are few or no barriers in communication between patient and pharmacist. In reality, there are often obstacles to overcome in the environment or within the pharmacist or patient. Examples of problems within the pharmacy environment that deter patient consultation include lack of privacy, interruptions, high work load, and insufficient staff. Barriers present within the pharmacist include lack of desire or skills to adequately counsel patients, stereotyping patients and problems, and difficulty maintaining concentration while counseling, especially when stress is a factor. A detailed analysis of these barriers is beyond the scope of this discussion but can be found in the references.[3] Barriers that the patient brings to the encounter

will be discussed here insofar as overcoming them relates to the clinical communication skills discussed.

The structured approach for patient consultation can be likened to knowing the road on which you are traveling. However, unforeseen events happen on every path and may arise at any time. Just as one must remove or negotiate around the obstacle on the highway, the pharmacist must recognize and manage barriers brought by the patient during the encounter for the consultation to reach the desired end. There are two types of barriers: functional and emotional.

1. Functional Barriers

These barriers include problems with hearing and vision that make it difficult for the patient to absorb information during the consultation. Also, language barriers and illiteracy are formidable obstacles to proper consultation. Recognizing these barriers is usually not difficult, as the signs of poor vision are easy to observe. So, too, will language problems become apparent early in the counseling process provided you use open-ended questions to probe patient understanding. Strategies specific to each barrier are needed when these problems are identified. For instance, moving to a quiet area, repeating information, and asking for feedback from the patient are important when hearing is a problem. Giving clear verbal instructions and using large-type print materials are helpful when the patient has vision difficulties. Using translators, picture diagrams, and involving English-speaking care givers are important when language problems exist.

2. Emotional Barriers

Emotional barriers are common in everyday interactions, including pharmacist–patient communication. When not handled properly, they give rise to further aggravation, break down communication, and thus inhibit effective consultation. Patients may express anger, hostility, sadness, depression, fear, anxiety, or embarrassment directly or indirectly during consultation with the pharmacist. They may also give the attitude of a "know-it-all," be suspicious of medications, or seem unmotivated or uninterested. Some of these barriers might be momentary, such as the frustration experienced when the prescription cannot be filled because the medication is unavailable at that time. On the other hand, the patient with a chronic pain syndrome may at various times be less attentive due to being uncomfortable or in pain. The attitude of the patient who "knows all" about his or her medications likely will not change over time. The patient with a terminal illness may be chronically depressed, uninterested, or feel hopeless about the benefits of therapy.

Unlike seeing the patient with a white cane and knowing that a vision problem exists, emotional barriers can be more difficult to discern. Since most patients will not say "I'm angry and frustrated about feeling so ill" or "I'm upset that my doctor didn't spend much time with me," their feelings surface in statements such as "I don't know why it takes all day to put a few pills in the bottle!" or "I don't know why I have to take this stupid medicine. Nothing seems to help anyway." Unfortunately, we usually respond to the content of the message (e.g., "I'll have this ready for you as soon as I can") without recognizing that there may be other issues behind the statement, issues that may impact on the encounter and more importantly, on the patient's decision to comply with therapy. It takes patience and practice to listen beyond the words, and this requires the skill of *reflective responding*.

When we respond with a reflection of what the patient is saying, thinking, or feeling, we let the person know we are truly listening and give the person the opportunity to admit to feelings, clarify thoughts, and bring forth information. Making a reflecting response initially is difficult for some pharmacists, because most of us have not been trained to use these skills. Reflective responding attempts to reflect in words what the patient is saying or feeling. The reflection may be based on the *content* or thought expressed by the patient, and/or the *feelings* associated with it that are often not outwardly expressed. Reflecting responses are especially called for when the patient is demonstrating emotions. Angry looks, pounding fists, averted eye contact, and head drooping all convey certain emotional states. Hesitating gestures or remarks such as "Well . . . I guess I could try it" suggest concerns that need to be gently brought to light.

The first step in effective reflective responding is to identify and label the emotional state. The four basic emotional states are *mad, sad, glad,* and *scared.* As you observe the patient during consultation, certain nonverbal or verbal signs (e.g., hesitating words) may suggest one of the four feeling states. The second step is to put the word describing the feeling state into a sentence to use as a response to the patient. Some basic structures for sentences include, "It sounds as if you are (frustrated, mad, happy)" or "I can see that you are (happy, confused, mad)." These remarks indicate to patients that you are truly attempting to understand their concerns; thus, the patient and his or her concerns remain the focus of the encounter.

To the patient who remarked, "I don't know why I have to take this. Nothing helps anyway," the pharmacist might determine that the nonverbal tone of voice and choice of words indicate the patient is disappointed with results of his therapy. Alternatively, he may be feeling hopeless about getting better. An appropriate reflecting response is, "It sounds as if you have been frustrated with the things you have tried." This statement neither judges nor advises. It allows the patient the opportunity to open up discussion of a difficult topic, if he so chooses. Contrast this with the following: "This is a good medicine, Joe, and I really think it will help." Although this may be true, maintaining the consultation on a technical, information-providing level avoids dealing with the underlying issues of the patient's fears.

Emotional barriers can occur at any time throughout the consultation, and they must be dealt with in order to put the patient in a receptive frame of mind. Embarrassment is a factor when vaginal preparations, condom use, and similar topics are the subject of the consultation. Observe for signs of embarrassment such as averted gaze or fidgeting, and respond with, "This can be hard to talk about, but it's important that we discuss . . ." Also, be matter-of-fact, move to a private space, and speak in a normal tone of voice to help alleviate the embarrassment.

When faced with patients' emotional outbursts, acknowledge their expressed feelings before continuing with the consultation. The initial use of reflecting responses will allow the consultation to proceed with both parties devoting attention to the primary issues of drug therapy and usage, rather than to interpersonal difficulties. Another important aspect of patient-focused care is compliance and disease monitoring.

COMPLIANCE AND DISEASE MONITORING

In no other situation is the pharmacist's role in monitoring and managing medication usage more vital than in the case of patients requiring chronic drug therapy, especially for diseases that are asymptomatic. Many factors contribute to the pharmacist's success in assuring beneficial outcomes. Among them are practice site, pharmacist competence, support of administration, and breadth of responsibilities, including in some cases prescriptive authority. Hatoum and Akhras have documented extensively the value of pharmacists' contributions to ambulatory care sites ranging from a community group practice to home health patients and others.[16]

The Indian Health Service has provided a full range of pharmaceutical care services to its patients for over three decades. Besides the traditional dispensing role, IHS pharmacists offer private consultations to all patients and have prescriptive authority for refilling chronic medications based on their assessment of the patient's needs.[17,18] Some pharmacists have been trained to provide primary medical care as pharmacist practitioners, and this movement has subsequently spread to other practice sites. Currently, several states have passed regulations that allow pharmacists to diagnose and prescribe.[17] Whether your practice is a sophisticated one such as those just described or a more typical one in community, hospital, or long-term care, providing pharmaceutical care to patients requiring chronic drug therapy can have significant positive outcomes. To effectively provide long-term pharmaceutical care, several important factors need to be considered.

Whose Disease Is It Anyway?

One of the common misperceptions held by health care professionals regarding a patient with a chronic disease is that the professional manages the patient's disease. Nothing could be further from the truth, and this medical myth is probably one of the major contributors to compliance problems among patients with chronic diseases. In the traditional medical care model, health care professionals perceive their roles to be in the diagnosis, treatment, and management of disease. As drug therapy managers, clinical pharmacists focus on blood levels, kinetic dosage calculations, and drug interactions. Guided by this focus on technical aspects of patient care, health care professionals often become frustrated and angry when patients do not follow instructions, or despite the provider's best efforts achieve only partially satisfactory results. In reality, the only time the professional manages the treatment is during the very limited time that patients encounter the health care delivery system during an office visit or while institutionalized in a hospital or long-term care facility. For the vast majority of time, the patient controls the treatment of his or her disease, especially those that require continuous medication. Failure to recognize this basic truth has created: (1) considerable tension in patient–provider relationships, (2) provider frustration and anger, (3) poor communication, (4) negative provider attitudes toward individual patients, (5) poor patient outcomes, (6) patient distrust of providers, and (7) legal consequences that have been a major contributor to rising health care costs.[19–22]

One author strongly suggests that non-compliance in diabetes mellitus is due in large part to the failure of providers to recognize that their goal is not treating the disease, but *helping the patient treat the disease.*[23] That contention is supported by current medical literature on compliance that links good communication and a partnership style of provider–patient relationship to increased satisfaction, compliance, and better patient outcomes.[22–25]

To be successful in assisting patients achieve good outcomes, the provider and pharmacist must eschew the traditional medical myth regarding who manages the disease and adopt a partnership approach, acting as facilitators to help patients manage their disease. That is, it is the *patient's* disease; the providers' job is to *help them manage it.*

Go Slow/Use Interactive Techniques

Patients can only absorb a limited amount of new information at each encounter. Too many times, in an attempt to do a thorough job, health care professionals inadvertently overwhelm the patient with information at or near the time of diagnosis or treatment initiation. Patients' active listening abilities last less than a minute during a monologue presentation, and they retain only a few pieces of information from a prolonged discussion and may miss key facts. In addition, a large volume of technical information may confuse or frighten patients, leading to the poor outcome that educational efforts are intended to prevent.[24]

Successful patient educators do two things: (1) give patients information in small manageable increments, and (2) actively involve the patient in the educational process by creating an interactive dialogue and using other hands-on approaches that are consistent with adult learning principles.[25] For the pharmacist dispensing the initial prescription, this entails verifying that the patient understands how to take the medicine and its most common side effects. For example, with hydrochlorothiazide 25 mg daily for hypertension, the pharmacist should verify that the patient knows what it is for, to take it once daily in the morning to prevent nighttime voiding, that it takes a while before any changes in blood pressure occur, and that the patient will notice increased urination the first week, which should lessen thereafter. Discussions about diet, exercise, and related issues can wait until later visits. Giving the patient a handout on hypertension and diuretics would be appropriate and can lead to questions and subsequent education at later visits or during a follow-up phone call.

Set the Stage for Future Encounters

Many providers initially explain to patients how they are going to monitor for disease control and progression so that subsequent questions, laboratory tests, and examinations are viewed by the patients as a normal part of their care. However, few providers follow a similar process regarding compliance. Therefore, without previous explanation, provider questions about compliance are likely to be associated with parental-type sanctions from the provider. To avoid this "punishment," patients may avoid disclosing compliance problems when asked. This all-too-common problem can be prevented by remembering who ultimately manages the disease and by using specific strategies during the *initial* patient contact. Explain that compliance is very important to successful outcomes, but that you know how hard it is to remember to take medication every day. Tell the patient that you expect that he or she will be like all patients and experience some difficulty remembering to take the medication. Ask the patient to keep track of those instances if possible, and further explain that you will be asking at each visit about the problems he or she has had with the medication so you can assist to better remember to take the medication. This can easily be done in association with explanations about how the progress of the disease will be monitored.

Monitoring and Education of the Patient at Return Visits

Organizing an effective approach to evaluating and educating patients with chronic diseases at return visits may be problematic in a busy practice setting. One simple way to look at all patients returning for follow-up of chronic diseases is to use the three Cs: *Control, Complications,* and *Compliance.* To evaluate the *control* of the chronic disease, couple objective findings (e.g., blood pressure or range of motion) with subjective findings from the consultation (e.g., reports of dizziness, nocturnal voiding, or degree of morning joint stiffness). *Complications* can occur both from disease progression and drug effects. As with the control parameters, a combination of subjective findings from the patient interview and objective findings from the health record or patient profile (e.g., physical examination findings and pertinent laboratory or other tests) can be used to quickly evaluate the presence of potential complications. For example, a patient with hypertension, diabetes mellitus, and osteoarthritis who takes captopril, chlorpropamide, and ibuprofen can be queried about the presence of cough, difficulty sleeping, and exercise tolerance. These questions are primarily directed at detecting congestive heart failure or renal failure due to hypertension and/or diabetes but also will help detect drug-related problems such as cough due to the angiotensin-converting enzyme (ACE) inhibitor and renal effects from ibuprofen. Checking recent laboratory values for serum creatinine, electrolytes, and blood glucose will help assess diabetes and hypertension and detect NSAID-induced renal impairment, excessive chlorpropamide dosage, and ACE inhibitor-induced hyperkalemia.

With regard to *compliance* problems, the pharmacist's actions can be divided into three steps: (1) *recognize* potential compliance problems, (2) *identify* probable causes of non-compliance, and (3) *manage* the problem with specific steps. This "RIM" model is a process that can be used by pharmacists to enhance patient compliance.[26] In this model (Table 2), subjec-

TABLE 2. Steps in the "RIM" Model for Compliance Counseling

Recognize Potential Non-compliance

• For objective evidence, use supportive compliance probes.
  Examples: *I noticed that this refill was due.*
  I'm concerned that you will not get the full benefits from your medication if it's not taken as prescribed.

• For subjective evidence, use reflecting responses.
  Examples: *It sounds as if you are worried about side effects.*
  So you feel that your medication is not working.

Identify/Categorize the Non-compliance
• *Knowledge deficits* are evidenced through a patient's statements, indicating a misunderstanding or lack of information.
• *Practical impediments* are revealed by a patient's description of lack of funds, inability to access the medication, forgetfulness, difficulty with a complicated dosing schedule, or an adverse reaction.
• *Attitudinal barriers* are disclosed by a patient's statements that highlight his or her lack of faith in medication.
Manage the Non-compliance
• *Knowledge deficits* are resolved by providing both verbal and written information, verifying the patient's understanding.
• *Practical impediments* are dealt with by providing corrective actions individualized for the problem (e.g., providing a dosing calendar developed with the patient, working with the physician to find easier dosing regimens, or using pill boxes). Adverse reactions require the use of the *Key Symptom Questions.*
• *Attitudinal barriers* are rectified by maintaining an understanding of the patient's view using empathy, open-ended questions, and universal statements.

tive and objective findings are used to detect potential compliance problems. First, the health record or patient profile is reviewed for objective evidence of potential non-compliance before talking with the patient. During profile review, three items should alert the pharmacist to potential compliance problems. The first and most common item is a discrepancy between the number of doses that should have been taken and the number of doses dispensed. Second, patients with incomplete refill requests (e.g., only one or two of multiple chronic medications due at the same time) raise suspicion for non-compliance. Third, the prescribing of a new medication for the same condition or one that may unknowingly be prescribed to offset adverse effects from another medication may indicate compliance problems. Patients often present to medical providers with new complaints. If the provider does not make the connection between the new symptom and the side effect, compliance or therapeutic problems may eventually occur. If patients taking ACE inhibitors present with new or repeat prescriptions for cough suppressants or antibiotics for bronchitis, the pharmacist should be alerted to consider the potential for ACE inhibitor-induced cough. In extreme cases, patients may stop the needed drug and continue with the drug used to treat the side effects, which is unnecessary and could pose risks in itself.

Care must be taken in interpreting these signs. Positive findings during profile or chart review call for further exploration before a definite compliance problem can be ascertained. In some cases there are rational explanations for the objective findings. Gaps in refills may be due to patients obtaining refills at another location, or the doctor may have told the patient to change the dosage schedule or to stop the drug altogether.

When the profile indicates potential non-compliance, the best approach is to begin consultation using the *Show-and-Tell* technique for refill prescriptions. The patient may provide one or more clues during consultation to confirm your suspicions. If not, the pharmacist must initiate a more direct approach using a *supportive compliance probe*. This is a specific type of statement that uses "I" language to describe specifically what the pharmacist sees and to ask a question to probe into the discrepancy. For example, "I noticed when I reviewed your profile that you hadn't had your prednisone refilled in about two weeks. I was concerned that there might have been some changes that I'm not aware of." This combination of "I noticed . . . and I'm concerned . . ." can be very effective in getting a dialogue started in a non-threatening manner. Another useful approach is the *universal statement,* such as, "Most of my patients have problems remembering to take every dose of their medication. What kinds of problems are you having?" Open the discussion of compliance problems with non-threatening language, and there is a greater likelihood that the patient will disclose problems.

During the consultation, the patient may provide the pharmacist with clues to compliance problems not revealed by patient record review. Indeed, patients may refill their medications on time but actually take only some of the doses. Patients who tell the pharmacist during the *Show-and-Tell* questioning that they are taking their medication differently than prescribed provide a strong indication of a potential compliance problem. Some clues may be obvious, such as when a patient asks, "Why do I have to keep taking this medicine?" This might be a "red flag," since it seems fairly clear that the patient wishes not to take the prescription. However, many statements are more subtle. Examples of these vague clues, called "pink flags," include: "My doctor says I *should* take it . . ." or "My doctor *wants* me to. . ." or "I'm *supposed* to be taking . . ." These are usually detected when the pharmacist asks the first two *Show-and-Tell* questions. Other "pink

flags" are more closely associated with the third question, such as when a long pause occurs during the patient's reply, which may indicate potential problems. For example, the question "What kinds of problems are you having with the medication?" may prompt the following "pink flag" responses: "Well . . . none, really," or a hesitation before saying "No, none." Reflecting responses discussed earlier in this chapter are appropriate in this situation. Such responses include "It seems as if you are not too sure about taking that," or "It sounds as if you think there may be a problem." These responses open the dialogue in a non-threatening manner and focus on the patient's perceptions or suggestion that a problem exists.

Patients may ask, "Does this medicine have any side effects?" or "What kind of side effects does this have?" or "Is this anything like (another specific drug)?" More often than not, pharmacists simply answer the question without really listening to the underlying concern. An appropriate response would be "Why do you ask?," especially if the patient looks hesitant or the intonation of the question suggests doubt about taking the medication. When the authors use this question, patients often disclose that a relative had it (or a similar medication) or the media has reported problems with the drug. These indirect experiences create enough doubt such that the patient wavers about taking the medication. Obviously, if the pharmacist uses the *Show-and-Tell* technique alone and does not *recognize* these "pink flags," the consultation will be in vain, for the patient will leave not having the underlying doubt resolved. Therefore, it is crucial to develop keen active listening skills to denote the presence of the "pink flags" and then use reflecting responses to probe into the problem.

During the *Show-and-Tell* questioning, patients may disclose symptoms that may indicate an adverse effect. This is sometimes a reason for premature discontinuation of treatment or for skipping doses. When such appears to be the case, use of the previously mentioned *Key Symptom Questions* will help identify the exact nature of the problem. Resolution of the problem will be dictated by its clinical urgency.

Once the presence of the compliance problem has been confirmed, further use of reflecting and other responses can identify the nature of the problem. Compliance problems can be categorized within three groups. The first is a *knowledge* deficit. In these cases, patients have insufficient information or skills or misinformation that prevents compliance. An example is the patient who put contraceptive jelly on toast, or the patient who was never shown or has forgotten how to use an inhaler. The second group involves *practical impediments* or barriers, such as complex drug regimens involving multiple drugs and/or different dosage schedules, difficulty in developing routines that facilitate medication compliance, difficulty in opening containers, or insufficient mental aptitude to comply. The final category is *attitudinal barriers*. Among the most difficult to identify and manage, these include patient beliefs about health, disease, and/or treatment that are inconsistent with the prescribed regimen. These may reflect differences in cultural beliefs.[27–29] As outlined by the health belief model, the patient's perceived severity of risk compared to the perceived benefit of treatment plays a large role in determining medication compliance.[28] Other factors such as patient desire to be in control and patient belief that he or she can successfully implement the recommended treatment also strongly influence compliance.[24] Finally, the most prevalent and potentially the most difficult belief differences to overcome are patients' *lay theories*.[28] Common lay theories held by patients include, "You need to give your body a rest from medicine or it will become immune to it," or "You only need to take medicine when you feel sick, not when you feel okay," or "If one dose is good, then two must be better."

Once the specific cause is identified, a specific strategy to manage that problem can be attempted. Most knowledge and skill deficiencies can be successfully corrected with education and/or training. Practical impediments respond well to specific measures such as simplifying regimens, use of easy-open containers, and enlisting the aid of a spouse or caregiver. Attitudinal issues tend to be the most complex and difficult to solve. Even lay theories, which would seem easily fixed by correcting misinformation, are extremely difficult to overcome because the nature of lay theories makes them highly resistant to change. Again, it takes practice, careful listening, repeated conversations with the patient, and a supportive climate for the patient to acknowledge one of these barriers. Patients will only do so when they feel the pharmacist will not denigrate them or argue against their beliefs. Partnership language and gentle confrontation on the facts are indicated. Repeated efforts to enlighten may, over time, change the view of the patient.

CONCLUSION

Contemporary pharmacy practice is changing at a very rapid pace. Pharmaceutical care, that which focuses on the patient's outcomes of drug therapy, is the founding principle for practitioners. For today's pharmacist, whether he or she practices in the community, hospital, or another setting, the delivery of quality pharmaceutical care involves the skills and techniques discussed in this chapter, as well as others that support the pharmacist–patient interaction and medication use process. As direct patient contact and responsibility for drug therapy outcomes become the main task for the pharmacist, the skills of interpersonal communication, medical history taking, patient medication consultation, plus compliance monitoring and enhancement become the "tools of the trade." The consistent application of a high level of interpersonal and applied clinical skills by the pharmacist will lead to optimal outcomes for the patient.

References

1. Bolton R. People Skills. New York, Simon & Schuster, 1979.
2. Gardner M, Boyce RW, Herrier RN. Pharmacist–Patient Consultation Program, Unit 1: An Interactive Approach to Verify Patient Understanding. New York, Pfizer, 1991.
3. Pharmacist–Patient Consultation Program, Unit 2: Counseling Patients in Challenging Situations. New York, Pfizer, 1993.
4. Meldrum H. Interpersonal Communication in Pharmaceutical Care. New York, Haworth Press, 1994.
5. Muldary TW. Interpersonal Relations for Health Professionals: A Social Skills Approach. New York, Macmillan, 1983.
6. Meade V. OBRA '90: How has pharmacy reacted? Am Pharm 1995;NS35:12–16.
7. Pugh CB. Pre-OBRA '90 Medicaid survey: How community pharmacy practice is changing. Am Pharm 1995;NS35:17–23.
8. Gardner M, Hurd PD, Slack M. Effect of information organization on recall of medication instructions. J Clin Pharm Ther 1989;14:1–7.
9. Morris LA, Grossman R, Barkdoll GL, et al. A survey of patient sources of prescription drug information. Am J Public Health 1984;74:1161–1162.
10. Lamb GC, Green SS, Heron J. Can physicians warn patients of potential side effects without fear of causing those side effects? Arch Intern Med 1994; 154:2753–2756.
11. Howland JS, Baker MG, Poe T. Does patient education cause side effects? A controlled trial. J Fam Pract 1990;31:62–64.
12. Gardner ME, Rulien N, McGhan WF, Mead RA. A study of patients' perceived importance of medication information provided by physicians in a health maintenance organization. Drug Intell Clin Pharm 1988;22:596–598.
13. Meldrum H, Hardy M. Challenges in communicating about risk. In: Communicating Risk to Patients: Proceedings of the Conference. Rockville, MD, United States Pharmacopeial Convention, 1995:36–49.
14. Billings JA, Stoeckle JD. The Clinical Encounter. Chicago, Year Book Medical Publishers, 1989.
15. Boyce RW, Herrier RN. Obtaining and using patient data. Am Pharm 1991;NS31:65–71.
16. Hatoum HT, Akhras K. 1993 Bibliography: A 32-year literature review on the value and acceptance of ambulatory care provided by pharmacists. Ann Pharmacother 1993;27:1106–1119.
17. Church RM. Pharmacy practice in the Indian Health Service. Am J Hosp Pharm 1987;44:771–775.
18. Herrier RN, Boyce RW, Apgar DA. Pharmacist-managed patient-care services and prescriptive authority in the U.S. Public Health Service. Hosp Formul 1990;25:67–68, 76–78, 80.
19. Beckman HS, Markakis KM, Suchman AL, Frankel RM. The doctor–patient relationship and malpractice: Lessons from plaintiff depositions. Arch Intern Med 1994;154:1365–1370.
20. Anderson LA, Zimmerman MA. Patient and physician perceptions of their relationship and patient satisfaction: A study of chronic disease management. Patient Educ Couns 1993;20:27–36.
21. DiMatteo MR. The physician–patient relationship: Effects on the quality of health care. Clin Obstet Gynecol 1994;37:149–161.
22. Viinamaki H. The patient–doctor relationship and metabolic control in patients with type 1 (insulin dependent) diabetes mellitus. Int J Psychiatry Med 1993;23:265–274.
23. Anderson RM. Is the problem of noncompliance all in our heads? Diabetes Educ 1985;11:31–34.
24. Herrier RN, Boyce RW. Compliance with prescribed drug regimens. In: Bressler R, Katz M, eds. Geriatric pharmacology. New York, McGraw-Hill, 1993:63–77.
25. Eraker SA, Kirscht JP, Becker MH. Understanding and improving patient compliance. Ann Intern Med 1984;100:258–268.
26. Pharmacist–Patient Consultation Program, Unit 3: Counseling to Enhance Compliance. New York, Pfizer, 1995.
27. Becker MH. Patient adherence to prescribed therapies. Med Care 1985; 23:539–555.
28. Leventhal H. The role of theory in the study of adherence to treatment and doctor–patient interactions. Med Care 1985;23:556–563.
29. Kübler-Ross E. On Death and Dying. New York, Macmillan, 1969.

PATIENT CASES

This section includes three scenarios with patient profiles and prescriptions that require counseling. First, review the profile and prescription and think about issues that may arise during the consultation. Then provide written answers to the questions asked. Use concepts from the preceding material on counseling strategies, as well as any other techniques you think are useful or have found useful through your own experience or by observing others in practice.

Case No. 1: Sally M. Johnson

NAME	Johnson, Sally M.	DATE 1/20/99	
ADDRESS	1862 Briar Court		
	Lansdale, PA 18018	AGE IF CHILD	

FULL DIRECTIONS FOR USE	Rx No. 148647
R_x	Date filled
Tamoxifen 10 mg	Cost
#60	Fee
Sig: i po BID	Total Price
	☐ Do not refill
	No. of refills authorized: 6

☐   IDENTIFY CONTENTS ON LABEL UNLESS CHECKED

☐   NON-PROPRIETARY EQUIVALENT UNLESS CHECKED

S. Mayer   M.D.

Patient Medication Profile

Name: Sally M. Johnson	Known Diseases	Allergies and Sensitivities	Additional Information
Address: 1862 Briar Court	s/p hysterectomy 9/90 with	Sulfa: rash	
Lansdale, PA 18018	estrogen replacement		
Telephone: 832-7358	s/p surgery, CA breast 12/95		
Date of Birth: 4/15/42			

Date	Rx No.	Medication	Strength	Quantity	Dosage Regimen	R.Ph.	Physician
07/18/97	83104	Premarin	0.625 mg	#100	1 QD	JD	Hepler
10/25/97	89436	Premarin	0.625 mg	#100	1 QD	HV	Hepler
12/04/98	145922	Tylox		#12	1–2 Q4H PRN	JD	Cavanaugh
12/04/98	145923	Dicloxacillin	250 mg	#40	2 QID	JD	Cavanaugh

Sally comes to the pharmacy alone to pick up the tamoxifen prescription. You have reviewed the profile and are ready to counsel her on the medication.

1. Before talking with the patient, what concerns do you have about counseling this patient? What else would you like to know about your patient?
2. How are you going to begin the consultation?
3. Listed below are three different responses by the patient to the first *Prime Question*. For each statement, consider what each statement reveals about what the patient knows or feels, and state what should happen next in the consultation.

   Patient Response A:*   *"He gave it to me after my surgery."*
   Patient Response B: *"I just had surgery for breast cancer."*
   Patient Response C: *"I know what it's for."*

4. Listed below are three different responses to the second *Prime Ques-*

tion. Consider what each tells you, and state what you would do next in the consultation.

Patient Response A: *"I'm going to take it twice a day."*
Patient Response B: *"It's on the label, isn't it?"*
Patient Response C: *"I don't remember. He didn't tell me."*

5. Listed below are three different responses to the third *Prime Question*. Consider what each tells you, and state what you would do next in the consultation.

Patient Response A: *"I hope it will keep my cancer in check."*
Patient Response B: *"The doctor says things look good, but I thought I heard something about uterine cancer?"*
Patient Response C: *"Nothing. I'm not sure anything is going to help me now."*

---

* Patient statements A, B, and C do not necessarily correspond throughout the consultation.

Case No. 2: Thomas Gordon

NAME	Gordon, Thomas	DATE	2/15/99
ADDRESS	38 Main Street		
	Muncie, IL	AGE IF CHILD	

FULL DIRECTIONS FOR USE		
R_x		Rx No. 82695
		Date filled
	Cephalexin 500 mg	Cost
	#40	Fee
	Sig: i po QID	Total Price

☐   Do not refill
No. of refills authorized: 0

☐   IDENTIFY CONTENTS ON LABEL UNLESS CHECKED

☐   NON-PROPRIETARY EQUIVALENT UNLESS CHECKED

B. Higley   M.D.

Patient Medication Profile

Date: 1/19/95

Name:	Thomas Gordon	Known Diseases:	Allergies/Sensitivities
Date of Birth:	01/10/48	Diabetes since 1994	NKA

Address: 38 Main Street, Muncie, IL   Telephone: 542-5016

Additional Information:

Notes:

Date	Rx No.	Medication	Strength	Quantity	Dosage	R.Ph.	M.D.
01/10/98	75243	Glipizide	10 mg	100	1 Q AM	EM	B. Higley
06/20/98	75243R	Glipizide	10 mg	100	1 Q AM	EM	B. Higley
10/28/98	75243R	Glipizide	10 mg	100	1 Q AM	JR	B. Higley
02/15/99	82695	Cephalexin	500 mg	40	1 QID	JR	B. Higley

Tom is a 50-year-old man with type 2 diabetes mellitus who is picking up an antibiotic for an infected cut on his arm. He owns his own construction company and is always "on the go." You are ready to counsel him about his antibiotic prescription.

1. What concerns do you have based on review of the patient's medication profile? What else would you like to know about your patient? Before talking with the patient, what concerns do you have about counseling this patient? What are the goals of the consultation?
2. How are you going to begin the consultation?
3. Listed below are Tom's responses to the *Prime Questions.* Consider what each response reveals about what the patient knows or feels, and state how you would address any concerns you detect.

Pharmacist: "What did the doctor tell you the medication was for?"
Tom: "He said he was giving me an antibiotic for this infection on my arm. It started as just a scratch, but it's gotten really bad."
Pharmacist: "How did the doctor tell you to take the medicine?"
Tom: "I don't know. He said it was on the label. I know I'm supposed to take it all."
Pharmacist: "What did the doctor tell you to expect?"
Tom: "I guess it will kill the infection and make the cut heal."

4. You have decided to ask about glipizide. Listed next is Tom's answer to your inquiry about the glipizide. Consider what the statement reveals, and state how you would address his concerns.

Tom: "Yeah, well, I'm really busy with my business and it's hard to remember to take it."

Case No. 3: William Hodges

NAME Hodges, William	DATE 7/12/99	
ADDRESS 4212 W. Mission Lane		
Albuquerque, NM 87546	AGE IF CHILD	
R_x FULL DIRECTIONS FOR USE	Rx No. 27021	
1. Digoxin 0.125 mg #45	Date filled	
Sig: 1 tab po Q AM on Sat M W F	Cost	
2 tab po Q AM on Tues Thurs Sun	Fee	
	Total Price	
2. Captopril 25 mg #180	☐ Do not refill	
Sig: 2 po TID	No. of refills authorized: 6	
☐ IDENTIFY CONTENTS ON LABEL UNLESS CHECKED		
☐ NON-PROPRIETARY EQUIVALENT UNLESS CHECKED		
	Ames M.D.	

Patient Medication Profile

Name: **William Hodges**		Known Diseases	Allergies and Sensitivities	Additional Information
Address: 4212 W. Mission Ln.		CABG s/p 1987	Penicillin	
Albuquerque, NM 87546		Angina		
Telephone: 505/425-7219		CHF		
Date of Birth: 3/22/36				

Date	Rx No.	Name of Med.	Strength	Quantity	Dosage Regimen	R.Ph.	Physician
04/20/99	18591	Digoxin	0.125 mg	45	1 Sat M W F 2 Sun T Th	BR	Ames
04/20/99	18592	K Tabs	10 mEq	60	2 QD	BR	Ames
04/20/99	18593	Furosemide	40 mg	15	½ tab QD	BR	Ames
04/20/99	18594	Nifedipine XL	30 mg	60	1 BID	BR	Ames
05/15/99	21052	Digoxin	0.125 mg	45	1 Sat M W F 2 Sun T Th	JC	Ames
05/15/99	21053	K Tabs	10 mEq	120*	2 QD	JC	Ames
05/15/99	21054	Furosemide	40 mg	30*	½ QD	JC	Ames
05/15/99	21055	Nifedipine XL	30 mg	60	1 BID	JC	Ames
6/16/99	24273	Digoxin	0.125 mg	45	1 Sat M W F 2 Sun T Th	DT	Ames
6/16/99	24274	K Tabs	10 mEq	60	2 QD	DT	Ames
6/16/99	24275	Furosemide	40 mg	15	½ QD	DT	Ames
6/16/99	24276	Captopril	25 mg	180	2 TID	DT	Ames

* Vacation supply

Bill is a 62-year-old man with an 8-year history of congestive heart failure secondary to an anterior wall myocardial infarction. Shortly after his recovery, he had a four-vessel coronary artery bypass graft performed. In addition to his prescription medications, he takes one baby aspirin daily to prevent re-infarction.

Bill has seen his physician today and brings in renewal prescriptions for digoxin and captopril (captopril replaced nifedipine due to lack of efficacy). His condition worsened enough that he had to cancel his June trip to Disneyland with his grandchildren.

1. Review the patient's profile. What concerns do you have based on your review of the patient profile? What are the goals of the consultation?
2. How are you going to begin the consultation?
3. Listed below are Bill's responses to *Show-and-Tell* questions. What do you notice?

   a. Digoxin
   Pharmacist: "What is this for?" (as he shows the patient the tablets)
   　　　Bill: "That's digoxin, my heart pill."
   Pharmacist: "How do you take it?"
   　　　Bill: "I take it once a day in the morning."
   Pharmacist: "What kind of problems are you having?"
   　　　Bill: "None. I'm doing great!"

   b. Captopril
   Pharmacist: "What is this for?" (as he shows the patient the tablets)
   　　　Bill: "Also for my heart."
   Pharmacist: "How do you take it?"
   　　　Bill: "Uh . . . two, three times a day."
   Pharmacist: "What kind of problems are you having?"
   　　　Bill: "None. . . . What kind of problems could this medicine cause?"

4. How should you respond to Bill's last question?
5. Bill tells you that captopril made him feel funny when he first started taking it. What should be your next response, and what technique should you now use?
6. The patient's response to your questions was:
   a. I felt real dizzy.
   b. It started about 24 hours after I started taking it.
   c. It was bad enough that I saw spots and almost fell.
   d. It happened primarily when I got up out of bed or from a chair.
   e. I tried getting up slowly and it only helped some, so I stopped it for a day and it went away. Then I started back at one pill twice a day for a couple of weeks. I'm back up to one pill three times a day and I'm not having any problems. I'm going to try to slowly increase it to what the doctor wants me to take. I mean to ask him about it, but I forget.
   f. I haven't noticed anything else except this new medicine seems to be working better than the other. I've got lots more energy and I can make that six-block walk to the store without getting winded.

What clinical assessment do you make from these responses?

7. Before taking action to correct the problem, what should you do now in the consultation?
8. What about the problem with his digoxin?
9. You need to call Dr. Ames. How would you phrase your comments to Dr. Ames regarding the two problems you detected?
10. What would you recommend to Dr. Ames?

CHAPTER 4

Documentation of Pharmacist Interventions

Timothy J. Ives, PharmD, MPH, FCCP, BCPS
Bruce R. Canaday, PharmD, BCPS, FASHP, FAPhA
Peggy C. Yarborough, MS, CDE, FAPP, FASHP, NAPP

INTRODUCTION

If there is no documentation, then it didn't happen! This philosophy is the standard in all health care settings as physicians, nurses, respiratory therapists, physical therapists, social workers, and other health care providers generate and maintain detailed notes regarding the patient's situation and their efforts to achieve the best possible outcomes for the patient. Documentation chronologically outlines the care the patient received and serves as a form of communication among health care providers, so that each practitioner involved knows what evaluation has occurred, what the plan for the patient's treatment is, and who will provide it. Furthermore, third-party payers require reasonable documentation from practitioners that assures that the services provided are consistent with the insurance coverage.[1] General principles for documentation include:

- A complete and legible record.
- Documentation for each encounter with a rationale for the encounter, physical findings, prior test results, assessment, clinical impression (or diagnosis) and plan for care.
- Identified health risk factors.
- The patient's progress, response to and changes in treatment, and revision of the original diagnosis/assessment.

Much of this documentation is derived from a systematic patient care process of evaluation that is standardized within each discipline. For example, physicians are taught to perform a history and physical examination based upon a standardized review of body systems and to document their results using a universally accepted, standardized, systematic process.

Several evaluation/documentation systems have been suggested for health care professionals. Over 30 years ago, the use of a Problem-oriented Medical Record was proposed,[2] and most physicians, nurse practitioners, physician associates, and other health care practitioners have been taught to write progress notes using the *Subjective, Objective, Assessment, Plan* (SOAP) format. Variations of this standard exist,[3] but the underlying process is the same. For example, institutional consultant notes often use an abbreviated version of the SOAP format. This abbreviated version usually includes Findings (i.e., subjective and objective information), Assessment (or Impression), and Diagnosis (or Recommendations). Historically, pharmacy has not had a corresponding standard approach to the evaluation and documentation of the patient's pharmacotherapy that is applicable to all types of pharmacy practice settings. Thus, pharmacy has not been as active as other disciplines in documenting its contributions to patient care.

IMPORTANCE OF DOCUMENTATION

Pharmaceutical care uses a process through which a pharmacist cooperates with a patient and other health care professionals in designing, implementing, and monitoring a therapeutic plan that will produce specific therapeutic outcomes for the patient.[4] This process involves three major functions:

1. Identifying potential and actual drug-related problems
2. Resolving actual drug-related problems
3. Preventing potential drug-related problems

These functions aid in the provision of patient care through the identification of medication-related problems, development of a pharmacotherapeutic plan to address the problems, and the ultimate resolution or prevention of those problems.

As described in Chapter 1, a systematic approach is used in this casebook to identify and resolve the medication-related problems of patients. These steps are summarized as follows:

1. Identification of real or potential medication-related problems
2. Determination of the desired therapeutic outcome
3. Determination of therapeutic alternatives
4. Design of an optimal pharmacotherapeutic plan for the patient
5. Identification of parameters to evaluate the outcome
6. Provision of patient counseling
7. Communication and implementation of the pharmacotherapeutic plan

The final step is crucial; the tenets of pharmaceutical care suggest that pharmacists should document, at the very least, the actual or potential medication-related problems identified, as well as the associated interventions that they desire to implement or have implemented. The pharmacist must adequately communicate his or her recommendations and actions to non-pharmacy health care practitioners (e.g., physicians, nurses), the patient or caregiver (e.g., parents), or other pharmacists. The goal is to provide a clear, concise record of the actual/potential problem, the thought process that led the pharmacist to select an intervention, and the intervention itself. Additionally, the ability to receive remuneration for services provided necessitates an acceptable documentation strategy.

TRADITIONAL DOCUMENTATION FORMAT: SOAP NOTES

In the SOAP note format, the subjective (S) and objective (O) data are recorded and then assessed (A) to formulate a plan (P). Subjective data include patient symptoms, things that may be observed about the patient, or information obtained about the patient. Subjective information is by nature descriptive and generally cannot be confirmed by diagnostic tests or procedures. Much of the subjective information is obtained by speaking with the patient while obtaining the medical history, as described in Chapter 1 (chief complaint, history of present illness, past medical history, family history, social history, medications, allergies, and review of systems). Important subjective information may also be obtained by direct interview with the patient after the initial medical history has been performed (e.g., a description of an adverse drug effect, rating of pain severity using standard scales).

A primary source of objective information (O) is the physical examination. Other relevant objective information includes laboratory values, serum drug concentrations (along with the target therapeutic range for each level), and the results of other diagnostic tests (e.g., ECG, x-rays, culture and sensitivity tests). Risk factors that may predispose the patient to a particular problem should also be considered for inclusion. The communication note should include only the pertinent positive and negative findings. Pertinent negative findings are signs and symptoms of the disease or problem that are not present in the particular patient being evaluated.

The assessment (A) section outlines what the practitioner thinks the patient's problem is, based upon the subjective and objective information acquired. This assessment often takes the form of a diagnosis or differential diagnosis. This portion of the SOAP note should include all of the reasons for the clinician's assessment. This helps other health care providers reading the note to understand how the clinician arrived at his or her particular assessment of the problem.

The plan (P) may include ordering additional diagnostic tests or initiating, revising, or discontinuing treatment. If the plan includes changes in pharmacotherapy, the rationale for the specific changes recommended should be described. The drug, dose, dosage form, schedule, route of administration, and duration of therapy should be included. The plan should be directed toward achieving a specific, measurable, goal or end point, which should be clearly stated in the note. The plan should also outline the efficacy and toxicity parameters that will be used to determine whether the desired therapeutic outcome is being achieved and to detect or prevent drug-related adverse events. Ideally, information about the therapy that should be communicated to the patient should also be included in the plan. The plan should be reviewed and referred to in the note as often as necessary.

AN ALTERNATIVE APPROACH TO DOCUMENTING DRUG-RELATED PROBLEMS AND PLANS

There is a pharmacist equivalent of a physician's progress note in a systematized approach for the construction and maintenance of a record reflecting the pharmacist's contributions to care.[5] This process includes provisions for the identification and assessment of actual or potential medication-related problems, description of a therapeutic plan, and appropriate follow-up monitoring of the problems. Although there is no current uniform documentation system for the profession of pharmacy, students are encouraged to try this system as they learn to document patient interventions and compare its effectiveness with the SOAP format. In this system, problems that have been identified are addressed systematically in a pharmacist's note under the headings *F*indings, *A*ssessment, *R*esolution, and *M*onitoring. The sections of the pharmacist's note can be easily recalled with the mnemonic "FARM."

Identification of Drug-related Problems

The first step in the construction of a FARM note is to clearly state the nature of the drug-related problem(s). Each problem in the FARM note should be addressed separately and assigned a sequential number. Understanding the types of problems that may occur facilitates identification of pharmacotherapy problems. Eight types of medication-related problems have been identified (see Chapter 1).[6] These problems include:

1. Untreated indications
2. Improper drug selection
3. Subtherapeutic dosage
4. Failure to receive drugs
5. Overdosage

6. Adverse drug events
7. Drug interactions
8. Drug use without indication

Use of a classification system such as this for the various types of medication-related problems offers at least two advantages. First, it presents a framework, applicable in any practice setting, to assure that the pharmacist has considered each possible type of problem. Second, categorization allows optimal data analysis and retrieval capabilities. Thus, problems as well as the interventions to resolve them can be stored in a standardized format in a computer. When later analysis of this information is needed, such as determining how much money was saved through an intervention, how outcomes were improved by the pharmacist, or how many problems of a certain type have occurred, the problems and interventions can be reviewed by groups rather than individually.

Documentation of Findings

Each statement of a drug-related problem should be followed by documentation of the pertinent findings (F) indicating that the problem may (potential) or does (actual) exist. Information included in this section should include a summary of the pertinent information obtained after collection and thorough assessment of the available patient information. Demographic data that may be reported include a patient identifier (name, initials, or medical record number), age, race (if pertinent), and gender. As noted earlier under the section on SOAP notes, medical information included in the note should include both subjective and objective findings that indicate a drug-related problem.

Assessment of Problems

The assessment (A) section of the FARM note includes the pharmacist's evaluation of the current situation (i.e., the nature, extent, type, and clinical significance of the problem). This part of the note should delineate the thought process that led to the conclusion that a problem did or did not exist and that an active intervention either was or was not necessary. If additional information is required to satisfactorily assess the problem and make recommendations, this data should be stated along with its source (e.g., the patient, pharmacist, physician). The severity or urgency of the problem should be indicated by stating whether the interventions that follow should be made immediately or within one day, one week, one month, or longer. The desired therapeutic outcome should be stated. This may include both short-term goals (e.g., lower blood pressure to < 140/90 mm Hg in a patient with primary hypertension) and long-term goals (e.g., prevent cardiovascular complications in that patient).

Problem Resolution

The resolution (R) section should reflect the actions proposed (or already performed) to resolve the drug-related problem based upon the preceding analysis. The note should convey that, after consideration of all appropriate therapeutic options, the option(s) considered to be the most beneficial was either carried out or suggested to someone else (e.g., the physician, patient, or caregiver). Recommendations may include non-pharmacologic therapy, such as dietary modification or assistive devices (e.g., canes, walkers); the rationale for this method of treatment should be described. If pharmacotherapy is recommended, a specific drug, dose, route, schedule, and du-

ration of therapy should be specified. It is not sufficient to simply provide a list of choices for the prescriber. Importantly, the rationale for selecting the particular regimen(s) should be stated. It is reasonable to include alternative regimens that would be satisfactory if the patient is unable to complete treatment with the initial regimen because of adverse effects, allergy, cost, or other reasons. If patient counseling is recommended, the information that will be included in the counseling session should be included. Conversely, if certain types of information will be withheld from the patient, the reasons for doing so should be stated. If no action is recommended or was taken, that should be documented as well. In this situation, the note serves as a record of the pharmacist's involvement in the patient's care. The pharmacist then has documentation that patient care activities were performed.

Monitoring for Outcomes

It is not enough, however, to only provide a clear, concise record of the nature of a problem, the assessment that led to the conclusion that a problem exists, and the selection of a plan for resolution of the problem. In the spirit of pharmaceutical care, the patient must not be abandoned after an intervention has been made. A plan for follow-up monitoring (M) of the patient must be documented and adequately implemented. This process is likely to include questioning the patient, gathering laboratory data, and performing the ongoing physical assessments necessary to determine the effect of the plan that was implemented to assure that it results in an optimal outcome for the patient.

Monitoring parameters to assess efficacy generally include improvement in or resolution of the signs, symptoms, and laboratory abnormalities that were initially assessed. The monitoring parameters used to detect or prevent adverse reactions are determined by the most common and most serious events known to be associated with the therapeutic intervention. Potential adverse reactions should be precisely described along with the method of monitoring. For example, rather than stating "monitor for GI complaints," the recommendation may be to "question the patient about the presence of dyspepsia, diarrhea, or constipation." The frequency, duration, and target end point for each monitoring parameter should be identified. The points at which changes in the plan may be warranted should be included. For example, in the case of a patient with dyslipidemia, one may recommend to "obtain fasting HDL, LDL, total cholesterol, and triglycerides after 3 months of treatment. If the goal LDL of < 100 mg/dL is not achieved with good compliance at 3 months, increase simvastatin to 40 mg po once daily. If goal LDL is achieved, maintain simvastatin 20 mg po once daily and repeat fasting lipoprotein profile annually."

SUMMARY

A SOAP or FARM progress note constructed in the manner described identifies each drug-related problem and states the pharmacist's *F*indings observed, an *A*ssessment of the findings, the actual or proposed *R*esolution of the problem based upon the analysis, and the parameters and timing of follow-up *M*onitoring. Either form of note should provide a clear, concise record of process, activity, and projected follow-up. When written for each medication-related problem, these notes should provide data in a standardized, logical system. In particular, FARM notes provide a convenient format for progress notes for all pharmacists, applicable to any practice setting.

SAMPLE CASE PRESENTATION

The following case presentation illustrates how such a system can be used in practice. Franklin Jones is a 9-year-old Caucasian male seen on rounds Monday morning, who was admitted the previous evening with a painful right ear and fever (T_{max} = 102°F). He has a 6-year history of asthma. At home, he uses Theo-Dur 300 mg twice daily and albuterol 2 puffs TID. The admitting physician noted no wheezing. A theophylline level on admission was 19 μg/mL. His white blood cell count was $16.0 \times 10^3/mm^3$ with 12% bands and no eosinophils. The physician's working diagnosis is otitis media. Upon admission Sunday night, orders were written for acetaminophen 325 mg po Q 6 H PRN temp >101°F and ciprofloxacin 500 mg po BID.

Construction of a SOAP Note

S: Pt complains of right ear pain.
O: Inflamed right TM, fever (T_{max} = 102°F). He has a 6-year history of asthma, well controlled on Theo-Dur 300 mg po BID and albuterol MDI 2 puffs TID. Chest clear to A & P. Theophylline level on admission (i.e., random) was 19 μg/mL. Admission WBC = 16,000 with a left shift. He was started last night on acetaminophen 325 mg po Q 6 H PRN temp > 101°F and ciprofloxacin 500 mg po BID.
A: Right otitis media, with inappropriate antibiotic selection.
P: D/C ciprofloxacin, and start co-trimoxazole 1 tablet po BID × 10 days. Reassess clinical condition on a daily basis. Follow temps every shift. Follow improvement in pain, changes in TMs. Monitor fever every shift, and obtain daily WBC count. Obtain a theophylline level if toxicity is suspected. Educate the patient to take each dose with a full glass of water and to complete the entire course of therapy.

Construction of a FARM Note

F: Franklin Jones is a 9 yo WM presenting with a right otitis media and fever (T_{max} = 102°F). He has a 6-year history of asthma, well controlled on Theo-Dur 300 mg po BID and inhaled albuterol 2 puffs TID. His chest was clear to A & P. Theophylline level on admission was 19 μg/mL. WBC on admission was 16,000 with a left shift. He was begun last night on aceta-minophen 325 mg po Q 6 H PRN temp > 101°F and ciprofloxacin 500 mg po BID.

Problem # 1: Chronic Asthma
A: Controlled on current medication.
R: Continue current condition daily.
M: Monitor clinical condition daily. Obtain theophylline level if exacerbation occurs.

Problem # 2: Right Otitis Media
A: Ciprofloxacin presents a problem for several reasons:
  1. The broad spectrum may lead to superinfection.
  2. It is not indicated in children due to risk of arthropathy and osteochondrosis.
  3. Ciprofloxacin may elevate serum theophylline levels, resulting in toxicity.

R: Discontinue ciprofloxacin. Begin sulfamethoxazole/trimethoprim 1 double-strength tablet po BID × 10 days.
M: Monitor clinical improvement in pain, TMs. Follow fever and WBC count daily.

Problem # 3: Fever
A: Fever is controlled on current medication.
R: Continue acetaminophen.
M: Monitor temperature every shift.

References

1. Documentation Guidelines for Evaluation and Management Services. Washington, DC, Health Care Finance Administration, August 1997.
2. Weed LL. Medical records that guide and teach. N Engl J Med 1968;278:593–600, 652–657.
3. Larimore WL, Jordan EV. SOAP to SNOCAMP: Improving the medical record format. J Fam Pract 1995;41:393–398.
4. Hepler CD, Strand LM. Opportunities and responsibilities in pharmaceutical care. Am J Hosp Pharm 1990;47:533–543.
5. Canaday BR, Yarborough PC. Documenting pharmaceutical care: Creating a standard. Ann Pharmacother 1994;28:1292–1296.
6. Strand LM, Morley PC, Cipolle RJ, et al. Drug-related problems: Their structure and function. Ann Pharmacother 1990;24:1093–1097.

SECTION 1

Cardiovascular Disorders

Robert L. Talbert, PharmD, FCCP, BCPS, Section Editor

1 CARDIOPULMONARY RESUSCITATION

▶ **A Near-death Experience** (Level II)

Tate N. Trujillo, PharmD
Donna S. Wall, PharmD, BCPS

▶ After completing this case study, students should be able to:

- Discuss possible causes for cardiac arrest.
- Outline medications used to treat cardiac arrest.
- List the pharmacologic actions of medications used in cardioversion.
- Outline the Advanced Cardiac Life Support (ACLS) guidelines.
- Identify appropriate parameters to monitor a patient who has just been cardioverted.

☀ PATIENT PRESENTATION

Chief Complaint
"I'm finally going to get my heart problem taken care of."

HPI
Joanna Rule is a 62 yo woman who was admitted this morning for coronary artery bypass surgery. Recently while on vacation, she was hospitalized for unstable angina. Upon returning she underwent cardiac catheterization, which showed multiple-vessel CAD. The patient has been followed for some time for chronic renal insufficiency related to membranous nephropathy.

While admitted for her cardiac catheterization, a right-sided Perma-Cath was placed followed by her first dialysis session. The Perma-Cath did not function during the second dialysis session. After trying to reposition the catheter, it was removed and replaced with another Perma-Cath.

PMH
ESRD (chronic membranous glomerulonephritis)
IV access difficulties
Anemia secondary to CRF
HTN
Hyperlipidemia
Type 2 DM—diet controlled
AMI × 2; coronary angioplasty 9 years ago
S/P appendectomy
S/P cholecystectomy
S/P hysterectomy

FH
Mother had HTN and died of an AMI at age 69; no information available for father; one brother at age 73 is alive with HTN and DM

SH
Smoker; quit 8 years ago; previously $1^1/_2$ ppd

ROS
Feels tired with frequent chest pain, fever, chills, nausea, and fatigue

Meds
Diltiazem CD 300 po Q HS
Nephrocaps 1 po QD
Atorvastatin 20 mg po QD
Furosemide 160 mg po QD

EC ASA 325 mg po QD (hold until after CABG)

Prochlorperazine 10 mg po TID PRN nausea

Nitroglycerin 0.4 mg SL PRN chest pain

PhosLo 667 mg 2 po PC

Nitroglycerin transdermal patch 0.4 mg QD at night and remove in AM

Acetaminophen 650 mg po QID PRN pain

Clonidine 0.2 mg po TID, but not before dialysis

All

IV Dye → worsened renal function (10 years ago)

PE

Gen

Obese Caucasian woman in NAD

VS

BP 168/106, P 86, T 37.9°C; dry wt 76.5 kg

Skin

Warm, dry

HEENT

PERRLA; EOMI; arteriolar narrowing on funduscopic exam; no hemorrhages, exudates, or papilledema; oral mucosa clear

Neck/LN

Supple with no JVD or bruits; no lymphadenopathy or thyromegaly

Chest

Mild bibasilar rales

CV

RRR; S_1, S_2 normal; no S_3 or S_4; no murmurs or rubs

Abd

Obese, soft, non-tender; (+) BS; no HSM

Genit/Rect

Stool heme (−)

MS/Ext

2+ pedal edema with palpable pulses; capillary refill <2 sec; age-appropriate strength and ROM

Neuro

A & O × 3, decreased sensation in lower legs, CN II → XII intact

Labs

Na 134 mEq/L	Hgb 9.3 g/dL	Ca 6.7 mg/dL
K 3.9mEq/L	Hct 28%	Mg 2.5 mg/dL
Cl 97 mEq/L	Plt 229 × 10³/mm³	Phos 5.5 mg/dL
CO_2 20 mEq/L	WBC 18.9 × 10³/mm³	Alb 2.5g/dL
BUN 86 mg/dL	79% PMNs	
SCr 11.1 mg/dL	1% Bands	
Glu 88 mg/dL	17% Lymphs	
	3% Monos	

ECG

NSR at a rate of 86 bpm

► Clinical Course

The patient subsequently underwent CABG. Postoperatively she was given a morphine PCA for pain control, cefuroxime 1.5 g IV Q 12 hours × 4 doses, and sliding scale insulin. She had an unremarkable course for 24 hours and was restarted on all preoperative medications except for nitroglycerin patch. Approximately 36 hours S/P CABG the patient developed multifocal PVCs that quickly changed to ventricular fibrillation. A code was called.

► Questions

Problem Identification

1. a. What actual and potential drug-related problems does this patient have just prior to the development of ventricular fibrillation?
   b. Discuss the possible causes for the development of ventricular fibrillation.

Desired Outcome

2. What are the short-term goals of pharmacotherapy for this patient?

Therapeutic Alternatives

3. a. What non-pharmacologic maneuvers should be undertaken immediately in a patient with ventricular fibrillation?
   b. What pharmacotherapeutic agents are available for the acute therapy of this patient's condition?

Optimal Plan

4. a. A pharmacist was not available to participate in this resuscitation effort. Assess the appropriateness of the treatment used to obtain a cardiac conversion in this patient (see Clinical Course on page 29).

► Clinical Course

Cardiopulmonary Resuscitation Record of Events and Orders

Time	BP	Spont. Resp.	Cardiac Rhythm	HR	Defib. (watt sec)	Rhythm after Defib.	Drugs Given
1320	188/56	10	VF	98	100	Torsades	
1321	150/46				200	Torsades	
1322	116/?				300	Agonal	
1325	88/?	10	Torsades		360	Agonal to Torsades	EPI 1 mg IVP Atropine 1 mg IVP Lidoc. 100 mg IVP
1332	302/133	10	SVT	160	360	SVT	
1338	160/84	10	SVT	180	360	NSR	Lidoc. 50 mg IVP
1347	133/50	10	NSR	96		Torsades to NSR with PVC	
1352						NSR with PVC	

Key: ?, not recorded; BP, blood pressure; Spont. Resp., spontaneous respirations; HR, heart rate; Defib., defibrillation; VF, ventricular fibrillation; EPI, epinephrine; IVP, intravenous push; Lidoc., lidocaine; SVT, supraventricular tachycardia; NSR, normal sinus rhythm; PVC, premature ventricular contraction.

b. *Upon conversion to normal sinus rhythm, what is your pharmacotherapeutic plan to maintain the patient's stability?*

Outcome Evaluation

5. *How should the patient be monitored to assess drug efficacy and to prevent and detect adverse effects? Describe how the therapy should be adjusted if adverse events occur.*

► Self-study Assignments

1. Compare and contrast the various modes of medical management of ventricular arrhythmias in ESRD patients.
2. Perform a literature search to determine the odds of surviving a cardiac arrest while hospitalized.
3. List medications that can be administered through an endotracheal tube.

► Clinical Pearl

During a cardiac arrest, a patient's potassium and glucose levels will increase dramatically due to the presence of acidosis; this may be further accentuated in the presence of renal failure.

References

1. Cummins RO, ed. Advanced Cardiac Life Support. American Heart Association, Dallas, TX, 1997.
2. Lopez LM, Scheife RT, eds. Acute management of ventricular arrhythmias: Focus on new developments. Pharmacotherapy 1997;17(2 Pt 2):56S–88S.

2   HYPERTENSION

► No More Time for Complacency   (Level I)

J. Edwin Underwood, Jr., PharmD

► After completing this case study, students should be able to:

- Establish goals for antihypertensive therapy and identify the complications of uncontrolled hypertension.
- Provide appropriate life-style modifications and antihypertensive therapy based on patient characteristics and concurrent disease states.
- Implement appropriate monitoring parameters for patients receiving antihypertensive therapy.
- Provide recommendations for modifying therapy in patients who do not respond to or are intolerant of the initial therapy.
- Counsel patients appropriately based on the particular antihypertensive they are receiving.

☼ PATIENT PRESENTATION

Chief Complaint
"My insurance has changed and I'm here to see my new primary care physician."

HPI
Thomas Kramer is a 61 yo man who presents to his new general internist for evaluation and follow up of his medical problems. He has no particular

complaints today. He recently saw his previous physician at another clinic for chronic sinus drainage and an ENT specialist for the same problem. He has been prescribed multiple antibiotics for this problem in the past. He reports a recent increase in shortness of breath with moderate exertion and bothersome nocturia. However, he states that he feels better today and just needs a check-up.

PMH

Chronic sinus drainage (S/P laryngoscopy)
Hypertension for approximately 8 years
"Malignant" mole removed 3 years ago
No history of heart disease, TB, or DM

FH

Father died of acute MI at age 73, mother deceased due to lung cancer at age 69 and had high blood pressure and "sugar"; brother (age 68) has HTN and high cholesterol; younger sister (age 52) has no known medical problems.

SH

He has been married for 39 years and has one son who is healthy. He quit smoking a pipe about 6 years ago. He states that his alcohol intake is "too much." He has recently retired and plays golf 1 to 2 times per week. He does not pay attention to sodium, fat, or carbohydrate content of foods ("I eat what I want"). His wife does most of the cooking, and he usually adds "a little" table salt to his foods. He denies ever being placed on any diet due to his medical conditions. He denies noncompliance with his medications.

Meds

Nasalide 2 sprays each nostril QD
Dyazide 25/50 mg po QD × 8 years
Sudafed 60 mg po Q 6 H PRN
Aleve 1 to 2 tablets po PRN elbow pain

All

NKDA

ROS

States that overall he is doing okay. Weight is up about 6 kg in the last year. No chest pain, SOB at rest, or hemoptysis; mild exertional SOB when climbing stairs. No N/V/D or blood in stool. Reports increasing urinary hesitancy over the past 6 months, straining to urinate, and frequent nocturia; no dysuria. Occasional tendinitis and left elbow pain that he self-treats with OTC naproxen.

PE

Gen
The patient is a WDWN, moderately obese Caucasian man in NAD.

VS
Average BP 150/98 (sitting), HR 56 (regular), RR 16, T 37.1°C; Ht 6′2″, Wt 96 kg, BMI = 27

HEENT
TM's clear throughout and no drainage; sclerae without icterus; EOMI; R pupil < L; funduscopy shows mild arteriolar narrowing with AV ratio 1:3; no hemorrhages, exudates, or papilledema (Keith-Wagener-Barker funduscopic class: grade I to II).

Neck
Supple without masses or bruits, no thyroid enlargement or lymphadenopathy

Lungs
A few basilar crackles; no wheezing

Heart
RRR (slow) with mild S_3

Abd
Soft and ND; mildly tender in suprapubic area; no masses, bruits, splenomegaly, hepatomegaly. Normal BS

Rectal/GU
Prostate 2+ (enlarged); prostate benign without nodules, induration, or asymmetry. Heme (−) stool. Normal penis and testes

Ext
No clubbing, cyanosis, or edema. Limited ROM of the left elbow

Neuro
No gross motor-sensory deficits present. CN II–XII intact. Negative Babinski

Labs (fasting)

Na 142 mEq/L	AST 35 U/L	Ca 9.7 mg/dL	Lipid Profile:
K 4.4 mEq/L	ALT 28 U/L	Mg 1.9 mEq/L	T. chol 290 mg/dL
Cl 101 mEq/L	Alk phos 88 U/L	Phos 4.2 mg/dL	HDL 29 mg/dL
CO_2 27 mEq/L	GGT 106 IU/L	Uric acid 8.7 mg/dL	LDL 181 mg/dL
BUN 22 mg/dL	T. bili 0.6 mg/dL	FBG 172 mg/dL	TG 400 mg/dL
SCr 1.5 mg/dL	T. prot 6.7 g/dL		

UA
Color clear, appearance amber, SG 1.010, pH 5.0, protein (−), RBC 0/hpf, WBC 1–2/hpf, no bacteria

ECG
Bradycardia, regular rhythm

Echocardiogram
Mild LVH with an EF of 45%; evidence of mild mitral regurgitation

▶ Questions

Problem Identification

1. a. Create a list of this patient's drug-related problems.

   b. Outline the steps for obtaining a proper blood pressure measurement. Please demonstrate if a cuff is available (see Figure 2–1).

   c. This patient has established disease and has already been diagnosed with hypertension. What evidence supports that his BP has been poorly controlled?

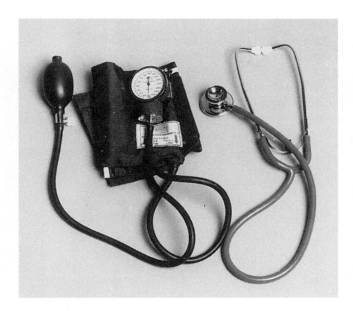

Figure 2-1. An aneroid sphygmomanometer (left) and stethoscope for evaluating blood pressure.

d. What pathophysiologic mechanisms might explain the etiology of the elevated BP in this patient?

e. Based on the most recent guidelines from JNC VI, classify this patient's hypertension.

Desired Outcome

2. *List the goals of antihypertensive therapy for this patient, including the desired BP range.*

Therapeutic Alternatives

3. *a. What non-pharmacologic therapies are necessary for this patient to obtain and maintain adequate BP reduction?*

   b. What reasonable pharmacotherapeutic options are available for controlling this patient's BP?

Optimal Plan

4. *a. Outline an appropriate regimen of specific life-style modifications for this patient.*

   b. Outline a specific and appropriate pharmacotherapy regimen for this patient, including drug, dosage form, dose, and schedule.

Outcome Evaluation

5. *Based on your recommendations, what parameters should be monitored after initiating these changes and throughout the treatment course?*

Patient Counseling

6. *Based on your recommendations, provide appropriate counseling to this patient.*

► Clinical Course

The patient returns for follow-up 2 months later. He states that he is walking 3 miles a day, following his dietary regimen, has cut down his alcohol intake to one to two glasses of wine each evening, has lost 6 pounds, and is taking his medications as prescribed. His average BP today is 122/76 mm Hg. His fasting blood glucose is 118 mg/dL, and his fasting lipid profile is improving: total cholesterol 250 mg/dL, HDL 35 mg/dL, LDL 139 mg/dL, triglycerides 380 mg/dL.

► Follow-up Questions

1. *What advice and counseling should you give the patient at this point in his therapy?*
2. *Suppose the patient now complains of intolerable adverse effects due to the current antihypertensive drug therapy. Outline an appropriate change to his current therapy.*
3. *Suppose the patient is tolerating the current drug therapy but has not achieved the desired BP control (average BP = 142/92 mm Hg). Outline an appropriate change to his current therapy.*

► Self-study Assignments

1. Outline the pharmacotherapeutic regimen you would recommend for a patient with same level of HTN as this patient on his initial visit, but with the following characteristics:

   - A patient with asthma
   - A patient with severe systolic dysfunction
   - A patient with major depression
   - A patient with severe coronary artery disease and angina pectoris
   - A patient with gout
   - A pregnant woman
   - A patient with chronic renal failure
   - A patient on a low fixed income

► Clinical Pearl

The mechanisms by which thiazide diuretics lead to glucose intolerance and dyslipidemia are complex and not fully understood, but there is little evidence that thiazide-induced dyslipidemia is maintained for more than 1 year after treatment is initiated.

References

1. Barry MJ, Fowler FJ, O'Leary MP, et al. The American Urological Association symptom index for benign prostatic hyperplasia. The Measurement Committee of the American Urological Association. J Urol 1992;148:1549–1557.
2. Joint National Committee on Prevention, Detection, Evaluation, and Treatment of High Blood Pressure. Sixth report. Arch Intern Med 1997;157:2413–2446.
3. Baba T, Ishizaki T. Recent advances in pharmacological management of hypertension in diabetic patients with nephropathy. Effects of antihypertensive drugs on kidney function and insulin sensitivity. Drugs 1992;43:464–489.

3 HYPERTENSIVE URGENCY

▶ **My Doctor Made Me Do It**   **(Level I)**

James J. Nawarskas, PharmD

▶ After completing this case study, students should be able to:

- Distinguish a hypertensive urgency from a hypertensive emergency.
- Identify treatment goals for a patient with a hypertensive urgency.
- Recommend an appropriate antihypertensive drug for a patient in a hypertensive urgency.
- List advantages and disadvantages of oral versus parenteral drug therapy for a patient with a hypertensive urgency.

☀ PATIENT PRESENTATION

Chief Complaint
"My doctor told me to come here because of my blood pressure."

HPI
Timothy McGinnis is a 72 yo man with a history of HTN (well-controlled on medication) who was undergoing pre-operative assessment by his primary care physician for a subtotal pancreatectomy when he was noted to have a BP of 230/127 mm Hg and a pulse of 101 bpm. The patient was referred to the urgent care center where two stories were obtained from the family regarding his BP medications. The patient stated that his gastroenterologist told him to stop taking the medications, but the patient's wife said that his cardiologist told him to discontinue the medications 3 months ago. The patient reports not taking any antihypertensive medications for "a couple of months."

PMH
HTN diagnosed about 25 years ago.
Chronic pancreatitis diagnosed about 10 years ago without associated malabsorption. No history of diabetes

FH
Father died in his 70s secondary to CHF, mother had HTN and died in her 80s from a stroke. Two brothers, 68 and 70 years old, both alive and both have HTN.

SH
Married, retired construction worker. States he used to smoke 1 ppd for about 40 years before quitting 10 years ago, and used to drink "several" alcoholic beverages daily (mostly beer) before cutting back when his endocrinologist diagnosed pancreatitis 10 years ago. He says he completely stopped drinking about a year ago.

ROS
Dull, abdominal pain that comes and goes; no headache, nausea, dizziness, loss of muscle control, or other signs of CNS damage; no palpitations, chest pain, or visual changes

Meds
Pancrease MT-16, 2 tablets po with meals and snacks
Zantac 150 mg po BID
Vicodin 2 tablets po PRN abdominal pain
Procardia XL 120 mg po QD, discontinued 2 months ago
Zestril 40 mg po QD, discontinued 2 months ago

All
NKDA

PE

Gen
The patient is a thin, elderly Caucasian man in NAD.

VS
BP 220/118, P 100, RR 20, T 36.8°C; Ht 68 in, Wt 59 kg

Skin
Cool to touch, good turgor

HEENT
PERRLA; EOMI; funduscopic exam revealed no hemorrhages, exudates, AV nicking, or papilledema; oropharynx clear

Neck/LN
Neck supple, no JVD, no bruits, no thyromegaly

Chest
CTA

CV
RRR, III/VI SEM at right upper sternal border, $S_2 > S_1$, no S_3 or S_4

Abd
Soft, tender, no guarding, (+) epigastric & rebound tenderness, (+) BS, liver span about 15 cm

Genit/Rect
Normal male genitalia, heme-negative stool

MS/Ext
Normal ROM, no CCE, pulses 3+ throughout

Neuro
A & O × 3, CN II–XII intact, motor/sensory normal, DTRs 2+

Labs

Na 141 mEq/L	Hgb 13.4 g/dL	AST 182 IU/L
K 4.1 mEq/L	Hct 43.1%	ALT 150 IU/L
Cl 102 mEq/L	WBC 8.9×10^3/mm^3	
CO_2 24 mEq/L	Plt 271×10^3/mm^3	
BUN 14 mg/dL		
SCr 1.1 mg/dL		
Glu 140 mg/dL		

UA
Negative for protein and blood with 2 to 5 WBCs/hpf and 0 to 2 casts/lpf

CXR
Enlarged heart, no infiltrates

ECG
NSR, rate 100, LVH by voltage criteria, no ST segment changes, no Q waves

Assessment
72 yo man with a history of HTN, chronic pancreatitis, and prior alcohol abuse presents to the urgent care center asymptomatic with a BP of 220/118 following a pre-operative evaluation for subtotal pancreatectomy. The elevated BP is likely due to discontinuation of antihypertensive treatment and is not accompanied by ECG changes.

▶ Questions

Problem Identification

1. a. *Create a list of the patient's drug-related problems.*
   b. *What classifies this patient's situation as a hypertensive urgency?*
   c. *How does this situation differ from a hypertensive emergency?*
   d. *How does this patient's underlying pancreatitis affect the severity of his hypertension?*
   e. *What other signs and symptoms are present that may be related to this patient's hypertension?*

Desired Outcome

2. a. *What are the goals of pharmacotherapy for this patient's hypertension?*
   b. *If this patient had a hypertensive emergency, how would the goals of treatment differ?*

Therapeutic Alternatives

3. a. *What non-drug therapies might be useful for this patient?*
   b. *What feasible pharmacotherapeutic alternatives are available for the treatment of this patient's hypertension?*
   c. *The attending physician requests that the medical resident write prescriptions for Procardia XL 120 mg po QD and Zestril 40 mg po QD (the patient's previous antihypertensive regimen) and discharge the patient from the urgent care center. The resident does not feel comfortable with this and proceeds to phone the patient's cardiologist, who wants the patient admitted. What do you think is the most appropriate course of action for this patient?*

Optimal Plan

4. *What drug, dosage form, schedule, and duration of therapy are best for this patient?*

Outcome Evaluation

5. *What clinical and laboratory parameters are necessary to evaluate your therapy for reducing this patient's blood pressure and monitoring for adverse events?*

Patient Counseling

6. *The patient received the treatment and monitoring regimen you recommended and is now ready to be discharged on Procardia XL 60 mg po QD and Zestril 20 mg po QD. What information will you provide to the patient to enhance compliance, ensure successful therapy, and minimize adverse effects?*

▶ Self-study Assignments

1. Write a one-page paper describing the pathophysiology of LVH in the setting of chronic hypertension.
2. List the clinical and laboratory monitoring parameters for a patient receiving nitroprusside.
3. Explain why prazosin is especially useful for treating hypertensive urgencies due to circulating catecholamines.

▶ Clinical Pearl

"True" hypertensive urgencies are based on medical history and clinical presentation, not solely on blood pressure readings.

References

1. Thach AM, Schultz PJ. Nonemergent hypertension. New perspectives for the emergency medicine physician. Emerg Med Clin North Am 1995;13:1009–1035.
2. Abdelwahab W, Frishman W, Landau A. Management of hypertensive urgencies and emergencies. J Clin Pharmacol 1995;35:747–762.
3. Joint National Committee on Prevention, Detection, Evaluation, and Treatment of High Blood Pressure. Sixth report. Arch Intern Med 1997;157:2413–2446.
4. Gales MA. Oral antihypertensives for hypertensive urgencies. Ann Pharmacother 1994;28:352–358.

4 HEART FAILURE

▶ The Pump Organist   (Level III)

Jon D. Horton, PharmD

▶ After completing this case study, students should be able to:

- Recognize the signs and symptoms of heart failure.
- Develop a pharmacotherapeutic plan for treatment of heart failure.
- Outline a monitoring plan for heart failure that includes both clinical and laboratory parameters.
- Initiate, titrate, and monitor β-adrenergic blocker therapy in heart failure when indicated.

☀ PATIENT PRESENTATION

Chief Complaint
"I've gained some weight and can only go up a half a flight of stairs without becoming winded."

HPI
Richard Anderson is a 65 yo man who presents to the ED after a routine visit to his endocrinologist for follow-up of his diabetes mellitus. The endocrinologist referred him to the local ED for evaluation and potential hospitalization. The patient states that he has been gaining weight and having progressively worsening dyspnea on exertion. His shortness of breath is often worse at night, forcing him to "sit bolt upright." He began utilizing three pillows at night one week ago. He is unable to complete physical exertion that had been completed one month ago without difficulty. This morning he became short of breath and diaphoretic after climbing a flight of stairs to his endocrinologist's office. When he saw his continuing care physician one week ago, he was in atrial fibrillation and was started on digoxin for rate control. Upon arrival in the ED, his sweating had resolved and his heart rate was in the range of 120 to 140 bpm.

PMH
Atrial fibrillation × 2 weeks
Type 2 DM × 15 years, untreated until 3 years ago; neuropathy × 2 years and retinopathy × 1 year
HTN × 20 years
Hypercholesterolemia (documented 6 months ago)
CVA 2 and 3 years ago
Recurrent TIAs × 4 years resistant to ASA and ticlopidine; started on warfarin 7 months ago with improvement

FH
Father died at age 65 of leukemia. Mother died in her 30's of unknown cause. One brother age 70 alive with DM.

SH
Retired musician who lives with his wife of 24 years. Prior to his CVAs, his hobby was repairing and playing antique pump organs. He has a 50 pack-year smoking history but reports quitting 22 years ago. He has a positive history for alcohol use, but states he "hasn't had a drop in 12 years."

Meds
Metformin 850 mg po TID
Glyburide 2.5 mg po BID
Pravastatin 10 mg po QD (LDL 112 mg/dL one month ago)
Lisinopril 2.5 mg po QD
Digoxin 0.125 mg po QD
Warfarin 7.5 mg po QD since his last admission 7 months ago because of repeated "mini-strokes." INR 1 week ago was 2.2

All
NKDA

ROS
Reports having headaches recently, but nothing that he would consider unusual or out of the ordinary. He is followed ophthalmologically and was told he had a small bleeding area in the back of one eye, but he states that this occurred prior to taking warfarin. Denies any recent chest pain. No chronic cough, but has had recent episodes of coughing spells without productivity. Complains of recent abdominal bloating and of being awakened the past four evenings to relieve his bladder. He reports some weakness in his right lower extremity but states that it is unchanged from his most recent stroke. He denies chronic joint pain.

PE

Gen
The patient is sitting up on the gurney in the ED in moderate distress.

VS
BP 150/95, P 100 to 150 (irregularly irregular), RR 22, T 35°C; Ht 71 in; Wt 103 kg (usual weight 93 kg)

Skin
Color pale and diaphoretic; no unusual lesions noted

HEENT
PERRLA, EOMI, fundi were not examined. He has a complete upper denture and about two-thirds of the teeth in the lower jaw are remaining and are in fair repair.

Neck
(+) JVD at 30 degrees (8 cm). Carotid bruit is not appreciated. No lymphadenopathy or thyromegaly.

Heart
Irregularly irregular rhythm, no rubs, variation in intensity of S_1 as expected. S_3 is appreciated at apex in lateral position. PMI displaced laterally and difficult to discern.

Thorax/Lungs
Respirations are even. There are fine crackles in both lung fields posteriorly noted 2/3 of the way up the lung fields. No CVAT.

Abd
Soft, NT/ND, (+) HJR, liver and spleen slightly enlarged, no masses, hypoactive bowel sounds

Genit/Rect
Guaiac (−), genital examination not performed

MS/Ext
2+ pitting pedal edema bilaterally, radial and pedal pulses are of poor intensity bilaterally, grip strength greater on left than right.

Neuro
A & O × 3, CNs intact. Some sensory loss in both LE below the knee. DTR 1+

Labs

Na 139 mEq/L	Hgb 12.6 g/dL	Mg 1.2 mEq/L	CK 20 IU/L
K 3.4 mEq/L	Hct 39.5%	Ca 8.8 mg/dL	CK-MB 0.8 IU/L
Cl 99 mEq/L	Plt 339 × 10³/mm³	AST 36 IU/L	PT 20.6 sec
CO_2 27 mEq/L	WBC 8.6 × 10³/mm³	ALT 43 IU/L	INR 2.8
BUN 20 mg/dL	70% PMNs	Alk phos 150 IU/L	TSH 1.42 μIU/mL
SCr 1.3 mg/dL	23% Lymphs	GGT 37 IU/L	Digoxin 1.0 ng/mL
Glucose 139 mg/dL	7% Monos	T. bili 0.2 mg/dL	HbA_{1c} 7.2%

ECG

Atrial fibrillation with a rapid ventricular response (see Figure 4–1); rate of 140, QRS 0.08. Diffuse non-specific ST-T wave changes. Low voltage

Chest X-ray

PA and lateral views (see Figure 4–2) show evidence of congestive failure with cardiomegaly, interstitial edema, and some early alveolar edema. There is a small right pleural effusion.

Assessment

Diabetic patient with new-onset congestive heart failure and atrial fibrillation with rapid ventricular response

▶ Clinical Course

RA was admitted to a step-down unit and placed on telemetry. A 2D echocardiogram was obtained to evaluate LV and valvular function (see Figure 4–3). The results showed severe left ventricular dilation and increased left atrial dimension, akinesia of the septum, and severe LV dysfunction. EF is estimated at 15% to 20%, with no visible clots.

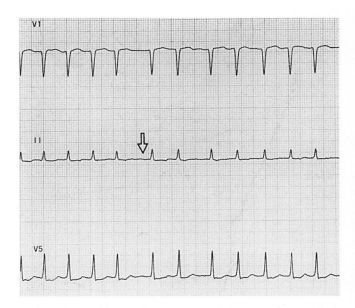

Figure 4–1. The ECG demonstrates low voltage in all leads. The arrow points out the absence of a P wave, which is observed in patients with atrial fibrillation. This ECG does not meet criteria for left ventricular hypertrophy (S in V1 + R in V5 > 35 mm).

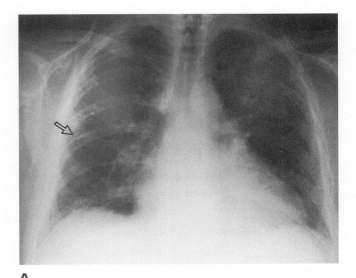

A

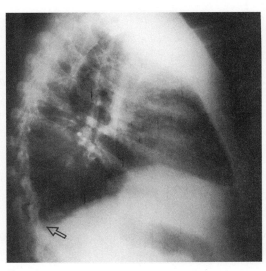

B

Figure 4–2. A. PA CXR demonstrates increased vascular markings representative of interstitial edema, with some early alveolar edema. The arrow points out fluid lying in the fissure of the right lung. Note the presence of cardiomegaly. **B.** Lateral view of CXR. Arrow points out the presence of pulmonary effusion.

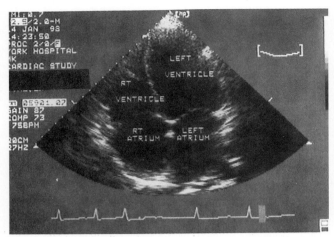 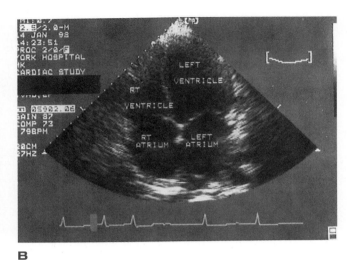

A   **B**

Figure 4–3. 2D echocardiogram. **A.** End systole. **B.** End diastole. Note the presence of severe left ventricular dilation and increased left atrial dimension in end diastole **(B)** that appear to be unchanged from the photographs of end systole **(A).** The ventricular septum appears to be in nearly the identical position in both films, thus representing akinesia.

► Questions

Problem Identification

1. a. *Create a list of this patient's drug-related problems.*
   b. *What signs and symptoms indicate the presence and severity of the patient's heart failure?*
   c. *What functional classification and hemodynamic subset is this patient upon presentation?*
   d. *Could any of this patient's problems have been caused by drug therapy?*

Desired Outcome

2. a. *What are the goals for the pharmacologic management of heart failure in this patient?*
   b. *Considering his other medical problems, what other treatment goals should be established?*

Therapeutic Alternatives

3. *What medications are indicated in the long-term management of this patient's heart failure?*

Optimal Plan

4. *What drugs, doses, schedules, and duration are best suited for the management of this patient?*

Outcome Evaluation

5. *What clinical and laboratory parameters are needed to evaluate the therapy for achievement of the desired therapeutic outcome and to detect and prevent adverse events?*

► Clinical Course

Over the next 3 days, the patient received maximal drug therapy and his condition improved. He was discharged on lisinopril 20 mg po QD, digoxin 0.25 mg po QD, furosemide 40 mg po QD, potassium chloride 40 mEq po QD, magnesium oxide 400 mg po QD, metformin 850 mg po TID, glyburide 2.5 mg po QD, warfarin 7.5 mg po QD, and pravastatin 20 mg po QD.

Patient Counseling

6. *What patient information should be provided to the patient about the medications used to treat his heart failure?*

► Clinical Course

Despite subsequent inpatient efforts to chemically convert the patient to sinus rhythm, he remained in atrial fibrillation. The Cardiology Service recommended outpatient DC cardioversion to try to improve cardiac output by reestablishing an effective atrial kick. An outpatient elective DC cardioversion failed. Despite 3 months of maximal drug therapy, the patient currently complains of episodic shortness of breath that he associates with "faster palpitations." A Holter monitor was placed, and the results suggested poor rate control. The current serum digoxin concentration is 1.8 ng/mL.

► Follow-up Questions

1. *What medications could be used to provide better rate control, and which of these alternatives would be most appropriate considering the patient's heart failure?*
2. *Outline a therapeutic plan for employing a β-blocking agent in this patient.*
3. *The patient was started on carvedilol at an appropriate starting*

dose. What information should be provided to the patient about common adverse effects? Describe how they should be managed if they occur.

▶ Clinical Course

The patient returns to your clinic site 3 weeks later stating that his palpitations seem to be better. However, he feels worse despite using the new medication as prescribed. You sense that there is potential for noncompliance with the carvedilol.

4. *What information should you convey to the patient about his current perspective on the usefulness of carvedilol?*

▶ Self-study Assignments

1. What vitamins and/or minerals should this patient consider supplementing based upon his chronic diuretic use?
2. This patient may develop diuretic resistance. Write a one-page paper describing what this phenomenon is and how it might be overcome.
3. Describe how you would evaluate and monitor this patient's quality of life.

▶ Clinical Pearl

The presence of pitting edema is associated with a substantial increase in body weight; it typically takes a weight gain of 10 pounds to result in the development of pitting edema.

References

1. Packer M, Bristow MR, Cohn JN, et al. The effect of carvedilol on morbidity and mortality in patients with chronic heart failure. N Engl J Med 1996;334: 1349–1355.
2. Vagelos R, Nojedly M, Willson K, et al. Comparison of low versus high dose enalapril therapy for patients with severe congestive heart failure (CHF). J Am Coll Cardiol 1991:275A. Abstract.
3. Hammill SC, Packer DL. Amiodarone in congestive heart failure: Unraveling the GESICA and CHF-STAT differences. Heart 1996;75:6–7. Editorial.

5 ISCHEMIC HEART DISEASE

▶ **Neither Hale Nor Hearty**   (Level II)

Amy J. Guenette, PharmD, BCPS

▶ After completing this case study, students should be able to:
- Identify modifiable risk factors for IHD and discuss the potential benefit to be derived by their modification in an individual patient.
- Optimize medical therapy in a patient with persistent angina considering response to present therapy and the presence of comorbidities.
- Assess clinical response to antianginal therapy by identifying relevant monitoring parameters for efficacy and adverse effects.
- Identify the relative risk/benefit profile of glycoprotein IIb/IIIa receptor antagonist therapy and apply it to an individual patient.

☼ PATIENT PRESENTATION

Chief Complaint
"I'm still getting my chest pains."

HPI
Roger Hale is a 65 yo man with a history of CAD, MI, and CABG × 3 vessels 7 years ago. He presents to the clinic today following his discharge from the hospital 1 month ago. During that admission, he underwent a cardiac catheterization for evaluation of increasingly frequent intermittent chest pain. The catheterization showed some progression of disease over previous studies but revealed no target lesions for intervention. The discharge summary indicated that his cardiologist decided to treat him medically, noting his intention to avoid β-blocker therapy due to the patient's asthma. Mr. Hale still complains of chest pain characteristic of his angina (substernal in location, crushing in character). He states that he thinks he might be able to walk a little farther than before he went to the hospital when his Procardia XL dose was increased. The pain, which he rates as approximately 7 or 8 on a scale of 1 to 10, comes on with exertion and subsides with rest. He avoids stairs, but says he can walk approximately 100 yards before he has to stop because of chest pain and fatigue. The pain occurs as often as he attempts this level of exertion. Mr. Hale frequently has some baseline shortness of breath due to his asthma, but that also worsens with exertion.

PMH
S/P CVA after last cath—some residual weakness in LUE
S/P cath 1 month ago; LVEF 45%
S/P MI 7 years ago; subsequently underwent CABG × 3
Asthma
HTN

FH
Father deceased at 72 from CVA; mother and sister deceased from cancer; brother deceased due to MI at age 57; four children, alive and well

SH
Married, lives with wife, nonsmoker, nondrinker

Meds
EC aspirin 325 mg po QD
Mavik 2 mg po QD
Imdur 60 mg po QD
Procardia XL 60 mg po QD
Dyazide 1 po QD
Albuterol MDI 2 puffs QID
Vanceril MDI 1 puff Q HS

All
NKDA; codeine intolerance (nausea/vomiting)

ROS
(+) chronic cough 2° asthma; (+) nocturnal coughing paroxysms; (−) fever/chills

(+) SOB, CP & fatigue on exertion; (−) orthopnea

(+) reduction in appetite with 10-lb weight loss over 2 months

(+) loose stools, (−) for melena or frank blood

(+) occasional LE cramps during sleep, (−) cramps on exertion

PE

Gen

Mr. Hale is an elderly male in NAD who appears somewhat fatigued.

VS

BP 130/68, P 88, RR 22, T 36.4°C; Ht 6'0", Wt 79 kg

Skin

Intact, no lesions

HEENT

TMs clear, nl landmarks, translucent; PEERLA; EOMI; white sclerae; conjunctiva non-edematous; funduscopic exam (+) AV nicking, (−) hemorrhages, exudates, or papilledema; no oral erythema or exudates

Neck

Supple, no masses; no JVD, lymphadenopathy, or thyromegaly

Lungs

Diffuse wheezes bilaterally, decreased breath sounds at bases, good inspiratory effort

CV

RRR, S_1, S_2 nl; no murmurs or gallops; PMI palpated at left 5th ICS, MCL

Abd

(+) BS, soft, NT/ND, no organomegaly

G/U

Heme (+) stool

Ext

No edema; pulses 2+ throughout; nl PROM throughout; nl AROM except for diminished AROM left wrist and hand

Neuro

A & O × 3, CN II–XII intact; (+) weakness of L hand 2° recent CVA; DTRs 2+ throughout (LUE slightly hyper-reflexive); diminished sensitivity to pinprick and 2-point discrimination on left hand, Babinski downgoing

Labs

Na 137 mEq/L	Hgb 11.8 g/dL	Chol 162 mg/dL
K 5.8 mEq/L	Hct 35.1%	LDL 99 mg/dL
Cl 103 mEq/L	Plt $187 \times 10^3/mm^3$	
CO_2 21 mEq/L	WBC $7.9 \times 10^3/mm^3$	
BUN 36 mg/dL	MCV 77 μm^3	
SCr 2.2 mg/dL	MCHC 29 g/dL	
Glu 98 mg/dL		

ECG
Sinus rhythm at 90 bpm, old AWMI, No ST–T wave changes noted

Assessment
Elderly gentleman with persistent exertional angina symptoms poorly controlled on present regimen

S/P CVA, receiving PT for LUE weakness

HTN—controlled

Asthma—mildly symptomatic on present regimen

▶ Questions

Problem Identification

1. a. What drug-related problems appear to be present in this patient?

   b. Could any of these problems potentially be caused or exacerbated by his current therapy? Would any additional information be helpful to you in making this judgment?

   c. What information presented in this case supports the diagnosis of ischemic heart disease and provides insight into the severity of this disease?

Desired Outcome

2. What are the goals of pharmacotherapy for IHD in this case?

Therapeutic Alternatives

3. a. Does this patient possess any modifiable risk factors for IHD? If so, would addressing them improve his condition?

   b. What pharmacotherapeutic options are available for treating this patient's IHD? Discuss the items in each class with respect to their relative utility in his care.

Optimal Plan

4. Given the patient information provided, construct a complete pharmacotherapeutic plan for optimizing his IHD management.

Outcome Evaluation

5. When the patient returns to the clinic in 2 weeks for his follow-up visit, how will you evaluate the response to his new antianginal regimen for efficacy and adverse affects?

Patient Counseling

6. What information will you communicate to the patient about his antianginal regimen to help him experience the greatest benefit and fewest adverse effects?

Clinical Course

Two months later, the patient's cardiologist is notified of his arrival at the ED of the local hospital. He is complaining of severe substernal chest pain that came on at rest. He rated the pain as 10/10 on presentation and said that it radiated to his left arm. He has received some relief with IV NTG and morphine. An echocardiogram reveals worsened anterior wall hypokinesis and an ECG revealed ST segment changes consistent with anterior wall ischemia. He is diagnosed with unstable angina and is taken to the cath lab. Catheterization reveals a high-grade lesion at the site of his LIMA (left internal mammary artery) to LAD graft. The previous film from 3 months ago showed a 50% occlusion at the same site. An angioplasty with concomitant abciximab therapy is planned.

Follow-up Questions

1. *What role does abciximab play in the setting of PTCA?*
2. *What is this patient's risk/benefit assessment for abciximab therapy?*
3. *Given the information provided, what changes, if any, would you make in the therapy for his other drug-related problems?*

Self-study Assignments

1. Design a pharmacotherapeutic plan for prevention of restenosis in patients undergoing stent placement.
2. Compare and contrast eptifibatide with abciximab with respect to mechanism and duration of action and efficacy and adverse effect profiles when used in acute coronary syndromes and PTCA.
3. Discuss the relative merits of using drugs with T-channel calcium blockade versus agents with L-channel activity.
4. Discuss strategies for avoidance or minimization of nitrate tolerance with the various nitrate preparations available.

Clinical Pearl

The presence of mild LV dysfunction is an important consideration in choosing antianginal therapy; but its presence does not necessarily preclude the use of agents with negative inotropic activity if they are instituted cautiously and carefully monitored.

References

1. EPIC investigators. Use of a monoclonal antibody directed against the platelet glycoprotein IIb/IIIa receptor in high-risk coronary angioplasty. N Engl J Med 1994;330:956–961.
2. EPILOG investigators. Platelet glycoprotein IIb/IIIa receptor blockade and low-dose heparin during percutaneous coronary revascularization. N Engl J Med 1997;336:1689–1696.
3. CAPTURE investigators. Randomised placebo-controlled trial of abciximab before and during coronary intervention in refractory unstable angina: The CAPTURE study. Lancet 1997;349:1429–1435.

6 ACUTE MYOCARDIAL INFARCTION

Not Just for Men Alone   (Level II)

B. Nhi Nguyen, PharmD
Robert B. Parker, PharmD

▶ After completing this case study, students should be able to:

- Determine the goals of pharmacotherapy for acute MI patients.
- Design an optimal therapeutic plan for management of acute MI and describe how the selected drug therapy achieves the therapeutic goals.
- Identify appropriate parameters to assess the recommended drug therapy for both efficacy and adverse effects.
- Provide appropriate patient counseling information to an acute MI patient.

PATIENT PRESENTATION

Chief Complaint
"I'm having pain in my chest, and I feel like I'm full of gas."

HPI
Lorraine Hunt is a 66 yo woman who is transferred to the ED from the Radiology Department, where she developed severe crushing, substernal chest pain prior to an IVP for renal calculi. The pain has lasted for 20 minutes. It is associated with mild SOB, diaphoresis, and radiation to the neck and both arms. In the ED, she had some decrease in her chest pain after taking three SL NTG tablets.

PMH
CABG × 2 (10 and 15 years ago)
CVA after her last CABG
HTN × 20 years
Type 2 DM
Hyperlipidemia
Hysterectomy 30 years ago; ovaries intact

FH
Father died of an MI at age 54; mother died of breast CA at age 80. She has one sister 61 yo alive and well and one brother 58 yo with HTN.

SH
No tobacco × 15 years; no ETOH × 15 years

ROS
Positive for some baseline CP for "some time"

All
NKDA

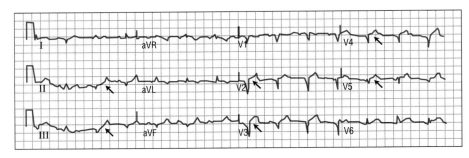

Figure 6–1. ECG taken on arrival in the ED showing ST segment elevation (arrrows) in leads V2 to V6 consistent with acute anterior myocardial infarction.

Meds

Metoprolol 100 mg po Q 12 H

Glyburide 10 mg po Q AM, 5 mg po Q PM

Folic acid 1 mg po QD

EC ASA 325 mg po QD

NTG SR 6.5 mg po TID

Gemfibrozil 600 mg po BID

PE

Gen

A & O woman, still with chest pain

VS

BP 130/78, P 82, RR 18, T 37.1°C; Ht 5′10″, Wt 86 kg

HEENT

PERRLA, EOMI, fundi benign, TMs intact

Neck

No bruits, mild JVD; no thyromegaly

Lungs

Few dependent inspiratory crackles, bibasilar rales, no wheezes

CV

PMI displaced laterally, nl S_1 and S_2, no S_3 or S_4, I/VI SEM @ LUSB

Abd

Soft, nontender, liver span ≈10–12 cm, no bruits

MS/Ext

Normal ROM; muscle strength on right 5/5 UE/LE, on left 4/5 UE/LE; pulses 2+, no femoral bruits or peripheral edema

Neuro

CN II–XII intact; DTRs decreased on left; Babinski (−)

Labs

Na 134 mEq/L	PO_4 2.4 mg/dL	Hgb 14.0 g/dL
K 4.4 mEq/L	Chol 214 mg/dL	Hct 44%
Cl 102 mEq/L	Trig 175 mg/dL	WBC $5.0 \times 10^3/mm^3$
CO_2 23 mEq/L	LDL 144 mg/dL	Plt $268 \times 10^3/mm^3$
BUN 15 mg/dL	HDL 35 mg/dL	PT 12.5 sec
Scr 1.0 mg/dL	CPK 68 U/L	aPTT 32.4 sec
Glu 266 mg/dL	CK-MB 1.1 IU/L	INR 1.0
Ca 9.8 mg/dL	CK-MB% ND*	HbA_{1c} 1 mo. ago 9.3%
Mg 2.0 mg/dL	Troponin I 0.0	

* ND, not determined.

ECG

2 to 5 mm ST segment elevation in leads V2 to V6 (see Figure 6–1).

Assessment

Acute anterior MI

▶ Questions

Problem Identification

1. a. *What findings in this patient's case history are consistent with acute myocardial infarction?*

    b. *What risk factors for the development of coronary artery disease are present in this patient?*

Desired Outcome

2. *What are the goals of pharmacotherapy in this patient?*

Therapeutic Alternatives

3. a. *What feasible pharmacotherapeutic alternatives are available to treat this patient?*

    b. *What non-pharmacologic alternative therapies might be used in this patient?*

Optimal Plan

4. *Based on the history and presentation, what drug therapy is indicated in this patient?*

Outcome Evaluation

5. *How should the recommended therapy be monitored for efficacy and adverse effects?*

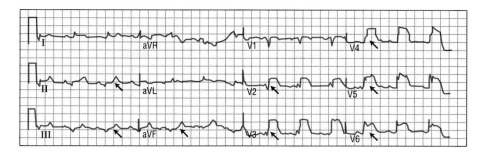

Figure 6–2. ECG taken during TPA infusion showing increasing ST segment elevation (arrows) in leads V2 to V6.

▶ **Clinical Course**

The patient received aspirin, IV nitroglycerin, captopril, and metoprolol. Approximately 1 hour after initiation of the TPA infusion, the patient's chest pain had improved but had not completely resolved, and the ECG showed increasing ST segment elevations in leads V1 to V6 (5 to 8 mm), and inferiorly (see Figure 6–2). With the ongoing chest pain and increasing ST elevations, she was taken to the cardiac catheterization laboratory for an emergent catheterization with rescue PTCA. The cath revealed the culprit lesion to be a severe proximal stenosis involving a saphenous vein graft (SVG) from the aorta to the left anterior descending artery. PTCA was performed followed by placement of a coronary artery stent. Because of residual thrombus in the distal portion of this SVG, abciximab was infused. Ejection fraction by echocardiogram 3 days post-infarct was 47%. The rest of the patient's hospital stay was uncomplicated, and she was discharged 8 days post-MI.

Patient Counseling

6. a. *What discharge medications would be most appropriate for this patient?*
    b. *What patient counseling information should you provide to this patient?*

▶ **Follow-up Question**

1. *This patient returns to the cardiology clinic in 6 weeks for a follow-up visit. She reports feeling fine. What interventions do you recommend at this time?*

▶ **Self-study Assignments**

1. The patient comes into your pharmacy and asks you if taking antioxidants or vitamins would do her heart any good. What would you tell her about antioxidants? Which ones would you recommend and why?
2. A 38 yo man with an established history of coronary artery disease is admitted to the CCU for his second MI. The attending physician wants to check *Chlamydia* titers and asks you for your drug therapy recommendations. What therapy would you recommend, and how would you monitor such therapy?
3. Perform a literature search and evaluate recent clinical trials using platelet glycoprotein II_B/III_A inhibitors in MI patients.

▶ **Clinical Pearl**

Signs of successful thrombolysis include disappearance of chest pain, reperfusion arrhythmias, resolution of ST segment changes, and early peak of cardiac isoenzymes.

References

1. Ryan TJ, Bauman WB, Kennedy JW, et al. ACC/AHA guidelines for percutaneous transluminal coronary angioplasty: A report of the American College of Cardiology/American Heart Association Task Force on Assessment of Diagnostic and Therapeutic Cardiovascular Procedures (Committee on Percutaneous Transluminal Coronary Angioplasty). J Am Coll Cardiol 1993;22:2033–2054.
2. Ryan TJ, Anderson JL, Antman EM, et al. ACC/AHA guidelines for the management of patients with acute myocardial infarction: A report of the American College of Cardiology/American Heart Association Task Force on Practice Guidelines (Committee on Management of Acute Myocardial Infarction). J Am Coll Cardiol 1996;28:1328–1428.
3. Schömig A, Neumann FJ, Kastrati A, et al. A randomized comparison of antiplatelet and anticoagulant therapy after the placement of coronary-artery stents. N Engl J Med 1996;334:1084–1089.
4. Pfeffer MA, Braunwald E, Moye LA, et al. Effect of captopril on mortality and morbidity in patients with left ventricular dysfunction after myocardial infarction. Results of the Survival and Ventricular Enlargement (SAVE) trial. N Engl J Med 1992;327:669–677.

7 VENTRICULAR TACHYCARDIA

▶ **Hello, 911 Operator?**   (Level III)

Ashesh J. Gandhi, PharmD

▶ After completing this case study, students should be able to:

- Understand the risk factors for development of ventricular tachycardia (VT).
- Differentiate VT from other cardiac arrhythmias.
- Select appropriate first-line and second-line therapies for treatment of VT.
- Monitor antiarrhythmic and other therapies used to treat VT.
- Discuss long-term approaches to prevention of recurrent VT.

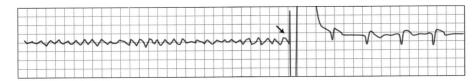

Figure 7–1. Rhythm strip showing ventricular fibrillation that was successfully defibrillated (arrow) to sinus rhythm. *(Photo courtesy of Jason Lazar, MD.)*

☼ PATIENT PRESENTATION

Chief Complaint
"Operator, I've had pains in my chest twice that shoot down into my left arm. I think I need the paramedics."

HPI
Paul Gates is a 41 yo man who has had minor chest pains in the past, and an exercise stress test done about 1 month ago was negative. Today he was watching TV at home when he felt a crushing pain in his chest that radiated to the left arm that was relieved by lying down. A few minutes later, he developed recurrent chest pain, grade 7/10 in pain intensity that again radiated to the left arm. The chest pain was associated with shortness of breath and diaphoresis. He then called 911. Upon arrival of the paramedics, he had an episode of sustained VT that degenerated into VF, and he passed out. He was defibrillated × 1 by the paramedics and was successfully resuscitated (see Figure 7–1). He was taken by ambulance to the ED at a community hospital, where he was found to have an acute anterior wall MI. He was treated with 100 mg TPA in an accelerated dose fashion. He still had recurrences of chest pain grade 6/10 in pain intensity not relieved with IV nitroglycerin and was emergently transferred to a university hospital for cardiac catheterization. The cardiac cath showed 100% mid and proximal LAD occlusion. He underwent rescue PTCA, and two coronary artery stents were placed in the mid and proximal LAD. He also received abciximab during PTCA/stent placement to prevent abrupt vessel closure. He was then admitted to the CCU.

PMH
HTN × 10 years

PSH
Appendectomy

FH
Father alive age 66 with angina; mother alive age 62 with arthritis; both paternal grandparents had CAD at age 70

SH
Works as a systems analyst for a large corporation; occasional cigar smoker

ROS
Negative except for complaints noted above

Meds
Quinapril 20 mg po QD (on admission)

All
NKDA

PE (Performed in the CCU)

Gen
WDWN male

VS
BP 125/75, P 89, RR 20, T 36.8°C

HEENT
PERRLA, EOMI, pink conjunctiva, AV nicking (Grade 1) on funduscopic exam

Neck
Supple, no JVD, no bruits

Chest
Occasional bibasilar crackles

CV
S_1 and S_2 normal; no S_3. No m/r/g

Abd
Soft, NT/ND. (+) bowel sounds

Ext
Right groin lines in place, no hematomas, 2+ peripheral pulses

Neuro
No focal neurologic deficits. CN II–XII intact

Labs

Na 133 mEq/L	Hgb 14.3 g/dL	Ca 8.4 mg/dL
K 3.8 mEq/L	Hct 44.6%	Mg 1.5 mEq/L
Cl 96 mEq/L	Plt 262 × 10³/mm³	aPTT 48.1 sec
CO_2 23.6 mEq/L	WBC 18.1 × 10³/mm³	PT 13.5 sec
BUN 16 mg/dL	Polys 89%	INR 1.2
SCr 1.1 mg/dL	Lymphs 9%	CPK 2171 IU/L
Glu 169 mg/dL	Monos 2%	CK-MB 196 IU/L
		LDH 281 IU/L

UA
Appearance: Yellow, hazy; SG 1.015; pH 7.5; protein 30 mg; glucose neg; ketones neg; Hgb 3+, WBC 2-5/hpf; RBC 5-10/hpf; epithelial cells occ; bacteria 1+; leukocyte esterase neg; urobilinogen 0.2 EU/dL; bilirubin neg

ECG
Day 1: HR 94 bpm; NSR; acute anterior wall MI; anterolateral ST segment elevations; Q waves in V1 to V3 (see Figure 7–2).

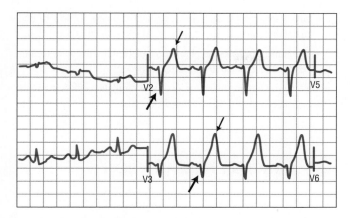

Figure 7–2. ECG leads V2 and V3 showing antero-lateral ST segment elevations (small arrows) and Q waves (large arrows), consistent with anterior wall myocardial infarction.

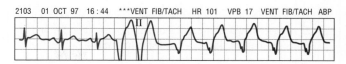

Figure 7–3. ECG (lead II) showing sustained ventricu-lar tachycardia.

▶ Clinical Course

During his hospitalization, he developed one episode of sustained asymptomatic VT with a BP of 70/40 mm Hg and HR of 105 bpm (see Figure 7–3). He also had multiple episodes of NSVT (8 to 10 beats) but still maintained his blood pressure and heart rate with no symptoms.

▶ Questions

Problem Identification

1. a. *What are the possible causes of sudden cardiac death and VT in this patient? What information presented in the case suggests these causes?*

   b. *How are VT and NSVT characterized on the ECG?*

Desired Outcome

2. *What are the goals of treatment for acute-onset VT?*

Therapeutic Alternatives

3. a. *What non-drug therapies may be useful for treating acute VT in this patient?*

   b. *What pharmacotherapeutic alternatives are available for the treatment of acute-onset VT?*

Optimal Plan

4. *What drug, dosage form, schedule, and duration of therapy are best for this patient for the treatment of acute-onset VT?*

Outcome Evaluation

5. *What monitoring parameters are necessary to evaluate the therapy for achievement of the desired therapeutic outcome and to prevent toxicity?*

▶ Clinical Course

The patient received the treatment you recommended with no further episodes of VT. The abciximab infusion (0.125 μg/kg/min) was subsequently discontinued. Other medications taken during the 3-day CCU hospitalization included heparin 500 units/hour by continuous IV infusion, nitroglycerin infusion 10 μg/min, aspirin 325 mg po QD, ticlopidine 250 mg po BID, metoprolol 50 mg po BID, quinapril 20 mg po QD, and magnesium chloride 2 g IV × 1. Heparin was discontinued on the second day, and warfarin 5 mg po QD × 1 month was initiated to prevent stent occlusion. Warfarin was overlapped with enoxaparin 30 mg SQ Q 12 H until the INR was therapeutic (target INR set at 1.8 to 2.0). The medication given for VT was discontinued after 2 days, and the patient was observed on telemetry. There was no recurrence of VT or NSVT after 3 days of telemetry observation, and the patient was then discharged on warfarin 5 mg po QD, EC ASA 325 mg po QD, ticlopidine 250 mg po BID, metoprolol 50 mg po BID, and quinapril 20 mg po QD.

Patient Counseling

6. *What information should be provided to the patient to enhance patient understanding and compliance upon discharge?*

▶ Follow-up Question

1. *Create a list of the patient's drug-related problems.*

▶ Self-study Assignments

1. Patients with recurrent sustained VT after an acute MI (even after correction of precipitating factors) are at a high risk of sudden cardiac death. These patients are often taken to the electrophysiology lab and tested for inducibility of VT and are then given some form of preventative therapy (e.g., antiarrhythmics or implantable cardiac defibrillators). However, in patients who have asymptomatic NSVT, it is still not clear what treatment approach should be taken. The Multicenter Automatic Defibrillator Implantation Trial (MADIT) was conducted in patients with coronary artery disease and NSVT to determine whether all patients with asymptomatic NSVT require long-term preventative therapy.[7] Look up this article and write a one-page paper on your assessment of the study results.

2. The ACC/AHA guidelines[8] on management of acute MI suggest that all patients should receive ACE inhibitor therapy within the first 24 hours as long as there are no contraindications. Patients with asymptomatic or symptomatic LV dysfunction after an acute MI typically receive ACE inhibitors indefinitely due to decreased mortality (ISIS-4, GISSI-3, SOLVD trials). However, what is the duration of ACE inhibitor therapy in patients who do *not* develop asymptomatic or symptomatic LV dysfunction after an acute MI?

▶ Clinical Pearl

After an MI, β-blockers are the most effective prophylactic interventions against VT/VF for most patients. The role of amiodarone is uncertain, but some patients at a higher risk of sudden cardiac death will require an implantable defibrillator device or other antiarrhythmic therapy.

References

1. Hazinski MF, Cummins RO, eds. 1997 Handbook of Emergency Cardiac Care for Healthcare Providers. Dallas, American Heart Association, 1996.
2. Yusuf S, Peto R, Lewis J, et al. β-blockade during and after myocardial infarction: An overview of the randomized trials. Prog Cardiovasc Dis 1985;27:335–371.
3. Joint National Committee on Prevention, Detection, Evaluation, and Treatment of High Blood Pressure. Sixth report. Arch Intern Med 1997;157:2413–2445.
4. MIAMI Trial Research Group. Metoprolol in acute myocardial infarction. Am J Cardiol 1985;56:1G–57G.
5. TIMI Study Group. Comparison of invasive and conservative strategies after treatment with intravenous tissue plasminogen activator in acute myocardial infarction: Results of the thrombolysis in myocardial infarction (TIMI) phase II trial. N Engl J Med 1989;320:618–627.
6. Dalen JE, Hirsh J, eds. Fourth ACCP Consensus Conference on Antithrombotic Therapy. Antithrombotic therapy in patients undergoing coronary angioplasty. Chest 1995;108(4 suppl):486S–501S.
7. Moss AJ, Hall WJ, Cannom DS, et al. Improved survival with an implanted defibrillator in patients with coronary disease at high risk for ventricular arrhythmia. Multicenter Automatic Defibrillator Implantation Trial Investigators. N Engl J Med 1996;335:1933–1940.
8. American College of Cardiology/American Heart Association Task Force on Practice Guidelines (committee on management of acute myocardial infarction). ACC/AHA guidelines for the management of patients with acute myocardial infarction. J Am Coll Cardiol 1996;28:1328–1428.

8   ATRIAL FIBRILLATION

▶ If It's Not Love, Head for the ER   (Level II)

Bradley G. Phillips, PharmD

▶   After completing this case study, students should be able to:

- Determine therapeutic goals for patients presenting with atrial fibrillation.

- Select appropriate pharmacotherapeutic regimens to achieve and maintain ventricular rate control in patients with atrial fibrillation.
- Recommend appropriate pharmacologic or other therapies to convert atrial fibrillation to normal sinus rhythm.
- Recognize how treatment for lone atrial fibrillation differs from that associated with identifiable underlying causes.

☀ PATIENT PRESENTATION

Chief Complaint
"I feel that my heart is beating too fast and I feel a bit dizzy."

HPI
Matthew Jacobson is a 63 yo man who presents to the ED with heart palpitations and dizziness. He first noticed the palpitations 3 hours ago while he was mowing his lawn. He describes the palpitations as a heavy fluttering sensation in his chest. The severity of his dizziness fluctuates; the dizziness was the worst when he was pushing his lawn mower. He has been seen in the medicine clinic for many years for his HTN and COPD and has a history of medication noncompliance.

PMH
HTN (uncontrolled due to noncompliance)
COPD × 15 years
BPH × 7 years

FH
Both parents had HTN; his mother died of a stroke at age 65, his father died after suffering an AMI at the age of 62. He has one brother who is alive and well.

SH
Mr. Jacobson is retired and lives at home with his wife. He smoked 1 ppd for 20 years and quit 3 years ago. He drinks 1 to 2 beers every other week.

Meds
Terazosin 10 mg po QD
Albuterol inhaler 2 puffs QID
Ipratropium bromide inhaler 2 puffs QID
Multivitamin 1 tablet po QD

All
NKDA

ROS
No headache, blurred vision, chest pain, or fainting spells; complains of occasional wheezes, but has no cough or SOB; no present difficulty with urination

PE

Gen
Cooperative overweight man in moderate distress

VS
BP 98/70 (supine), P 140 (irregular), RR 20, T 36.3°C; Ht 5'11", Wt 93 kg

Skin
Cool to touch, normal turgor and color

HEENT
PERRLA, EOMI; funduscopic exam reveals mild arteriolar narrowing but no hemorrhages, exudates, or papilledema

Neck
Supple, no carotid bruits; no lymphadenopathy or thyromegaly

Pulm
Inspiratory and expiratory wheezes bilaterally without rales or rhonchi

CV
Tachycardia with irregular rate; varying S_1, S_2; no S_3 or S_4; no m/r/g

Abd
NT/ND, (+) BS; no organomegaly

Genit/Rect
Stool heme (−); prostate slightly enlarged and smooth

MS/Ext
Pulses 2+, full ROM, no CCE

Neuro
A & O × 3; CN II–XII intact. DTR 2+, negative Babinski

Labs (non-fasting)

Na 140 mEq/L	Hgb 15.2 g/dL	Ca 9.1 mg/dL
K 4.2 mEq/L	Hct 48%	Mg 2.1 mEq/L
Cl 99 mEq/L	Plt 293 × 10³/mm³	
CO_2 24 mEq/L	WBC 12.1 × 10³/mm³	
BUN 23 mg/dL	Polys 71%	
SCr 1.5 mg/dL	Bands 2%	
Glu 125 mg/dL	Lymphs 24%	
	Monos 3%	

ECG
Atrial fibrillation, ventricular rate 144, no LVH

Chest X-ray
No infiltrates, mild thoracic overinflation

Assessment
New-onset atrial fibrillation
Hypotension: Hold BP meds until rhythm disturbance is corrected and BP is stabilized
COPD: Continue current medications
BPH: Hold terazosin due to low BP and arrhythmia

► Questions

Problem Identification

1. a. *List and prioritize the patient's drug-related problems.*
   b. *Does this patient have "lone" atrial fibrillation?*
   c. *Considering his presenting signs and symptoms, how would you characterize the severity of this patient's atrial fibrillation? State the rationale for your answer.*

Desired Outcome

2. *What are the acute goals for pharmacotherapy in this case?*

Therapeutic Alternatives

3. *Describe the benefits and risks of drugs that can be used to achieve and maintain ventricular rate control in patients with atrial fibrillation.*

Optimal Plan

4. *Which agent and dosage regimen would you recommend to achieve and maintain control of this patient's ventricular response rate?*

► Clinical Course

The drug regimen that you recommended to control the ventricular response was initiated. The rate prior to drug administration was 131 beats per minute with a BP of 101/71 mm Hg. His baseline rhythm recorded just prior to drug therapy administration is shown in the top portion of Figure 8–1. The patient's rhythm and vital signs were monitored over the next 15 minutes. At 15 minutes, his rhythm showed atrial fibrillation with a ventricular response of 95 bpm and he had a BP of 108/83 mm Hg (see bottom portion of Figure 8–1). He stated that he felt better and did not notice the fluttering in his chest any longer. A continuous infusion of the same drug was initiated to maintain the patient's ventricular response rate. He also received heparin 5000 units by IV bolus and was started on a heparin infusion of 1000 units per hour. Shortly thereafter, the Cardiology Service arrives in the ED to evaluate the patient. The team decides to admit him to a telemetry bed for further evaluation with plans to perform cardioversion.

Outcome Evaluation

5. *How would you monitor and adjust the IV infusion to control his ventricular response rate?*

► Follow-up Questions

1. *Is it possible that the drug therapy you recommended to control the ventricular response rate will also convert his atrial fibrillation to normal sinus rhythm?*
2. *If the cardiology team decides to chemically cardiovert the patient, why is it important to first control his ventricular rate?*
3. *Assuming that the patient is successfully cardioverted, should the therapy you prescribed to control his ventricular response be prescribed long term?*

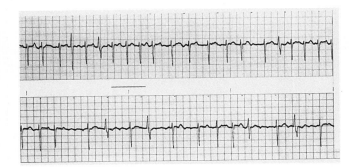

Figure 8–1. Rhythm recorded just prior to (top) and 15 minutes after (bottom) the administration of drug therapy. Top rhythm depicts atrial fibrillation with a ventricular response rate of 131 bpm. Bottom rhythm depicts atrial fibrillation with a rate of 95 bpm. Atrial fibrillation is characterized in each rhythm strip by the absence of atrial "p" waves and an irregular ventricular response (intervals between each QRS complex vary irregularly).

▶ Self-study Assignments

1. Outline the antiarrhythmic drug regimen you would recommend to convert this patient's atrial fibrillation to normal sinus rhythm.
2. If this patient develops atrial fibrillation again, which antiarrhythmic drug and regimen would you recommend to maintain normal sinus rhythm chronically?
3. After successful cardioversion, would you recommend that this patient be prescribed aspirin or warfarin therapy? If so, give specific recommendations on which agent you would recommend along with monitoring parameters for efficacy and toxicity.
4. Give your recommendations for treating this patient's hypertension and on the wisdom of restarting terazosin for managing his BPH.

▶ Clinical Pearl

In atrial fibrillation, the ventricular rate must be controlled prior to chemical cardioversion so that paradoxical increases in ventricular response and subsequent hemodynamic instability do not occur.

References

1. Prystowsky EN, Benson W, Fuster V, et al. Management of patients with atrial fibrillation. A statement for healthcare professionals from the Subcommittee on Electrocardiography and Electrophysiology, American Heart Association. Circulation 1996;93:1262–1277.
2. Seto TB, Taira DA, Tsevat J, et al. Cost-effectiveness of transesophageal echocardiographic-guided cardioversion: A decision analytic model for patients admitted to the hospital with atrial fibrillation. J Am Coll Cardiol 1997;29:122–130.
3. Roberts SA, Diaz C, Nolan PE, et al. Effectiveness and costs of digoxin treatment for atrial fibrillation and flutter. Am J Cardiol 1993;72:567–573.
4. Phillips BG, Gandhi AJ, Sanoski CA, et al. Comparison of intravenous diltiazem and verapamil for the acute treatment of atrial fibrillation and atrial flutter. Pharmacotherapy 1997;17:1238–1245.

9 HYPERTROPHIC CARDIOMYOPATHY

▶ Having a Big Heart Is Not Always a Good Thing   (Level I)

Laura A. Bartels, PharmD

▶ After completing this case study, students should be able to:

- Describe the risk factors for hypertrophic cardiomyopathy (HCM).
- Differentiate the benefits and side effects of pharmacologic treatments for HCM.
- Advise and counsel patients on the appropriate use of medications used to treat HCM.
- Design monitoring parameters for achievement of the desired therapeutic outcomes while minimizing adverse effects of medications used to treat HCM.

☼ PATIENT PRESENTATION

Chief Complaint
"I've been short of breath this past week at school, and the school nurse suggested I see my doctor right away. He sent me to see you."

HPI
John Lawrence is a 17 yo senior in high school who presents to a cardiologist's office after referral by his PMD. He was in a normal state of health for the past 17 years but over the past week he has become very tired and short of breath while awake and at night. This has progressed to the point where he can no longer talk without gasping for air. Yesterday, he experienced a slight pressure on his chest and lightheadedness with a "flip flop feeling" which happened when he participated in his gym class. Resting with two pillows to elevate his head relieved this pressure. The school nurse was called to assess John's health, and she dismissed him from class so that he could see his private physician immediately.

PMH
No known health problems. John had a viral-like URI at age 12 and right ear infections at ages 3 and 4.

FH
Father died last year of sudden cardiac death at the age of 45. Mother has a heart murmur. Younger brother age 15 is in good physical health. Older brother died suddenly at the age of 19 of unknown causes.

SH
John is very popular at school and is well liked by others. He dates a few girls at school and claims not to be sexually active. He comes from an upper socioeconomic background. He doesn't drink alcohol, smoke, or use any recreational drugs. He claims that is "un-cool" with the friends he

hangs out with. He and his friends play baseball every day after school because he is on the varsity team this year. His home life was difficult this past year due to the death of his father and remembering him in thought. John claims that, for the most part, he has a very caring and close family.

ROS
(+) for fatigue, palpitations with feelings of lightheadedness, occasional chest pain upon exertion, dyspnea, and orthopnea. Worsening shortness of breath for the past week. No fever or hemoptysis

Meds
No regular medications; occasional aspirin, ibuprofen, and Tylenol use for headaches, aches, and pains

All
NKDA

PE

Gen
John is a 17 yo male gasping for breath after walking into the doctor's office.

VS
BP 130/95, P 80, RR 23, T 37.0°C; Wt 83.9 kg, Ht 6'2"

HEENT
PERRLA, EOMI, fundi benign, TMs intact

Neck
A brisk carotid upstroke can be felt.

Lungs
Bibasilar crackles noted upon auscultation in the lower quarter of the lung fields; RLL and LLL dull to percussion posteriorly; wheezes noted without auscultation.

CV
RRR, S_1 with slight systolic murmur of variable intensity is heard along the left sternal border and at the apex; S_2 present and clearly audible, slight S_4 gallop present. MR II/VI. Effects of Valsalva maneuver—increased murmur intensity during peak strain phase (II) and decrease in late strain release phase (IV).

Abd
Soft, NT/ND; normal and reactive bowel sounds

Ext
Radial pulses 4+ bilaterally; pedal pulses 3+ bilaterally; extremities are slightly cool to the touch.

Rect
Guaiac (−)

Neuro
A & O × 3; without focal deficits

Labs
Na 135 mEq/L	Hgb 14.5 g/dL	aPTT 28.3 sec
K 4.7 mEq/L	Hct 45%	PT 10 sec
Cl 101 mEq/L	Plt $310 \times 10^3/mm^3$	INR 1.1
CO_2 22 mEq/L	WBC $8.8 \times 10^3/mm^3$	
BUN 19 mg/dL	PMNs 75%	
SCr 1.2 mg/dL	Bands 5%	
Glu 120 mg/dL	Lymphs 15%	
	Monos 5%	

Chest X-ray
Subtle left ventricular enlargement; pulmonary venous engorgement is noted.

ECG
Increased QRS voltage and T wave inversion changes in the lateral precordial leads (V4 to V6)

Two-dimensional Echocardiography
Hypertrophy noted; asymmetric wall thickness; sparkling or granular appearance of walls; normal cavity size. Slightly dilated left atrium; hyperdynamic LV function (EF > 70%); thickened, elongated anterior leaflet

Doppler Echocardiography
Slight mitral regurgitation at times. Mitral inflow: diastolic dysfunction pattern with impaired relaxation; low normal end-diastolic dimension. Septal wall thickness of 16 mm. Septal to posterior wall thickness ratio of 1.5:1

Assessment
17-year-old male with hypertrophic cardiomyopathy requiring relief of his shortness of breath

▶ Questions

Problem Identification
1. *What signs and symptoms indicate the presence or severity of the patient's HCM?*

Desired Outcome
2. *What are the goals of pharmacotherapy in this case?*

Therapeutic Alternatives
3. a. *What non-drug therapies might be useful for this patient?*
   b. *What feasible pharmacotherapeutic alternatives are available for the treatment of HCM?*

Optimal Plan

4. *What drug, dosage form, dose, and schedule, and duration of therapy are the best for this patient?*

Outcome Evaluation

5. *What clinical and laboratory parameters are necessary to evaluate the therapy for achievement of the desired therapeutic outcome and to detect or prevent adverse effects?*

Patient Counseling

6. *What information should be provided to the patient to enhance compliance, ensure successful therapy, and minimize adverse effects?*

▶ Clinical Course

It has been 1 week since John's diagnosis, and he has responded well to his therapy with no complaints. His diary shows that his heart rate has been between 70 and 110 bpm this entire week with a normal blood pressure. Today his vital signs in the clinic are BP 120/85, HR 76, RR 16, T 37.2°C.

▶ Follow-up Question

1. *Are any adjustments in his medication dosage warranted at this time?*

▶ Clinical Pearl

In general, the earlier the onset of clinical findings in HCM, the worse the prognosis. In younger individuals the first manifestation may be sudden death; patients who live beyond the age of 35 usually have a better long-term prognosis.

▶ Self-study Assignments

1. When a patient with HCM arrives at your pharmacy or clinic, what questions would you ask to assess his or her therapy?
2. Perform a literature search and make a chart to ascertain the pharmacodynamic responses that a patient with HCM may have in relation to drug therapy.
3. Perform a literature search to ascertain when the initiation of anticoagulation should begin in the disease course of HCM.

References

1. Maron BJ, Roberts WC. Hypertrophic cardiomyopathy. In: Schlant RC, Alexander RW, eds. Hurst's The Heart, 8th ed. New York, McGraw-Hill, 1994:1621–1635.
2. Koga Y, Ogata M, Kihara K, et al. Sudden death in hypertrophic and dilated cardiomyopathy. Jpn Circ J 1989;53:1546–1556.
3. Maron BJ, Bonow RO, Cannon RO III, et al. Hypertrophic cardiomyopathy. Interrelations of clinical manifestations, pathophysiology, and therapy. N Engl J Med 1987;316:780–789, 844–852.
4. Martin AB, Garson A, Perry JC. Prolonged QT interval in hypertrophic and dilated cardiomyopathy in children. Am Heart J 1994;127:64–70.
5. Hopf R, Kaltenbach M. Management of hypertrophic cardiomyopathy. Annu Rev Med 1990;41:75–83.
6. Rosing DR, Idanpaan-Heikkila U, Maron BJ, et al. Use of calcium channel blocking drugs in hypertrophic cardiomyopathy. Am J Cardiol 1985;55:185B–195B.
7. Pollick C. Disopyramide in hypertrophic cardiomyopathy. II. Noninvasive assessment after oral administration. Am J Cardiol 1988;62:1252–1255.

10   DEEP VEIN THROMBOSIS

▶ From San Diego to Portland   (Level I)

Nannette A. Sageser, PharmD

▶ Upon completing this case study, students should be able to:

- Recognize the signs and symptoms of deep vein thrombosis (DVT) and any predisposing risk factors.
- Develop a therapeutic plan that includes the initiation of low-molecular-weight heparin (LMWH) and oral warfarin therapy in suitable patients.
- Titrate a patient's oral warfarin therapy based on daily INR values.
- Appropriately counsel patients receiving oral warfarin therapy.

☀ PATIENT PRESENTATION

Chief Complaint
"Since yesterday, I have had increased swelling and pain in my left lower leg that won't go away."

HPI
Alex Lelander is an 83 yo gentleman with a PMH significant for LLE DVT and a recent long car trip, traveling from San Diego to Portland. He is on vacation visiting his younger brother. He was in his usual state of good health when he noted that his left lower leg started aching, swelling, and feeling warm to the touch. He ignored this, thinking that it would eventually go away. Upon awakening this morning, the symptoms were still present. He asked his brother to drive him to the nearest emergency room. His previous DVT was 5 to 6 years ago, and he has a history of postphlebitic syndrome in the LLE.

PMH
Previous DVT × 1, diagnosed 6 years ago
Duke's B colon CA, s/p right hemicolectomy 7 years ago
BPH × 20 years
Hypothyroidism × 23 years

FH
Father died at age 62 from cancer; mother had high blood pressure and arthritis and died at age 95 from CVA. He has one brother age 70, alive and well.

SH

Patient quit tobacco 25 years ago; quit alcohol 10 years ago, but recently had some heavy drinking with his brother while visiting. His brother drinks heavily at night. Patient is retired and lives in San Diego. He has no wife or children.

ROS

(+) Non-productive cough over past week, (−) shortness of breath, chest pain, diaphoresis or hemoptysis; (+) nocturia and recent history of reduced frequency of urination; (−) polyuria, dysuria, or hematuria; (+) continued pain/pressure in left lower leg and swelling of calf about "double" the normal size, sock feels tight on left calf; (−) for swelling or pain in RLE

Meds

Levoxyl 75 μg po QD
Hytrin 2 mg po Q HS
Denies any herbal product or OTC drug use

All

NKDA; codeine causes nausea

PE

Gen

This is a well nourished, well appearing man in NAD.

VS

BP 105/66, P 67, RR 16, T 96.8°F, Wt 80 kg, O_2 sat 93% on RA

HEENT

PERRLA, EOMI, oropharynx is clear with no lesions, TMs are normal bilaterally

Neck/LN

Supple with full range of motion; no thyromegaly, carotid bruits, JVD, or lymphadenopathy

Chest

Lungs clear except for bibasilar rales that clear with inspiration, no wheezing

Cardiac

Regular rate with an occasional extra beat; no murmurs or S_3.

Abd

Soft, NT/ND, BS (+)

Rectal

Enlarged prostate with heme-negative brown stool

Ext

LLE with increased calf circumference (6 cm larger than right calf) with slight ankle swelling and non-pitting nature; (+) Homan's sign with a palpable cord

Neuro

Cranial nerves II to XII intact; 5/5 strength throughout; DTRs are symmetrical throughout with normal cerebellar exam.

Labs

Na 141 mEq/L	Hgb 14.2 g/dL	T. bili 0.4 mg/dL	PT 13.4 sec
K 4.1 mEq/L	Hct 42.0%	AST 18 IU/L	aPTT 28.8 sec
Cl 105 mEq/L	WBC $7.8 \times 10^3/mm^3$	LDH 452 IU/L	INR 1.36
CO_2 28 mEq/L	Plt $108 \times 10^3/mm^3$	Alk Phos 73 IU/L	TSH 4.34 μIU/mL
BUN 13 mg/dL	Ca 8.0 mg/dL	GGT 23 IU/L	
SCr 1.2 mg/dL	Phos 2.4 mg/dL	A/G ratio 0.9	
Glu 105 mg/dL			

ABG

pH 7.42, pco_2 40 mm Hg, po_2 89 mm Hg, bicarbonate 25 mEq/L, BE 1.2

UA

Straw colored, clear, SG 1.015, pH 7.5, glucose (−), bilirubin (−), ketones (−), blood (−), protein (−), nitrites (−)

Chest X-ray

Clear; normal lung fields; negative for infiltrates

ECG

NSR with occasional PVCs; intraventricular conduction delay in leads I, III, and V6 with no ischemic changes

VQ Scan

No apparent bilateral mismatched segmental defects; low probability for pulmonary embolus

Doppler Ultrasound

LLE ultrasound shows decreased venous flow in region of the left anterior tibial vein, with evidence of old phlebitis.

Assessment

LLE DVT of the left anterior tibial vein, no evidence of PE. Consults to Home Care and pharmacist-managed anticoagulation service for teaching, initiation, and management of heparin/warfarin therapy

---

▶ Questions

Problem Identification

1. a. Create a list of the patient's drug-related problems.
    b. What risk factors for DVT are present in this patient?
    c. What subjective and objective evidence is suggestive of a lower extremity DVT?

Desired Outcome

2. What are the immediate and long-term therapeutic goals for this patient?

Therapeutic Alternatives

3. a. *What are the therapeutic alternatives for the initial anticoagulation management of this patient?*

   b. *What alternatives are available if this patient were to have a history of heparin-induced thrombocytopenia (HIT)?*

▶ Clinical Course

The physician decided that this patient would be a good candidate for outpatient treatment of DVT. The patient is willing to come back each day for daily PT/INR monitoring, and his prescription benefit will cover the cost of the LMWH. The nurse from Home Care taught the patient how to self-administer the LMWH. He gave himself the first SQ injection prior to discharge from the ED. The anticoagulation clinic pharmacist educated the patient on warfarin therapy and scheduled the patient for daily PT/INRs at the pharmacist-managed anticoagulation clinic. The patient was then discharged to home with the following prescriptions: enoxaparin 80 mg (1 mg/kg) SQ Q 12 H (5-day minimum), and Coumadin 5 mg po QD or as directed by the anticoagulation pharmacist. The patient was instructed to start Coumadin 5 mg po that evening with the second dose of enoxaparin. Coumadin dosing (per pharmacist) and platelet counts over the next 6 days were as follows:

Day	INR	Coumadin Dose	Platelet Count
1	1.02	5 mg	$108 \times 10^3/mm^3$
2	1.26	5 mg	$113 \times 10^3/mm^3$
3	1.47	7.5 mg	
4	2.30	5 mg	$123 \times 10^3/mm^3$
5	2.95	2.5 mg	
6	2.56	2.5 mg	$160 \times 10^3/mm^3$

Enoxaparin was discontinued on day 6 of therapy. The patient was continued on the following Coumadin dose: 5 mg po on Monday, Wednesday, and Friday and 2.5 mg po on Tuesday, Thursday, Saturday, and Sunday. The patient had an appointment to see his PCP one week after starting this regimen. The physician ordered a PT/INR without notifying the anticoagulation clinic pharmacist. Protime came back subtherapeutic with an INR of 1.85. The PCP informed the patient of the level and instructed him to increase his dose of warfarin to 5 mg po QD. The patient was then rescheduled for repeat PT/INR in 4 weeks.

Optimal Plan

4. *Do you agree with the above plan made by the patient's PCP? If not, what would you recommend at this point in therapy?*

Outcome Evaluation

5. *What clinical and laboratory monitoring parameters should be assessed to ensure the efficacy and safety of chronic warfarin therapy in this patient?*

Patient Counseling

6. *What information should be provided to the patient to enhance compliance and minimize adverse effects of warfarin therapy?*

▶ Self-study Assignments

1. Develop a plan for using vitamin K to reverse the effect of warfarin if the patient should become overanticoagulated and experience a hemorrhagic event.

2. Set up a patient assistance program in your institution or clinic for patients who cannot afford the cost of enoxaparin or warfarin therapy.

3. Outline the pros and cons of patient self-testing with the Coagu-check protime monitor, and discuss the feasibility of implementing such a program.

▶ Clinical Pearl

Many patients can be started on 5 mg of warfarin when initiating therapy. The traditional 10-mg "loading dose" can lead to overshooting of the therapeutic range.

References

1. Hull RD, Raskob GE, Rosenbloom D, et al. Optimal therapeutic level of heparin therapy in patients with venous thrombosis. Arch Intern Med 1992;152:1589–1595.

2. Raschke RA, Reilly BM, Guidry JR, et al. The weight-based heparin dosing nomogram compared with a "standard care" nomogram: A randomized controlled trial. Ann Intern Med 1993;119:874–881.

3. Chaffee BJ. Low-molecular-weight heparins for treatment of deep vein thrombosis. Am J Health-Syst Pharm 1997;54:1995–1999.

4. Oertel LB. Managing maintenance therapy. In: Ansell JE, Oertel LB, Wittkowsky AK, eds. Managing Oral Anticoagulation Therapy: Clinical and Operational Guidelines. Gaithersburg, MD, Aspen, 1997:4B-3:1–3:4.

11   PULMONARY EMBOLISM

▶ The Clot Thickens   (Level I)

Amy L. Seybert, PharmD
Ted L. Rice, MS, BCPS

▶ After completing this case study, students should be able to:

- Identify signs and symptoms of pulmonary embolism.

- Recognize risk factors predisposing a patient to pulmonary embolism.

- Design an appropriate pharmacotherapy regimen for the treatment of pulmonary embolism.

- Recommend patient counseling for anticoagulation therapy.

☼ PATIENT PRESENTATION

Chief Complaint

"My chest hurts when I cough or take a deep breath."

HPI

Carol Pelungi is a 22 yo woman who presents to the ED following 12 days of illness. She states that approximately 2 weeks prior to admission she awoke with a sore throat, called her doctor, and received penicillin. The patient notes that in the morning of the second day of illness, she had acute onset of sharp, constant left-sided pleuritic chest pain and left-sided mid-back pain. The pain was made worse with laying flat, deep inspiration, and exercise. She became short of breath while talking. She also reports that pleuritic chest pain improves when seated. The patient has since had a mild cough productive of clear sputum tinged with bright red blood. Denies fever and chills. States the cough is worse in the morning and in the evening. Says she had been seen at an outside hospital and diagnosed with bronchitis and possible pericarditis. The penicillin was changed to ciprofloxacin and Percocet was added. She returned to the outside hospital as the pain persisted and prevented sleep. The ciprofloxacin dose was increased from 250 to 500 mg po BID. Review of records from the hospital, however, reveal no ECG evidence for pericarditis. Chest x-ray, which was performed 3 days prior to presentation here, was read as normal by the radiologist. The patient presents complaining of continued pleuritic pain and cough.

PMH

Ovarian cyst that was drained 4 years ago

PSH

Tonsillectomy 2 years ago

SH

Denies tobacco, alcohol, or other drug use. She is a single student, living alone, no pets, and is sexually active.

ROS

No headache, blurred vision. No auditory complaints. No abdominal pain. No lightheadedness. No extremity or neurologic complaints. All other systems are negative, except for complaints noted in HPI.

Meds

Lo/Ovral × 3 years
Ciprofloxacin 500 mg po BID
Percocet 1 to 2 tabs po Q 6 H PRN

All

Sulfa→rash

PE

Gen
Well-developed young woman appearing somewhat anxious

VS
BP 110/64, HR 110, RR 24; T 37.9°C; Wt 63 kg; Ht 5′4″. O_2 sat 99% on room air

HEENT
Atraumatic; PERRLA; sclerae anicteric; TMs clear; oropharynx moist and pink, without erythema or exudate

Neck
No JVD, no lymphadenopathy; trachea midline; no thyromegaly

CV
RRR; no m/r/g

Lungs
There is some reproducible tenderness in the left lower costal margin; scattered inspiratory rales that clear with cough

Abd
Soft, NT/ND; normoactive bowel sounds

Rect
Normal sphincter tone; heme-negative stool

Ext
Well perfused, no CCE; normal distal pulses; negative Homan's sign; LE are without palpable cords, tenderness, and warmth; patient has a port wine stain on LLE

Neuro
A & O × 3; nonfocal exam; CN II–XII intact; DTRs 2+, Babinski ↓

Labs

Na 139 mEq/L	Hgb 11.5 g/dL	aPTT 24 sec
K 4.2 mEq/L	Hct 33.9 %	PT 12.0 sec
Cl 103 mEq/L	Plt 284 × 10^3/mm^3	INR 0.9
CO_2 27 mEq/L	WBC 7.8 × 10^3/mm^3	
BUN 11 mg/dL		
SCr 0.7 mg/dL		

Chest X-ray

Small left pleural effusion with possible left basal consolidation

ECG

Sinus tachycardia at 110 bpm with a normal axis, normal intervals, and normal ST segments

Lower Extremity Venous Doppler Studies

Negative

Assessment

R/O PE vs. pneumonia

Plan

Initiate empiric treatment for both possible etiologies of the patient's complaints. Order VQ scan and possible angiogram.

▶ Questions

Problem Identification

1. a. *What risk factors for the development of a pulmonary embolus are present in this patient?*
   b. *What subjective and objective evidence is suggestive of a pulmonary embolus in this patient? (See Figure 11–1).*

Desired Outcome

2. *What are the goals of therapy for this patient?*

Therapeutic Alternatives

3. a. *What non-pharmacologic therapeutic alternatives are available for the acute treatment of pulmonary embolism?*

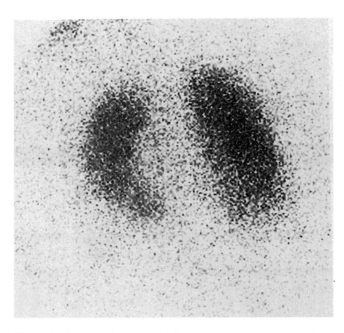

Figure 11–2. Xenon ventilation scan, posterior view. Asymmetry in ventilation due to elevation of diaphragm and decreased volume of the left hemithorax.

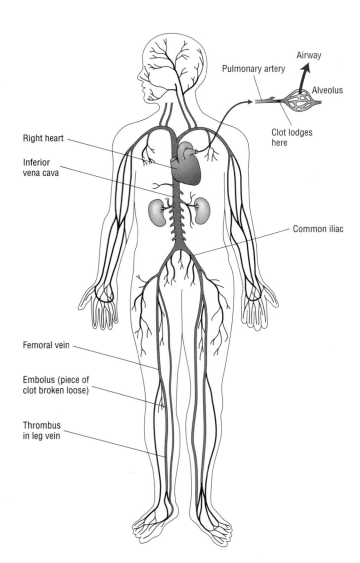

Figure 11–1. Development of pulmonary embolism. *(Reprinted with permission from Mulvihill ML,* Human Diseases: A Systemic Approach, *4th ed. Norwalk, CT, Appleton & Lange, 1995.)*

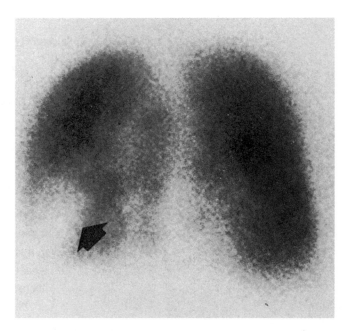

Figure 11–3. Perfusion lung scan, left posterior oblique view. Focal segmental perfusion defect at the left costophrenic angle, consistent with pulmonary embolism.

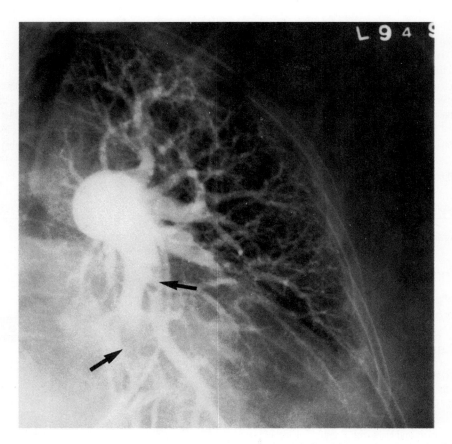

Figure 11–4. Anterior view of the left lung. Catheterization of the left pulmonary artery via the femoral vein and inferior vena cava. Emboli to basilar segments of the left lower lobe (arrows).

b. *What pharmacotherapeutic alternatives are available for the acute treatment of pulmonary embolism?*

Optimal Plan

4. a. *Design a pharmacotherapeutic plan for the empiric treatment of pulmonary embolism in this patient.*

▶ Clinical Course

In the ED, the patient was started on erythromycin for a possible pneumonia and the regimen that you recommended for empiric treatment of PE. She was then admitted for further work-up of possible PE.

V/Q scan report. Perfusion abnormality in the left base. There is a marked discrepancy between the perfusion defect and ventilation of the left lung, indicating an intermediate probability for pulmonary embolus (see Figures 11–2 and 11–3).

Pulmonary angiogram report. Consistent with pulmonary emboli in the left lower lobe pulmonary arteries (see Figure 11–4).

b. *Based on the new information, what additions or changes need to be made to the current therapy?*

Outcome Evaluation

5. a. *What monitoring parameters should be used to assess efficacy and toxicity of anticoagulation?*

▶ Clinical Course

The following table is a summary of heparin/warfarin dosing (by the physician) in this patient:

Day #	Heparin Dose	Warfarin Dose	aPTT	PT/INR
1	5000 units loading dose, then 1100 units/hr constant infusion	—	(6 hr after starting heparin infusion) 32 sec	12.1 sec/1.0
2	1500 units/hr constant infusion, then rate decreased to 1400 units/hr constant infusion	5 mg	(6 hr after change to 1500 units/hr) 90 sec (6 hr after change to 1400 units/hr) 76 sec	Not done Not done
3	1300 units/hr constant infusion	5 mg	(with A.M. labs) 70 sec	14.4 sec/1.2
4	1300 units/hr constant infusion	5 mg	(with A.M. labs) 68 sec	19.0 sec/1.7
5	Discontinued	5 mg	32 sec	23.2 sec/2.2

b. *What is your assessment of the appropriateness of these inter-ventions?*

Patient Counseling

6. *What medication counseling about warfarin should this patient receive at the time of hospital discharge?*

▶ **Self-study Assignments**

1. Perform a literature search to obtain information about various treatment strategies for IV heparin administration, and prepare written recommendations for the safest and most effective method of administration.
2. Review recent clinical trials and assess the potential benefits of low-molecular-weight heparin in the treatment of pulmonary embolism.
3. Prepare a written document summarizing the primary literature on the use of thrombolytics in the treatment of pulmonary embolism.
4. Describe the alternative methods of birth control that could be used by this patient and provide patient counseling on these methods.

▶ **Clinical Pearl**

Weight-based heparin dosing results in more rapid achievement of therapeutic aPTT than standard dosing and results in fewer recurrent episodes of venous thromboembolism.

References

1. Price H. Deaths from venous thromboembolism associated with combined oral contraceptives. Lancet 1997;350:450.
2. Rosing J, Tans G, Nicolaes GA, et al. Oral contraceptives and venous thrombosis: Different sensitivities to activated protein C in women using second- and third-generation oral contraceptives. Br J Haematol 1997;97:233–238.
3. Goldhaber SZ, Grodstein F, Stampfer MJ, et al. A prospective study of risk factors for pulmonary embolism in women. JAMA 1997;277:642–645.
4. Raschke RA, Reilly BM, Guidry JR, et al. The weight-based heparin dosing nomogram compared with a "standard care" nomogram. A randomized controlled trial. Ann Intern Med 1993;119:874–881.
5. Simonneau G, Sors H, Charbonnier B, et al. A comparison of low-molecular-weight heparin with unfractionated heparin for acute pulmonary embolism. N Engl J Med 1997;337:663–669.
6. Goldhaber SZ. Contemporary pulmonary embolism thrombolysis. Chest 1995; 107(1 suppl):45S–51S.
7. Hylek EM, Heiman H, Skates SJ, et al. Acetaminophen and other risk factors for excessive warfarin anticoagulation. JAMA 1998;279:657–662.

12   CHRONIC ANTICOAGULATION

▶ **A Delicate Balance**   (Level II)

Beth Bryles Phillips, PharmD

▶ After completing this case study, students should be able to:

- List the goals of oral anticoagulant therapy in preventing recurrent thromboembolism.
- Recognize common drug–drug interactions associated with warfarin therapy.
- Assess patients on chronic warfarin therapy.
- Appropriately educate patients about chronic warfarin therapy.

☼ PATIENT PRESENTATION

Chief Complaint
"I'm here to get my blood drawn."

HPI
Keith Waters is a 59 yo man with a history of recurrent DVT × 3, PE × 1, and GERD who presents to the clinic for follow-up of his chronic anticoagulant therapy. The most recent DVT and PE occurred 2 years ago, at which time he was started on warfarin therapy. He uses a pillbox to organize his warfarin therapy and states that he has not missed any doses in the last month. He reports having a nosebleed 3 days ago which is quite unusual for him. It lasted for about 5 minutes and has not recurred. He does not drink alcohol of any kind and he tries to avoid foods containing vitamin K. When asked if he had started any new medications, he reports that he recently started taking vitamin E about 4 weeks ago because his wife read that it prevents heart attacks. He also reports taking a few doses of pseudoephedrine 30 mg last week for a cold but is no longer taking this medication. Except for the recent cold, he denies being ill in the past month. His weight has also

been stable over the past 3 months. His use of OTC antacids has increased over the last 3 weeks due to increasing heartburn. He reports that his symptoms are not adequately controlled because he works during the day and is not able to use the antacids often enough. He states the heartburn has worsened despite wearing loose-fitting clothing, elevating the head of his bed, eating several small meals instead of three large meals, and avoiding chocolate, spicy, fatty, and caffeine-containing foods.

PMH

DVT × 3 (2, 8, and 12 years ago)
PE × 1 (2 years ago)
GERD
S/P LLE cellulitis (2 years ago)
Obesity

FH

Mother died at age 75 due to CVA; father alive and well

SH

(−) EtOH—patient has not had any alcohol since starting chronic warfarin therapy
(+) Smoking, 1 ppd

ROS

(+) For epistaxis and LE edema
(−) For CP, SOB, leg pain, bruises, or change in color of stool or urine

Meds

Warfarin 5 mg po QD
Vitamin E 1000 IU po QD
Mylanta II PRN
Pepcid AC 10 mg po PRN

All

NKDA

PE

Gen

Pleasant, obese man in NAD

VS

BP 119/74, HR 59, RR 12, T 35.7°C; Wt 119.2 kg, Ht 73″

Skin

Normal turgor and color; warm; no rashes

HEENT

PERRLA, EOMI; disks flat; fundi with no hemorrhages or exudates

Neck/LN

No lymphadenopathy, thyromegaly, or carotid bruits

Lungs

CTA bilaterally

CV

RRR; normal S_1 and S_2; no S_3 or S_4; no m/r/g

Abd

Obese, non-tender, (+) BS

Genit/Rect

Deferred

Ext

1+ edema in right LE; no clubbing or cyanosis

Neuro

A & O × 3; CN II–XII intact; DTR 2+; Babinski negative

Labs

Date	PT/INR	Warfarin Dose
Today	39/3.5	5 mg QD
1 mo ago	31/2.7	5 mg QD
2 mo ago	28/2.5	5 mg QD
3 mo ago	28/2.5	5 mg QD
4 mo ago	16/2.1	5 mg QD
5 mo ago	18/2.4	5 mg QD
6 mo ago	28/2.5	5 mg QD

Assessment

Recurrent thromboembolism (TBE) requiring chronic anticoagulation with a target INR of 2.0 to 3.0
GERD
Postphlebitic syndrome

▶ Questions

Problem Identification

1. a. Identify this patient's drug-related problems.
   b. Do any signs or symptoms indicate that this patient is over-anticoagulated?
   c. What questions would you ask this patient to assess his current warfarin therapy?

Desired Outcome

2. What are the goals of oral anticoagulant therapy in this patient?

Therapeutic Alternatives

3. a. What medications other than warfarin could be used to prevent recurrent thromboembolism in this patient?
   b. Because the patient is experiencing symptoms of GERD, the physician would like to prescribe a medication to relieve his symptoms. He would like to initiate therapy with an H_2-receptor antagonist (H2RA), but he thinks there are drug interactions with these agents and warfarin. Instead, he is consider-

ing a proton pump inhibitor (PPI) because his under- stand-
ing is that these agents do not interact with warfarin. He asks
you if this is correct and if you could recommend an appro-
priate agent. What would you recommend?

Optimal Plan

4. *Based on today's laboratory result, what is your recommenda-*
   tion for this patient's warfarin therapy?

Outcome Evaluation

5. *How will you monitor this patient's warfarin therapy?*

Patient Counseling

6. *What information should this patient know about his warfarin*
   therapy?

► Clinical Course

Upon return to clinic 2 weeks later, the patient reports that he has stopped taking the vitamin E and he is still taking warfarin 5 mg once daily. His PT and INR are 27 sec and 2.3. He has had no medication changes since the last visit. He has not taken any OTC medications and there have been no significant changes in his diet. He denies signs or symptoms of bleeding and states that he has not missed any of his warfarin doses.

► Follow-up Question

1. *Based on this information, what are your recommendations for*
   his warfarin therapy?

► Self-study Assignments

1. There are several mechanisms by which drugs may interact with warfarin. What are the major mechanisms of these interactions? Give examples of drugs that interact by each mechanism.
2. Antibiotics are a common cause of drug–drug interactions with warfarin. Which antibiotics are likely to interact with warfarin? Which antibiotics are reasonable alternatives to these drugs?

► Clinical Pearl

When assessing warfarin therapy, it is important not only to ask about any changes in prescription medications but OTC and any alternative therapies a patient may be taking as well.

References

1. Hirsh J, Dalen JE, Deykin D, et al. Oral anticoagulants: Mechanism of action, clinical effectiveness, and optimal therapeutic range. Chest 1995;108(4 suppl): 231S–246S.
2. Unge P, Svedberg E, Nordgren A, et al. A study of the interaction of omeprazole and warfarin in anticoagulated patients. Br J Clin Pharmacol 1992;34;509–512.
3. Gibaldi M. Stereoselective and isozyme-selective drug interactions. Chirality 1993;5:407–413.
4. Corrigan JJ, Ulfers LL. Effect of vitamin E on prothrombin levels in warfarin-induced vitamin K deficiency. Am J Clin Nutr 1981;34:1701–1705.
5. Schrogie JJ. Coagulopathy and fat-soluble vitamins. JAMA 1975;232:19.
6. Corrigan JJ. The effect of vitamin E on warfarin-induced vitamin K deficiency. Ann NY Acad Sci 1982;393:361–368.
7. Kim JM, White RH. Effect of vitamin E on the anticoagulant response to warfarin. Am J Cardiol 1996;77:545–546.

13 ISCHEMIC STROKE

► Brain Attack   (Level II)

Susan R. Winkler, PharmD, BCPS
Mark S. Luer, PharmD

► After completing this case study, students should be able to:

- Identify and provide patient education on the risk factors for ischemic stroke.
- Discuss the various treatment options available for acute ischemic stroke.
- Develop an appropriate patient-specific therapeutic plan for the acute treatment of ischemic stroke.
- Develop an appropriate therapeutic plan for the outpatient management of a patient with ischemic stroke.

☼ PATIENT PRESENTATION

Chief Complaint
"I can't move my right arm and leg."

HPI
John Gaines is a 67 yo man who was brought into the ED complaining of weakness in the right arm and leg and slurred speech. He stated that he awoke at 5:00 A.M. and went into the kitchen for a snack. He then went back to bed but awoke at 6:30 A.M. unable to move his right arm and leg, causing him to fall from bed. His daughter heard the "thump" and found him on the floor somewhat confused. She immediately called the paramedics. Approximately 2 weeks prior, he had an episode of right arm weakness that lasted approximately 2 minutes.

PMH
Hypercholesterolemia
HTN
Seizure disorder (generalized tonic-clonic seizures of unknown etiology); last seizure 2 years ago

FH
Non-contributory

SH
Smokes 1 ppd × 47 years; h/o alcohol abuse

ROS

Slight headache, c/o double vision and slurred speech, no CP or SOB

Meds

Phenytoin 300 mg po Q HS

Lovastatin 60 mg po Q HS

All

NKDA

PE

Gen

WDWN right-handed, thin, African-American man; appears slightly anxious

VS

BP 174/94, P 101, RR 22, T 37.2°C; Wt 64 kg, Ht 5′ 10″

Skin

Warm, dry

HEENT

PERRLA; no nystagmus; (+) diplopia; funduscopic exam reveals (+) arteriolar narrowing; no exudates, hemorrhages, or papilledema

Neck/LN

No carotid bruits; no lymphadenopathy; normal thyroid

Chest

Lungs clear

CV

RRR; S_1, S_2 normal, no S_3, (+) S_4

Abd

NT/ND; no HSM

Genit/Rect

Deferred

MS/Ext

Good pulses throughout; no CCE

Neuro

A & O × 2, not oriented to time; (+) dysarthria; CN II–XII intact

Motor: RUE: 3/5 LUE: 5/5

RLE: 3/5 LLE: 5/5

Sensory: Normal pin-prick and light touch

DTRs: 2+ throughout; Babinski normal

Labs

Na 143 mEq/L	Hgb 17.6 g/dL	Chol 333 mg/dL
K 4.2 mEq/L	Hct 51.5%	Phenytoin 18.6 mg/L
Cl 101 mEq/L	Plt $240 \times 10^3/mm^3$	
CO_2 21 mEq/L	WBC $6.7 \times 10^3/mm^3$	
BUN 23 mg/dL	PTT 22.0 sec	
SCr 1.2 mg/dL	PT 11.4 sec	
Glu 105 mg/dL		

ECG

Normal rhythm; tachycardia with a rate of 101 bpm

Brain CT Scan

Normal; no evidence of hemorrhage

Carotid Ultrasound

Normal flow

Assessment

Acute ischemic stroke in the left hemisphere in a 67 yo man with HTN, hypercholesterolemia, and seizure disorder

▶ Questions

Problem Identification

1. a. Create a list of the patient's drug-related problems.
   b. What risk factors for acute ischemic stroke are present in this patient?
   c. What signs and symptoms indicate the presence of an acute ischemic stroke?

Desired Outcome

2. What are the initial and long-term goals of pharmacotherapy in this case?

Therapeutic Alternatives

3. a. What non-drug therapies might be useful for this patient?
   b. What feasible pharmacotherapeutic alternatives are available for the treatment of acute ischemic stroke?

Optimal Plan

4. What initial therapy would you recommend for this patient?

Outcome Evaluation

5. What clinical and laboratory parameters are necessary to evaluate the chosen therapy for achievement of the desired effect and to detect or prevent adverse effects?

▶ Clinical Course

The patient is now 5 days post-stroke and is ready for discharge from the hospital.

Patient Counseling

6. What information should be provided to the patient about the secondary preventive therapy you recommended?

▶ Follow-up Questions

1. *What non-drug therapies might be useful for preventing recurrent stroke in this patient?*
2. *What feasible pharmacotherapeutic alternatives are available for the secondary prevention of acute ischemic stroke?*
3. *What drug, dosage form, dose, schedule, and duration of therapy would you recommend for the secondary prevention of acute ischemic stroke in this patient?*
4. *How should the therapy you recommended be monitored?*
5. *In addition to the management of the ischemic stroke, what other therapeutic interventions should be undertaken for this patient?*

▶ Self-study Assignments

1. Perform a literature search and evaluate the role of ticlopidine and clopidogrel in the secondary prevention of ischemic stroke.
2. Review the trials involving thrombolytics for acute stroke treatment. Pay particular attention to the inclusion and exclusion criteria used in each of the trials. Write a one-page paper summarizing your conclusions about the safety and efficacy of these agents for treatment of acute ischemic stroke.

References

1. Camarata PJ, Heros RC, Latchaw RE. "Brain attack": The rationale for treating stroke as a medical emergency. Neurosurgery 1994;34:144–158.
2. National Institute of Neurological Disorders and Stroke rt-PA Stroke Study Group. Tissue plasminogen activator for acute ischemic stroke. N Engl J Med 1995;333:1581–1587.
3. Chimowitz WI, Kokinos J, Strong J, et al. The warfarin–aspirin symptomatic intracranial disease study. Neurology 1995;45:1488–1493.
4. CAPRIE Steering Committee. A randomised, blinded, trial of clopidogrel versus aspirin in patients at risk of ischaemic events (CAPRIE). Lancet 1996;348: 1329–1339.

14   HYPERLIPIDEMIA: PRIMARY PREVENTION

▶ What, Me Worry?   (Level I)

Laura A. Bartels, PharmD

▶ After completing this case study, students should be able to:

- Determine goal LDL, HDL, and total cholesterol concentrations for the primary prevention of coronary heart disease (CHD) in hyperlipidemia patients.
- Identify hyperlipidemia patients who are candidates for therapeutic interventions.
- Recommend appropriate pharmacotherapy for primary prevention of CHD in patients with hyperlipidemia.
- Design monitoring parameters to achieve the desired therapeutic outcomes while minimizing adverse effects.
- Counsel patients on the dosing, administration, adverse effects, need for compliance, and goals of their pharmacotherapy.

☀ PATIENT PRESENTATION

Chief Complaint

"I'm here for my appointment with the doctor because I was told that my cholesterol was high at my last visit."

HPI

Alfred Newman is a 55 yo man who was noted to have a total cholesterol of 275 mg/dL by finger-stick analysis at his community pharmacy screening program 2 months ago. One month later he gave the results to his doctor during a routine visit for follow-up of his hypertension. His fasting lipoprotein levels at the time of this visit revealed the following: total cholesterol 268 mg/dL, triglycerides 150 mg/dL, HDL-cholesterol 30 mg/dL, and LDL-cholesterol 208 mg/dL. At this time, his physician advised him to see a dietitian and to return for another fasting lipid profile in one month. Alfred has been advised several times in the past 10 years to see a dietitian and to take better care of himself by eating right and entering a smoking cessation program and exercise program. Alfred went the first time to the dietitian but failed to comply with the other programs. Alfred mentions to the doctor that he will try harder in the next month to comply but he states he doesn't have a strong "will-power" to do so. One month later, the results of his profile show the following: total cholesterol 260 mg/dL, triglycerides 148 mg/dL, HDL-C 32 mg/dL, and LDL-C 198 mg/dL. Alfred tells his doctor that he needed to cheat on his diet a little and that he couldn't make it to the smoking cessation and exercise programs.

PMH

HTN for the past 10 years
PUD 1 year ago

FH

Father died of an MI at age 54; mother, age 82, is alive with type 2 DM. An older brother died 2 years ago of an MI at age 55. He has one younger brother age 48 with HTN and hyperlipidemia and a sister age 42 with depression and no knowledge of her cholesterol levels.

SH

Drinks 2 or 3 vodka martinis every day after work and smokes a pack of cigarettes every day.

ROS

(+) For occasional headache in the morning; no chest pain, SOB, abdominal pain, melena, or recent changes in bowel or bladder habits

Meds

Procardia XL 90 mg po Q AM
Zestril 10 mg po Q AM
HCTZ 25 mg po Q AM
Occasional Tylenol use PRN
MVI one tablet po QD

All

NKDA

PE

Gen

Patient is an obese man who wears glasses. He is in no acute distress.

VS

BP 140/95, P 76, RR 13, T 37.2°C; Ht 5'7", Wt 128 kg

Skin

Warm and dry, normal turgor, no lesions/tumors/moles

HEENT

PERRLA; EOMI; funduscopic exam reveals mild arteriolar narrowing, with AV ratio 1:3; no hemorrhages, exudates, or papilledema (Keith-Wagener-Barker funduscopic class: grade II); TMs intact; oral mucosa clear

Neck/LN

Neck supple with no lymphadenopathy. Normal thyroid

Lungs/Thorax

Diffuse wheezing bilaterally

CV

RRR, no murmurs, normal S_1 and S_2; no S_3 or S_4

Abd

(+) BS, liver and spleen not palpable

Genit/Rect

Guaiac (−), normal prostate

Ext

2+ pedal edema, pulses 2+ throughout

Neuro

A & O × 3; reflexes bilaterally equal; memory intact; coordination and gait normal; CN II to XII intact

Labs (fasting)

Na 142 mEq/L	AST 36 IU/L
K 4.6 mEq/L	ALT 31 IU/L
Cl 109 mEq/L	Alk Phos 105 IU/L
CO_2 26 mEq/L	T. Bili 1.0 mg/dL
BUN 20 mg/dL	TSH 3.2 μIU/mL
SCr 1.2 mg/dL	
Glu 95 mg/dL	

UA

SG 1.017; no protein, glucose, or ketones

Assessment

Patient is a 55 yo man with high LDL-C and multiple other risk factors for CHD.

▶ Questions

Problem Identification

1. a. Create a drug-related problem list for this patient.
   b. What signs, symptoms, and laboratory values indicate the presence and severity of hyperlipidemia in this patient?
   c. In addition to an elevated LDL-cholesterol, what other risk factors does this patient have for the development of coronary heart disease (CHD)?
   d. What additional information is needed to satisfactorily assess this patient?

Desired Outcome

2. What is the desired therapeutic outcome for this patient?

Therapeutic Alternatives

3. a. What non-drug therapies might be useful in the initial management of this individual?
   b. What feasible pharmacologic alternatives are available?

Optimal Plan

4. What drug, dosage form, dose, schedule, and duration of therapy are the best for this patient?

Outcome Evaluation

5. What clinical and laboratory parameters are necessary to evaluate the therapy for achievement of the desired therapeutic outcome and to detect or prevent adverse effects?

Patient Counseling

6. What information should be provided to the patient to enhance compliance, ensure successful therapy, and minimize adverse effects?

▶ Clinical Course

The dietician instituted a Step I diet low in saturated fat, total fat, and cholesterol. The patient was requested to decrease his alcohol intake to one ounce of alcohol per day during this time. Subsequent compliance with diet was determined to be acceptable by a diary after 6 months of follow-up, and the patient also lost 15 pounds. He reported no adverse effects from the medication you recommended. Pharmacy refill records demonstrated good compliance with medication regimen. Liver function tests obtained at 6 and 12 weeks revealed AST and ALT values within the normal range (<40 IU/L). A fasting lipid profile 6 months after these interventions were initiated revealed the following values:

Lipid Fraction	Value (mg/dL)
Total Cholesterol	200
Triglycerides	95
HDL-Cholesterol	40
LDL-Cholesterol	141

▶ Follow-up Question

1. *What is your assessment of the effectiveness of the interventions? Is any other type of pharmacologic intervention required at this time?*

▶ Clinical Pearl

In patients with hyperlipidemia who are at high risk for the development of CHD, lowering LDL-cholesterol level reduces CHD events and CHD mortality; dietary modification and pharmacotherapy should be implemented in all high-risk patients.

▶ Self-study Assignments

1. Perform a literature search and provide a written summary of recent research demonstrating the benefit of primary prevention with drug therapy in high-risk patients.
2. Describe how home cholesterol testing would be helpful in monitoring a patient's compliance with diet and pharmacotherapy.
3. Explain in your own words how to use a home cholesterol testing kit to a patient (see Figure 14–1).

References

1. Pollare T, Lithell H, Berne C. A comparison of the effects of hydrochlorothiazide and captopril on glucose and lipid metabolism in patients with hypertension. N Engl J Med 1989;321:868–873.
2. National Cholesterol Education Program. Second report of the expert panel on detection, evaluation, and treatment of high blood cholesterol in adults (adult treatment panel II). Circulation 1994;89:1333–1445.
3. Pazzucconi F, Mannucci L, Mussoni L, et al. Bezafibrate lowers plasma lipids, fibrinogen and platelet aggregability in hypertriglyceridemia. Eur J Clin Pharmacol 1992;43:219–223.

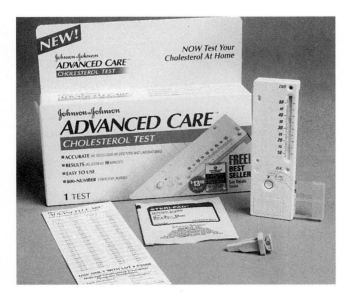

Figure 14–1. Non-prescription device for home testing of blood cholesterol levels.

4. Holme I. Cholesterol reduction and its impact on coronary artery disease and total mortality. Am J Cardiol 1995;76:10C–17C.
5. Lennernas H, Fager G. Pharmacodynamics and pharmacokinetics of the HMG-CoA reductase inhibitors. Similarities and differences. Clin Pharmacokinet 1997;32:403–425.
6. Dart A, Jerums G, Nicholson G, et al. A multicenter, double-blind, one-year study comparing safety and efficacy of atorvastatin versus simvastatin in patients with hypercholesterolemia. Am J Cardiol 1997; 80:39–44.

15 HYPERLIPIDEMIA: SECONDARY PREVENTION

▶ The Mushroom Hunter   (Level I)

Kjel A. Johnson, PharmD, BCPS

▶ After completing this case study, students should be able to:

- Provide goal lipid levels for secondary prevention of cardiovascular events in patients with CAD.
- Choose appropriate antihyperlipidemic agents and initial doses for patients with CAD.
- Titrate drug doses based upon fasting lipid profiles to achieve appropriate goals.

☀ PATIENT PRESENTATION

Chief Complaint
"My back and hip hurts."

HPI
Paul Brown is a 53 yo man with chronic stable angina who was referred to the Pharmacy Coronary Artery Disease Clinic because of difficulty in controlling his dyslipidemia. He presents for his first visit this morning with complaints of back and hip pain. He admits to falling onto his left side 2 days ago while looking for wild mushrooms in the woods. Nevertheless, he is concerned that this pain may be an atypical manifestation of his cardiac pain. His dyslipidemia was discovered at a follow-up visit several months after he had an MI 11 years ago. A review of his past medical history shows a baseline LDL in the range of 160 mg/dL before the institution of gemfibrozil 5 years ago.

PMH
S/P MI 11 years ago that was treated with cardiac catheterization and PTCA
Chronic stable angina for the past 10 years, currently graded as Canadian CV Class I
Dyslipidemia × 11 years
Ulcerative colitis × 7 years
HTN × 25 years
Adenomatous colonic polyps

FH

Mother alive, with HTN and PVD at age 75; father died at 62 of "heart disease." The patient is an only child.

SH

Smoked cigarettes 1 ppd × 30 years, quit 10 years ago after MI. Denies regular use of alcohol but admits to several drinks a week. Admits to lack of exercise and a sedentary life-style. He works at an electronics store as a manager and lives at home with his wife and stepchild. He reports eating out several times a week with his wife.

ROS

No complaints of recent chest pain, diarrhea, or blood in his stool

Meds

Gemfibrozil 600 mg po BID
Vitamin E 400 IU po BID
Quinapril 20 mg po QD
Nitroglycerin 0.4 mg SL PRN
ASA 325 mg po QD
Sulfasalazine 500 mg po, 2 Q AM, 1 Q PM

All

NKDA

PE

Gen

Patient is in mild pain and is holding his lower left side; appears older than stated age.

VS

BP 130/88, P 58, RR 18, Wt 85 kg, Ht 5'8"

Skin

Dry, but with normal turgor

HEENT

Funduscopic exam reveals no hemorrhages or arterial narrowing

Neck/LN

Neck supple, without lymphadenopathy or thyromegaly

Lungs/Thorax

Clear; no CVAT or spinal tenderness; does have pain and tenderness on left side that waxes and wanes upon breathing or movement of the left arm

CV

NSR; normal S_1, S_2; no S_3 or S_4

Abd

(+) BS, somewhat hyperactive

Genit/Rect

Guaiac (−), normal prostate

Other Systems

Not evaluated at this time

Labs

12-hour fasting lipid levels measured by portable lipid analyzer (see Figure 15–1)

T. chol 229 mg/dL	SCr 1.2 mg/dL
TG 341 mg/dL	K 3.6 mEq/L
HDL-C 21 mg/dL	Glu 110 mg/dL
LDL-C 140 mg/dL	AST 25 IU/L
	ALT 22 IU/L

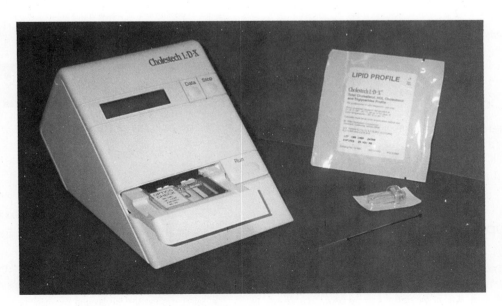

Figure 15–1. The Cholestech LDX lipid profile monitor.

UA
Negative for WBC and RBC; specific gravity 1.025

ECG
Evidence of old anterior-lateral MI (small Q waves in V2 and V3). No ST segment changes evident at this time

---

► Questions

Problem Identification

1. a. *Create a list of the patient's drug-related problems.*
   b. *What signs, symptoms, or laboratory tests indicate presence or severity of this individual's hyperlipidemia?*
   c. *What additional information is needed to satisfactorily assess this patient's dyslipidemia?*

Desired Outcome

2. *What is the desired therapeutic outcome for this patient?*

Therapeutic Alternatives

3. a. *What non-drug therapies may be used in the management of this patient's dyslipidemia?*
   b. *What feasible pharmacologic alternatives are available for the treatment of this individual's dyslipidemia?*

Optimal Plan

4. *What drug doses, schedules, and duration of therapy are best suited for management of this patient's dyslipidemia?*

Outcome Evaluation

5. *What parameters should be assessed to determine the effectiveness and adverse effects of the therapy you recommended?*

Patient Counseling

6. *What information should be provided to the patient about his new therapy?*

► Clinical Course

The patient is initiated on the therapy you recommended and returns to the clinic in 6 weeks for a fasting lipid panel. The results are as follows: total cholesterol 199 mg/dL, HDL-C 25 mg/dL, LDL-C 118 mg/dL, and TG 280 mg/dL. AST is 32 IU/L and ALT is 28 IU/L.

► Follow-up Questions

1. *Based on this new information, what interventions, if any, should be made at this time?*
2. *If the patient's goal lipid levels cannot ultimately be obtained with the maximum dose of the initial agent chosen, what therapeutic options are available?*

► Self-study Assignments

1. Are elevations in triglycerides associated with adverse outcomes? What data support or refute these associations?
2. Perform a literature search for recent information on the effect of reductase inhibitors in reducing the risk of stroke.

► Clinical Pearl

Each doubling of the dose of any reductase inhibitor beyond the initial starting dose reduces LDL by an additional 6 mg/dL from that starting dose. Therefore, estimated starting doses can be calculated based upon the patient's required LDL reduction.

References

1. National Cholesterol Educational Program. Second report of the expert panel on detection, evaluation, and treatment of high blood cholesterol in adults (adult treatment panel II). Circulation 1994;89:1333–1445.
2. Scandinavian Simvastatin Survival Study Group. Randomised trial of cholesterol lowering in 4444 patients with coronary heart disease: The Scandinavian Simvastatin Survival Study (4S). Lancet 1994;344:1383–1389.
3. Sacks FM, Pfeffer MA, Moye LA, et al. The effect of pravastatin on coronary events after myocardial infarction in patients with average cholesterol levels. Cholesterol and Recurrent Events Trial investigators. N Engl J Med 1996;335:1001–1009.
4. Tonkin A, et al. Long-term intervention with pravastatin in ischemic disease (LIPID Study). American Heart Association Meeting, November 1997, Orlando.
5. Jones P, Kafonek S, Laurora I, et al. Comparative dose efficacy study of atorvastatin versus simvastatin, pravastatin, lovastatin, and fluvastatin in patients with hypercholesterolemia (the CURVES study). Am J Cardiol 1998;81:582–587.

16   PERIPHERAL VASCULAR DISEASE

► The Colors of the Flag   (Level II)

Susan D. Bear, BS, PharmD

► Upon completing this case study, the student should be able to:

- Describe the pathophysiology of Raynaud's phenomenon.
- Identify subjective and objective findings consistent with the diagnosis of Raynaud's phenomenon.
- Recommend appropriate nonpharmacologic strategies to minimize the frequency and severity of Raynaud's exacerbations.
- Select a pharmacotherapeutic regimen for the treatment of Raynaud's phenomenon.

☀ PATIENT PRESENTATION

Chief Complaint

"I'm vomiting and I can't keep anything down. My joints hurt and I ache all over."

HPI

Jane Alexander is a 67 yo woman admitted with a 6-month history of weight loss, anorexia, fatigue, weakness, decreased appetite, intermittent diarrhea, GERD, and painful aching joints and fingers.

PMH

NIDDM × 4 years controlled by diet alone
Hypothyroidism
Chronic arthritis associated with systemic sclerosis
Hypercholesterolemia
HTN
S/P lumpectomy in 1988 for breast CA

FH

Mother died at age 98 from metastatic melanoma and father died at age 62 from an intracranial hemorrhage. Two sisters, both living, are hypothyroid. One brother who suffered from diabetes and PUD is deceased; another brother is living with heart disease.

SH

Widowed with one child; smoked 2 ppd × 52 years, (−) tobacco × 2 years; (−) alcohol

ROS

Positive for dry eyes, dry mouth, arthralgias of neck and hands, painful and swollen knees, headaches, reflux symptoms, diarrhea, vomiting, and fatigue. She notes numbness and pallor followed by cyanosis of fingers when exposed to cold and rubor and painful burning upon re-warming.

Meds

Synthroid 0.1 mg po QD
Zocor 5 mg po QD
Inderal LA 60 mg po QD
HCTZ 50 mg po QD
Advil 200 mg po PRN (patient states 12 to 14 tablets per day in the last 10 to 14 days)

All

NKDA

PE

Gen

Awake, alert, tired-appearing female in NAD

VS

BP 130/74, HR 78, RR 18, T 98.7°F; Wt 57 kg, Ht 65″

Skin

Facial skin with diffuse tightening and absence of wrinkles, contracted oral orifice, smooth and shiny hidebound skin on fingers proximal to the MCP joint accompanied by decreased ROM, areas of ulceration on fingertips

HEENT

Dry mucous membranes; (−) JVD

Neck/LN

Neck painful to full ROM

Lungs/Thorax

CTA

Breasts

Atrophic; (−) lumps or masses; lumpectomy scar evident

CV

RRR with II/VI systolic murmur at the apex; (−) S_3, S_4 appreciated; carotids bilaterally palpable; (−) carotid bruit auscultated

Abd

Mild distention and epigastric tenderness; (+) bowel sounds

Genit/Rect

Hemoccult (+) × 3

Ext

(−) Rash, (+) limited ROM right shoulder, (+) swollen knees bilaterally

Neuro

Eye movements normal, facial muscle strength normal with normal facial symmetry, facial skin is taut, jaw opening and closing strength are normal, visual fields are full to confrontation. Skin on fingertips is quite taut and flexion is difficult; grip strength is adequate and finger abduction is fairly strong. Patient is able to ambulate slowly, but must use hands to push off to stand from a seated position

Labs

Na 140 mEq/L	Hgb 9.2 g/dL	WBC 12.5 × 10³/mm³	CK 1530 IU/L	TSH 4.8 μIU/mL
K 4.1 mEq/L	Hct 29.1%	Neutros 84%	CK-MB 76 IU/L	Free T_4 0.7 ng/dL
Cl 100 mEq/L	RBC 3.33 × 10⁶/mm³	Lymphs 9%	%MB 5%	B_{12} 144 pg/mL
CO_2 26 mEq/L	Plt 585 × 10³/mm³	Monos 7%	LDH 659 IU/L	Folate 2.5 ng/mL
BUN 55 mg/dL	MCV 87 μm³	Eos 0%	Alb 2.8 g/dL	ESR 92 mm/hr
SCr 1.5 mg/dL	MCH 27.7 pg	Basos 0%	T. chol 150 mg/dL	RA 30 IU
Glu 139 mg/dL	MCHC 31.8 g/dL		Trig 140 mg/dL	ANA (+) speckled
Ca 9.6 mg/dL				fluorescence
Mg 1.8 mg/dL				
Phos 4.6 mg/dL				

HOSPITAL DAY 2 DIAGNOSTIC INFORMATION:

24-hour Urine Collection
SCr 1.4 mg/dL, urine creatinine 45 mg/dL, total volume 1325 mL, CLcr 30 mL/min.

Other Tests
Urinalysis, urine cultures, and stool cultures were negative.

Chest X-ray
WNL

ECG
Sinus rhythm

Endoscopy
GE reflux with stricture, erosive esophagitis, diffuse gastritis, loss of mucosal folds, esophageal hypomotility

Colonoscopy
Diverticula noted in sigmoid and rectum; (−) internal hemorrhoids or polyps

EMG
Nerve conduction consistent with an active inflammatory process

Assessment
Systemic sclerosis
Raynaud's phenomenon
Renal insufficiency
GERD with stricture, erosive esophagitis, gastritis
Anemia with heme (+) stool
Malabsorption syndrome
Controlled hypercholesterolemia
Controlled primary hypothyroidism
Controlled hypertension
Controlled NIDDM

▶ Questions

Problem Identification

1. a. Create a list of this patient's drug-related problems.
    b. What signs, symptoms, and laboratory values indicate the presence of Raynaud's phenomenon?
    c. Could any of the patient's peripheral vascular symptoms have been caused by drug therapy?

Desired Outcome

2. What are the goals of therapy for this patient's Raynaud's phenomenon?

Therapeutic Alternatives

3. a. What non-drug therapies could be useful for the treatment of the patient's painful symptoms associated with exacerbation of Raynaud's phenomenon?
    b. What pharmacotherapeutic alternatives are available for the treatment of Raynaud's disease?

Optimal Plan

4. a. What drug, dose, and schedule would be most appropriate for treaing this patient's Raynaud's phenomenon?
    b. In addition to initiating the new therapy that you suggested for control of the patient's peripheral vascular symptoms, what other adjustments would you make to her current drug regimen?

Outcome Evaluation

5. What clinical and laboratory parameters are needed to evaluate the patient's therapy for achievement of therapeutic goals and avoidance of adverse events?

Patient Counseling

6. What information should be provided to the patient to enhance compliance, ensure successful therapy, and minimize adverse events?

▶ Self-study Assignments

1. Provide therapy recommendations for the treatment of chronic arthritis and the painful joint symptoms experienced by this patient with systemic sclerosis. What drug classes should not be used and why?
2. Assume that the patient has used pseudoephedrine in the past for nasal congestion. If she requires a nasal decongestant in the future, should this drug be recommended?

▶ Clinical Pearl

An occupational therapist can be instrumental in instructing patients with Raynaud's phenomenon about life-style and occupational modifications to minimize trigger exposure and restrictions on activities of daily living.

References

1. Bolster MB, Maricq HR, Leff R. Office evaluation and treatment of Raynaud's phenomenon. Cleve Clin J Med 1995;62:51–61.
2. Belch JJ, Ho M. Pharmacotherapy of Raynaud's phenomenon. Drugs 1996;52:682–695.
3. Ferro CJ, Webb DJ. The clinical potential of endothelin receptor antagonists in cardiovascular medicine. Drugs 1996;51:12–27.
4. Wigley FM, Flavahan NA. Raynaud's phenomenon. Rheum Dis Clin North Am 1996;22:765–781.

17 HYPOVOLEMIC SHOCK

▶ **A Glass Half Full** (Level II)

Brian L. Erstad, PharmD, FASHP, FCCM

▶ After completing this case study, students should be able to:

- Develop a plan for implementing fluid or medication therapies for treating a patient in the initial stages of shock.
- Outline the major parameters used to monitor hypovolemic shock and its treatment.
- List the major disadvantage of using isolated hemodynamic recordings such as blood pressure measurements for monitoring the progression of shock.
- Compare and contrast fluids and medications used for treating hypovolemic shock.

☀ PATIENT PRESENTATION

Chief Complaint
Bill Hobbs is a 47 yo male admitted for fatigue and diarrhea.

HPI
Four days PTA, Mr. Hobbs had become nauseated and did not feel like eating. Although the nausea resolved after a couple of days, he began to have diarrhea, which led him to continue his avoidance of food intake. The diarrhea, in conjunction with increasing fatigue and lack of substantial fluid intake for 2 days, prompted his physician to hospitalize him for further evaluation and to temporarily stop his tacrolimus therapy (10 mg po BID); other medications were continued.

PMH
S/P orthotopic liver transplantation 6 months PTA for sarcoidosis involving the liver; the transplant was complicated by an adrenal vein hemorrhage that required reoperation for ligation
Diabetes mellitus post-transplant
Moderate cellular rejection on recent biopsy

FH
Noncontributory

SH
Does not smoke, drink EtOH, or use illicit drugs

ROS
Patient has had a recent increase in weight over past month (6 kg), although this has decreased by 2 kg in the past few days. Hearing intact with no vertigo. No dizziness or fainting episodes. Colorless sputum. No chest pain or dyspnea, but heart has been "racing." Has not had a bowel movement for 3 days; no vomiting, abdominal pain or cramping. No musculoskeletal pain or cramping

Meds
Prednisone 2.5 mg po every M, W, F
Mycophenolate mofetil 250 mg po every day
Fluconazole 50 mg po every M, W, F
Acyclovir 400 mg po BID
Famotidine 20 mg po BID

All
NKDA

PE

Gen
WDWN, but somewhat anxious man in mild distress

VS
BP 84/58 (baseline 135/85), but possible orthostatic changes not determined, HR 132 (baseline 80), RR 16, T 37°C; admission wt 78 kg

Skin
Pale color (including nail beds) and dry, but not cyanotic; no lesions

HEENT
Normal scalp/skull; conjunctiva pale and dry with clear sclerae; PERRLA, dry oral mucosa; remainder of ophthalmologic exam not performed

Neck/LN
Supple, no lymphadenopathy or thyromegaly

Lungs/Thorax
Decreased breath sounds since last exam

CV
RRR; S_1 and S_2 normal; apical pulse difficult to palpate; no m/r/g

Abd
Symmetrical with bulging flanks due to recent marked increase in ascites; palpable fluid wave; bowel sounds present; no tenderness or masses; scar from transplant evident.

Genit/Rect
Normal male genitalia; prostate smooth, not enlarged; no hemorrhoids noted; stool heme-negative

MS/Ext
No deformities with normal ROM; 2–3 + leg edema; no ulcers or tenderness

Neuro
Mild muscular atrophy with weak grip strength; CN II–XII intact; 2 + reflexes throughout; Babinski downgoing

Labs

Na 118 mEq/L	Hgb 11.9 g/dL	Phos 6.3 mg/dL
K 4.3 mEq/L	Hct 34.3%	AST 86 IU/L
Cl 83 mEq/L	Plt $51 \times 10^3/mm^3$	ALT 59 IU/L
CO_2 25 mEq/L	WBC $6.3 \times 10^3/mm^3$	T. bili 1.6 mg/dL
BUN 66 mg/dL	PT 12.1 sec	Alk phos 83 IU/L
SCr 3.0 mg/dL	PTT 33 sec	
Glu 137 mg/dL		

Other

I/O 1260/350 for first 14 hours of hospitalization

Ultrasound of abdomen ordered with possible paracentesis planned

Stool cultures negative for gastroenteric pathogens; O & P negative; negative *Clostridium difficile* titer

Normal response to synthetic ACTH adrenal stimulation testing

Assessment

Volume depletion/dehydration, possible nephrotoxicity from medications

---

► Questions

Problem Identification

1. a. Create a list of the patient's drug-related problems.
   b. What information (signs, symptoms, laboratory values) indicates the presence or severity of hypovolemic shock?

Desired Outcome

2. What are the goals of pharmacotherapy in this case?

Therapeutic Alternatives

3. a. What non-drug therapies might be useful for this patient?
   b. What feasible pharmacotherapeutic alternatives are available for treatment of shock?

Optimal Plan

4. What drug, dosage form, dose, schedule, and duration of therapy are best for this patient?

Outcome Evaluation

5. What clinical and laboratory parameters are necessary to evaluate the therapy for achievement of the desired therapeutic outcome and to detect or prevent adverse events?

Patient Counseling

6. What information should be provided to the patient to enhance compliance, ensure successful therapy, and minimize adverse effects?

► Clinical Course

All cultures were negative and there was no other evidence of infection. However, the patient had a complicated clinical course since inadequate fluids were given due to concerns about fluid overload. Paracenteses were performed every few days to remove accumulated ascitic fluid; this led to further vascular depletion with decreased renal perfusion. After approximately 10 days, the patient had to be admitted to the ICU for renal failure precipitated by inadequate vascular expansion. However, there was no evidence of progressive organ rejection after resolution of the renal failure, and the tacrolimus was eventually restarted.

► Follow-up Question

1. Why might this patient have changes in urine output, heart rate, and other parameters that are consistent with volume depletion even though he has edema on physical examination and his admission weight was indicative of volume overload?

► Clinical Pearl

While interstitial fluid accumulation in the lungs possibly leading to pulmonary edema is a concern, other sites of fluid accumulation such as the legs should not preclude adequate intravascular expansion, which is necessary to avoid organ hypoperfusion and subsequent dysfunction.

► Self-study Assignments

1. Search the literature and be able to discuss the results of comparative trials involving crystalloids and colloids for plasma expansion.
2. Write a two-page report comparing the advantages and limitations of each type of fluid for the plasma expansion indication.

References

1. Vermeulen LC Jr, Ratko TA, Erstad BL, et al. A paradigm for consensus. The University Hospital Consortium guidelines for the use of albumin, nonprotein colloid, and crystalloid solutions. Arch Intern Med 1995;155:373–379.
2. Schierhout G, Roberts I. Fluid resuscitation with colloid or crystalloid solutions in critically ill patients: A systematic review of randomised trials. BMJ 1998;316:961–964.

SECTION 2
Respiratory Disorders
Robert L. Talbert, PharmD, FCCP, BCPS, Section Editor

18   ACUTE ASTHMA

▶ **Living With Restricted Spaces**   (Level I)

Daniel T. Kennedy, PharmD, BCPS
Ralph E. Small, PharmD, FCCP, FASHP, FAPhA

▶ After completing this case study, students should be able to:

- Recognize the signs and symptoms of acute asthma.

- Describe pharmacologic and non-pharmacologic alternatives for the treatment of acute asthma according to patient signs and symptoms.

- Develop a pharmaceutical care plan for the treatment of acute asthma, including therapeutic end points, dosage regimens, monitoring parameters, and follow-up.

- Provide discharge counseling on the appropriate use of metered dose inhalers and peak flow meters as well as the role of different medications for the treatment of asthma.

☀ PATIENT PRESENTATION

Chief Complaint
"When I woke up, I couldn't breathe."

HPI
Jake Johnson is a 20 yo man who was brought to the ED this evening via EMS after the jail staff reported that he had SOB secondary to an asthma attack. The patient was given 2 albuterol nebs (5 mg each) and 0.5 mg SQ epinephrine en route to the hospital (see Figure 18–1). His asthma attack was thought to be exacerbated by strong paint fumes at the jail. Mr. Johnson refused nasal trumpet en route and did not wish to be intubated upon presentation to the ED. Patient has been on prednisone taper to be completed in 1 week for a recent exacerbation; however, Mr. Johnson is breathing too hard to expound on this. He reported "breathing fine" earlier in the day. He does not monitor his peak flows at the jail. Medication adherence is reported to be adequate, as the prison staff watches Mr. Johnson as he takes his medications. His last dose of Theo-Dur and MDIs was earlier in the day.

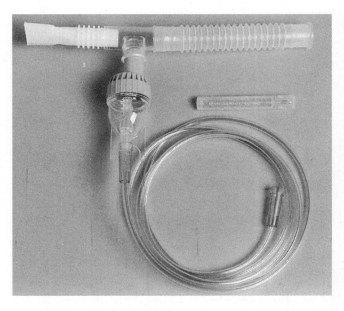

Figure 18–1. Nebulizer tubing used to administer inhaled β$_2$-agonist pharmacotherapy.

PMH
Asthma S/P 5 intubations; last event 14 months ago
Laryngeal dyskinesis possibly secondary to GERD
H/O seizure disorder; last event 1 year ago
Depression

FH
Noncontributory

SH
Currently an incarcerated convicted felon. Denies EtOH, tobacco use, and IVDA. Marital status: single

ROS
No complaints of weakness, fatigue, fever, or pain of any kind. Recent heartburn has been a concern for the patient. Cough and wheezing upon presentation to the ED

Meds
Guaifenesin 15 mL po QID PRN
Doxepin 200 mg po Q HS
Prednisone 10 mg po QD (to be continued one more week)
Theo-Dur 200 mg po BID
Atrovent MDI 2 puffs QID
Azmacort MDI 2 puffs QID
Albuterol MDI 2 puffs BID–QID PRN
Omeprazole 20 mg po QD

All
NKDA

PE

Gen
WDWN man in acute respiratory distress, labored breathing, using accessory muscles

VS
BP 113/47, pulsus paradoxus 14 mm Hg, P 129, RR 26, T 36.8°C; Wt 81 kg, Ht 6′3″

Skin
Warm and dry, no cyanosis

HEENT
NC/AT, EOMI, PERRLA, O/P clear, difficulty in speaking

Neck
Neck supple; no bruits, JVD, or lymphadenopathy

Chest
Bilateral decreased breath sounds, tight air movement, high-pitched wheezes bilaterally

CV
RRR, normal S_1 and S_2, no m/r/g

Abd
Bowel sounds present, soft, NTND

Rectal
Deferred

Ext
No CCE, peripheral pulses 2+

Neuro
Alert and oriented × 3, CN II–XII grossly intact, DTRs 2+

Labs

Na 145 mEq/L	Hgb 14.7 g/dL	AST 25 IU/L	Ca 9.7 mg/dL
K 3.2 mEq/L	Hct 45%	ALT 22 IU/L	Mg 1.9 mg/dL
Cl 105 mEq/L	Plt 324 × 10^3/mm^3	Alk Phos 64 IU/L	Phos 3.5 mg/dL
CO_2 29 mEq/L	WBC 10.4 × 10^3/mm^3	T. bili 0.1 mg/dL	Theoph 6.3 mg/L
BUN 13 mg/dL	70% PMNs	Alb 4.4 g/dL	
SCr 1.1 mg/dL	4% Bands		
Glu 118 mg/dL	22% Lymphs		
	4% Monos		

Peak Flow
150 L/min (baseline at last office visit 480 L/min)

ABG
pH 7.36, pco_2 42 mm Hg, po_2 188 mm Hg, HCO_3^- 23 mEq/L, O_2 sat 95% on 100% FIo_2

ECG
Sinus tachycardia

Chest X-ray
No pneumonia, (+) pneumomediastinum on L heart border most likely due to barotrauma of acute asthma attack

Assessment
Acute asthma attack probably secondary to exposure to paint fumes

---

▶ Questions

Problem Identification

1. a. Create a list of the patient's drug related problems.
   b. What information (signs, symptoms, laboratory values) indicates the severity of the acute asthma attack?

Desired Outcome

2. What are the goals of pharmacotherapy in this case?

Therapeutic Alternatives

3. a. What non-drug therapies might be useful for this patient?
   b. What feasible pharmacotherapeutic alternatives are available for the treatment of acute asthma?
   c. What psychosocial considerations are applicable to this patient?

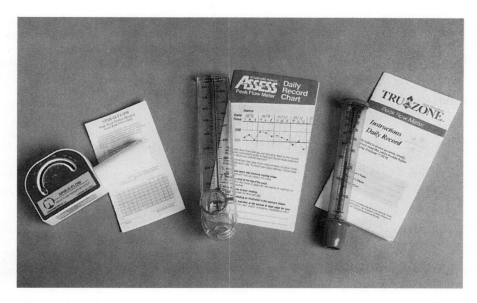

Figure 18–2. Examples of peak flow meters for assessing asthma control.

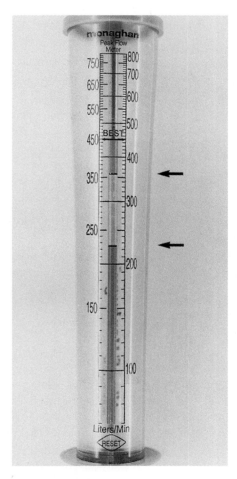

Figure 18–3. Scale of a peak flow meter. A reading in the green zone (above the top arrow) indicates that breathing is at least 80% of the patient's maximum flow rate (450 L/min). The yellow zone (between the arrows) indicates 50% to 80%, and the red zone (below the bottom arrow) indicates <50% of the patient's maximum flow rate.

Optimal Plan

4. a. *What drug, dosage form, dose, schedule, and duration of therapy are best for this patient?*

▶ Clinical Course

Within 6 hours of admission, Mr. Johnson's PEF increased to >70% and was maintained for >24 hours with the plan you recommended. Only mild wheezing and minimal shortness of breath were reported and the patient stated "I feel much better." As treatment continued, the patient further improved and the decision was made to discharge the patient to jail.

b. *What pharmacotherapy would you recommend for this patient upon discharge?*

Outcome Evaluation

5. a. *What are the long-term goals of asthma therapy for this patient?*
   b. *What will you monitor to assess the efficacy of asthma pharmacotherapy in this patient?*
   c. *What will you monitor to assess the side effects of drug therapy?*
   d. *What laboratory tests or other objective measures are necessary to monitor therapy?*

Patient Counseling

6. *Describe the information that should be provided to this patient regarding inhaler technique, the differences between quick-relief and long-term-control medications, and the use of a peak flow meter (see Figures 18–2 and 18–3).*

▶ Follow-up Question

1. *What other actions could be taken to control the factors contributing to this patient's asthma severity?*

▶ Self-study Assignments

1. Conduct a literature search to determine the relationship between asthma and GERD.
2. Research the efficacy of albuterol via nebulization versus MDI in acute asthma.
3. Develop a specific action plan for an asthmatic in your pharmacy.
4. Determine the benefit of guaifenesin in the treatment of chronic asthma.

▶ Clinical Pearl

It is imperative that every persistent asthmatic be placed on an inhaled corticosteroid at the optimal dose.

References

1. National Asthma Education and Prevention Program. Expert Panel Report 2: Guidelines for the Diagnosis and Management of Asthma. Bethesda, National Institutes of Health, 1997. www.nhlbi.nih.gov/nhlbi/nhlbi

2. Idris AH, McDermott MF, Raucci JC, et al. Emergency department treatment of severe asthma. Metered-dose inhaler plus holding chamber is equivalent in effectiveness to nebulizer. Chest 1993;103:665–672.
3. Mandelberg A, Chen E, Noviski N, et al. Nebulized wet aerosol treatment in emergency department—Is it essential? Comparison with large spacer device for metered-dose inhaler. Chest 1997;112:1501–1505.
4. Ratto D, Alfaro C, Sipsey J, et al. Are intravenous corticosteroids required in status asthmaticus? JAMA 1988;260:527–529.
5. Murphy DG, McDermott MF, Rydman RJ, et al. Aminophylline in the treatment of acute asthma when beta-2-adrenergics and steroids are provided. Arch Intern Med 1993;153:1784–1788.
6. Kerstjens HA, Brand PL, Hughes MD, et al. A comparison of bronchodilator therapy with or without inhaled corticosteroid therapy for obstructive airways disease. N Engl J Med 1992;327:1413–1419.

19 CHRONIC ASTHMA

▶ A Tale of Cats, Colds, Compliance, and Corticosteroids (Level I)

Dennis M. Williams, PharmD, FASHP, FCCP, BCPS

▶ After completing this case study, students should be able to:

- Recognize uncontrolled asthma.
- Identify potential causes of poorly-controlled asthma.
- Describe a self-management plan and action plan for improving control of asthma.
- Recommend a rational, comprehensive approach to management of persistent asthma.

☼ PATIENT PRESENTATION

Chief Complaint
"My asthma is acting up and I have missed too much school."

HPI
Randi Kerney is a 20 yo woman who presents to the student health service physician complaining of increased shortness of breath, wheezing, poor exercise tolerance, and a head cold for 4 days. She began monitoring her peak flow rates twice daily and implemented an action plan that included albuterol nebulizations. However, she recently replaced her nebulizer machine and felt that it wasn't working as well as her previous one. She notes that the time to complete her nebulizer treatments has increased from 6 to 8 minutes to 12 to 15 minutes with the new machine.

PMH
Moderate persistent asthma for 12 years; she has been hospitalized twice in the past two years for asthma exacerbations and has been to the ED four times in the past 9 months.
Perennial allergic rhinitis

FH

Both parents living; mother 52 years old with HTN; father 58 years old with COPD (50 pack-year smoking history); one sibling age 24 in apparent good health

SH

No alcohol or tobacco use; sexually active for 2 years with the same boyfriend. Patient is a college sophomore history major and lives in a dormitory with her non-smoking roommate. Her boyfriend has a cat in his apartment.

Meds

Proventil HFA MDI 2 puffs PRN
Azmacort MDI 3 puffs TID
Beconase Inhalation Aerosol (nasal) 1 spray each nostril TID
Albuterol nebulization 2.5 mg in 3 mL NS PRN
Serevent MDI 2 puffs BID
Ortho Novum 7/7/7 one tablet po QD

Compliance with above regimen is variable; she refills her OC and Serevent regularly on schedule but is typically a few weeks late on the steroid nasal and oral inhaler; patient obtains a Proventil HFA MDI approximately every 6 to 8 weeks. She frequently misses the midday dose of the steroid medications and experiences discomfort from the nasal spray.

All

Aspirin (urticaria and wheezing)
Cats (wheezing)

ROS

Unremarkable except for nasal stuffiness and heartburn. Patient also reports that she wakes up at least twice a week with shortness of breath and wheezing, and occasionally feels chest tightness in the morning.

PE

Gen

Anxious-appearing Caucasian female in apparent distress with audible wheezing, unable to speak in complete sentences due to dyspnea. Suprasternal muscle retractions noted.

VS

BP 148/88, P 105, RR 28, T 38.2°C; Wt 58 kg

Skin

No rashes or bruises

HEENT

EOMI; PERLA; fundi benign, no hemorrhages or exudates; TMs intact; nasal mucosa boggy

Neck

Supple, no adenopathy or thyromegaly

Lungs

Diffuse wheezes bilaterally on exhalation and occasionally on inspiration

Breasts

Nontender without masses

CV

Tachycardia, regular rhythm; no murmurs, rubs, or gallops

ABD

Soft, NT/ND; bowel sounds active

Ext

Normal ROM; pulses 3+ throughout; no CCE

Neuro

CNs intact; no focal or sensory defects

Labs

Na 132 mEq/L	Hgb 12 g/dL	WBC $8.0 \times 10^3/mm^3$
K 4.4 mEq/L	Hct 36%	67% PMNs
Cl 102 mEq/L	Plt $180 \times 10^3/mm^3$	2% Bands
CO_2 26 mEq/L		20% Lymphs
BUN 22 mg/dL		8% Eos
SCr 0.9 mg/dL		3% Monos
Glu 104 mg/dL		Pulse ox 88% (on RA)

Nasal Smear

Numerous eosinophils

Chest X-ray

Hyperinflated lungs; no infiltrates

Peak Flow

130 L/min (baseline 340 L/min)

Assessment

20-year-old woman with moderate to severe exacerbation of asthma likely precipitated by viral upper respiratory infection.

▶ Clinical Course

The patient is admitted for treatment with oxygen, inhaled bronchodilators, and oral prednisone (60 mg/day initially, followed by a slow taper to discontinuation over 10 days). After 2 days, she is significantly improved. Her lungs are clear without wheezing; her respiratory rate is 18; and her pulse oximetry is 94%. Her peak flow has improved to 270 L/min, and she is discharged home with a new nebulizer.

▶ Questions

Problem Identification

1. a. *Create a list of the patient's drug-related problems.*
   b. *What information indicates the presence of uncontrolled chronic asthma and an acute asthma exacerbation?*
   c. *Could any of the patient's problems have been caused by drug therapy?*

Desired Outcome

2. *What are the goals of pharmacotherapy in this case?*

Therapeutic Alternatives

3. a. *What non-drug therapies might be useful for this patient?*
   b. *What feasible pharmacotherapeutic alternatives are available for treatment of this patient's chronic asthma?*

Optimal Plan

4. a. *Outline an optimal plan of treatment for this patient's chronic asthma.*
   b. *What alternatives would be appropriate if the initial therapy fails?*

Outcome Evaluation

5. *What clinical and laboratory parameters are necessary to evaluate the therapy for achievement of the desired therapeutic effect and to detect or prevent adverse effects?*

Patient Counseling

6. *What information should be provided to enhance compliance, ensure successful therapy, and minimize adverse effects?*

▶ Clinical Course

With the institution of the changes you recommended, the patient's asthma is well controlled. She is questioned about her new nebulizer and reports that it is working well. Over the next several months, she notes only occasional nighttime symptoms that are responsive to albuterol. She has needed to initiate her action plan (of increased β agonist and inhaled corticosteroid use) only twice in the past seven months.

▶ Self-study Assignments

1. If this patient became pregnant, what impact would this have on her asthma control and therapy?
2. If this patient continues to take inhaled corticosteroids when she is postmenopausal, what can be done to minimize the problem of osteoporosis?
3. What recommendations can you make about stepping down her current regimen?
4. What ongoing monitoring is necessary as her medications are tapered or discontinued?
5. What role would immunotherapy play for her asthma and allergies?

▶ Clinical Pearl

All patients with persistent forms of asthma should receive influenza vaccine annually. It is well established that viral respiratory infections, including influenza, are a common trigger of asthma exacerbations in children and adults.

References

1. Clinical Practice Guidelines. Expert Panel Report 2: Guidelines for the Diagnosis and Management of Asthma. NIH pub. no. 97-4051. April 1997. Also available on the Internet at http://www.nhlbi.nih.gov/nhlbi/lung/asthma/prof/asthgdln.htm.
2. Haahtela T, Jarvinen M, Kava T, et al. Effects of reducing or discontinuing inhaled budesonide in patients with mild asthma. N Engl J Med 1994;331: 700–705.
3. Gross NJ. Leukotriene modifiers: What place in asthma management? J Resp Dis 1998;19:245–261.
4. Greening AP, Ind P, Northfield M, et al. Added salmeterol versus higher-dose corticosteroid in asthma patients with symptoms on existing inhaled corticosteroid. Lancet 1994;344:219–224.

20 CHRONIC OBSTRUCTIVE LUNG DISEASE

▶ Waiting to Exhale   (Level II)

Daren L. Knoell, PharmD

▶ After completing this case study, students should be able to:

- Differentiate the signs and symptoms of chronic bronchitis, emphysema, and mixed obstructive lung disease.
- Identify the importance of nonpharmacologic therapy in patients with COLD.
- Identify the association between cigarette smoking, lung disease, and the importance of smoking cessation strategies.
- Educate patients on the proper use of inhaled medications and determine which patients may benefit from spacers and/or holding chambers.
- Describe the relationship between α_1-antitrypsin deficiency and the development of emphysema.

☀ PATIENT PRESENTATION

Chief Complaint
"I could barely breathe, and my cough was worse, so I went to the emergency room."

HPI
William Marley is a 64 yo man with COLD and asthma who is admitted to the hospital after presenting to the ED with a 3-day history of progressive

shortness of breath, cough, and increased production of clear sputum, but without fever or night sweats. The patient's wife recalls that prior to this episode, he complained of weakness and myalgias. He treated himself at home with albuterol MDI but had increasing respiratory distress despite multiple puffs. Upon arrival to the ED, he was noted to have decreased breath sounds and was unable to speak full sentences. In the ED, he was placed on 4 L oxygen via face mask and given nebulized Atrovent and albuterol treatments. Solu-Medrol 60 mg IV and erythromycin 500 mg IV were given, and he was transferred to the floor.

PMH

COLD × 5 years
Asthma for as long as he can remember
Alcoholic cirrhosis × 5 years
HTN × 20 years

His respiratory symptoms are often worse in the fall but usually respond well to inhaled bronchodilators. He states that he is compliant as long as his wife reminds him to take his medications. He admits that he does not like to use the Atrovent because it gives him blurred vision; he uses the open-mouth technique and does not currently use a spacer or holding chamber (see Figure 20–1). The patient lacks coordination and demonstrates poor overall MDI technique. He last visited his PCP approximately 1 month ago at which time his hypertension medication was changed from Dyazide to nadolol.

FH

Father died of MI at age 65. Mother is alive and also has COLD.

SH

Married × 35 years; wife is alive and in good health. Retired construction worker, installed insulation as part of his job. Currently drinks several beers every day, but used to drink the equivalent of a fifth of hard liquor every day up until 2 years ago. Has smoked cigarettes 1 ppd for over 40 years. He is willing to consider smoking cessation, especially since his daughter re-cently moved back into their home and now makes him smoke outside. No history of IVDA.

ROS

(+) Shortness of breath with cough productive of clear sputum; (+) weakness and myalgias. Denies chest pain, fever, or night sweats

Meds

Theo-Dur 100 mg po BID
Albuterol MDI 2 puffs QID PRN
Atrovent MDI 2 puffs BID
Nadolol 40 mg po QD
Furosemide 20 mg po QD

All

NKDA

PE

Gen

Thin elderly male somewhat improved and now in moderate respiratory distress after receiving treatment in the ED

VS

BP 160/95, P 140, RR 34, T 37.9°C; pulsus paradoxus 12 mm Hg; Wt 65 kg, Ht 5′7″

Skin

Warm, dry, (+) jaundice

HEENT

PERRLA, EOMI; icteric sclerae; AV nicking on funduscopic exam; no hemorrhages or exudates; TMs intact; oropharynx clear

Neck/LN

(+) JVD; no lymphadenopathy or thyromegaly

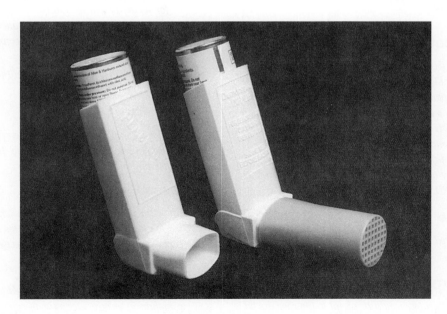

Figure 20–1. Metered-dose inhalers with (right) and without (left) a spacer device attached.

Lungs
Diffuse inspiratory and expiratory wheezes bilaterally, no rales or rhonchi

CV
RRR; normal S_1; accentuated S_2 sound, no S_3 or S_4

Abd
(+) Hepatosplenomegaly, (+) fluid wave; (+) tenderness and distention; (−) superficial veins

Genit/Rect
Testicular atrophy; heme (−) stool

MS/Ext
Cyanotic nail beds; no clubbing; 1+ bilateral ankle edema; pulses 2+ throughout

Neuro
A & O × 3; CN II–XII intact; DTRs 2+; Babinski downgoing; no encephalopathic findings

Labs

Na 130 mEq/L	Hgb 13.0 g/dL	AST 248 IU/L	ABG on 6 L O_2 by NC
K 2.7 mEq/L	Hct 39.5%	ALT 212 IU/L	pH 7.30
Cl 109 mEq/L	Plt 245 × 10³/mm³	T. bili 3.2 mg/dL	po_2 100 mm Hg
BUN 14 mg/dL	WBC 8.0 × 10³/mm³	PT 13.2 sec	pco_2 55 mm Hg
SCr 0.9 mg/dL	PMNs 65%	Alb 3.0 g/dL	HCO_3 25 mEq/L
Glu 110 mg/dL	Bands 3%	Theoph 9.0 mg/L	Sao_2 98%
	Lymphs 27%		
	Monos 5%		

Pulmonary Function Tests
Prebronchodilator FEV_1 = 800 mL
Postbronchodilator FEV_1 = 1000 mL
Diffusion capacity (DLco) = 71% predicted (from tests performed 6 months ago)

Chest X-ray
Flattened diaphragm; loss of peripheral vascular markings; no effusions or infiltrates noted

ECG
ST depression, flattened T-waves

Assessment
This is a thin elderly man with acute respiratory insufficiency secondary to an acute exacerbation of COLD and/or asthma. He also has hypokalemia, acute respiratory acidosis, and a history of HTN and liver disease.

Meds Initiated After Transfer to Floor
Theo-Dur 100 mg po BID
Albuterol nebulized solution 1 mL of 0.5% solution (5 mg) in 3 mL NS Q 4 H
Atrovent MDI 4 puffs QID
Solu-Medrol 60 mg IV Q 6 H
Erythromycin 500 mg IV Q 6 H
Furosemide 20 mg po QD
Oxygen 2L via nasal cannula

► Questions

Problem Identification

1. a. Create a list of this patient's drug-related problems prior to treatment in the ED.
   b. What signs, symptoms, and laboratory data provide evidence that this patient is experiencing a COLD exacerbation? Based on the evidence, is his presentation more consistent with emphysema or chronic bronchitis?
   c. What additional information do you need to satisfactorily assess the adequacy of COLD treatment in this patient before he presented to the ED?

Desired Outcome

2. What are the desired goals for the treatment of this patient's COLD?

Therapeutic Alternatives

3. a. What non-drug therapies would be useful to improve this patient's COLD symptoms?
   b. What feasible pharmacotherapeutic alternatives are available for the treatment of COLD in this patient, particularly those that can be continued as an outpatient?
   c. Should home oxygen therapy be considered for the patient at this time?
   d. Is this patient a candidate for $α_1$-antitrypsin (Prolastin) therapy?

Optimal Plan

4. Develop a complete outpatient regimen for the treatment of COLD in this patient, including dose, route, frequency, and duration for therapy.

Outcome Evaluation

5. What clinical and laboratory parameters are necessary to evaluate the therapy for achievement of the desired therapeutic outcome and to detect or prevent adverse effects?

Patient Counseling

6. What information should be provided to the patient to enhance compliance, ensure successful therapy, and minimize adverse effects?

Self-study Assignments

1. Describe and compare the expectations for deterioration in pulmonary function in normal healthy adults and smokers with emphysema. In particular, emphasis should be placed on expected patterns of change in DLco, FEV_1, and FVC and general health over time in years.
2. If this patient were to have an abnormally low serum α_1-antitrypsin level, describe why additional phenotyping would be necessary. Furthermore, define what implications the results would have if the patient were designated as homozygous ZZ, heterozygous MZ, or heterozygous SZ at the α_1-antitrypsin allele.
3. Search the Internet (see suggested site in References at end of chapter) for supplementary materials on smoking cessation guidelines for patients and health care providers. Study these materials and use them to work with an actual patient in the outpatient setting. Document your findings over time while working with this patient. The patient may be you.

Clinical Pearl

Spacer devices and holding chambers are not interchangeable. Although both are designed to improve drug deposition in the airway, only the holding chamber avoids the need for the patient to coordinate actuation with inhalation.

References

1. Ferguson GT, Cherniack RM. Management of chronic obstructive pulmonary disease. N Engl J Med 1993;328:1017–1022.
2. Nelson HS. Beta-adrenergic bronchodilators. N Engl J Med 1995;333:499–506.
3. MacDonald JL, Johnson CE. Pathophysiology and treatment of alpha 1-antitrypsin deficiency. Am J Health-Syst Pharm 1995;52:481–489.
4. Toogood JH. Helping your patients make better use of MDIs and spacers. J Resp Dis 1994;15:151–166.
Suggested Internet site: Agency for Health Care Policy and Research, http://www.ahcpr.gov/clinic/

21 RESPIRATORY DISTRESS SYNDROME

The Breath of Life (Level II)

Jennifer L. Schoelles, PharmD
Robert J. Kuhn, PharmD

After completing this case study, students should be able to:

- Identify the common signs and symptoms of respiratory distress syndrome (RDS) in the neonate.
- Recommend appropriate dosing and administration of surfactants for patients with RDS.
- Devise a monitoring plan for patients with RDS who are receiving pulmonary surfactants.
- Recognize the similarities and differences in the surfactants currently available.
- Appreciate the pharmacoeconomic impact that the use of surfactants may have on premature infants in the first 5 years of life.

PATIENT PRESENTATION

Chief Complaint
Premature infant with difficulty breathing

HPI
Tanner Williams is a 34-week gestation, 1930-g infant born to a G_1P_{2-0-2} single African-American mother (editor's note: G is the number of pregnancies; 2-0-2 means 2 infants delivered, 0 abortions, and 2 living children). He was the first born of twins. Apgar scores were $7_1 8_5$. Tanner's mother had a benign prenatal course until she developed pre-eclampsia at 32 weeks' gestation.

Maternal History
19 yo woman with worsening pre-eclampsia and twin gestation with breech vertex presentation. She had high blood pressure (138/90 in clinic that day and 166/78 in the hospital), 3+ proteinuria, and 4+ pitting edema the day of delivery. She received IV magnesium sulfate before delivery but did not receive betamethasone. She denies a history of alcohol, tobacco or drug abuse, is HIV negative, and has no known history of any Group B streptococcus infection or colonization.

Birth History
Tanner was brought to the resuscitation area with a weak cry, appeared cyanotic, and had decreased tone. He was bulb suctioned, dried, stimulated, and received blow-by O_2 and positive pressure breaths administered by bag mask. He cried after 1.5 minutes and received deep suctioning. He pinked up on O_2 but had grunting, flaring and retractions. Tanner was brought to the Neonatal Intensive Care Unit (NICU) for prematurity and respiratory distress syndrome, where he was intubated due to continuing respiratory distress. Ventilating settings upon admission to the NICU: Rate = 60, MAP = 8, PAP = 16, PEEP = 4, IT = 0.3, FIo_2 = 100%.

ROS
Apgar scores taken at 1 minute and 5 minutes after birth:

Apgar Scores (0–2)	1 Minute	5 Minutes
Heart rate	2	2
Respiratory effort	2	2
Activity	1	2
Reflexes	1	1
Skin color	1	1
TOTAL	7	8

Meds
None

All
NKDA

PE
Upon arrival to the NICU:

Gen
Premature infant of 34-week gestation, weight = 1935 g

VS
BP 71/39, HR 161, RR 38, T 36.3°C

Skin
Pink and well perfused

HEENT
Anterior fontanel flat and soft; sagittal sutures patent; normocephalic; unable to evaluate eyes due to antibiotic ointment; nasal flaring despite intubation and mechanical ventilation; oral pharynx normal

Neck
Supple, no masses, clavicles intact

Chest
Symmetric, mild to moderate subcostal/intercostal retractions, lungs clear bilaterally with ventilation

CV
RSR, no murmur, pulses +2/4, capillary refill time 2 seconds

Abd
Soft, no organomegaly, umbilical vein and umbilical artery catheters in place

Genit/Rect
Testicles descended bilaterally, normal phallus, anus patent

Spine
Straight and intact

Ext
Bilateral hip clicks, symmetric extremities

Labs
Obtained 3–4 hours after birth, except as noted:

			VBG (at birth)
Hgb 17.1 g/dL	WBC $12.9 \times 10^3/mm^3$	Na 124 mEq/L	
Hct 52.1 %	PMNs 59 %	K 4.3 mEq/L	pH 7.23
Plt $204 \times 10^3/mm^3$	Bands 1%	Glu 123 mg/dL	pco_2 55 mm Hg
MCV 106 μm^3	Lymph 26%	Bili 2.3 mg/dL	po_2 65 mm Hg
MCH 34.7 pg	Mono 14 %		O_2 Sat 88%
MCHC 32.8 g/dL	NRBC 6%		BE −6.1 mEq/L
RDW 17.0%			HCO_3 22 mEq/L

Chest X-ray
Diffuse reticular granular pattern and slightly enlarged heart, probably artifact secondary to a large thymus gland, air bronchograms noted consistent with surfactant deficiency

Impression
Respiratory failure/respiratory distress/surfactant deficiency; rule out sepsis; preterm male twin A at 34 weeks' gestation

---

▶ Questions

Problem Identification

1. a. *What risk factors does this patient have for developing respiratory distress syndrome (RDS)?*
   b. *What signs, symptoms, and other data indicate that this patient needs to be treated for RDS?*

Desired Outcome

2. *What are the goals of treatment in neonates who have RDS?*

Therapeutic Alternatives

3. *What pharmacologic and non-pharmacologic treatments are available for RDS?*

Optimal Plan

4. a. *What pharmacotherapeutic drug regimen (including dose and administration information) would you recommend for treating RDS in this patient?*
   b. *What adjunctive care or supportive pharmacotherapy is needed in the management of RDS in this patient?*

Outcome Evaluation

5. *What monitoring parameters should be used to evaluate therapy in this infant?*

Patient Counseling

6. *What information about surfactants should be provided to the infant's parents?*

▶ Follow-up Question

1. *What measures could have been used prenatally with the patient's mother to prevent or decrease the severity of RDS?*

▶ Clinical Pearl

The appropriate, early use of surfactants since their introduction has cut mortality from RDS in half.

Self-study Assignments

1. Perform a literature search to obtain information comparing the efficacy of different surfactant preparations.
2. Investigate the differences in cost, storage, expiration, and administration of the two products currently available in the United States.

References

1. Halliday HL. Natural vs synthetic surfactants in neonatal respiratory distress syndrome. Drugs 1996;51:226–237.
2. Ishisaka DY. Exogenous surfactant use in neonates. Ann Pharmacother 1996;30:389–398.
3. Soll RF. Surfactant therapy in the USA: Trials and current routines. Biol Neonate 1997;71(suppl 1):1–7.
4. Taketomo CK, Hodding JH, Kraus DM. Pediatric dosing handbook, 4th ed. Hudson, OH, Lexi-Comp, 1997.

22 CYSTIC FIBROSIS

Blood, Sweat, Lungs, and Gut   (Level I)

Robert J. Kuhn, PharmD

After completing this case study, students should be able to:

- Identify signs and symptoms of common problems in patients with cystic fibrosis (CF).
- Develop a monitoring plan for antimicrobial therapy in the treatment of acute pulmonary exacerbation in CF.
- Devise treatment strategies for common complications of drug therapy in patients with CF.
- Provide counseling on aerosolized medications in patients with CF, including appropriate instructions for dornase alfa and inhaled tobramycin.

PATIENT PRESENTATION

Chief Complaint
As reported by his mother: "Shortness of breath, increasing cough and sputum production, and decreased energy"

HPI
Eric Conley is a 9 yo male with a long history of CF diagnosed at 4 weeks of age. He had been doing well until 2 weeks ago when he developed shortness of breath, pulmonary congestion, and severe fatigue. Mother reported increasing cough productive of very dark-colored sputum, but no fever. The patient has had a decreased appetite and has lost 2 pounds. His oxygen saturation at home was 96% but is now 88% in clinic. Mother initially took him to clinic 5 days ago for the same symptoms and was given ciprofloxacin 500 mg po BID and an increased dose of inhaled tobramycin TID. His prednisone was increased from 5 mg to 10 mg po QD, and his

mother was instructed to call or return if no improvement was seen. The patient now presents 5 days later with worsening respiratory symptoms.

PMH
Significant for 11 hospitalizations for acute pulmonary exacerbations of CF since his diagnosis.
H/O allergic bronchopulmonary aspergillosis, recently under control with treatment; last hospitalization was 8 weeks ago
Pancreatic insufficiency requiring supplementation with 1491 units/kg/meal of lipase to maintain weight gain
Pulmonary changes c/w long-standing CF with bronchiectasis and two episodes of hemoptysis

FH
Both parents are alive and well. Eric has one sister who had a recent cold and upper respiratory infection. Two maternal uncles died at ages 13 and 17 from CF.

SH
Eric attends third grade but has been homebound the last 2 months. Lives with his mother, father, and sister. They have city water and no pets; father smokes, but only outside of the home.

ROS
Patient complains of severe back pain, especially when coughing. Reduced ability to perform usual daily activities due to SOB. No vomiting, abdominal pain, or complaints of abnormal stool odor or character

Meds
Aerosolized tobramycin 80 mg TID
Cromolyn sodium 20 mg via nebulizer BID
Albuterol 0.5 mL with 3 mL 0.9% NaCl TID via nebulizer
Pulmozyme 2.5 mg via nebulizer QD
Azmacort 4 puffs BID
Prednisone 10 mg po QD
Creon 20, two with meals and one with snack
Ferrous sulfate 300 mg po QD
ADEK one tablet po QD

All
NKDA

PE

Gen
A pleasant, cooperative 9-year-old boy who has shortness of breath with his oxygen cannula removed during the exam

VS
BP 110/70, P 144, RR 44, T 36.9°C; Wt 59 lb. Oxygen saturation 95% with 1.5 L of oxygen; 88% on room air

HEENT
EOMI, PERRL; nares with dried mucus in both nostrils; no oral lesions, but secretions noted in the posterior pharynx

Neck/LN
Supple; no lymphadenopathy or thyromegaly

Lungs

Crackles heard bilaterally in the upper lobes greater than in the lower lobes

Heart

RRR without murmurs

Abd

Ticklish during exam; (+) bowel sounds; abdomen soft and supple. No steatorrhea noted

MS/Ext

Clubbing noted with no cyanosis; capillary refill <2 seconds

Neuro

Eric is alert and awake; CNs intact; somewhat uncooperative with the full neurologic exam

Labs

Na 138 mEq/L	Hgb 15.4 g/dL	WBC $20.1 \times 10^3/mm^3$	AST 24 IU/L
K 4.5 mEq/L	Hct 45.2%	61% Neutros	ALT 22 IU/L
Cl 102 mEq/L	MCV 91 μm^3	32% Bands	LDH 330 IU/L
CO_2 27 mEq/L	MCH 31.1 pg	6% Lymphs	GGT 42 IU/L
BUN 10 mg/dL	MCHC 34 g/dL	1% Monos	T. Prot 8.3 g/dL
SCr 0.7 mg/dL		Ca 4.6 mEq/L	Alb 3.8 g/dL
Glu 188 mg/dL		Phos 4.6 mEq/L	

Urine Drug Screen

Negative

Sputum Culture Results

Organism A: *Pseudomonas aeruginosa*
Organism B: *Pseudomonas aeruginosa*
Organism C: *Pseudomonas aeruginosa*—mucoid strain
Organism D: *Staphylococcus aureus*
Organism E: *Staphylococcus aureus*
Organism F: *Aspergillus* species

PFTs

FEV_1 56% of predicted, FVC_1 80% of predicted

Chest X-ray

Bronchiectatic and interstitial fibrotic changes consistent with CF. No difference noted from previous exam 8 weeks ago

▶ Questions

Problem Identification

1. a. *Identify this patient's drug-related problems.*
   b. *What information indicates the disease severity and the need to treat his CF pharmacologically?*
   c. *Could any of his problems be caused by drug therapy?*

Desired Outcome

2. *What are the goals of pharmacotherapy in this case?*

Therapeutic Alternatives

3. a. *What non-drug therapies might be useful for this patient?*
   b. *What therapeutic alternatives are available for treatment of this patient's acute pulmonary exacerbation?*

Optimal Plan

4. a. *What drugs, dosage form, dose, schedule and duration of therapy are best for this patient?*

▶ Clinical Course

Serum tobramycin concentrations drawn after the fourth dose of tobramycin 80 mg infused over 30 minutes were 5.9 $\mu g/mL$ collected 1 hour after the end of the infusion, and a trough concentration just before the dose of 0.4 $\mu g/mL$.

   b. *Based on this new information, evaluate his drug therapy and suggest modification if necessary.*

Outcome Evaluation

5. *What clinical and laboratory parameters are necessary to evaluate the therapy?*

Patient Counseling

6. *What information should you provide the patient regarding the administration of aerosolized drug therapy? The patient will be going home on aerosolized tobramycin, dornase alfa, albuterol, and cromolyn sodium.*

▶ Self-study Assignments

1. What potential problem is associated with the use of very-high-dose pancreatic enzyme in patients with CF? What dosage guidelines should be followed to minimize any potential risk?
2. What are the recommendations for the administration of high-dose ibuprofen in patients with CF? When would you suggest that serum concentrations be drawn, and what levels are thought to be necessary to optimize therapy in a patient with CF?
3. Perform a literature search to determine the progress of gene therapy in CF.

4. What is the preferred treatment of acute bronchopulmonary aspergillosis in patients with CF? What long-term therapy is indicated?

► Clinical Pearl

Low doses of ibuprofen may increase the migration of neutrophils and inflammatory mediators in the lung and exacerbate the progression of lung disease. Care should be taken to evaluate the use of PRN ibuprofen in CF patients.

References

1. Saiman L, Campbell P, Burns J, et al. TOBI Consensus Conference. North American Cystic Fibrosis Conference, Nashville, October 1997.
2. Konstan MW, Byard PJ, Hoppel CL, et al. Effect of high-dose ibuprofen in patients with cystic fibrosis. N Engl J Med 1995;332:848–854.

SECTION 3

Gastrointestinal Disorders

Joseph T. DiPiro, PharmD, FCCP, Section Editor

23 GASTROESOPHAGEAL REFLUX DISEASE

► **More Than Garden-variety Heartburn**   (Level I)

Meredith L. Rose, PharmD

► After completing this case study, students should be able to:

• Identify typical and atypical symptoms associated with gastroesophageal reflux disease (GERD).

• Define the treatment goals for GERD.

• Describe both non-pharmacologic and pharmacologic approaches to the treatment of GERD.

• Develop an individualized treatment plan for a patient with GERD, taking into consideration the efficacy, safety, and cost of available agents.

• Understand the role of maintenance therapy in the treatment of GERD.

☀ PATIENT PRESENTATION

Chief Complaint

"About an hour after I eat, I get this burning pain in the middle of my chest, and sometimes it feels like my food won't go down; like I can't swallow it."

HPI

Roberta Woodson is a 70 yo woman with a significant history of GERD. She presents to clinic today for a routine follow-up visit. The patient reports that over the past month she has experienced increasing episodes of postprandial heartburn along with a variable degree of dysphagia. She has required daily use of antacids (in addition to her usual H_2-receptor antagonist) for symptom relief. The patient also experiences frequent nocturnal awakenings secondary to epigastric discomfort despite sleeping with 3 pillows. She feels as if her frequent episodes of heartburn prevent her from doing routine activities and living a normal life.

PMH

GERD × 10 years
HTN × 30 years
Paroxysmal SVT
Hiatal hernia (see Figure 23–1)
Atypical chest pain
Postmenopausal since the age of 50

FH

Father died at age 68 from CAD; mother died at age 74 from DM; two siblings with "heart disease"

SH

Patient is widowed and lives alone; she is a retired waitress and enjoys backyard gardening in the spring and summer months. (+) EtOH – history of "heavy" alcohol abuse in past; current alcohol consumption reported at 5 to 6 beers/week; 60 pack-year smoking history; currently smokes ½ ppd. She is a retired waitress and enjoys backyard gardening in the spring and summer months.

Meds

Verapamil 120 mg po TID
Hydrochlorothiazide 25 mg po QD
Famotidine 20 mg po Q HS
Fibercon 500 mg po QD
Amphogel 15 mL PRN upset stomach

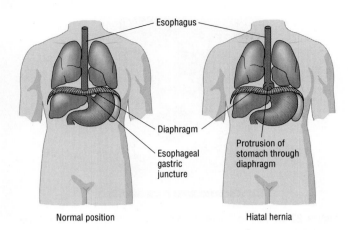

Esophagus

Diaphragm

Esophageal gastric juncture

Protrusion of stomach through diaphragm

Normal position

Hiatal hernia

Figure 23–1. Schematic representation of hiatal hernia. *(Reprinted with permission from Mulvihill ML,* Human Diseases: A Systemic Approach, *4th ed. Norwalk, CT, Appleton & Lange, 1995.)*

All

NKA

ROS

(−) HA, dizziness, visual changes, tinnitus or vertigo; (−) SOB, cough, PND; (+) frequent episodes of non-radiating substernal CP which she describes as burning in nature; (−) N/V/D, BRBPR, or dark/tarry stools; (+) frequent constipation; (−) urinary frequency, dysuria, nocturia, or hematuria, (−) recent weight loss.

PE

Gen

The patient is a nervous-appearing, elderly, African-American female who looks her stated age.

VS

BP 150/90, P 80, RR 16, T 97.8°F, Ht 5′5″, Wt 69.8 kg

Skin

No rashes or lesions noted

HEENT

PERRLA, EOMI, no arterial narrowing or A-V nicking; pink, moist mucus membranes; gums without swelling or ulceration; tonsils absent; oropharynx clear; patient wears dentures

Neck

No thyromegaly, lymphadenopathy, or JVD

Lungs

CTA

CV

RRR, normal S_1 and S_2; no S_3 or S_4; II/VI SEM at the apex

Breasts

Symmetrical; no lumps or masses detected; nipples without discharge

Abd

Normoactive BS, soft, NT/ND; no HSM

Genit/Rect

Vulva normal; dry vaginal mucosa; no palpable rectal masses; brown stool without occult blood

Ext

No CCE

Neuro

A & O × 3, CN II–XII intact; 5/5 strength in upper and lower extremities bilaterally

Labs

Na 140 mEq/L	Hgb 12.5 g/dL	*Fasting Lipid Profile*
K 3.2 mEq/L	Hct 37.3%	T. chol 233 mg/dL
Cl 95 mEq/L	RBC 4.3×10^6/mm³	LDL 153 mg/dL
CO_2 30 mEq/L	WBC 6.8×10^3/mm³	HDL 68 mg/dL
BUN 9 mg/dL		Trig 77 mg/dL
SCr 0.7 mg/dL		
Glu (fasting) 92 mg/dL		

ECG

Atrial tachycardia at 98 bpm with nonspecific ST-T wave changes that are not new

Stress Thallium (6 mo ago)

Very low probability of coronary artery disease

Assessment

Elderly woman with a significant history of GERD who presents with worsening of symptoms over the past month

► Questions

Problem Identification

1. a. *Develop a list of this patient's drug-related problems.*
   b. *What clinical information indicates worsening symptoms of GERD in this patient?*
   c. *What symptom(s) indicates the possible severity of the patient's GERD? Are the symptoms classic or atypical?*
   d. *What factors may be contributing to the patient's symptoms of GERD? (Refer to Figure 23–2 for a depiction of possible causes of esophagitis.)*

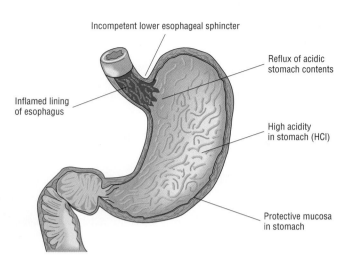

Figure 23–2. Various causes of esophagitis. *(Reprinted with permission from Mulvihill ML, Human Diseases: A Systemic Approach, 4th ed. Norwalk, CT, Appleton & Lange, 1995.)*

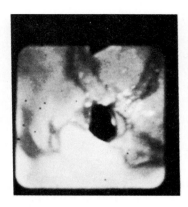

Figure 23–3. An endoscopic photograph of erosive esophagitis. The streaks are erosions, and the thick white material is exudate. *(Reprinted with permission from Gitnick G, et al. Principles and Practice of Gastroenterology and Hepatology, 2nd ed. Norwalk, CT, Appleton & Lange, 1994.)*

Desired Outcome

   2. *What are the goals of pharmacotherapy for this patient's GERD?*

Therapeutic Alternatives

   3. a. *What non-pharmacologic therapies or life-style modifications might be useful in the management of this patient's GERD?*
      b. *What pharmacotherapeutic alternatives are available for the treatment of this patient's GERD?*

Optimal Plan

   4. *Based upon the patient information provided, design an individualized pharmacotherapeutic plan for the management of this patient's GERD.*

Outcome Evaluation

   5. *What clinical and/or laboratory parameters should be evaluated at the patient's next follow-up appointment in order to assess for therapeutic response and to detect or prevent adverse effects?*

Patient Counseling

   6. *How will you educate the patient about her GERD therapy in order to enhance compliance, minimize adverse effects, and promote successful therapeutic outcomes?*

▶ Clinical Course

Ms. Woodson underwent an upper endoscopy that revealed multiple erosive lesions in the distal esophagus (Savary–Miller classification: II/IV; see Figure 23–3). There was no evidence of ulceration, obstruction, or stricture. The patient was treated with an 8-week course of omeprazole 20 mg daily for her symptoms of GERD and then switched back to famotidine 20 mg at bedtime. While on omeprazole therapy, the patient's burning sensation and dysphagia resolved. Approximately 3 months after discontinuation of the omeprazole, the patient reported that her GERD symptoms had returned and that she was again suffering from frequent postprandial and nocturnal reflux episodes.

▶ Follow-up Questions

   1. *What is the role of maintenance therapy for the management of this patient's continued GERD symptoms?*
   2. *What maintenance therapies could be recommended for the long-term management of GERD in this patient?*

▶ Self-study Assignments

   1. Develop an algorithm for the diagnosis and treatment of both uncomplicated and complicated GERD.
   2. How do omeprazole and lansoprazole compare in terms of efficacy and cost for the treatment of GERD?
   3. Perform a literature search to evaluate the effects of long-term PPI therapy for the management of GERD. Is the hypergastrinemia associated with long-term acid suppression associated with an increased risk of gastrointestinal cancer?
   4. Discuss the role of fundoplication in the management of GERD. How does it compare to medical management?

▶ Clinical Pearl

GERD can have a profound effect on a patient's quality of life and sense of well-being. In fact, GERD impacts a patient's quality of life more than duodenal ulcer, untreated hypertension, mild congestive heart failure, angina, and menopause.[4]

References

1. Collen MJ, Abdulian JD, Chen YK. Gastroesophageal reflux disease in the elderly: More severe disease that requires aggressive therapy. Am J Gastroenterol 1995;90:1053–1057.

2. DeVault KR, Castell DO. Current diagnosis and treatment of gastroesophageal reflux disease. Mayo Clin Proc 1994;69:867–876.

3. Sandmark S, Carlsson R, Fausa O, et al. Omeprazole or ranitidine in the treatment of reflux esophagitis. Results of a double-blind, randomized, Scandinavian multicenter study. Scand J Gastroenterol 1988;23:625–632.

4. Dimenas E, Glise H, Hallerback B, et al. Quality of life in patients with upper gastrointestinal symptoms: An improved evaluation of treatment regimens? Scand J Gastroenterol 1993:28:681–687.

24 PEPTIC ULCER DISEASE

▶ ## Stamping Out an Infectious Disease   (Level I)

Marie A. Chisholm, PharmD
Mark W. Jackson, MD, FACG

▶ After completing this case study, students should be able to:

- Construct a pharmaceutical care plan and evaluate pharmacotherapeutic outcomes for peptic ulcer disease (PUD) based on patient-specific information.

- Assess anti-ulcer regimens to detect and prevent adverse drug events.

- Understand the role of *Helicobacter pylori* in PUD and recommend appropriate regimens to eradicate this organism.

- Counsel patients suffering from PUD on which medications to avoid.

☀ PATIENT PRESENTATION

Chief Complaint
"My stomach has been hurting for over a month."

HPI
Wylean Cane is a 42 yo woman who presents to the clinic complaining of epigastric pain for over 1 month and feeling weak for 10 days. Her pain is non-radiating and occurs to the right of her epigastrium. This pain occurs daily, wavers in intensity, and increases at night and between meals. The patient states that ingesting food or antacids seems to decrease the severity of the pain. In addition to being constipated for over 1 week, she noticed 4 days ago that she was having black, tarry bowel movements. She does not have any history of PUD or GI bleeding, and has not experienced anorexia, weight loss, nausea, or vomiting.

PMH
HTN × 6 years
Hypothyroidism × 8 years
Type 2 DM × 9 years
Occasional back pain

FH
Her father died at age 77 from colon cancer and her mother died at age 65 from CHF. She has three siblings who are alive and well.

SH
Presently employed as a postal worker. She is married, and she and her husband Arnold have one daughter, Annette, who is 20 years old. She smokes approximately one-half pack of cigarettes per day and drinks two to three cans of beer per week.

Meds
Procardia XL 30 mg po QD
Synthroid 100 mcg po QD
DiaBeta 5 mg po QD
Aspirin 2 tablets PRN back pain (she remembers taking at least 25 tablets over the last month)
Tums 2 tablets po PRN abdominal pain

All
NKDA

ROS
Unremarkable except for complaints noted above

PE

Gen
Well-nourished woman in slight distress

VS
BP 142/82 right arm, seated; P76; RR 16 reg; T 37.5°C; Ht 5'0", Wt 87 kg (80 kg 3 months ago)

Skin
Warm and dry

HEENT
PERRLA; EOMI; discs flat; no AV nicking, hemorrhages, or exudates

Chest
Clear to A & P

CV
S_1 and S_2 normal; no murmurs, rubs, or gallops

Abd
Normal bowel sounds and mild epigastric tenderness; liver size normal; no splenomegaly or masses observed

GU
Pelvic exam normal and uterus is intact. LMP 2 weeks ago

Rect
Non-tender; melenic stool found in rectal vault; stool heme (+)

Ext
Normal ROM

Neuro
CN II–XII intact, DTRs 2+ throughout

Labs

Na 142 mEq/L	Hgb 10.5 g/dL	Ca 10.1 mg/dL
K 4.6 mEq/L	Hct 29%	Mg 2.0 mEq/L
Cl 104 mEq/L	Plt $210 \times 10^3/mm^3$	Phos 4.0 mg/dL
CO_2 26 mEq/L	WBC $7.5 \times 10^3/mm^3$	Alb 4.0 g/dL
BUN 10 mg/dL	MCV 74 μm^3	TSH 2.0 μIU/mL
SCr 1.0 mg/dL	Retic 0.3%	Total T_4 RIA 8.0 μg/dL
FBG 98 mg/dL	Fe 49 μg/dL	Free T_4 1.8 ng/dL

Peripheral Blood Smear

Positive for microcytic anemia

► Questions

Problem Identification

1. a. Create a list of the patient's drug-related problems.
   b. What information (signs, symptoms, tests, and laboratory values) indicates the presence of peptic ulcer disease?

► Clinical Course (Part 1)

An EGD revealed a 7-mm ulcer in the roof of the duodenum (see Figure 24–1). The ulcer base is clear and without evidence of active bleeding. Inflammation of the antrum and the stomach was detected and biopsied. Refer to Figure 24–2 for common anatomic sites of peptic ulcerations.

Desired Outcome

2. What are the goals for treating this patient's PUD?

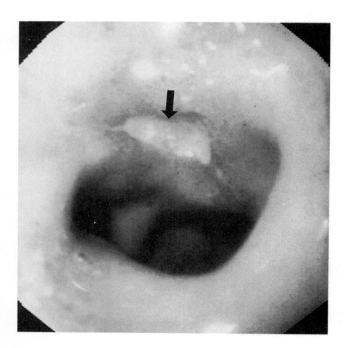

Figure 24–1. Endoscopy showing a 7-mm ulcer in the bulb of the duodenum (arrow).

Therapeutic Alternatives

3. a. Considering this patient's presentation, what non-pharmacologic alternatives are available to treat her PUD?
   b. In the absence of information about the presence of Helicobacter pylori, what pharmacologic alternatives are available to treat duodenal ulcers?

Optimal Plan

4. Based on the patient's presentation and the current medical assessment, design a pharmacotherapeutic regimen to treat her duodenal ulcer and anemia.

Outcome Evaluation

5. What clinical and laboratory parameters are necessary to evaluate the therapy for achievement of the desired therapeutic outcomes and to detect or prevent adverse effects?

Patient Counseling

6. What information should be provided to the patient to ensure successful therapy, enhance compliance, and minimize adverse effects?

► Clinical Course (Part 2)

At the time of endoscopy a biopsy of the gastric mucosa was taken and indicated the presence of inflammation and abundant H. pylori-like organisms (see Figure 24–3).

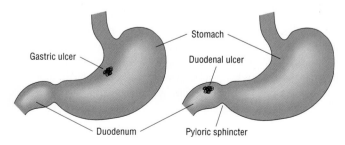

Figure 24–2. Common anatomic sites of peptic ulcers. (Reprinted with permission from Mulvihill ML, Human Diseases: A Systemic Approach, 4th ed. Norwalk, CT, Appleton & Lange, 1995.)

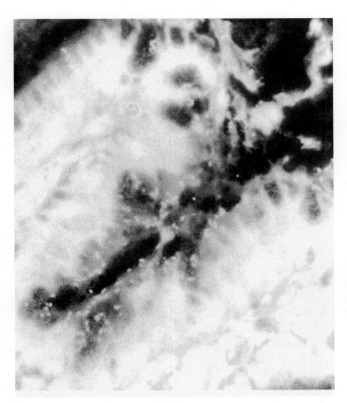

Figure 24–3. *Helicobacter pylori* organisms fluoresce above gastric epithelial cells.

Follow-up Questions

1. *What is the significance of this new finding?*
2. *Based on this new information, how would you modify your goals for treating this patient's PUD?*
3. *What pharmacotherapeutic alternatives are available to achieve the new goals?*
4. *Design a pharmacotherapeutic regimen for this patient's ulcer that will accomplish the new treatment goals.*
5. *How should the PUD therapy you recommended be monitored for efficacy and adverse effects?*
6. *What information should be provided to the patient about her therapy?*

Self-study Assignments

1. Describe the advantages and limitations of diagnostic tests available to detect *H. pylori*.
2. After performing a literature search on *H. pylori* eradication therapy, compare the efficacy of proton pump inhibitors plus *H. pylori* antimicrobial therapy versus H$_2$-receptor antagonists plus *H. pylori* antimicrobial therapy.

Clinical Pearl

Studies have indicated that the 1-year recurrence rates of duodenal ulcer decreases from 70% to 90% with antisecretory agents to <15% after eradication of *H. pylori* infection.

References

1. Peterson WL. *Helicobacter pylori* and peptic ulcer disease. N Engl J Med 1991;324:1043–1048.
2. Graham DY. *Helicobacter pylori*: Its epidemiology and its role in duodenal ulcer disease. J Gastroenterol Hepatol 1991;6:105–113.
3. Soll AH. Consensus conference. Medical treatment of peptic ulcer disease. Practice guidelines. JAMA 1996;275:622–629.

25 STRESS ULCER PROPHYLAXIS/UPPER GI HEMORRHAGE

▶ Prophylaxis Offers No Guarantee (Level I)

Steven V. Johnson, PharmD, BCPS
Christine L. Solberg, PharmD, BCPS, CSPI

▶ After completing this case study, students should be able to:

- Identify risk factors associated with stress gastritis/ulceration and to determine which critically ill patients should receive pharmacologic prophylaxis.
- Provide appropriate pharmacologic alternatives including agent, route of administration, and dose for the prevention of stress induced gastritis/ulceration.
- Identify and implement monitoring parameters for their recommended stress gastritis/ulceration prophylactic regimens.
- Discuss the pharmacologic approaches to the management of stress ulcer-induced bleeding.

☀ PATIENT PRESENTATION

Chief complaint
"Terrible pain everywhere around my stomach"

HPI
Benjamin Jones is a 57 yo man who presents to the ED complaining of increasing abdominal pain over the last 24 hours. He noticed diffuse abdominal pain yesterday that was initially relieved by Percocet that he had left over from a previous prescription. This morning he rated his pain as a 10 on a 1 to 10 scale, with radiation to his back. He reports several vomiting episodes (yellow-green in color) in the last day and that his last BM was about 48 hours ago.

PMH
HTN
CAD; S/P MI 8 years ago

CHF; EF 15% to 20% by transesophageal echocardiogram 4 years ago
COPD
GI bleed secondary to NSAIDs 5 years ago
S/P cholecystectomy
S/P appendectomy

FH
Father died of "heart attack" at age of 55 and mother is in "good health"

SH
Patient is self-employed as a carpenter. Smokes cigarettes 1 ppd, which is down from a couple of years ago. He had previously smoked 2 ppd for 25 years.

ROS
Patient is nauseated with labored breathing; some confusion is noted when speaking with him. No complaints of chest pain, increased weakness, fatigue, or recent weight gain

Meds
Furosemide 40 mg po BID
Digoxin 0.25 mg po QD
Amlodipine 5 mg po QD
Enalapril 10 mg po BID
Atrovent inhaler 2 puffs QID
Albuterol inhaler PRN
Colace 100 mg po BID

All
PCN (hives)

PE

Gen
Middle-aged gentleman in obvious distress with difficulty breathing and significant abdominal pain

VS
BP 105/65, P 120, RR 26, T 37.9°C; Ht 70″, Wt 71 kg

Skin
Warm, dry

Neck/LN
Supple; no JVD or bruits; no lymphadenopathy or thyromegaly

HEENT
PERRL, EOMI; fundi benign; nares patent; TMs intact

LUNG
Decreased breath sounds bilaterally with both inspiratory and expiratory wheezes bilaterally; no rales or rhonchi

CV
S_1, S_2 normal; sinus tachycardia with S_3, S_4

Abd
Firm, with diffuse tenderness to light palpation; no bowel sounds appreciated

Genit/Rect
Normal male genitalia; stool heme negative

Neuro
A & O × 2; somewhat confused

Labs
Na 138 mEq/L	Hgb 14.1 g/d
K 3.8 mEq/L	Hct 40.8%
Cl 101 mEq/L	WBC $10.7 \times 10^3/mm^3$
CO_2 28 mEq/L	Plt $203 \times 10^3/mm^3$
BUN 13 mg/dL	Digoxin 0.5 ng/mL
Scr 1.4 mg/dL	
Glu 160 mg/dL	

ABG
pH 7.26, $Paco_2$ 59 mm Hg, Pao_2 95 mm Hg

Abdominal X-ray
Demonstrates free air

▶ Clinical Course

The patient was taken to the operating room for an exploratory laparotomy and was found to have a perforation of his cecum near the ileocecal valve. The surgeons noted minimal soilage, and the patient underwent a right hemicolectomy with a primary anastamosis. A central line was placed intra-operatively. He received 7 liters of lactated Ringer's solution and 2 units of whole blood during the operation. He was taken to the surgical ICU post-operatively, mechanically ventilated and hemodynamically stable. He received antibiotic prophylaxis with clindamycin 900 mg IV Q 8 H plus aztreonam 1 g IV Q 8 H beginning before surgery and continuing for 24 hours after surgery to prevent surgical wound infection. Six hours post-operatively, his vital signs are BP 120/75, P 95, and CVP 14. Breath sounds are decreased bilaterally with bilateral rales now present. His urine output has been 60 to 80 mL/hr for the past 6 hours.

▶ Questions

Problem Identification

1. a. The resident asks for your recommendations about the patient's chronic medications. Specifically, he would like to know which agents should be restarted post-operatively and why. Secondly, he inquires as to which of these agents are available intravenously.

▶ Clinical Course

Two days post-operatively, the patient is improving but remains mechanically ventilated. Faint bowel sounds are now present but he is still NPO and requiring continuous NG suction. In addition to the medications restarted on your recommendation, he is also receiving lorazepam 4 mg IV Q 6 H, morphine 2 mg/hr by continuous IV infusion, and heparin 5000 unit SQ Q 8 H. Recorded NG aspirate pH 2.0.

   b. List all of the patient's drug related problems at this point in his hospital course (include both potential and actual drug related problems).
   c. What are the risk factors for developing stress gastritis/ulceration in critically ill patients?
   d. Do the risk factors that this patient has warrant prophylactic therapy to prevent stress ulceration?

Desired Outcome

2. What are the goals of pharmacotherapy for prevention of stress gastritis and ulceration?

Therapeutic Alternatives

3. Discuss the pharmacologic options available for the prophylaxis of stress ulceration in critically ill patients.

Optimal Plan

4. What would you recommend for stress ulcer prophylaxis in this patient?

Outcome Evaluation

5. What clinical parameters should be monitored to assess the effectiveness of this regimen?

▶ Clinical Course

The following morning you note that the pH readings for the past two nursing shifts (16 hours) have been 2.0 and 3.0, respectively, on the therapy you recommended. The nurse notes that the NG aspirate is guaiac positive. You check the medication administration record and determine that all prescribed doses of therapy have been administered. Of note, the team thinks that he may be extubated later today with the possibility of moving him to the floor tomorrow. Morning labs: Na 141 mEq/L, K 4.3 mEq/L, BUN 12 mg/dL, SCr 1.5 mg/dL, Glu 180 mg/dL, WBC 11.2 × 10³/mm³, Hgb 11.4 g/dL.

▶ Follow-up Questions

1. Based on the above information, what action should be taken to improve the patient's prophylaxis regimen?

▶ Clinical Course

Bloody NG returns and a drop in BP to 90/50 mm Hg are now noted by the nurse. His HR is 125 bpm, but he remains in NSR. Hgb is 10.1 g/dL. Two 500-mL saline flushes were given and resulted in an increase in his blood pressure to 115/80 mm Hg. His heart rate decreased to 105 bpm. Once he was determined to be hemodynamically stable, an EGD was performed. The gastroenterologist visualized multiple small gastric lesions that are oozing blood.

2. If a saline administration were insufficient to restore the patient's baseline hemodynamic status, what therapy should be administered next?

3. What pharmacologic therapy would you suggest at this time?

▶ Clinical Course

Three days later the NG aspirate has cleared of blood but remains guaiac positive. He has received a total of 3 units of PRBC and is hemodynamically stable and extubated. Active bowel sounds are documented, and enteral feedings have been initiated and are being tolerated at 3/4 of the goal rate. Hgb 11.3 g/dL, BP 135/85 mm Hg, HR 85 to 90 bpm.

4. What medication changes, if any, would you recommend at this time?

▶ Self-study Assignments

1. How should omeprazole be administered to patients who cannot swallow intact capsules? Can it be administered via a nasogastric or nasojejunal feeding tube?
2. Discuss the administration of sucralfate to renally compromised patients who may be at risk for aluminum accumulation.
3. Identify pharmacologic agents whose absorption may be reduced by the concomitant administration of sucralfate.
4. List the dosage adjustments that must be made for H₂-receptor antagonists given to renally compromised patients.
5. Discuss whether or not sucralfate use for stress ulcer prophylaxis decreases the incidence of nosocomial pneumonia in comparison to the use of H₂-receptor antagonists.

▶ Clinical Pearl

For agents administered through a nasogastric tube, check to see if the patient is currently on active suction. If so, NG suction should be held for at least 30 to 60 minutes after the administration of any medication to prevent suctioning out significant amounts of the drug.

References

1. Tryba M, Cook D. Current guidelines on stress ulcer prophylaxis. Drugs 1997;54:581–596.
2. Cook DJ, Fuller HD, Guyatt GH, et al. Risk factors for gastrointestinal bleeding in critically ill patients. Canadian Critical Care Trials Group. N Engl J Med 1994; 330:377–381.
3. Cook D, Guyatt G, Marshall J, et al. A comparison of sucralfate and ranitidine for the prevention of upper gastrointestinal bleeding in patients requiring mechanical ventilation. N Engl J Med 1998;338:791–797.
4. Heiselman DE, Hulisz DT, Fricker R, et al. Randomized comparison of gastric pH control with intermittent and continuous intravenous infusion of famotidine in ICU patients. Am J Gastroenterol 1995;90:277–279.
5. Siepler JK, Trudeau W, Petty DE. Use of continuous infusion of histamine₂-receptor antagonists in critically ill patients. Drug Intell Clin Pharm 1989;23(suppl): S40–S43.

26 ULCERATIVE COLITIS

▶ **The School Teacher's Lament**   (Level I)

Nancy S. Yunker, PharmD
Ralph E. Small, PharmD, FCCP, FASHP, FAPhA

▶ After completing this case study, students should be able to:

- Identify the common signs and symptoms of ulcerative colitis.

- Describe treatment options for an acute episode of ulcerative colitis and recommend a specific treatment plan for a patient that includes the medication, dosing regimen, potential side effects, and monitoring parameters.

- Develop a pharmacotherapeutic plan for an ulcerative colitis patient whose disease is in remission.

- Educate other health care professionals on recent advances in the pharmacotherapy of ulcerative colitis.

☀ PATIENT PRESENTATION

Chief Complaint
"I've got blood in my stool and feel very weak."

HPI
Frederick Johnson is a 31 yo man who presents to the ED with the chief complaint of BRBPR and weakness. He was in his usual state of health until 4 days ago when he noticed BRBPR and an increased frequency of bowel movements (4 to 5 each day). He describes bowel urgency and states that each bowel movement contains approximately 1 tablespoonful of blood; no bleeding is noted between bowel movements. He states that he has been weak for approximately 2 days. He has not traveled outside the city, been hospitalized, or received antibiotics recently.

PMH
HTN

FH
Non-contributory

SH
Works as a school teacher; lives alone. No alcohol; quit smoking 1 year ago.

ROS
Negative for lightheadedness, previous episodes of rectal bleeding or spraying of toilet with blood, N/V, and muscle stiffness/soreness. Positive for occasional mild abdominal soreness.

Meds
Hydrochlorothiazide 25 mg po QD
Felodipine 5 mg po QD

All
Sulfa drugs (rash/hives)

PE

Gen
A & O, pleasant, healthy-appearing Caucasian man in NAD; appears pale

VS
At 8 A.M.:
  BP (lying down) 160/63 mm Hg, P 61 bpm
  BP (standing) 157/65 mm Hg, P 89 bpm
  RR 20 bpm, T 37.0°C, Pulse oximetry 96% on RA
  Wt 81.2 kg (usual weight 83.0 kg), Ht 5′ 8½″

Skin
No lesions; warm, adequate turgor

HEENT
PERRLA; EOMI; negative for iritis, uveitis, and conjunctivitis; funduscopic exam shows no AV nicking, hemorrhages, or exudates; moist mucous membranes; TMs intact

Lungs
CTA, no rales or rhonchi

CV
RRR, normal S_1 and S_2; no S_3, S_4

Abd
BS (+), soft, NTND, no palpable mass, no liver or spleen enlargement

Rectal
Somewhat tender; no hemorrhoids, fissures, or lesions by anoscopy; heme (+)

MS/Ext
No CCE; pulses 2+; normal ROM; normal strength bilaterally

Neuro
A & O × 3; CN II–XII intact; DTRs 2+

Labs
At 8:00 A.M.:

Na 139 mEq/L	Hgb 10.9 g/dL	WBC 6.8×10^3/mm³	AST 32 IU/L
K 3.2 mEq/L	Hct 33.4%	PMNs 52%	ALT 30 IU/L
Cl 92 mEq/L	Plt 298×10^3/mm³	Bands 5%	Alk phos 40 IU/L
CO_2 31 mEq/L	MCV 82 μm³	Lymphs 36%	T. Bili 0.5 mg/dL
BUN 26 mg/dL	MCH 28 pg	Basos 1%	PT 12.0 sec
SCr 1.2 mg/dL	MCHC 32.6 g/dL	Monos 6%	INR 1.0
Glu 162 mg/dL			Ca 8.5 mg/dL
			Po_4 4.4 mg/dL

▶ Clinical Course

The patient received 1 liter of 0.9% saline with KCl 30 mEq over 4 hours starting at 9:00 A.M. Vital signs at 1:00 P.M. were as follows: BP (lying down) 155/82 mm Hg, P 62 bpm; BP (standing) 158/84 mm Hg, P 64 bpm. Repeat laboratory tests at 2:00 P.M. were as follows:

Na 137 mEq/L

K 3.5 mEq/L

Cl 97 mEq/L

CO_2 28 mEq/L

BUN 11 mg/dL

SCr 1.0 mg/dL

Glu 119 mg/dL

Hgb 10.0 g/dL

Hct 31.3%

Plt 262×10^3/mm^3

MCV 82 μm^3

MCH 26.2 pg

MCHC 32 g/dL

WBC 6.2×10^3/mm^3

ED assessment:

1. GI bleed; patient is stable after volume repletion
2. D/C to home with instructions to return to ED or PCP if symptoms return
3. Referral to GI clinic for endoscopy

Follow-up Evaluation

Colonoscopy (2 days after discharge from the ED): Adequate preparation. Diagnoses: (1) edema, erythema, crypt abscesses with mild oozing of blood; continuous from rectum to mid transverse colon, c/w moderate ulcerative colitis; (2) small internal hemorrhoids; (3) biopsy negative for cancer; (4) histology: distorted crypt architecture, mixed acute and chronic inflammation in the lamina propria, PMNs in the surface epithelium; no granulomas noted.

Assessment

Ulcerative colitis

Questions

Problem Identification

1. a. List all of the patient's drug-related problems, including those existing at his initial presentation to the ED.
   b. List the signs, symptoms, and laboratory values that indicate the presence and severity of ulcerative colitis; also include pertinent negative findings.
   c. Could the manifestations of the patient's ulcerative colitis have been precipitated by any event?

Desired Outcome

2. What are the short- and long-term pharmacotherapeutic goals for this patient?

Therapeutic Alternatives

3. a. What non-drug therapies might be useful for this patient?
   b. What feasible pharmacotherapeutic alternatives should be considered for the treatment of ulcerative colitis?

Optimal Plan

4. a. Based on your current assessment of the patient's disease severity, recommend an appropriate drug regimen.
   b. What alternatives should be considered if the patient fails to respond to initial therapy?

Outcome Evaluation

5. What clinical and laboratory parameters are necessary to evaluate the therapy for achievement of the desired therapeutic outcome and to detect or prevent adverse effects?

Patient Counseling

6. What information should be provided to the patient to enhance adherence, ensure successful therapy, and minimize adverse effects?

Clinical Course

The patient successfully completed the initial course of therapy and returns to the physician 8 weeks later for follow up. He states adherence with his therapeutic regimen, describes his bowel habits as normal, and has no complaints of weakness or abdominal/rectal tenderness. The repeat Hgb today is 13.1 g/dL.

Follow-up Questions

1. Considering this new information, what therapeutic intervention(s) do you recommend at this time?
2. What additional information should be provided to the patient?

Self-study Assignments

1. Review the literature comparing mesalamine and sulfasalazine preparations regarding efficacy, adverse effects, and cost.
2. Perform a literature search to determine what new therapies are being evaluated for ulcerative colitis.
3. Conduct a literature search to determine which quality of life instruments have been used to assess ulcerative colitis patients. Write a summary that includes the results that have been reported.

Clinical Pearl

Pentasa and Asacol carry FDA approval for the active treatment of mild to moderate, symptomatic, ulcerative colitis. However, studies have also shown these agents to be effective for maintaining remission of this disease.

References

1. Motley RJ, Rhodes J, Ford GA, et al. Time relationships between cessation of smoking and onset of ulcerative colitis. Digestion 1987;37:125–127.

2. Kornbluth A, Sachar DB. Ulcerative colitis practice guidelines in adults. American College of Gastroenterology, Practice Parameters Committee. Am J Gastroenterol 1997;92:204–211.

3. Sandborn WJ, Tremaine WJ, Offord KP, et al. Transdermal nicotine for mildly to moderately active ulcerative colitis: A randomized, double-blind, placebo-controlled trial. Ann Intern Med 1997;126:364–371.

4. Guyatt G, Mitchell A, Irvine EJ, et al. A new measure of health status for clinical trials in inflammatory bowel disease. Gastroenterology 1989;96:804–810.

5. Thomas GA, Rhodes J, Mani V, et al. Transdermal nicotine as maintenance therapy for ulcerative colitis. N Engl J Med 1995;332:988–992.

27   NAUSEA AND VOMITING

▶ Jill's Bicycle and Other Cycles   (Level II)

Amy J. Becker, PharmD

▶ After completing this case study, students should be able to:

- Develop a regimen of prophylactic antiemetics based on the emetogenic risk associated with cancer chemotherapeutic agents.

- Design a treatment regimen for anticipatory, breakthrough, and delayed nausea and vomiting.

- Design a monitoring plan to assess the effectiveness of an antiemetic regimen.

- Advise patients and caregivers on the reason for antiemetics, their appropriate use, and management of side effects.

- Recommend appropriate alternative antiemetic strategies based on patient-specific conditions such as response to the initial regimen and side effects.

☀ PATIENT PRESENTATION

Chief Complaint
"I've been vomiting for 2 days."

HPI
Jill Jackson is a 36 yo premenopausal woman who comes to the cancer center clinic 2 days after her first cycle of chemotherapy because of nausea and vomiting that started approximately 18 hours after her chemotherapy. She was diagnosed with Stage I infiltrating ductal carcinoma of the right breast 1 month ago and underwent a lumpectomy at that time. The current plan is for her to receive 8 cycles of the revised CMF chemotherapy regimen along with radiation therapy. Revised CMF consists of cyclophosphamide 600 mg/m^2 IV over 1 hour, methotrexate 40 mg/m^2 IV push, and fluorouracil 600 mg/m^2 IV push, all given on the same day and repeated every 21 days. Her antiemetics prior to her first cycle consisted of granisetron 2 mg po and dexamethasone 12 mg po 30 minutes before her chemotherapy. She was given prescriptions for prochlorperazine and lorazepam to be used for breakthrough nausea and vomiting. She states that she did not have the prescriptions filled because she was not expecting to have problems with nausea or vomiting.

PMH
Migraine headaches × 12 years
Lactose intolerance
Appendectomy at age 15

FH
Maternal grandmother had breast cancer, maternal great grandmother had uterine cancer

SH
Married. No children. Works as a journalism instructor at a local college. No alcohol or tobacco use. Physically very active. Runs 18 to 20 miles per week and bicycles to work

ROS
Complains of nausea, vomiting, epigastric discomfort, headache (migraine), fatigue. Denies fever, abdominal pain, diarrhea, change in stool color (i.e., melena), GU complaints, weakness, SOB, numbness or tingling in extremities

Meds
Propranolol LA 80 mg po QD
Midrin 2 po PRN migraine
Calcium carbonate 1.25 g po QD
Phosphate and hydroxyapatite 118 mg (purchased at the local health food store)

All
Sulfa (hives); dairy products (bloating, diarrhea)

PE

Gen
WDWN woman in moderate distress

VS
BP 110/75, P 100, RR 16, T 37°C; Wt 58 kg (60.5 kg 2 days ago), Ht 67"

Skin
Warm, dry, decreased turgor. No rashes or petechiae. Well-healing incisions in R axilla and R breast

HEENT
PERRLA, EOMI, fundi benign, TMs intact, mucous membranes dry

Neck/LN
Thyroid NL. No adenopathy. Post-op scarring R axilla

Lungs/Thorax
Lungs clear to auscultation

Breasts
Post-op scarring on R

CV
RRR, no m/r/g

Abd
Soft, non-tender, no HSM, appendectomy scar

Genit/Rect
Genital exam not done. Rectal NL, stool guaiac negative

MS/Ext
No R arm edema. Pulses 3+ throughout

Neuro
No visual abnormalities, cranial nerves intact, DTRs 2+

Labs
Na 146 mEq/L
K 3.1 mEq/L
Cl 94 mEq/L
CO_2 32 mEq/L
BUN 30 mg/dL
SCr 1.1 mg/dL
Glu 71 mg/dL
T. bili 0.7 mg/dL

Hgb 13.6 g/dL
Hct 43%
Plt $190 \times 10^3/mm^3$
WBC $3.4 \times 10^3/mm^3$
48% PMNs
0% Bands
43% Lymphs
6% Monos
2% Eos
1% Basos

Assessment
Dehydration and hypokalemia secondary to chemotherapy-induced emesis vs. migraine-associated nausea and vomiting

► Questions

Problem Identification

1. a. Create a list of this patient's drug-related problems.
   b. What are this patient's risk factors for nausea and vomiting?

Desired Outcome

2. What are the goals of therapy in this case?

Therapeutic Alternatives

3. a. What non-drug therapies may be useful to prevent nausea and vomiting?
   b. What pharmacologic alternatives may be helpful for the acute treatment of this patient?
   c. What therapeutic alternatives should be considered prior to her next cycle of chemotherapy to prevent future episodes of nausea and vomiting?

Optimal Plan

4. a. Design a plan for the treatment of acute nausea and vomiting in this patient.
   b. Design a plan for the prevention of nausea and vomiting in this patient.

Outcome Evaluation

5. a. State how you will determine whether the antiemetic regimen you recommended for her acute treatment has been effective.
   b. Describe the information you will need to assess the efficacy and adverse effects of the prophylactic antiemetic regimen prior to each future course of chemotherapy.

Patient Counseling

6. How would you counsel this patient on her antiemetic regimen?

► Clinical Course

After treatment according to your recommendations, Mrs. Jackson reports that she has not vomited for several hours and no longer feels nauseated. She will be coming back to the clinic in 3 weeks for her next course of CMF and she is fearful that she will again experience severe nausea and vomiting. In response to your counseling, she states that she feels less anxious. She agrees to take lorazepam prior to her clinic visit and the scheduled antiemetics after her next course of chemotherapy.

When she returns in 3 weeks, her physician follows your advice regarding antiemetics before and after her chemotherapy. Your follow-up phone call the next day confirms that she is taking her medications as instructed. She is experiencing no nausea or vomiting and no side effects of her antiemetics.

► Self-study Assignments

1. Compare the indications and costs of the newest 5-HT_3 antagonist, dolasetron, with ondansetron and granisetron.
2. Perform a literature search on the impact of corticosteroids on control of chemotherapy-induced nausea and vomiting.
3. Develop a plan for educating patients about the potential benefit or harm that could result from their use of unconventional therapies for nausea and vomiting.

► Clinical Pearl

Even though none of the individual components of a chemotherapy regimen are considered highly emetogenic, the combination may increase the potential for nausea and vomiting. When a steroid is included in the chemotherapy regimen, that potential may be decreased.

References

1. Hesketh PJ, Kris MG, Grunberg SM, et al. Proposal for classifying the acute eme-togenicity of cancer chemotherapy. J Clin Oncol 1997;15:103–109.
2. Osoba D, Zee B, Pater J, et al. Determinants of postchemotherapy nausea and vomiting in patients with cancer. Quality of Life and Symptom Control Commit-tees of the National Cancer Institute of Canada Clinical Trials Group. J Clin On-col 1997;15:116–123.
3. Grunberg SM, Hesketh PJ. Control of chemotherapy-induced emesis. N Engl J Med 1993;329:1790–1796.
4. Nolte MJ, Berkery R, Pizzo B, et al. Assuring the optimal use of serotonin antago-nist antiemetics: The process for development and implementation of institu-tional antiemetic guidelines at Memorial Sloan-Kettering Cancer Center. J Clin Oncol 1998;16:771–778.

28 DIARRHEA

▶ Accentuation of Evacuation   (Level I)

Marie A. Abate, PharmD
Charles D. Ponte, BS, PharmD, BCPS, CDE, FAPhA, FASHP, FCCP

▶ After completing this case study, students should be able to:

- Identify the common causes of acute diarrhea.
- Establish primary goals for the treatment of acute diarrhea.
- Recommend appropriate non-drug therapy for patients experiencing acute diarrhea.
- Explain the place of drug therapy in the treatment of acute diarrhea and recommend appropriate products.

☀ PATIENT PRESENTATION

Chief Complaint
"I have diarrhea and I haven't been able to eat because of an upset stomach."

HPI
Linda Cunis is a 28 yo woman who presents to the Family Practice Center with nausea, vomiting, and diarrhea. She had been well until 2 days ago, when she began to experience severe nausea approximately 2 hours after eating three pieces of cheese pizza for supper. The pizza had been ordered from a local restaurant. The nausea persisted, and she subsequently vom-ited three times with some relief. As the evening progressed, she still felt "bad" and took some Maalox to settle her stomach. She began to feel achy and warm. Her temperature at the time was 101.5°F. She has continued to have nausea, vomiting, and a mild fever. She has not tolerated solid foods but has been able to keep down small amounts of fluid. Since yesterday, she has had 6 to 8 liquid stools. She has not noticed any blood in the bowel movements. A friend brought her to the clinic because she was becoming weak and dizzy when she tried to stand up. She denies recent travel, antibi-otics, laxative use, excessive caffeine intake, or an eating disorder.

PMH
Type 2 DM × 5 years

FH
Noncontributory

SH
No tobacco use; drinks an occasional beer socially; has about two cups of coffee daily. Works as a computer software specialist for a local pharmaceu-tical manufacturer. Sexually active with one partner

ROS
Lightheadedness especially upon standing, denies sore throat, ear pain, or nasal discharge. Denies coughing or congestion. Frequent bouts of nausea. Frequent loose stools associated with some cramping. Decreased urination; no pain upon urination. Complains of generalized fatigue, mild aching

Meds
Glyburide 5 mg po BID × 3 years
Metformin 500 mg po TID × 6 months
Multivitamins one po QD
Ortho-Cyclen one po QD

All
Penicillin → maculopapular rash over chest and arms 5 years ago
Molds → watery eyes, sneezing

PE

Gen
Patient is an ill-appearing Caucasian woman in moderate distress.

VS
BP 110/70, P 80 (supine); BP 95/60, P 100 (standing), RR 16, T 38°C; Ht 5'4", Wt 116 lb

Skin
Slightly warm to touch

HEENT
Dry mucous membranes, non-erythematous TMs, PERRLA, no fundus-copic changes, slight erythema in throat

Neck/LN
Without masses, lymphadenopathy, or thyromegaly

Chest
Clear to A & P

CV
RRR without rubs, murmurs or gallops

Abd
Diffuse tenderness, no guarding or rebound, without organomegaly, non-distended, active bowel sounds

Genit/Rect
Gyne exam deferred; slightly heme (+) stool in the rectal vault; no gross blood, small internal hemorrhoids

MS/Ext
Normal muscle strength, no CCE

Neuro
A & O × 3; CN II to XII intact; decreased patellar reflex, otherwise normal reflexes, normal sensory and motor function

Labs

Na 138 mEq/L	Hgb 12.5 g/dL	AST 35 IU/L
K 3.5 mEq/L	Hct 35%	ALT 30 IU/L
Cl 100 mEq/L	Plt $350 \times 10^3/mm^3$	
CO_2 25 mEq/L	WBC $10.0 \times 10^3/mm^3$	
BUN 20 mg/dL	30% PMNs	
SCr 1.1 mg/dL	68% Lymphs	
Glu 200 mg/dL	2% Monos	

UA
Clear, dark amber; SG 1.028; pH 6.0; trace protein; glucose 2+; acetone (−), bilirubin (−), blood (−); microscopic: 0 to 2 WBC/hpf, 0 to 2 RBC/hpf, several hyaline casts

Serum Pregnancy Test
Negative

Assessment
Probable viral gastroenteritis
Diabetes mellitus

Plan
Admit to hospital for observation and acute therapy for diarrhea

▶ Questions

Problem Identification

1. a. Create a list of the patient's drug-related problems.
   b. What signs and symptoms does this woman have that indicate the presence or severity of the diarrhea?
   c. What questions should you ask the patient or members of the medical team to obtain the additional information needed for a complete assessment of this patient?
   d. Could any of this patient's problems have been caused by drug therapy?
   e. What are other possible causes of this patient's diarrhea?

Desired Outcome

2. What are the goals of therapy for this patient?

Therapeutic Alternatives

3. a. What types of non-drug therapy should be considered for this patient?
   b. What feasible pharmacotherapeutic alternatives are available for treatment of diarrhea in this patient?

Optimal Plan

4. What non-drug interventions and specific pharmacotherapeutic regimens would you recommend for treating this patient's diarrhea?

Outcome Evaluation

5. What clinical and laboratory parameters are necessary to evaluate the diarrhea therapy for achievement of the desired outcome and to detect or prevent adverse effects?

Patient Counseling

6. What information should be provided to this patient to enhance adherence, ensure successful therapy, and minimize adverse effects?

▶ Follow-up Questions

1. How should this patient's diabetes be managed while she is being treated in the hospital?
2. What interventions would you recommend for her diabetes control if the patient remains hyperglycemic after resolution of this acute illness and resumption of her normal medications?

▶ Clinical Course

The treatment and monitoring plan you recommended was initiated upon admission to the hospital. The patient's vomiting stopped during the evening of day 1, and the patient had no further episodes of diarrhea past midnight. On the morning of day 2, her orthostasis had resolved, her temperature was normal, the IV fluids were stopped, and she received clear liquids by mouth for breakfast and lunch, with the addition of gelatin and crackers for dinner. Her stool cultures were negative. On day 3, her diet was advanced to solid foods for breakfast, her diabetes medications were restarted, insulin started on admission was discontinued, and the patient was discharged in the late morning.

▶ Self-study Assignments

1. Identify the infectious causes of diarrhea. Design an effective pharmacotherapy treatment regimen for each cause.
2. Provide recommendations for the prevention of traveler's diarrhea.
3. Describe whether or not antidiarrheal products can be safely recommended for use in very young children (<3 yo) and if so, the specific products that could be used.
4. Describe when oral rehydration products should be used, and recommend a specific product and dosage for young or older patients who present with mild to moderate diarrhea and minimal dehydration.

▶ Clinical Pearl

Dehydration and electrolyte imbalances are major concerns with diarrhea, particularly when accompanied by nausea and vomiting; repletion and maintenance of body water and electrolytes are primary treatment goals.

References

1. Camilleri M. Gastrointestinal problems in diabetes. Endocrinol Metab Clin North Am 1996;25:361–378.
2. DuPont HL, Ericsson CD, DuPont MW, et al. A randomized, open-label comparison of nonprescription loperamide and attapulgite in the symptomatic treatment of acute diarrhea. Am J Med 1990;88(suppl 6A):20S–23S.

29 PEDIATRIC GASTROENTERITIS

▶ Dihydrogen Monoxide and Other Critical Elements   (Level II)

William McGhee, PharmD
Basil J. Zitelli, MD, FAAP

▶ After completing this case study, students should be able to:

• Recognize the signs and symptoms of diarrhea with dehydration and be able to assess the severity of the problem.

• Recommend appropriate oral rehydration therapy (ORT) products and treatment regimens for varying degrees of dehydration severity.

• Understand the limited role of antidiarrheal products for the treatment of acute diarrhea in children and be able to educate parents on their appropriate use.

• Properly assess the effectiveness of ORT therapy using both clinical and laboratory parameters.

• Identify the signs and symptoms indicating severe dehydration that requires referral to an ED for immediate IV volume replacement.

☀ PATIENT PRESENTATION

Chief Complaint
James Robinson is a 5-month-old infant who presented to the ED with a 5-day history of fever, vomiting, and diarrhea.

HPI
The patient was in good health when 5 days prior to presentation he felt warm to his mother and did not eat as well as usual. He normally takes between 6 and 8 ounces of Similac with iron formula every 4 to 6 hours. The mother introduced rice cereal into his diet 2 weeks prior to the onset of symptoms. The mother did not take the child's temperature but gave acetaminophen, one dropperful every 6 hours, when he felt warm.

In the evening of the first day of illness, James vomited shortly after feeding. The emesis was nonbloody and nonbilious. He continued to vomit after each feeding for the next three meals and was more irritable than usual. Four days prior to presentation, James developed loose, watery stools after each attempt at feeding and several times between feeds. The stools did not appear to contain blood or mucous.

Vomiting and diarrhea continued, and three days prior to presentation the mother called her pediatrician who recommended 12 hours of clear liquids given in frequent but small amounts. The mother gave a variety of clear liquids, including water, Pedialyte, Jell-O water, and flat Coca-Cola. The vomiting stopped, but the diarrhea continued despite these measures. Fever was intermittent, and the child became more lethargic. The mother continued the clear fluids that her doctor had recommended.

On the day of presentation, the mother stated that James was irritable, sleepy, and had a decreased number of wet diapers. She noted that his lips appeared dry. James is in day care, and other day care mates have had similar illnesses recently. At a doctor's appointment 7 days prior to presentation, his weight was 7.1 kg.

PMH
Born at 37 weeks' gestation; uncomplicated labor, pregnancy, and delivery. Hospitalized at 2 months of age for fever and possible sepsis

ROS
Small patches of eczema over the nape of his neck. History of a heart murmur heard at 2 months of age (mother didn't know what the doctors meant when they called it "innocent"). Immunizations are up-to-date, including hepatitis B vaccine. Development is age-appropriate.

All
No known allergies

FH
Mother is 24 yo, in good health; Father is 26 yo, in good health. A 2 yo sibling recently had diarrhea that lasted for 3 days but had no vomiting or fever.

SH
James lives with his parents and sibling; they have one dog and use a city water supply.

PE

Gen
Patient is ill appearing, lying limply in his mother's lap, sleepy, but arousable.

VS
BP 90/58, P 140, RR 34, T 38.5°C; Weight 6.5 kg

Skin
Pink, decreased skin turgor, capillary refill 2–3 seconds

HEENT
TMs gray and translucent; nose with crusted secretions; lips dry and cracked; tongue dry; anterior fontanelle and eyes sunken

Neck/LN
Normal

Lungs/Thorax
Tachypneic and hyperpneic; no retractions; no crackles or wheezes

Heart
Tachycardia; no murmur noted; pulses were normal

Abd
Scaphoid; active bowel sounds; soft, nontender; no masses or organomegaly

Genit/Rect
Normal circumcised male; testes descended; greenish, watery stool in the diaper

MS/Ext
Normal

Neuro
Sleepy but arousable; irritable when awake; no focal deficits noted

Labs

Na 138 mEq/L	Hgb 13.6 g/dL
K 4.6 mEq/L	Hct 42%
Cl 110 mEq/L	WBC $13.0 \times 10^3/mm^3$
CO_2 13 mEq/L	49% Polys
BUN 24 mg/dL	5% Bands
SCr 0.5 mg/dL	27% Lymphs
Glu 84 mg/dL	17% Monos
	2% Basos

UA
Normal except for specific gravity of 1.028

Assessment
1. Typical viral gastroenteritis, probably rotavirus infection
2. Dehydration with metabolic acidosis

▶ Questions

Problem Identification

1. a. *Create a list of the patient's drug-related problems.*
   b. *What information (signs, symptoms, laboratory values) indicates the presence or severity of gastroenteritis?*

Desired Outcome

2. *What are the goals of pharmacotherapy in this case?*

Therapeutic Alternatives

3. a. *What non-drug therapies might be useful for this patient?*
   b. *What feasible pharmacotherapeutic alternatives are available for treatment of this patient's diarrhea?*

Optimal Plan

4. *What drug(s), dosage forms, schedule, and duration of therapy are best for this patient?*

Outcome Evaluation

5. *What clinical and laboratory parameters should be monitored to evaluate therapy for achievement of the desired therapeutic outcome?*

Patient Counseling

6. *What information should be provided to the child's parents to enhance compliance, ensure successful therapy, and minimize adverse effects?*

▶ Self-study Assignments

1. In children with diarrhea and dehydration, in what circumstances would antimicrobial therapy be considered?
2. What is the role of drug therapy in the prevention of diarrhea when traveling to some foreign countries?
3. What barriers exist to the widespread implementation of ORT, especially by parents? How can these barriers be overcome? (Hint: Explore the advantages of ORT versus IV rehydration therapy.)
4. Write a two-page paper describing the role of the community-based pharmacy practitioner in the care of patients with pediatric gastroenteritis and dehydration.

▶ Clinical Pearl

Oral rehydration therapy is equivalent to IV therapy in rehydrating children with gastroenteritis and mild to moderate dehydration. Oral rehydration therapy is the preferred treatment in these patients, and antidiarrheal and antimicrobial therapies are rarely necessary.

References

1. Duggan C, Santosham M, Glass RI. The management of acute diarrhea in children: Oral rehydration, maintenance, and nutritional therapy. MMWR 1992;41(RR-16):1–20.
2. Provisional Committee on Quality Improvement, Subcommittee on Acute Gastroenteritis. Practice parameter: The management of acute gastroenteritis in young children. Pediatrics 1996;97:424–435.
3. Snyder J. The continuing evolution of oral therapy for diarrhea. Semin Pediatr Infect Dis 1994;5:231–235.

30 CONSTIPATION

▶ **Bound to Be Slow**   (Level I)

Barbara L. Kaltenbach, PharmD
Beth Bryles Phillips, PharmD

▶ After completing this case study, students should be able to:

- Recommend an appropriate pharmacotherapeutic plan for the treatment of constipation.
- Identify medications that can exacerbate constipation.
- Describe the advantages and disadvantages of each class of laxatives.
- Educate patients regarding laxative therapy.

☀ PATIENT PRESENTATION

Chief Complaint
"I'm feeling very full and bloated and I'm having trouble going to the bathroom."

HPI
Eleanor Powell is a 74 yo woman who presents to the geriatric clinic for an initial visit. She complains of infrequent bouts of constipation over the last several years, but claims that the problem has gotten worse over the last several months. She reports often going 5 to 6 days without having a bowel movement and feels that she has to strain most of the time. She was evaluated in the GI clinic 3 weeks ago to determine if other disease states could be causing the constipation. A colonoscopy to rule out irritable bowel syndrome (IBS) and a barium enema to rule out diverticulosis and malignancy were unremarkable. Upon recommendation of the GI pharmacist, she tried Metamucil powder, but after having taken two doses, reports that she could not continue therapy because she didn't like the taste and the powder form.

She also states that she has had heartburn in recent months for which she has been taking an occasional Pepcid AC. She reports using piroxicam for headache occasionally and, rarely, for arthritis-like pain in her hands. She reports feeling less depressed now than she has in the past and states that she uses diazepam for "nerves." She stated that she was started on imipramine for insomnia but it did not work very well, so she started taking two tablets instead of one tablet at bedtime and added OTC Sominex tablets. She admits that she does nap throughout the day and does not get very good sleep at night.

PMH
HTN
Parkinson's disease
Depression with anxiety
H/O difficulty sleeping
S/P total hip replacement 5 years ago
S/P CVA × 2, last episode 5 years ago; no residual deficits
H/O breast cancer, S/P mastectomy 16 years ago
S/P TAH/BSO at age 26

FH
Father and mother both died in their mid-80s of heart disease.

SH
(−) Alcohol or tobacco use; (+) caffeine use, 1 cup of coffee each AM; widowed × 1 year, has 2 daughters, both healthy

ROS
(+) For constipation, bloating, heartburn, occasional headache, and difficulty with sleep. She denies hip pain, dizziness, weakness, or difficulty getting up from a chair.

Meds
Piroxicam 10 mg Q 3 D
Dyazide 1 po BID
K-Dur 20 mEq po BID
Diazepam 2 mg po TID
Permax 0.5 mg po TID
Prozac 20 mg po TID
Imipramine 25 mg po Q HS (patient is actually taking 2 tablets Q HS)
Pepcid AC 10 mg po PRN heartburn
Sominex tablets 1 po PRN sleep

All
IV contrast dye (renal insufficiency)

PE

VS
BP 150/76, P 85, RR 18, T 37.2°C; Ht 62″, Wt 62 kg

Skin
Normal skin turgor and color

HEENT
PERRLA and EOM full without nystagmus, sclerae clear, fundi show flat disks with no hemorrhages or exudates; external auricular canal clear; TMs normal; oropharynx well hydrated, no drooling

Neck/LN
Supple, no lymphadenopathy or JVD; no thyromegaly or bruits

CV
Regular rate and rhythm, normal S_1 and S_2

Pulm
CTA & P

Abd
No hepatomegaly, splenomegaly, or masses; (+) tenderness without evidence of peritonitis; ND; normoactive bowel sounds

Rectal
No fissures, hemorrhoids, or strictures; large amount of stool in rectal vault

MS/Ext

No clubbing, 1+ pretibial edema, intact peripheral pulses, normal ROM in extremities, slight intention tremors in both upper extremities, decreased strength in both LE, no cogwheeling/rigidity

Neuro

Alert and oriented × 3, CN II–XII symmetric and intact, DTRs 2+, cerebellar ataxia, mildly depressed affect; no bradykinesia, dysarthria, postural instability

Labs

Na 137 mEq/L	Hgb 15.7 g/dL
K 3.8 mEq/L	Hct 46%
Cl 99 mEq/L	Plt 252 × 10^3/mm^3
CO_2 24 mEq/L	WBC 7.1 × 10^3/mm^3
BUN 19 mg/dL	Ca 9.3 mg/dL
SCr 1.4 mg/dL	TSH 1.48 μIU/mL
Glu 153 mg/dL	Free T$_4$ 0.89 ng/dL

▶ Questions

Problem Identification

1. a. *Develop a list of this patient's drug-related problems.*
   b. *What signs or symptoms in this patient indicate the presence of constipation?*
   c. *Does the patient have any medical conditions that could contribute to her constipation?*

▶ Clinical Course

A neurology consult to evaluate the past diagnosis of Parkinson's disease took place the same day. The neurologist concluded that her tremors are the result of her past CVAs. Because the patient has no other signs of Parkinson's disease (i.e., no bradykinesia, cogwheel rigidity, postural instability, drooling, and shuffling gait) and Permax had no improvement on the tremors, Parkinson's disease was ruled out. Permax was discontinued.

   d. *What information is necessary to adequately assess a report of constipation by a patient?*

Desired Outcome

2. *What are the goals of pharmacotherapy in treating constipation?*

Therapeutic Alternatives

3. a. *What non-pharmacologic measures can be used to treat constipation?*
   b. *What pharmacotherapeutic alternatives are available for the treatment of constipation?*

Optimal Plan

4. *What would be the most appropriate pharmacologic agent, formulation, dose, schedule, and duration of therapy for this patient?*

Outcome Evaluation

5. *What would you monitor in this patient to ensure that the desired therapeutic outcome has been achieved, and to detect or prevent adverse events?*

Patient Counseling

6. *What information should be provided to a patient receiving a bulk-forming laxative to enhance compliance, ensure successful therapy, and minimize adverse events?*

▶ Follow-up Question

1. *Is the patient's current regimen for insomnia appropriate? What recommendations can you make to optimize this regimen?*

▶ Self-study Assignments

1. Develop pharmacotherapeutic plans for the drug-related problems you identified in question 1a.
2. Suggest an optimal bowel regimen, along with appropriate alternatives, for different patient populations, such as pediatric or pregnant patients.
3. Create a list of drugs that could potentially cause or exacerbate constipation in a patient. Based on what these drugs are likely to be treating, determine what options you have, such as recommending an alternate agent or reducing the dose.
4. Suggest an appropriate bowel regimen and examine its advantages and disadvantages for patients on long-term opiate therapy (e.g., cancer or burn patients), where alternative agents or dosage reductions may not be feasible.

▶ Clinical Pearl

Appropriate diet and exercise play an important role in the treatment and prevention of constipation and should always be a part of the therapeutic plan for a patient with this condition.

Reference

1. Harari D, Gurwitz JH, Minaker KL. Constipation in the elderly. J Am Geriatr Soc 1993;41:1130–1140.

31   CIRRHOTIC ASCITES

▶ A Pint Is a Pound   (Level I)

Joette M. Meyer, PharmD

▶ After completing this case study, students should be able to:

- Identify signs and symptoms of cirrhosis and its complications.
- Develop a diuretic regimen for patients with ascites.
- Recommend appropriate monitoring for the diuretic regimen.
- Counsel patients on pharmacologic and non-pharmacologic therapy to control ascites and prevent further decompensation of their liver disease.

☼ PATIENT PRESENTATION

Chief Complaint
"My belly is swelling up."

HPI
Hector Quintana is a 47 yo Hispanic man with a history of hepatitis C and alcoholic cirrhosis admitted to the hospital from the outpatient clinic with abdominal swelling, 15-pound weight gain over the past 2 weeks, diffuse abdominal pain, fatigue, lethargy, and mild confusion. He has been approved for liver transplantation and is on the waiting list.

PMH
Cirrhosis secondary to alcohol and Hepatitis C diagnosed 5 years ago by liver biopsy
H/O of multiple upper GI bleeds secondary to esophageal varices
H/O spontaneous bacterial peritonitis (SBP) 5 years ago
IDDM

FH
No liver disease; otherwise noncontributory

SH
Recently divorced, living with his teen-age daughter and girlfriend. Unemployed for the past 7 years; previously worked in a liquor store. Receives Medicaid and SSI. History of ethanol abuse, quit 5 years ago. Previously drank three 6-packs of beer/day × 18 years. History of IVDA (heroin), quit 5 years ago

Meds
Human 70/30 Insulin 44 units SQ Q AM and 20 units SQ Q PM
Lactulose 15 mL po QD
H/O interferon-alfa 3 million units SQ 3 times/week × 6 months

All
None

ROS
Increasing abdominal girth and weight gain; vague abdominal pain. No fever, chills, nausea, vomiting, cough, chest pain, or shortness of breath

PE

Gen
Alert and oriented man in NAD; slow to answer questions, poor historian

VS
BP 118/56, P 85, R 20, T 97.2°C; current weight is 61.7 kg, Ht 5′6″

Skin
(+) Spider angiomata on chest, no apparent jaundice

HEENT
Icteric sclera, PERRL, EOMI, TMs intact; O/P moist, no erythema, no lesions

Neck/LN
Supple, (−) JVD; thyroid palpable, no nodules

Chest
CTA bilaterally, good air exchange bilaterally, (+) gynecomastia

CV
RRR, normal S_1 and S_2, no S_3, S_4, or murmurs

Abd
Distended, firm, slightly tender; (+) shifting dullness; hepatomegaly; spleen not palpated; bowel sounds present; no guarding or rebound tenderness

GU/Rect
Heme negative stool, external genitalia normal

MS/Ext
Slight asterixis, no lesions or edema, no palmar erythema, no deficit in extremities

Neuro
A & 0 × 3, slow to answer questions, normal tone and reflexes, CNs grossly intact

Labs

Na 137 mEq/L	Hgb 13.5 g/dL	AST 105 IU/L	T. prot 5.6 g/dL
K 4.4 mEq/L	Hct 39.1%	ALT 87 IU/L	Alb 2.5 g/dL
Cl 108 mEq/L	Plt 83 × 10³/mm³	Alk Phos 224 IU/L	Ca 8.7 mg/dL
CO_2 23 mEq/L	WBC 4.5 × 10³/mm³	LDH 169 IU/L	Mg 1.7 mg/dL
BUN 7 mg/dL	PT 15.6 sec	T. bili 2.7 mg/dL	Phos 2.4 mg/dL
SCr 0.5 mg/dL	PTT 45.4 sec	D. bili 0.9 mg/dL	HCV PCR 9597 copies/mL
Glu 241 mg/dL		HIV negative	AFP 9.8 IU/mL

Child–Pugh Score
11, "C" classification

Diet
Patient has been instructed to follow a 2-g sodium diet, unrestricted protein

Assessment

End-stage liver disease with cirrhosis due to alcohol and hepatitis C complicated by variceal bleeding, SBP and encephalopathy. Now presenting with worsening ascites. R/O recurrent SBP

▶ Clinical Course

A large volume paracentesis was performed and 5 L of fluid was removed. Cell count: 200 WBC with 13% neutrophils; albumin <1.0 g/dL; protein <3.0 g/dL; no growth on culture. A 24-hour urine collection was completed that showed sodium excretion of 50 mEq/day.

▶ Questions

Problem Identification

1. a. Create a list of the patient's drug-related problems.
   b. What information (signs, symptoms, laboratory values) indicates the presence or severity of ascites secondary to liver cirrhosis? (See Figure 31–1.)

Desired Outcome

2. What are the goals of pharmacotherapy for the management of ascites in this case?

Therapeutic Alternatives

3. a. What non-drug therapies might be useful for this patient?
   b. What feasible pharmacotherapeutic alternatives are available for treatment of cirrhotic ascites?

Optimal Plan

4. a. What drug, dosage form, dose, schedule, and duration of therapy are best for this patient?
   b. What pharmacologic alternatives would be appropriate if the initial therapy fails or cannot be used?

Outcome Evaluation

5. What clinical and laboratory parameters are necessary to evaluate the therapy for achievement of the desired therapeutic outcome and to detect or prevent adverse effects?

Patient Counseling

6. What information should be provided to the patient to enhance compliance, ensure successful therapy, and minimize adverse effects?

Additional Case Questions

1. How serious a condition is SBP, and what pharmacologic alternatives are available for its prevention?
2. What pharmacologic alternatives are available for the secondary prevention of variceal bleeding?
3. How can pharmacologic therapy be optimized to control hepatic encephalopathy in this patient?

▶ Self-study Assignments

1. Compare the pharmacokinetics and pharmacodynamics of the diuretics used in the treatment of cirrhotic ascites. Explain the rationale for using furosemide and spironolactone in combination.
2. Discuss the pros and cons of using fluoroquinolone antibiotics as prophylaxis against SBP, and identify high-risk patients who would benefit from this therapy.

▶ Clinical Pearl

Sodium restriction and bedrest alone reduce ascites in only about 10% to 20% of patients. The combination of sodium restriction and diuretics improves ascites in 90% to 95% of patients.

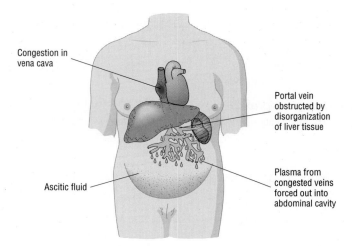

Figure 31–1. Development of cirrhotic ascites.
(Reprinted with permission from Mulvihill ML, Human Diseases: A Systemic Approach, 4th ed. Norwalk, CT, Appleton & Lange, 1995.)

Labels: Congestion in vena cava; Portal vein obstructed by disorganization of liver tissue; Ascitic fluid; Plasma from congested veins forced out into abdominal cavity

References

1. D'Amico G, Morabito A, Pagliaro L, et al. Survival and prognostic indicators in compensated and decompensated cirrhosis. Dig Dis Sci 1986;31:468–475.
2. Runyon BA. Refractory Ascites. Semin Liver Dis 1993;13:343–351.
3. Gatta A, Angeli P, Caregaro L, et al. A pathophysiologic interpretation of unresponsiveness to spironolactone in a stepped-care approach to the diuretic treatment of ascites in nonazotemic cirrhotic patients. Hepatology 1991;14:231–236.

4. Fogel MR, Sawhney VK, Neal EA, et al. Diuresis in the ascitic patient: a random-ized controlled trial of three regimens. J Clin Gastroenterol 1981;3(suppl 1):73–80.

5. Perez-Ayuso RM, Arroyo V, Planas R, et al. Randomized comparative study of ef-ficacy of furosemide versus spironolactone in nonazotemic cirrhosis with ascites. Relationship between the diuretic response and the activity of the renin-aldosterone system. Gastroenterology 1983;84(5 Pt 1):961–968.

6. Roberts LR, Kamath PS. Ascites and hepatorenal syndrome: Pathophysiology and management. Mayo Clin Proc 1996;71:874–881.

7. Bhuva M, Granger D, Jensen D. Spontaneous bacterial peritonitis: An update on evaluation, management, and prevention. Am J Med 1994;97:169–175.

8. Tito L, Rimola A, Gines P, et al. Recurrence of spontaneous bacterial peritonitis in cirrhosis: Frequency and predictive factors. Hepatology 1988;8:27–31.

9. Merkel C, Marin R, Enzo E, et al. Randomised trial of nadolol alone or with isosorbide mononitrate for primary prophylaxis of variceal bleeding in cirrhosis. Gruppo-Triveneto per L'ipertensione portale. Lancet 1996;348:1677–1681.

32 ESOPHAGEAL VARICES

▶ **The Ultimate Price for a Shot and a Beer**   (Level I)

Cesar Alaniz, PharmD

▶ After completing this case study, students should be able to:

- List nonpharmacologic options for the management of patients with bleeding esophageal varices.

- Recommend appropriate pharmacologic therapy for the control of bleeding esophageal varices.

- Provide appropriate patient counseling for patients receiving therapy for portal hypertension.

☀ PATIENT PRESENTATION

Chief Complaint
"I've been vomiting blood since yesterday."

HPI
Bill Rice is a 71 yo man with a history of alcoholic cirrhosis who was in his usual state of health until 3 months ago when he experienced an upper GI bleed that was managed at an outside hospital. According to the patient's wife, an EGD was performed at that time, which revealed esophageal varices. However, the bleeding episode was managed without banding or sclerotherapy. Approximately 2 weeks later, he had a repeat episode of upper GI bleeding and had an EGD performed with successful sclerotherapy. Two weeks ago he was seen in the outpatient clinic for routine evaluation where he had uneventful banding of varices. Now he presents to the ED after hav-ing 2 episodes of hematemesis this afternoon. He describes lightheadedness and weakness, without CP, SOB, melena, BRBPR, or hematuria.

PMH
Cirrhosis s/p variceal bleed × 2
IDDM × 10 years
Osteoporosis (compression fractures)
RLL pneumonia 3 to 4 years ago
6 cm AAA repair 3 to 4 years ago
No history of spontaneous bacterial peritonitis

FH
No history of liver disease, DM, or CAD

SH
Retired factory worker with 4 children. Quit EtOH 12 to 15 years ago; had been drinking 2 or 3 beers with 1 or 2 shots approximately 3 or 4 times per week for many years. Quit smoking 8 years ago; had smoked 1 to 2 PPD prior for many years.

ROS
Negative except for complaint noted above

Meds
Isosorbide dinitrate 10 mg po TID
Prevacid 20 mg po QD
Propranolol 10 mg po TID
NPH Human Insulin 30 units Q AM and 30 units Q PM

All
Amoxicillin → Diarrhea

PE

Gen
Well-nourished male lying comfortably in bed in NAD

VS
BP 139/67, P 107, RR 20, T 99.2°F; no orthostatics performed due to near syncopal episode with standing

HEENT
PERRLA, dry mucous membranes, edentulous posteriorly, telangectasias on nose

Neck/LN
Neck supple, no masses

Lungs/Thorax
Few angiomata with telangiectasias; no caput medusae, no gynecomas-tia

CV
Reg S_1, S_2; no S_3; no MR appreciated

Abd
Soft, no distension. Well-healed midline scar. Moderate-to-large, easily reducible ventral hernia. No palpable or pulsatile masses. No fluid wave, no shifting dullness. Liver edge non-palpable, no splenomegaly detected. No rebound or guarding

Rect
Heme negative at this point

Ext

Warm, 1+ edema, bruises and abrasions on left arm (fell 1 week ago); symmetric pulses

Neuro

A & O × 3, CN II–XII intact, no asterixis

Labs (on admission)

Na 137 mEq/L	Hgb 12 g/dL	AST 33 IU/L	Protein 6.9 g/dL
K 4.9 mEq/L	Hct 35%	ALT 27 IU/L	Alb 3.0 g/dL
Cl 103 mEq/L	WBC $11.3 \times 10^3/mm^3$	Alk phos 36 IU/L	Ca 8.8 mg/dL
CO_2 25 mEq/L	Plt $151 \times 10^3/mm^3$	LDH 274 IU/L	Phos 8.8 mg/dL
BUN 22 mg/dL	aPTT 20.1 sec	T. bili 1.0 mg/dL	
SCr 1.1 mg/dL	PT 13 sec	D. bili 0.1 mg/dL	
Glu 153 mg/dL	INR 1.5		

Chest X-ray

No pulmonary edema

ECG

NSR; no ST changes; no Q waves

Abdominal Ultrasound

Performed the day after admission. There is a small amount of ascites surrounding the liver but there are no focal deep fluid collections of ascites. The spleen is generous in size but of unremarkable echotexture.

Assessment

71 yo male with history of chronic alcohol use, cirrhosis, varices, IDDM, and osteoporosis who presents with upper GI bleed likely variceal in origin

---

▶ Questions

Problem Identification (see Figure 32–1)

1. a. *Create a list of the patient's drug-related problems.*
   b. *What information supports the diagnosis of bleeding esophageal varices, and what indicates the relative severity of disease?*

Desired Outcome

2. *What are the goals for managing this patient's clinical condition?*

Therapeutic Alternatives

3. a. *What non-pharmacologic interventions should be considered for this patient (see Figure 32–2)?*
   b. *What pharmacologic interventions should be considered for this patient's current condition?*

Optimal Plan

4. *What pharmacotherapeutic plan should be outlined for managing the patient's current problems?*

Outcome Evaluation

5. *What clinical and laboratory parameters should be followed to evaluate therapeutic interventions and to minimize the risk of adverse effects?*

Patient Counseling

6. *What information should be provided to the patient about his medication therapy?*

▶ Self-study Assignments

1. Compare the pharmacy costs of continuous infusions of octreotide, vasopressin, and vasopressin plus nitroglycerin.
2. Describe how β-blocking agents and nitrates decrease portal hypertension.

▶ Clinical Pearl

When used for management of bleeding esophageal varices, continuous infusion doses of octreotide greater than 50 µg/hr should not be used because they have not been studied in clinical trials.

References

1. Saeed ZA, Stiegmann GV, Ramirez FC, et al. Endoscopic variceal ligation is superior to combined ligation and sclerotherapy for esophageal varices: A multicenter prospective randomized trial. Hepatology 1997;25:71–74.
2. Grace ND. TIPS: The long and short of it. Gastroenterology 1997;112:1040–1043.
3. Bernard B, Lebrec D, Mathurin P, et al. Beta-adrenergic antagonists in the prevention of gastrointestinal rebleeding in patients with cirrhosis: A meta-analysis. Hepatology 1997;25:63–70.

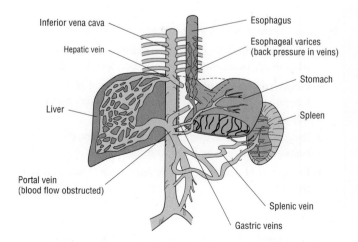

Figure 32-1. Anatomic relationships among intestinal veins affected by alcoholic cirrhosis. *(Reprinted with permission from Mulvihill ML, Human Diseases: A Systemic Approach, 4th ed. Norwalk, CT, Appleton & Lange, 1995.)*

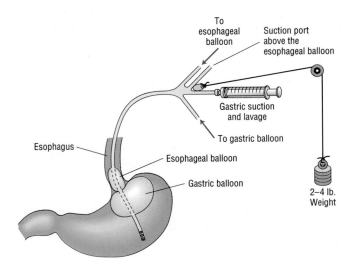

Figure 32-2. Sengstaken–Blakemore tube. A gastric balloon is inflated with 200 to 300 mL air and weights pull it snugly against the gastroesophageal junction. Then the esophageal balloon is inflated with 50 to 200 mL ait to produce tamponade with a balloon pressure of 30 to 40 mm Hg. Gastric suction is possible with the balloon inflated. Suction above the esophageal balloon prevents bronchopulmonary aspiration of oral secretions. *(Reprinted with permission from Gitnick G, et al. Principles and Practice of Gastroenterology and Hepatology, 2nd ed. Norwalk, CT, Appleton & Lange, 1994.)*

33   HEPATIC ENCEPHALOPATHY

▶ **People, Places, and Time**   **(Level I)**

Nancy P. Lam, PharmD, BCPS

▶ After completing this case study, students should be able to:

- Identify and correct the precipitating factors associated with the development of hepatic encephalopathy in a cirrhotic patient.
- Recommend appropriate non-pharmacologic and pharmacologic intervention for a cirrhotic patient who develops hepatic encephalopathy.
- Design a plan for monitoring the efficacy and adverse effects of recommended treatments for hepatic encephalopathy.
- Provide patient counseling for those receiving treatment for hepatic encephalopathy.

☀ PATIENT PRESENTATION

Chief Complaint (obtained from patient's daughter)
"Dad is very confused and not able to recognize anyone at home."

HPI
Michael Perez is a 55 yo Spanish-speaking man who was brought to the ED by his daughter because of confusion and disorientation. The daughter states that her father was well until about 2 days ago when he became confused about time and place. This morning, the patient could not respond to her questions appropriately, and he did not recognize her.

PMH
End-stage liver disease (ESLD) diagnosed 5 years ago secondary to chronic viral hepatitis C and heavy alcohol use. He has been admitted multiple times for hepatic encephalopathy, uncontrolled ascites, and esophageal variceal bleeding.

FH
Father died at age 50 from liver disease of unknown etiology; mother died of heart disease. One brother is alive and well.

SH
Unemployed. History of heavy alcohol use, quit 5 years ago when ESLD was diagnosed. History of IVDU 20 years ago. Divorced with two daughters and a son. Lives with the daughter who brought him to the hospital

ROS
Confused; no apparent pain or discomfort

Meds
Spironolactone 100 mg po QD
Furosemide 40 mg po QD
MVI 1 tablet po QD
Propranolol 20 mg po BID
Lactulose 30 mL po BID
Lorazepam 1 mg po Q HS
Ibuprofen 400 mg po Q 6 H PRN pain
Patient has a history of noncompliance with his diet and medications.

All
No known drug or food allergies

PE

Gen
Cachectic, dehydrated, and jaundiced Hispanic male who is disoriented to time, place and people

VS
BP 118/70, P 83 (supine); BP 90/60, P 105 (standing); RR 20, T 38°C; Ht 5′5″, Wt 60 kg (per patient's daughter)

Skin
Decreased skin turgor; dry; jaundiced; spider angiomata on face and upper body; (+) palmar erythema

HEENT
PERRLA; TMs intact; EOMI; fundi benign; dry mucous membranes; icteric sclerae

Lungs
Decreased breath sounds in left lower lobe

CV

RRR; S_1 and S_2 normal; no S_3 or S_4

Abd

Soft, non-tender; (+) fluid wave; prominent veins observed on abdomen; massive girth; liver palpable 9 cm below the right costal margin; spleen not palpable

Rect

Heme (−) stool

Ext

2+ pitting edema to the knees in both LE; good pulses throughout

Neuro

Confused; not oriented to time, place and people; (+) asterixis; CN II–XII intact; DTRs 2+

Labs

Na 130 mEq/L	Hgb 10.0 g/dL	WBC $5.0 \times 10^3/mm^3$	AST 57 IU/L	Ca 8.9 mg/dL
K 2.8 mEq/L	Hct 28%	48% PMNs	ALT 69 IU/L	Mg 1.2 mg/dL
Cl 108 mEq/L	MCV 76 μm^3	2% Bands	Alk phos 151 IU/L	Phos 4.5 mg/dL
CO_2 24 mEq/L	MCHC 30%	3% Eos	T. bili 2.4 mg/dL	PT 15.7 sec
BUN 40 mg/dL	Retic 0.3%	38% Lymphs	D. bili 0.6 mg/dL	aPTT 40 sec
SCr 1.5 mg/dL	Plt $70 \times 10^3/mm^3$	9% Monos	Alb 2.3 g/dL	
Glu 90 mg/dL			NH_3 100 $\mu g/dL$	

Assessment

Hepatic encephalopathy

► Questions

Problem Identification

1. a. Create a list of the patient's drug-related problems.
   b. What information presented indicates the presence of hepatic encephalopathy in this patient?
   c. What precipitating factors in this patient could potentially cause hepatic encephalopathy?
   d. What additional information is needed to satisfactorily assess the hepatic encephalopathy of this patient?

Desired Outcome

2. What are the general principles for the management of hepatic encephalopathy and desired therapeutic outcomes?

Therapeutic Alternatives

3. a. What non-drug interventions are important before initiating pharmacotherapeutic agents for the treatment of hepatic encephalopathy?
   b. What pharmacotherapeutic alternatives are available for the treatment of hepatic encephalopathy? Include the mechanism of action of each drug in your answer.

Optimal Plan

4. Outline a pharmacotherapeutic plan that is most suitable for this patient. Include the drug, dosage form, dose, schedule, and duration of treatment.

Outcome Evaluation

5. How would you monitor the efficacy and adverse effects of the treatment you recommended? (See Figure 33–1.)

► Clinical Course

Five days after beginning treatment with the regimen you recommended, the patient is responding positively, and the dose has been titrated appropri-

Number Connection Test 1.

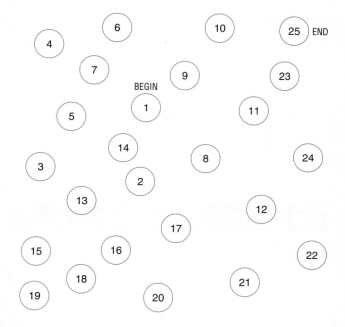

Figure 33–1. Number Connection Test part A (NCT-A): Measures cognitive motor abilities. Subjects have to connect the numbers printed on paper consecutively from 1 to 25, as quickly as possible. Errors are not counted, but patients are instructed to return to the preceding correct number and then carry on. The test score is the time the patient needs to perform the test, including the time needed to correct all errors. A low score represents a good performance. *(Reprinted with permission from reference 4.)*

ately. He is oriented to time, place, and people, and only slight asterixis is detected. The plan is to discharge the patient home tomorrow.

Patient Counseling

6. *What medication-related information should be provided to the patient about his therapy upon discharge?*

▶ Self-study Assignments

1. Perform a literature search to assess the efficacy and the potential role of flumazenil in the treatment of hepatic encephalopathy.
2. List the amino acid contents in the commercially available oral and parenteral formulations of branched-chain amino acid products; determine the cost of these products in your area.

▶ Clinical Pearl

The development of acute encephalopathy in a cirrhotic patient is usually associated with one or more precipitating factors. Identification and prompt correction of them are important components of the management of hepatic encephalopathy.

References

1. Cordoba J, Blei AT. Treatment of hepatic encephalopathy. Am J Gastroenterol 1997;92:1429–1439.
2. Riordan SM, Williams R. Treatment of hepatic encephalopathy. N Engl J Med 1997;337:473–479.
3. Fabbri A, Magrini N, Bianchi G, et al. Overview of randomized clinical trial of oral branched-chain amino acid treatment in chronic hepatic encephalopathy. JPEN 1996;20:159–164.
4. Quero JC, Schalm SW. Subclinical hepatic encephalopathy. Semin Liver Dis 1996;16:321–328.

34 ACUTE PANCREATITIS

▶ Cuts Like a Knife   (Level II)

Charles W. Fetrow, PharmD
Maria Yaramus, PharmD

▶ After completing this case study, students should be able to:

- Recognize signs, symptoms, and laboratory abnormalities commonly associated with acute pancreatitis.
- Describe potential systemic complications associated with acute pancreatitis.
- Recommend appropriate analgesic, nutritional, and enzyme therapy for patients with acute pancreatitis.
- Outline monitoring parameters to assist in realization of desired pharmacotherapeutic outcomes.

☀ PATIENT PRESENTATION

Chief Complaint
"It feels like I've got a knife through my stomach."

HPI
Gerald Sherman is a 59 yo man who presents to the ED because of intense mid-epigastric pain radiating to the back. He states that he has had sharp, intermittent epigastric/abdominal pain for 3 to 4 weeks, which has been increasing in severity and duration over the last 3 days.

PMH
Pneumonia 4 years ago that resolved with appropriate antimicrobial therapy
S/P open-reduction internal fixation of left femur secondary to MVA 18 years ago

FH
Father died at age of 75 from complications related to CVA; mother approximately 70 years of age, alive and well. One brother, also alive and without significant illness

SH
Married with 2 children. Employed as an electrician. Denies any smoking or alcohol consumption

Meds
Multiple vitamin 1 po QD
Extra-strength Tylenol several doses per day started recently PRN pain

All
NKDA

ROS
States that he has been feeling "overheated" and has experienced periodic bouts of nausea and vomiting for the past 3 to 4 days. Also describes an approximate 15-pound weight loss over the past 2 months secondary to anorexia and intense postprandial pain. He has noted a reduction in the frequency of bowel movements. No complaints of diarrhea or blood in the stool; no knowledge of any prior history of uncontrolled blood sugars

PE

Gen
The patient seems restless and in moderate distress but otherwise is a well-appearing, well-nourished male who looks his stated age.

VS
BP 100/68, P 118, RR 30, T 38.5°C; Wt 68 kg, Ht 5'8"

HEENT
PEERLA, EOMI, oropharynx pink and clear, oral mucosa dry

Skin
Dry with poor skin turgor; some skin tenting noted

Neck/LN
Supple; no bruits, lymphadenopathy, or thyromegaly

Cor
Sinus tachycardia; no murmurs, rubs, or gallops

Lungs
Bilateral basilar rales

Abd
Mildly distended with active but diminished bowel sounds; (+) guarding; pain is elicited on light palpation of mid-epigastric region. No rebound tenderness, masses, or HSM.

Ext
Extremities are warm and well perfused. Good pulses present in all extremities.

Rect
Normal sphincter tone; no bright red blood or masses visible; stool is guaiac negative; prostate may be slightly enlarged.

Neuro
Patient is A & O × 3; neuro exam essentially benign; CN II to XII intact; strength is equal bilaterally in all extremities.

Labs

Na 130 mEq/L	Hgb 18 g/dL	AST 349 IU/L	Ca 8.0 mg/dL
K 3.9 mEq/L	Hct 52%	ALT 154 IU/L	Mg 1.8 mEq/L
Cl 95 mEq/L	WBC $16.2 \times 10^3/mm^3$	Alk phos 275 IU/L	Phos 2.3 mg/dL
CO_2 23 mEq/L	Neutros 70%	LDH 225 IU/L	Trig 1182 mg/dL
BUN 32 mg/dL	Bands 5%	T. bili 0.7 mg/dL	Repeat Trig 1021 mg/dL
SCr 1.4 mg/dL	Eos 1%	Alb 3.3 g/dL	
Glu 399 mg/dL	Basos 1%	Prealb 19 mg/dL	
	Lymphs 21%	Amylase 2244 IU/L	
	Monos 2%	Lipase 1548 IU/L	

UA
Color yellow; turbidity clear; SG 1.010; pH 7.0; glucose >1000 mg/dL; bilirubin (−); ketones (−); Hgb (−); protein (−); nitrite (−); crystals (−); casts (−); mucous (−); bacteria (−); urobilinogen: 0.2 EU/dL; WBC 0–5/hpf; RBC 0/hpf; epithelial cells: 0–10/hpf

Chest X-ray
AP view of chest shows the heart to be normal in size. The lungs are clear without any infiltrates, masses, effusions, or atelectasis

Abd Ultrasound
Non-specific gas pattern; no dilated bowel. Questionable opacity/abnormality of common bile duct. Cannot rule out gallstone/obstruction

ECG
Sinus tachycardia; rate 140 bpm

Assessment
Acute pancreatitis precipitating hyperglycemia
R/O choledocholithiasis

▶ Questions

Problem Identification (see Figure 34–1)

1. a. *What signs, symptoms, and laboratory tests are consistent with the diagnosis of acute pancreatitis?*
   b. *What are the likely etiologies that may explain the development of acute pancreatitis in this case?*
   c. *Construct a drug-related problem list for this patient.*

Desired Outcome

2. *What are the desired goals of therapy for this patient?*

Therapeutic Alternatives

3. *What therapies may be instituted to achieve the goals outlined above? Provide a rationale for each therapy.*

Optimal Plan

4. *Develop a pharmacotherapeutic care plan for this patient.*

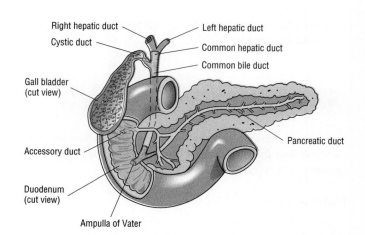

Figure 34-1. Anatomic relationship between the pancreas and other digestive organs. *(Reprinted with permission from Mulvihill ML. Human Diseases: A Systemic Approach, 4th ed. Norwalk, CT, Appleton & Lange, 1995.)*

Outcome Evaluation

5. *Outline monitoring parameters for efficacy and adverse effects of therapy for pain management.*

▶ Clinical Course

TPN is instituted after 24 hours. After several days of improvement in the hospital, the patient develops a WBC count of $20.4 \times 10^3/mm^3$ with neutrophils 77%, bands 11%, eosinophils 1%, basophils 0%, lymphocytes 7%, and monocytes 4%. He has a temperature of 39.8°C and is noted to be orthostatic (BP 128/76 sitting, 98/60 standing) with a glucose of 675 mg/dL. He has also experienced several episodes of diarrhea and steatorrhea.

▶ Follow-up Questions

a. *What potential etiologies might explain this patient's fever and relapsing acute pancreatitis?*
b. *What are the new treatment goals for this patient?*
c. *Given this new information, what therapeutic interventions should be considered for this patient?*
d. *How should these new therapies be monitored for efficacy and adverse effects?*

Patient Counseling

6. *The patient is being discharged today after a prolonged hospital course. The attending physician would like you to talk with the patient about his discharge medications. What information should be provided?*

▶ Self-study Assignments

1. Describe the pathophysiology through which autodigestion of the pancreas occurs.
2. Investigate the experimental use of CCK-receptor blockers, octreotide, and cytokine antagonists for their potential to improve outcomes related to acute pancreatitis.
3. Compose a list of drugs thought to aggravate or give rise to drug-induced pancreatitis.

▶ Clinical Pearl

More expensive microencapsulated pancreatic enzyme products have not consistently been shown to be superior to standard therapeutic doses of the less expensive, non-enteric coated dosage forms.[4]

References

1. Steinberg W, Tenner S. Acute pancreatitis. N Engl J Med 1994;330:17:1198–1210.
2. Pederzoli P, Bassi C, Vesentini S, et al. A randomized multicenter clinical trial of antibiotic prophylaxis of septic complications in acute necrotizing pancreatitis with imipenem. Surg Gynecol Obstet 1993;176:480–483.
3. Lankisch PG. Enzyme treatment of exocrine pancreatic insufficiency in chronic pancreatitis. Digestion 1993;54 (suppl 2):21–29.
4. Tenner S, Levine RS, Steinberg WM. Drug treatment of acute and chronic pancreatitis. In: Lewis JH, ed. A Pharmacologic Approach to Gastrointestinal Disorders. Baltimore, Williams & Wilkins, 1994:311–340.

35 VIRAL HEPATITIS

▶ The Lady With the Ankle Tattoo   (Level I)

Nancy P. Lam, PharmD, BCPS

▶ After completing this case study, students should be able to:

- Develop a treatment plan for patients with chronic hepatitis.
- Evaluate the clinical and laboratory end points for treatment of chronic hepatitis C.
- Develop a plan for monitoring efficacy and adverse effects of interferon treatment in chronic hepatitis C.
- Provide patient counseling for patients with chronic hepatitis C receiving interferon treatment.

PATIENT PRESENTATION

Chief Complaint
"I was told that my liver tests are abnormal."

HPI
Jean Berry is a 35 yo woman with no significant past medical history except for hypothyroidism. She has been referred by her family doctor to the liver clinic for assessment of her abnormal liver enzymes. The patient states that she has been very healthy and that her thyroid problem has been well controlled. Her only complaint is occasional fatigue, which she attributes to her busy work schedule. She has no past history of liver problems, except that about 2 years ago she was told that she had elevated liver tests, but no further work-up was done at that time.

PMH
Hypothyroidism
Blood transfusion 15 years ago after an MVA

FH
No known family history of liver disease. Both parents and two siblings are alive and well.

SH
Married for 3 years; no children. Non-smoker; denies illicit drug or inhalant use; denies heavy use of alcohol. Employed as a marketing manager for a computer firm, which requires occasional travel to the Far East

ROS
Denies any signs or symptoms of liver diseases except for occasional fatigue. No changes in urine color or history of icteric sclerae or skin

Meds

Levothyroxine 0.1 mg po QD
MVI 1 tablet po QD

All

No known drug or food allergies

PE

Gen

Obese woman in NAD

VS

BP 110/80, P 70, RR 18, T 37.1°C; Wt 75 kg; Ht 5'3"

Skin

No obvious icterus; no spider angiomata or palmar erythema

HEENT

PERRLA; EOMI; sclerae anicteric; funduscopic exam normal; TMs intact

Neck/LN

Neck supple; no lymphadenopathy or thyromegaly; no carotid bruits

Lungs

Normal breath sounds

CV

RRR, S_1, S_2 normal; no S_3 or S_4

Abd

Liver span 10 cm; spleen not palpable; no evidence of ascites

MS/Ext

No CCE; peripheral pulses 2+ throughout; normal ROM; a small tattoo close to the left ankle

Neuro

A & O × 3; CN II–XII intact; DTRs 2+

Labs

Obtained 2 weeks ago from patient's family physician:

Na 140 mEq/L	Hgb 12.5 g/dL	TSH 1.5 μIU/mL
K 3.9 mEq/L	Hct 36.9%	HIV negative
Cl 102 mEq/L	Plt $200 \times 10^3/mm^3$	
CO_2 24 mEq/L	WBC $8.0 \times 10^3/mm^3$	
BUN 12 mg/dL	68% PMNs	
SCr 1.0 mg/L	1% Bands	
Glu 120 mg/dL (non-fasting)	23% Lymphs	
	8% Monos	

Liver function tests and hepatitis screen values were compared with those obtained about 2 years ago:

	2 Years Ago	2 Weeks Ago
AST	80 IU/L	100 IU/L
ALT	60 IU/L	110 IU/L
GGT	40 IU/L	45 IU/L
Alk phos	93 IU/L	96 IU/L
T. bili	0.5 mg/dL	0.6 mg/dL
PT	12.4 sec	12.3 sec
Alb	3.7 g/dL	3.7 g/dL
ANA	Not done	(−)
HBsAg	(−)	(−)
Anti-HAV	Not done	(−)
Anti-HCV	(+)	(+)
HCV RNA (bDNA assay)	Not done	3.4 mEq/mL
HCV genotype	Not done	1b

Liver Biopsy

Performed 2 weeks ago. Moderate degree of fibrosis and inflammation consistent with chronic hepatitis.

Assessment

Chronic hepatitis C

▶ Questions

Problem Identification

1. a. Create a list of patient's drug-related problems.
   b. What physical findings, laboratory values, or medical history information suggests the presence of chronic hepatitis C virus (HCV) infection?

Desired Outcome

2. What are the goals of treatment of chronic HCV infection?

Therapeutic Alternatives

3. a. What non-pharmacologic measures should be considered for this patient?

   b. What pharmacotherapeutic alternatives are available for treatment of this patient?
   c. Does this patient have any concurrent medical conditions that are considered contraindications to receiving the treatments discussed in the previous question?

Optimal Plan

4. a. Design a pharmacotherapeutic plan for this patient. Include the drug, dose, schedule, and duration of therapy.
   b. Outline a plan for vaccination against other forms of viral hepatitis for this patient.

Outcome Evaluation

5. a. How should the therapy you recommended be monitored for efficacy and adverse effects?

b. *Which baseline parameters of this patient have been suggested as predictors of poor response to the treatment you recommended?*

c. *What actions can be taken if the patient develops intolerable adverse effects to the treatment you recommended?*

Patient Counseling

6. *What information should be provided to this patient regarding her treatment?*

▶ Clinical Course

Ms. Berry has been on the treatment you recommended for 12 weeks. Overall, she tolerates the treatment well without any significant adverse effects. The laboratory tests from her week 12 visit revealed the following: AST 90 IU/L, ALT 100 IU/L, and qualitative HCV RNA test (+).

▶ Follow-up Question

1. *Based on this new information, what changes, if any, would you recommend for the treatment of chronic hepatitis C for this patient?*

▶ Self-study Assignments

1. Estimate the cost of a 12-month course of interferon treatment for chronic hepatitis C. Include the cost of syringes and needles, monthly clinic visits, and laboratory tests.

2. Perform a literature search to compare the differences in the biological properties of interferon alfacon-1 versus interferon alfa-2a and 2b.

3. Perform a literature search on the efficacy of interferon in the treatment of acute hepatitis C infection. Write a brief paper summarizing the results, and provide your conclusion about the effectiveness of this treatment.

▶ Clinical Pearl

The course of chronic hepatitis C infection and treatment response can be adversely affected by alcohol consumption. Patients should limit consumption to less than one drink per day, and total abstinence from alcohol is strongly recommended.

References

1. National Institutes of Health Consensus Development Conference Panel Statement. Management of hepatitis C. Hepatology 1997;26(suppl 1):2S–10S.
2. Poynard T, Leroy V, Cohard M, et al. Meta-analysis of interferon randomized trials in the treatment of viral hepatitis C: Effects of dose and duration. Hepatology 1996;24:778–789.
3. Davis GL, Lau JY. Factors predictive of a beneficial response to therapy of hepatitis C. Hepatology 1997;26(3 suppl 1):122S–127S.
4. Keeffe EB, Hollinger FB, Consensus Interferon Study Group. Therapy of hepatitis C: Consensus interferon trials. Hepatology 1997;26(3 suppl 1):101S–107S.

SECTION 4 ··

Renal and Genitourinary Tract Disorders

Gary R. Matzke, PharmD, FCP, FCCP, Section Editor

36 DRUG-INDUCED ACUTE RENAL FAILURE

▶ **Unintended Consequences**   (Level II)

  Mary K. Stamatakis, PharmD

▶ After completing this case study, students should be able to:

- Evaluate common clinical and laboratory findings in a patient with acute renal failure.

- Develop a pharmacologic plan for the treatment of acute renal failure.

- Assess appropriateness of aminoglycoside serum concentrations in relation to efficacy and toxicity.

- Provide recommendations to prevent development of aminoglycoside-induced acute renal failure.

- Adjust dosage regimens, as appropriate, based on a patient's creatinine clearance.

☀ PATIENT PRESENTATION

Chief Complaint
Not available

HPI
The renal consult team has been asked to see James Edwards, a 71 yo man who originally presented to the hospital with symptoms of CHF which neces-sitated aortic and mitral valve replacement surgery. His surgery was compli-cated by a 1-hour hypotensive episode, with BP as low as 70/50. Three days post-op, the patient was found to have purulent drainage from the surgical site that required reexploration of the sternal incision site and mediastinal debridement. At this time, the patient was also found to have a Serratia bac-teremia (blood cultures × 4 positive for *Serratia marcescens,* sensitive to gentamicin, piperacillin, and ciprofloxacin) and presumed mediastinitis and was started on gentamicin and piperacillin. He has currently completed day 25 of a 6-week course of antibiotics for presumed *Serratia* mediastinitis. An increase in BUN and creatinine from baseline and volume overload have been noted over the past week. He is now 28 days post-surgery.

PMH
Type 2 DM
Gout
HTN
Atrial fibrillation

FH
Father with type 2 DM

SH
(−) Smoking, occasional EtOH, retired coal miner (9 years ago)

ROS
Currently complains of cough, trouble breathing, arthritis, and difficulty sleeping. No fever or chills

Meds
Gentamicin IVPB × 25 days (see table for dosages)
Piperacillin 3 g IVPB Q 4 H × 25 days
Colace 100 mg po BID
Prazosin 2 mg po TID

Furosemide 40 mg IV Q 12 H × 2 days
Digoxin 0.25 mg po QD
Allopurinol 100 mg po QD
Ranitidine 150 mg po Q 12 H
Meperidine 25 mg IM Q 4–6 H PRN
Sliding scale insulin

All
NKDA

PE

Gen
A & O × 3

VS
BP 154/70, P 80, RR 26, T 37.7°C, Current Wt 84 kg (baseline Wt 78 kg), Ht 69″

HEENT
PERRLA, EOMI, poor dentition

Neck/LN
(−) JVD

Chest
Basilar crackles, inspiratory wheeze

CV
S_1, S_2, normal, no S_3, irreg rhythm

Abd
Soft, non-tender, (+) BS, (−) HSM

Genit/Rect
(−) Masses

MS/Ext
2+ Ankle/sacral edema

Neuro
Grossly intact, no focal deficits noted

Labs (Current)

Na 138 mEq/L   Hgb 9.0 g/dL   Ca 8.5 mg/dL
K 3.8 mEq/L   Hct 27.5%   Mg 2.0 mg/dL
Cl 104 mEq/L   Plt 263 × 10^3/mm³   Phos 4.7 mg/dL
CO_2 25 mEq/L   WBC 9.9 × 10^3/mm³
BUN 52 mg/dL   (BUN 15 mg/dL on admission)
SCr 3.2 mg/dL   (SCr 1.3 mg/dL on admission)
Glu 146 mg/dL

			Renal Function and Gentamicin Serum Concentrations During Hospitalization			
Post-op Day	SCr (mg/dL)	BUN (mg/dL)	Gentamicin Conc. Peak[a]	(μg/mL) Trough[b]	Gentamicin Dosages	
3	1.4	15			160 mg × 1, then 120 mg Q 12 H	
5	1.2	22	4.5	1.2	↑ to 160 mg Q 12 H	
7	1.4	21				
10	1.4	22	8.1	2.1	↓ to 240 mg Q 24 H	
14	1.2	21				
17	1.4	26	9.6	1.0	↓ to 180 mg Q 24 H	
21	1.7	27				
24	2.4	38	7.4	2.6	↓ to 180 mg Q 48 H	
26	2.9	44				
28	3.2	52				

[a] Levels drawn 30 minutes after a 30-minute infusion.
[b] Levels drawn immediately before the next dose.

I/O and Daily Weights		
Day	I/O	Wt (kg)
3 days ago	3100 mL/1100 mL	N/A
2 days ago	3250 mL/1050 mL	83
Yesterday	2850 mL/1250 mL	N/A
Today	N/A	84

UA
Color, yellow; character, hazy; glucose (−); ketones (−); SG 1.020; pH 5.0; protein 30 mg/dL; coarse granular casts 5–10/lpf; WBC 5–10/hpf; RBC 2–5/hpf; no bacteria; nitrite (−); blood small; osmolality 325 mOsm; urinary sodium 77 mEq/L; creatinine 63 mg/dL.

Assessment
Acute renal failure and volume overload

Plan
Monitor creatinine daily to assess change in renal function. Fluid restriction and maximize IV diuretics to put him in negative fluid balance. He needs to lose 6 to 7 kg body water to return to his usual weight of 78 kg.

Questions

Problem Identification

1. a. *Create a list of the patient's drug-related problems.*
   b. *What information (signs, symptoms, laboratory values) indicates the presence or severity of each problem?*
   c. *What additional laboratory information would assist in the assessment of this patient?*
   d. *Could any of the patient's problems have been caused by drug therapy?*
   e. *What risk factors did the patient have for gentamicin-induced acute renal failure?*

Desired Outcome

2. *What are the goals of pharmacotherapy in this case?*

Therapeutic Alternatives

3. a. *What non-drug therapies might be useful for this patient?*
   b. *What pharmacotherapeutic alternatives are available for treatment of the acute renal failure in this patient?*

Optimal Plan

4. *What drug recommendations are optimal at this point?*

Outcome Evaluation

5. *What clinical and laboratory parameters are necessary to evaluate the therapy for achievement of the desired therapeutic outcome and to detect or prevent adverse effects?*

Patient Counseling

6. *What information should be provided to the patient to enhance compliance, ensure successful therapy, and minimize adverse effects?*

Additional Case Questions

1. *Based on the patient's creatinine clearance of 21 mL/min, do any of his medications require dosage adjustment?*
2. *What therapeutic interventions can decrease the likelihood of developing gentamicin-induced nephrotoxicity?*
3. *When assessing fractional excretion of sodium (FE_{Na}), what influence do previous dosages of furosemide have on interpretation of the results?*

▶ Self-study Assignments

1. Based on the original set of gentamicin plasma concentrations obtained (peak 4.5 μg/mL drawn 30 minutes after a 30 minute infusion, trough 1.2 μg/mL drawn immediately before the next dose) on the dosing regimen of gentamicin 120 mg IVPB Q 12 H, calculate his pharmacokinetic parameters and determine an appropriate dosage regimen for Mr. Edwards that would have avoided elevated trough concentrations.
2. Develop a treatment plan to minimize the occurrence of a drug–drug interaction between gentamicin and piperacillin.

3. Review the literature to determine if once-daily dosing of aminoglycosides has been shown to decrease the incidence of nephrotoxicity.
4. Calculate the appropriate dosage of digoxin for this patient given a trough digoxin concentration of 2.7 ng/mL.

▶ Clinical Pearl

There is a strong correlation between aminoglycoside clearance and creatinine clearance. If a patient's renal function deteriorates, a similar decline will be seen in aminoglycoside clearance.

References

1. Appel GB. Aminoglycoside nephrotoxicity. Am J Med 1990;88(suppl 3C): 16S–20S.
2. Matzke GR, Frye RF. Drug administration in patients with renal insufficiency. Minimizing renal and extrarenal toxicity. Drug Saf 1997;16:205–231.
3. Ellison DH. The physiologic basis of diuretic synergism: Its role in treating diuretic resistance. Ann Intern Med 1991;114:886–894.
4. Chertow GM, Sayegh MH, Allgren RL, et al. Is the administration of dopamine associated with adverse or favorable outcomes in acute renal failure? Am J Med 1996;101:49–53.
5. Lam YW, Banerji S, Hatfield C, et al. Principles of drug administration in renal insufficiency. Clin Pharmacokinet 1997;32:30–57.

37 PROGRESSION OF CHRONIC RENAL DISEASE

▶ The American Patient   (Level III)

Reina Bendayan, PharmD
Winnie M. Yu, PharmD, BCPS

▶ After completing this case study, students should be able to:

- Differentiate acute renal failure from chronic renal failure.
- Identify risk factors for progression of renal disease.
- Recognize potential comorbid or pathologic conditions that are frequently associated with chronic renal insufficiency.
- Recommend non-pharmacologic and pharmacologic interventions to alter the rate of progression of renal disease.
- Counsel a patient on the common medications prescribed for chronic renal insufficiency.

☼ PATIENT PRESENTATION

Chief Complaint
"I'm here to check the results of my urine test."

HPI

Rob Brandon is a 52 yo man with diabetes mellitus who visited his PCP 2 weeks ago for a routine examination. His laboratory tests revealed a serum creatinine of 1.6 mg/dL, which was elevated over his baseline of 1.3 mg/dL 1 year ago. A 24-hr urine collection was performed last week, and he was scheduled to return to clinic today for further evaluation of his kidney function. He states that he has not been checking his blood glucose at home because his machine is not working. However, he asserts that he has been taking his medications faithfully.

PMH

Type 2 DM × 16 years (failed glyburide, currently on insulin)
HTN × 2 years
Hypercholesterolemia × 5 years (non-compliant with diet)

FH

His father had DM and died in an MVA 3 years ago; his mother had HTN and died at the age of 50 secondary to MI.

SH

A high school teacher, married with 1 child (24 yo). No tobacco use but occasional alcohol (2 or 3 beers on weekends). Usual diet includes eggs and sausages for breakfast, turkey sandwiches for lunch, and pasta and salad for dinner

ROS

Occasional headaches; no c/o polyuria, polydipsia, polyphagia, sensory loss, or visual changes. No dysuria, flank pain, hematuria, pedal edema, CP, or SOB

Meds

Humulin N 35 units SQ Q AM, 20 units SQ Q PM (for 5 years)
Humulin R 12 units SQ Q AM, 8 units SQ Q PM
Hydrochlorothiazide 25 mg po QD (× 2 years)
Pravastatin 40 mg po QD (× 5 years; on current dose for 1 year)
Acetaminophen 650 mg po Q 6 H PRN headaches

All

Sulfa (anaphylaxis)

PE

Gen

The patient is a moderately obese African-American man in NAD

VS

BP 150/95 sitting and standing in both arms, HR 76, RR 16, T 37.2°C; Wt 88.5 kg, Ht 5'8"

Skin

Warm, dry

HEENT

PERRLA, EOMI, fundi revealed microaneurysms consistent with diabetic retinopathy, no retinal edema or vitreous hemorrhage. TMs intact. Oral mucosa moist with no lesions

Neck/LN

Supple; no cervical adenopathy or thyromegaly

Lungs/Thorax

CTA

CV

Heart sounds are normal

Abd

NT; no masses or organs palpable. No abdominal bruits

Gent/Rect

Normal rectal exam; prostate benign; heme (−) stool

MS/Ext

No CCE

Neuro

A & O × 3; CNs intact; normal DTRs

Labs (2 weeks ago, fasting)

		Fasting Lipid Profile
Na 140 mEq/L	Hgb 12.2 g/dL	T. chol 225 mg/dL
K 4.8 mEq/L	Hct 36.5%	Trig 135 mg/dL
Cl 108 mEq/L	WBC $10.8 \times 10^3/mm^3$	LDL 152 mg/dL
CO_2 26 mEq/L	Plt $148 \times 10^3/mm^3$	HDL 46 mg/dL
BUN 27 mg/dL	Ca 9.3 mg/dL	
SCr 1.6 mg/dL	Phos 2.5 mg/dL	
Glu 194 mg/dL	Uric acid 6.9 mg/dL	
$HgbA_{1c}$ 9%		

UA (1 wk. ago)

1+ glucose, (−) ketones, > 3+ protein, (−) leukocyte esterase & nitrite; (−) RBC; 2–5 WBC/hpf

24-Hour Urine Collection

Total urine volume 2.1 L, urine creatinine 60 mg/dL, urine albumin 680 mg/24 hr

Assessment

52-year-old man newly diagnosed with diabetic nephropathy

► Questions

Problem Identification

1. a. *Create a list of the patient's drug-related problems.*
   b. *What are the signs and symptoms of diabetic nephropathy, diabetes mellitus, hypertension, and hypercholesterolemia in this patient?*
   c. *Calculate this patient's creatinine clearance (CLcr in mL/min) using the following data: 1) baseline CLcr from 1 year ago; 2) current CLcr using the SCr from 2 weeks ago; 3) current CLcr using the data from the 24-hr urine collection.*

Discuss whether (2) and (3) provide good estimates of the patient's GFR.

Desired Outcome

3. *What are the goals of pharmacotherapy for the management of the patient's renal insufficiency, diabetes, hypertension, and hypercholesterolemia?*

Therapeutic Alternatives

3. a. *What non-pharmacologic therapies might be useful to control this patient's medical conditions?*
   b. *What are the pharmacotherapeutic alternatives for the prevention of renal disease progression and the management of diabetes mellitus, hypertension, and hyperlipidemia in this patient?*

Optimal Plan

4. *What drug regimens would provide optimal therapy for this patient's current medical problems?*

Outcome Evaluation

5. *Outline the clinical and laboratory parameters necessary to evaluate the efficacy and safety of the recommended regimens for the patient's nephropathy, diabetes mellitus, hypertension, and hypercholesterolemia.*

Patient Counseling

6. *What information should be provided to the patient to ensure successful therapy and minimize adverse effects of the antihypertensive and insulin therapy?*

► Clinical Course

The plan you recommended is implemented, and the patient returns to his PCP 1 month later. His blood pressure is 145/90 mm Hg (sitting and standing) and HR is 90 bpm. He has no new complaints and reports tolerating his new medications well. He also states that he has been watching his diet and has been using Cardia Salt (46% NaCl, 54% K/Mg salt) in his meals for the last 5 days. His laboratory results are BUN 30 mg/dL, SCr 1.6 mg/dL, Na 142 mEq/L, K 5.4 mEq/L, Cl 110 mEq/L, CO_2 28 mEq/L, Glu 135 mg/dL.

► Follow-up Questions

1. *What new or persistent drug-related problems does this patient have?*
2. *What changes, if any, would you recommend in the patient's drug regimen?*

► Self-study Assignments

1. Discuss the role of diuretic therapy in patients with normal renal function compared to those with creatinine clearance values <20 mL/min.
2. Review and compare the effects of antihypertensive agents on renal blood flow and glomerular filtration rate in patients with hypertension and diabetic nephropathy.

► Clinical Pearl

Normotensive patients with type 2 diabetes and persistent microalbuminuria should be treated with an ACE inhibitor to slow the progression of diabetic nephropathy.

References

1. Walser M. Assessing renal function from creatinine measurements in adults with chronic renal failure. Am J Kidney Dis 1998;32:23–31.
2. Pedrini MT, Levey AS, Lau J, et al. The effect of dietary protein restriction on the progression of diabetic and nondiabetic renal diseases: A meta-analysis. Ann Intern Med 1996;124:627–632.
3. Klahr S, Levey AS, Beck GJ, et al. The effects of dietary protein restriction and blood pressure control on the progression of chronic renal disease. Modification of Diet in Renal Disease Study Group. N Engl J Med 1994;330:877–884.
4. Midgley JP, Matthew AG, Greenwood CM, et al. Effect of reduced dietary sodium on blood pressure: A meta-analysis of randomized controlled trials. JAMA 1996; 275:1590–1597.
5. Joint National Committee on Prevention, Detection, Evaluation, and Treatment of High Blood Pressure. The sixth report of the Joint National Committee on Prevention, Detection, Evaluation, and Treatment of High Blood Pressure. Arch Intern Med 1997;157:2413–2446.
6. Stefanick ML, Mackey S, Sheehan M, et al. Effects of diet and exercise in men and postmenopausal women with low levels of HDL cholesterol and high levels of LDL cholesterol. N Engl J Med 1998;339:12–20.

38 END-STAGE RENAL DISEASE

► A Return to the Machine   (Level II)

James D. Coyle, PharmD

► Upon completing this case study, students should be able to:

- Assess all available information to identify medication-related problems in an end-stage renal disease patient on hemodialysis.
- State the desired therapeutic outcomes of each problem.
- List therapeutic alternatives for managing each problem.
- Develop a plan for managing each problem that includes plans for monitoring patient response to interventions.
- Outline a plan for helping the patient understand and effectively implement medication-related interventions.

☼ PATIENT PRESENTATION

Chief Complaint
"My kidney doesn't work anymore."

HPI

John Brooks is a 64 yo man who presented to the outpatient dialysis center for staff-assisted hemodialysis. His ESRD is secondary to a congenital kidney defect and long-standing HTN. He received a cadaveric renal transplant approximately 15 years ago, but the transplant has recently been rejected. He had an AV Gore-Tex graft placed in his left forearm 17 days prior to this first dialysis session.

PMH

Congenital kidney defect diagnosed at age 19 as a result of a HTN work-up. He was dialyzed for 3 years prior to his transplant 15 years ago.

FH

Mother died of cancer at age 93. Status of father unknown. Two brothers in good health. Three daughters in good health.

SH

Lives by himself. Employed full-time doing light maintenance work (currently on sick-leave). Relates that his daughters "care about me, but don't do enough to help me out." Occasional social alcohol use. Minimal caffeine consumption. No tobacco use.

ROS

Negative except for dry, itchy skin; feeling tired and weak over past several weeks; loss of appetite, with frequent N & V over past week; constipation; and swelling in feet and lower legs. No other complaints related to central or peripheral nervous system or cardiovascular system. Wears glasses for reading and driving.

Meds

Atenolol 50 mg po QHS
Paxil 10 mg ½ tab po QD
Restoril 30 mg po QHS

All

PCN (upper body rash after oral PCN approximately 10 years ago)

PE

Gen

The patient is a WDWN African-American man in NAD who appears his stated age.

VS

BP 170/100, P 82, RR 16, T 98.3°F; Ht 70″, Wt 72.5 kg

Skin

Dry, scaly arms and legs are noted

Ext

Mild bilateral foot/ankle edema
The remainder of the PE was WNL.

Labs

Na 142 mEq/L	Hgb 9.3 g/dL	AST 16 IU/L	T. chol 228 mg/dL	Iron 90 μg/dL
K 5.3 mEq/L	Hct 27.9%	ALT 21 IU/L	HDL 33 mg/dL	TIBC 275 μg/dL
Cl 110 mEq/L	RBC $3.41 \times 10^6/mm^3$	LDH 371 IU/L	LDL 149 mg/dL	T. sat. 33%
CO_2 20 mEq/L	MCV 81.7 μm³	Alk phos 124 IU/L	Chol/HDL 6.9	Ferritin 349 ng/mL
Anion gap 18	MCHC 33.4%	T. bili 0.5 mg/dL	Trig 229 mg/dL	Aluminum 14 μg/L
BUN 120 mg/dL	WBC $6.9 \times 10^3/mm^3$	D. bili 0.3 mg/dL	Ca 8.6 mg/dL	PTH 1835 pg/mL
SCr 9.2 mg/dL		T. prot 6.1 g/dL	Phos 7.4 mg/dL	Osm 308 mOsm/kg
Glu 85 mg/dL		Alb 3.6 g/dL	Urate 5.5 mg/dL	

Mr. Brooks' nephrologist provided the following dialysis prescription:

Dialyze 3.5 hours per session, 3 times per week
Dry weight: 67.5 kg
Dialyzer: Fresenius F80
Blood flow rate: 400 mL/min
Dialysate flow rate: 500 mL/min
Dialysate: Bicarbonate
Na 145 mEq/L, K 2.0 mEq/L, Ca 2.5 mEq/L, HCO_3^- 35 mEq/L
Heparin: 2000 unit bolus, then 500 units/hr until 1 hour before termination

---

▶ Questions

Problem Identification

1. a. *Create a list of this patient's medication-related problems.*
   b. *What information (signs, symptoms, laboratory values) indicates the severity of this patient's end-stage renal disease?*

Desired Outcome

2. *State the goal of pharmacotherapy with respect to each problem identified.*

Therapeutic Alternatives

3. *What therapeutic options are available for each of this patient's*

medication-related problems? Indicate the advantages and disadvantages of each option.

Optimal Plan

4. Which of the available therapeutic options identified in question 3 would you recommend for this patient? Provide a rationale for each recommendation. Include the name, dosage form, dose, schedule, and duration of therapy for any drugs recommended.

Outcome Evaluation

5. What clinical and/or laboratory parameters would you recommend to evaluate the desired and undesired consequences of each of your recommended interventions?

Patient Counseling

6. What information should be provided to the patient to enhance compliance, ensure successful therapy, and minimize adverse effects?

▶ Self-study Assignments

1. Assume that Mr. Brooks presents as above except that his serum iron is 45 μg/dL, serum ferritin is 72 ng/mL, MCV is 70 μm^3, and MCHC is 27%. Develop a therapeutic plan, including a monitoring plan, to treat his anemia under this scenario.
2. Compare the content and cost of a variety of water-soluble vitamin supplements appropriate for use by ESRD patients. Select the product you would recommend for use by your patients.
3. Mr. Brooks has a form of dyslipidemia that is commonly seen in ESRD patients (borderline-high cholesterol, slightly low HDL, borderline-high LDL, cholesterol/HDL ratio indicating increased risk, and borderline-high triglycerides). Assess the clinical significance of this dyslipidemia and, if appropriate, your recommendations for its treatment.
4. Assume that Mr. Brooks develops an infection that requires tobramycin. Develop a therapeutic plan for the use of tobramycin in this patient, including a monitoring plan.

▶ Clinical Pearl

Epoetin is an important but not sufficient requirement for normal red blood cell production—ya gotta have iron, too!

References

1. NKF-DOQI clinical practice guidelines for the treatment of anemia of chronic renal failure. National Kidney Foundation—Dialysis Outcomes Quality Initiative. Am J Kidney Dis 1997;4(suppl 3):S192–S240.
2. Gennari FJ, Rimmer JM. Acid–base disorders in end-stage renal disease. Semin Dial 1990;3:81–85.
3. Summary of the second report of the National Cholesterol Education Program (NCEP) Expert Panel on Detection, Evaluation, and Treatment of High Blood Cholesterol in Adults (Adult Treatment Panel II). JAMA 1993;269:3015–3023.
4. Fishbane S, Ungureanu VD, Maesaka JK, et al. The safety of intravenous iron dextran in hemodialysis patients. Am J Kidney Dis 1996;28:529–534.
5. Felsenfeld AJ. Considerations for the treatment of secondary hyperparathyroidism in renal failure. J Am Soc Nephrol 1997;8:993–1004.
6. Robertson KE, Mueller BA. Uremic pruritus. Am J Health-Syst Pharm 1996;53:2159–2170.

39 RENAL TRANSPLANTATION

▶ Frank's New Kidney   (Level II)

Marie A. Chisholm, PharmD
Tana R. Bagby, PharmD
Laura Mulloy, DO

▶ After completing this case study, students should be able to:

- Develop therapeutic plans for the complications associated with renal transplantation.
- Counsel renal transplant patients about the importance of adhering to their medication regimens.
- Counsel renal transplant patients on medication therapy and possible adverse effects to medications.
- Assess renal transplant patients to detect adverse drug events.

⚬ PATIENT PRESENTATION

Chief Complaint
"I'm just here for my regular check-up."

HPI
Franklin Parks is a 61 yo man who presents to the renal transplant clinic today for a routine clinic visit.

PMH
6 months S/P cadaveric renal transplantation
ESRD secondary to polycystic kidney disease diagnosed 15 years ago
HTN × 25 years
Hypothyroidism × 3 years

FH
Mother is 78 yo with HTN; father died in 1981 from renal failure secondary to PCKD. Mr. Parks is married and has 3 sons who are alive and well.

SH
Drinks 2 beers per week. He does not smoke cigarettes but has a history of intermittent tobacco use. He has no history of IVDA.

ROS
Unremarkable

Meds
Cyclosporine 250 mg po BID (last dose taken last night at 2000)
Prednisone 10 mg po QD
Mycophenolate mofetil 1500 mg po BID

Levothyroxine 0.15 mg po QD
Procardia XL 60 mg po QD

All
NKDA

PE

Gen
WDWN African-American male in NAD.

VS
BP 164/86 right arm, seated; P 90 reg; RR 21; T 38.3°C; Ht 68″, Wt 89 kg

Skin
Warm and dry

HEENT
PERRLA; EOMI; disks flat, no AV nicking, hemorrhages, or exudates

Chest
CTA & P

CV
Normal S_1 and S_2; no m/r/g

Abd
Soft, NT, with a palpable, nontender graft with no bruit; liver size normal

Ext
No CCE; normal ROM

Neuro
A & O × 3; CN II–XII intact; DTRs 2+ throughout

Labs
At 0800 today:

Na 140 mEq/L	Ca 8.9 mg/dL	WBC $8.1 \times 10^3/mm^3$	CSA 305 ng/mL^a
K 4.1 mEq/L	UA 6.0 mg/dL	Neutros 64%	*Fasting Lipid Profile*
Cl 103 mEq/L	Hgb 17.8 g/dL	Lymphs 24%	T. chol 260 mg/dL
CO_2 27 mEq/L	Hct 51%	Monos 10%	HDL-C 50 mg/dL
BUN 20 mg/dL	RBC $5.39 \times 10^6/mm^3$	Eos 1%	LDL-C 192 mg/dL
SCr 1.2 mg/dL	Plt $196 \times 10^3/mm^3$	Basos 1%	Trig 90 mg/dL
FBS 125 mg/dL			

^{a} Cyclosporine monoclonal fluorescence polarization immunoassay (FPIA) on whole blood (therapeutic range 150 to 400 ng/mL)

Assessment
Post-renal transplant erythrocytosis

▶ Questions

Problem Identification

1. a. Create a list of the patient's drug-related problems.
   b. What information (signs, symptoms, laboratory values) indicates the presence or severity of post-transplant erythrocytosis?

Desired Outcome

2. What are the goals of pharmacotherapy for this patient?

Therapeutic Alternatives

3. a. What non-drug therapies might be useful for this patient?
   b. What feasible pharmacotherapeutic alternatives are available for treating the post-transplant erythrocytosis?
   c. What feasible pharmacotherapeutic alternatives are available for treating the patient's dyslipidemia?

Optimal Plan

4. Based on the patient's presentation and the current assessment, design a pharmacotherapeutic regimen to treat this patient's erythrocytosis and dyslipidemia.

Outcome Evaluation

5. What clinical and laboratory parameters are necessary to evaluate the therapy for achievement of the desired therapeutic outcome and to detect or prevent adverse effects?

Patient Counseling

6. What information should be provided to the patient about his medication therapy to enhance compliance, ensure successful therapy, and minimize adverse effects?

▶ Clinical Course

The treatment plan you recommended was implemented. Two months later, Mr. Parks returns complaining that his hands have been shaking uncontrollably for the last 2 days.

Meds
Cyclosporine 250 mg po BID (last dose taken last night at 2000)
Prednisone 10 mg po QD
Mycophenolate mofetil 1500 mg BID
Levothyroxine 0.15 mg QD
Procardia XL 60 mg po QD
Enalapril 5 mg po QD
Lovastatin 20 mg po QD
Tagamet HB 100 mg, 6 to 8 tablets daily PRN heartburn

PE
Unremarkable except for tremors in his upper extremities

VS
BP 150/78, P 90, RR 21, T 38.3°C, Wt 89 kg

Labs

At 0800 today:

Na 143 mEq/L	Hgb 15.6 g/dL	Ca 8.2 mg/dL
K 4.4 mEq/L	Hct 47%	CSA 432 ng/mL
Cl 98 mEq/L	RBC $4.98 \times 10^6/mm^3$	
CO_2 26 mEq/L	Plt $180 \times 10^3/mm^3$	
BUN 21 mg/dL	WBC $7.5 \times 10^3/mm^3$	
SCr 1.4 mg/dL		
FBS 114 mg/dL		

▶ Follow-up Questions

1. *Based on this new information, can you propose any potential cause for the patient's tremors?*
2. *Design a pharmacotherapeutic plan to resolve the patient's tremors.*
3. *What clinical or laboratory parameters should be monitored?*
4. *What new information should be provided to the patient about his medications?*

▶ Self-study Assignments

1. Write a paper describing the most promising treatments for post-renal transplant erythrocytosis.
2. Write a paper describing the efficacy and safety of daclizumab, cyclosporine, and prednisone therapy compared to cyclosporine and prednisone therapy for preventing kidney transplant rejection.

▶ Clinical Pearl

Post-renal transplant erythrocytosis occurs in up to 22% of renal transplant patients and can result in serious thrombotic complications.

References

1. Lezaic V, Djukanovic LJ, Pavlovic-Kentera V, et al. Factors inducing posttransplant erythrocytosis. Eur J Med Res 1997;2:407–412.
2. Gaston RS, Julian BA, Curtis JJ. Posttransplant erythrocytosis: An enigma revisited. Am J Kidney Dis 1994;24:1–11.
3. Perazella MA, Bia MJ. Posttransplant erythrocytosis: Case report and review of newer treatment modalities. J Am Soc Nephrol 1993;3:1653–1659.
4. MacGregor MS, Rowe PA, Watson MA, et al. Treatment of postrenal transplant erythrocytosis. Long-term efficacy and safety of angiotensin-converting enzyme inhibitors. Nephron 1996;74:517–521.
5. Expert Panel on Detection, Evaluation, and Treatment of High Blood Cholesterol in Adults. Summary of the second report of the National Cholesterol Education Program (NCEP) expert panel on detection, evaluation, and treatment of high blood cholesterol in adults (adult treatment panel II). JAMA 1993;269:3015–3023.
6. Midtvedt K, Stokke ES, Hartmann A. Successful long-term treatment of posttransplant erythrocytosis with losartan. Nephrol Dial Transplant 1996;11:2495–2497.

40 CHRONIC GLOMERULONEPHRITIS

▶ Annie Brown's Battle With Lupus (Level III)

Melanie S. Joy, PharmD

▶ After completing this case study, students should be able to:

- Identify the risk factors for renal disease progression in a patient with lupus induced glomerulonephritis.
- Recognize laboratory and urinalysis abnormalities associated with lupus nephritis.
- Identify treatment options that are available for lupus-induced diffuse proliferative glomerulonephritis.
- Recognize the clinical significance of glucocorticoid-induced complications and recommend appropriate treatment options.
- Provide patient counseling regarding drug therapy for lupus nephritis and its complications.

☀ PATIENT PRESENTATION

Chief Complaint
"I have pain in my hips and lower back."

HPI
Annie Bryant is a 23 yo woman with a history of diffuse proliferative glomerulonephritis (DPGN) due to SLE, which decreased in activity after two courses of IV cyclophosphamide (10 and 6 years ago). During recent follow-up nephrology clinic appointments, urinalyses have demonstrated recurrent microscopic hematuria.

PMH
Lupus-induced DPGN × 10 years
History of oligomenorrhea
HTN
Hypercholesterolemia
Recent quantitative bone mineral density revealed decreased density of the spine and hip
S/P tonsillectomy as a child

SH
The patient works as an executive assistant. She drinks alcohol socially. There is no history of tobacco or illicit drug use.

FH
Paternal grandmother and two aunts also have SLE. No family history of DM, HTN, CVA, or MI

ROS
Complains of arthralgias and pain around the hip and lower back. Denies rash, fever, chills, nausea, vomiting, symptoms of Raynaud's phenomenon, pleuritic chest pain, or shortness of breath

Meds
Prednisone 15 mg po QD (with fluctuating doses over the past 10 years)
Atenolol 25 mg po QD
Clonidine patch 0.2 mg weekly

All
Gemfibrozil (rash) and cefadroxil ("swelling")

PE

Gen
WDWN Caucasian woman in NAD

VS
BP 160/115, P 64, RR 18, T 36.5°C; Wt 49 kg

Skin
Small papules over the PIPs and MCPs of first and second digits bilaterally. No alopecia

HEENT
NC/AT; clear sclerae, fundi show copper wiring alone; oropharynx is clear without exudates; no oral or nasal ulcers

Neck/LN
No cervical, supraclavicular, or axillary adenopathy; normal thyroid

Lungs
CTA bilaterally

CV
RRR; normal S_1, S_2; no m/r/g

Abd
Soft, nontender, without hepatosplenomegaly

MS/Ext
No synovitis; pulses are 2+ and equal without bruits; no clubbing or cyanosis; trace pedal edema; (+) pain during hip extension and flexion

Neuro
A & O × 3; CN II–XII are grossly intact; strength is 5/5 in all 4 extremities; 2+ DTRs in all 4 extremities

Labs

Na 144 mEq/L	Hgb 10.4 g/dL	AST 25 IU/L	Chol 400 mg/dL
K 4.2 mEq/L	Hct 31.7%	ALT 23 IU/L	LDL 204 mg/dL
Cl 110 mEq/L	Plt 318 × 10³/mm³	Alk phos 54 IU/L	HDL 34 mg/dL
CO_2 26 mEq/L	WBC 8.9 × 10³/mm³	GGT 27 IU/L	C3 75 mg/dL
BUN 45 mg/dL	Ca 7.8 mg/dL	T. bili 0.2 mg/dL	C4 22 mg/dL
SCr 2.2 mg/dL	Mg 2.1 mg/dL	Alb 2.5 g/dL	DS DNA Ab positive
Glu 71 mg/dL	Phos 5.1 mg/dL		

UA
Dip stick demonstrates 3+ Hgb, >250 RBCs. Microscopic examination reveals 10 RBC/hpf, some are dysmorphic; 2 waxy casts and 3 finely granular casts, oval fat bodies

24-hr Urine Collection
Urine protein 603 mg/dL, creatinine 54.5 mg/dL, volume 2151 mL. Results 6 months ago were urine creatinine 81 mg/dL, volume 1200 mL, with SCr 1.2 mg/dL

Renal Biopsy
Features of lupus-induced DPGN are present, with an increased chronicity score and a decreased activity score. There is persistent hypercellularity in >50% of the glomeruli. 50% of the glomeruli are globally sclerotic, and there is advanced tubular atrophy and interstitial fibrosis.

DEXA Scan
BMD of the spine (L1-L2) measured 0.763 g/cm² (T score 2.58 SD below the mean). Total BMD of the proximal right femur measured 0.719 g/cm² (T score 2.14 SD below the mean)

Assessment
1. Active lupus-induced DPGN with nephrotic syndrome
2. HTN
3. Corticosteroid-induced osteoporosis
4. Hypercholesterolemia

▶ Questions

Problem Identification

1. a. *Create a list of this patient's drug-related problems.*
   b. *What information obtained from the medical history, physical examination, and laboratory analysis indicates the presence of glomerulonephritis?*
   c. *What information indicates complications from the disease itself or long-term treatment?*
   d. *Calculate the patient's measured creatinine clearance (CLcr) from the present 24-hour urine collection and compare that to the Clcr 6 months ago to assess the rate of progression of renal failure.*
   e. *What other risk factors for renal disease progression does this patient have?*
   f. *Describe the possible glomerular lesions attributable to SLE in this patient.*
   g. *What is the typical clinical presentation of SLE, and which attributes are present in this patient?*

Desired Outcome

2. *What are the pharmacotherapy goals for this patient's lupus nephritis?*

Therapeutic Alternatives

3. *What treatment alternatives are available for achieving the goals related to lupus nephritis and its complications?*

Optimal Plan

4. *Based on the available therapeutic options, design a pharmacotherapeutic plan for the management of lupus nephritis and its complications.*

Outcome Evaluation

5. *Outline a clinical and laboratory monitoring plan for each of the patient's drug-related problems.*

Patient Counseling

6. *What should the patient be told regarding the drug therapy she is to receive to treat her condition and its complications?*

▶ **Clinical Course**

At the 3-month visit, the patient complained of nausea and vomiting. Labs: SCr 1.2 mg/dL, AST 17 IU/L, ALT 11 IU/L, Alk phos 41 IU/L, GGT 19 IU/L, amylase 182 IU/L, lipase 253 IU/L. Urinalysis results: Ucr 65 mg/dL, urinary protein 458 mg/dL, volume 1510 mL; CLcr 57 mL/min. A mild pancreatitis, possibly due to mycophenolate mofetil, was suspected due to the elevated amylase and lipase values and concurrent symptoms of nausea and vomiting. The dose of mycophenolate was decreased from 1000 mg BID to 500 mg BID.

▶ **Self-study Assignments**

1. What effects on the immune system do each of the various therapies for lupus-induced DPGN have?
2. What is the role of hyperlipidemia in progression of renal disease and what therapies may be effective?
3. What are the current recommendations regarding prevention of corticosteroid-induced osteoporosis?
4. What alternatives to mycophenolate mofetil exist if intolerable GI side effects continue and/or hepatic function worsens in this patient?

▶ **Clinical Pearl**

Severe forms of glomerular disease are manifest clinically as nephrotic range proteinuria, declining creatinine clearance, hematuria with dysmorphic red blood cells, presence of urinary casts, hypertension, edema, and hypercholesterolemia.

References

1. Klahr S, Levey AS, Beck GJ, et al. The effects of dietary protein restriction and blood-pressure control on the progression of chronic renal disease. Modification of Diet in Renal Disease Study Group. N Engl J Med 1994;330:877–884.
2. Merkel F, Netzer KO, Gross O, et al. Therapeutic options for critically ill patients suffering from progressive lupus nephritis or Goodpasture's syndrome. Kidney Int Suppl 1998;64:S31–S38.
3. Jennette JC, Falk RJ. Diagnosis and management of glomerular diseases. Med Clin North Am 1997;81:653–677.
4. Levey AS, Lan SP, Corwin HL, et al. Progression and remission of renal disease in the Lupus Nephritis Collaborative Study. Results of treatment with prednisone and short-term oral cyclophosphamide. Ann Intern Med 1992;116:114–123.
5. Steinberg AD, Steinberg SC. Long-term preservation of renal function in patients with lupus nephritis receiving treatment that includes cyclophosphamide versus those treated with prednisone only. Arthritis Rheum 1991;34:945–950.
6. Remuzzi G, Tognoni G, for the GISEN Group. Randomised placebo-controlled trial of effect of ramipril on decline in glomerular filtration rate and risk of terminal renal failure in proteinuric, non-diabetic nephropathy. Lancet 1997;349:1857–1863.
7. Massy ZA, Kasiske BL. Hyperlipidemia and its management in renal disease. Curr Opin Nephrol Hypertens 1996;5:141–146.
8. Recommendations for the prevention and treatment of glucocorticoid-induced osteoporosis. American College of Rheumatology Task Force on Osteoporosis Guidelines. Arthritis Rheum 1996;39:1791–1801.

41 SYNDROME OF INAPPROPRIATE ANTIDIURETIC HORMONE RELEASE

▶ **An Out-of-Body Experience** (Level I)

Rex W. Force, PharmD, BCPS
Jonathan D. Hubbard, DO

▶ After completing this case study, students should be able to:

- Identify the etiologies of hyponatremia and specifically the syndrome of inappropriate antidiuretic hormone (SIADH) release.
- Recognize risk factors for the development of hyponatremia and SIADH.
- Understand the importance of assessing osmotic and fluid status in patients with hyponatremia.
- Recommend appropriate therapy and alternative treatments for SIADH.
- Counsel patients on treatment options, proper administration of selected treatments, and observed side effects.

☀ PATIENT PRESENTATION

Chief Complaint
"I feel like I'm out of my body!"

HPI

Sarah Malanowski is a 48 yo woman who presents to the ED with nausea, headache, body aches, chills, and weakness which began about 18 hours PTA. She is accompanied by her husband, who stated that she had become progressively more confused and disoriented. The patient stated that she has never felt this way before. Shortly after presentation to the ED she experienced a generalized tonic-clonic seizure that lasted approximately one minute. She was given 1 gram of phenytoin IV. Post-ictally, she immediately became combative and agitated. She was given 5 mg of diazepam IV every 5 minutes × 4 (total of 20 mg) with no resolution of her agitation. At that time, 75 mg of chlorpromazine IM was administered, which resulted in rapid sedation.

PMH

Fibromyalgia
Headaches
Seasonal allergies
S/P tubal ligation

FH

Mother died at 83 and had no chronic medical problems. Father is living with Alzheimer's disease and diabetes at age 81.

SH

Married with no children. Denies smoking or alcohol consumption. Employment history is unknown.

ROS

Difficult to obtain due to decreased mental status. Husband states that she is healthy except for her headaches and occasional allergy symptoms.

Meds

Multivitamins
Black cohosh, licorice, grapeseed extract, and other herbal products (husband can't recall all the names)

All

NKDA

PE

Gen

Pre-ictal: A & O × 3 but disoriented about recent events. Patient appears her stated age and is of ideal body weight. Post-ictally she was agitated and then somnolent and disoriented.

VS

BP 148/85, P 97, RR 60, T 35.6°C

Skin

Diaphoretic centrally and very warm; no lesions or rashes noted

HEENT

NC/AT; EOMI; pupils equal at 4 mm with decreased response to light; no strabismus, nystagmus, or conjunctivitis; TMs WNL bilaterally

Neck/LN

Supple without lymphadenopathy, masses, goiter, or bruits

Lungs/Chest

Clear to A & P bilaterally with decreased inspiratory effort

CV

RRR; no m/r/g

Abd

Soft, NT/ND w/o masses or organomegaly; decreased bowel sounds in all four quadrants

Genit/Rect

Deferred

MS/Ext

Normal ROM; muscle strength 5/5 and equal bilaterally; pulses 2+ throughout; no CCE; capillary refill <2 sec

Neuro

CN II to XI intact; no focal or lateralizing signs; DTRs 2/4 and equal bilaterally; sensory intact; negative Babinski

Labs

Na 115 mEq/L	Ca 9.4 mg/dL	T. chol 165 mg/dL
K 2.9 mEq/L	Phos 2.3 mg/dL	TG 52 mg/dL
Cl 78 mEq/L	Uric acid 2.0 mg/dL	T4 7.1 μg/dL
CO_2 28 mEq/L	AST 95 IU/L	Serum osm 231 mOsm/kg
BUN 13 mg/dL	ALT 61 IU/L	
SCr 0.9 mg/dL	T. bili 0.7 mg/dL	
Glu 146 mg/dL	LDH 270 IU/L	

UA

SG 1.010, pH 7.0, leukocyte esterase (−), nitrite (−), protein (−), ketones (−), urobilinogen nl, bilirubin (−), blood (−), glucose 100 mg/dL, spot urine sodium 117 mEq/L, osmolality 323 mOsm/kg

ECG

Incomplete right BBB and sinus tachycardia

CT Head

Subtle low density in the left operculum at the gray-white matter junction; very likely an artifact, but subtle changes secondary to old ischemic disease, tumor, or old contusion are possible; no acute hemorrhage is present.

Chest X-ray

Normal except for scoliosis

Assessment

SIADH, electrolyte disturbances, and seizure in an otherwise healthy woman taking no prescription medications

► Questions

Problem Identification

1. a. *Create a list of the patient's drug-related problems.*
   b. *What information (signs, symptoms, laboratory values) indicates the presence or severity of SIADH as the cause of her hyponatremia?*
   c. *Could any of the patient's problems have been caused by drug therapy?*

Desired Outcome

2. *What are the goals of pharmacotherapy in this case?*

Therapeutic Alternatives

3. a. *What non-drug therapies might be useful for this patient?*
   b. *What pharmacotherapeutic alternatives are available for the treatment of hyponatremia?*

Optimal Plan

4. *What drug dosage form, dose, schedule and duration of therapy are most appropriate for initial treatment of this patient?*

Outcome Evaluation

5. *What clinical parameters are necessary to evaluate the therapy for achievement of the desired therapeutic outcome and to detect or prevent adverse effects?*

Patient Counseling

6. *What information should be provided to the patient to enhance compliance, ensure successful therapy, and minimize adverse effects?*

► Clinical Course

The patient received treatment you recommended, and her serum electrolytes normalized over the next 48 hours. At that time, the patient admitted to taking one of her husband's metolazone 5-mg tablets for what she called "fluid retention" on the day prior to her initial presentation.

► Follow-up Question

1. *Does this information alter your assessment of the patient's drug-related problems?*

► Self-study Assignments

1. Calculate this patient's serum osmolality.
2. Are phenothiazines appropriate in the treatment of agitated post-ictal patients?
3. Perform a literature search to determine the possible medicinal benefits of black cohosh, grapeseed extract, and herbal licorice.

► Clinical Pearl

Excessive serum concentrations of osmotically active substances such as glucose may cause hyponatremia due to movement of water from the intracellular compartment to extracellular spaces in an attempt to normalize osmolality. For each 100 mg/dL increase in serum glucose concentration, sodium will decrease by about 1.6 mEq/L.

References

1. Sterns RH. Severe symptomatic hyponatremia: Treatment and outcome. A study of 64 cases. Ann Intern Med 1987;107:656–664.
2. Fried LF, Palevsky PM. Hyponatremia and hypernatremia. Med Clin North Am 1997;81:585–609.
3. Mulloy AL, Caruana RJ. Hyponatremic emergencies. Med Clin North Am 1995;79:155–168.
4. Laureno R, Karp BI. Myelinolysis after correction of hyponatremia. Ann Intern Med 1997;126:57–62.

42 HYPOKALEMIA AND HYPOMAGNESEMIA

► Double Trouble   (Level II)

Denise R. Sokos, PharmD
W. Greg Leader, PharmD

► After completing this case study, students should be able to:

- Identify potential causes of electrolyte disorders given a patient case history.
- Select the appropriate route of administration and dose of electrolyte replacement therapy specific for a patient.
- Monitor patients receiving electrolyte replacement therapy for efficacy and toxicity.

☼ PATIENT PRESENTATION

Chief Complaint

"I've had vomiting and diarrhea for 3 days with belly pain and I feel weak."

HPI

Joanne Reynolds is a 45 yo woman who is a regular visitor to the ED because of abdominal pain, nausea, vomiting, and diarrhea. Two days ago she was seen in the ED because of emesis. Tonight, she presents with dull, band-like abdominal pain, 2 to 3 days in duration. The pain is unlike the pancreatitis pain that she has frequently. The pain does not radiate to the back and is not associated with N/V. She has had no emesis since admission. She also complains of intermittent diarrhea for a long time and a chronic cough with whitish sputum. She has lost 3 pounds in the last week and about 12 pounds in the last 4 months.

PMH
Chronic pancreatitis (s/p stent placement twice in the pancreatic duct)
Alcoholic hepatitis
Type 2 DM
Pneumonia 2 months ago
Hx leg cramps

FH
Unknown

SH
She lives with her husband. She had one son who was murdered last year. EtOH abuse (currently reports drinking one pint of whiskey every 3 days); 45 pack-year smoker, currently still smoking

ROS
No hematemesis or melena. No complaints of chest pain or respiratory difficulties (dyspnea, PND, orthopnea). She has intermittent headaches, but none currently; also has intermittent polyuria and polydipsia. Denies dysuria and incontinence. States that she has had some generalized muscle weakness for the last few days

Meds
Glipizide 20 mg po BID
Pancrelipase 2 po QID with meals
MVI 1 po QD
Quinine sulfate 260 mg po PRN for leg cramps
Ibuprofen 200 mg po Q 6 H PRN

All
NKDA

PE

Gen
The patient is A & O × 3. She is cooperative but tearful.

VS
Supine BP 130/90, P 90; Upright BP 108/69, P 110; RR 20, T 36.9°C; Ht 5′6″, Wt 75 kg

Skin
Normal appearing, no abnormal moles. Skin warm, dry; no spider angiomata

HEENT
PERRLA, EOM intact and full; no nystagmus. Disc demarcation clear; no A-V nicking, exudates, or papilledema. Nares patent, throat not red, and no exudate. Dry mucous membranes. TMs intact

Neck/LN
Jugular vein flat; no lymphadenopathy; thyroid smooth and not enlarged

Lungs
Clear breath sounds bilaterally; a few crackles at the base of the right lung

Breasts
Non tender; no lumps or discharge

CV
RRR; normal S_1 and S_2; no murmurs; apical pulse at fourth intercostal space

Abd
Soft, slight RUQ and LUQ tenderness to deep palpation; no fluid wave or shifting dullness; liver palpable 4 cm below the RCM. Spleen not palpable. (+) BS in all 4 quadrants

Genit/Rect
GU deferred. Rect: no polyps, heme (−) stool; no hemorrhoids

Ext
No CCE or tenderness. Pulses palpable bilaterally. Full ROM in all extremities

Back
No CVA tenderness

Neuro
CN II–XII intact. Muscle strength 5/5 in upper and lower extremities. DTR 2+ throughout. Plantars downgoing

Labs

Na 139 mEq/L	Ca 7.5 mg/dL	Amylase 81 IU/L
K 2.5 mEq/L	Mg 0.5 mEq/L	Lipase <10 IU/L
Cl 123 mEq/L	Phos 1.8 mEq/L	
CO_2 22 mEq/L	AST 153 IU/L	
BUN 5 mg/dL	ALT 92 IU/L	
SCr 0.5 mg/dL	T. bili 0.3 mg/dL	
Glu 305 mg/dL	Alb 2.6 g/dL	

ABG
pH 7.42, $Paco_2$ 37 mm Hg, Pao_2 79 mm Hg, bicarbonate 24 mEq/L on room air.

ECG
NSR, no U waves, no ischemic changes.

Assessment
Admit as observation to inpatient service.
1. Chronic abdominal pain
2. Chronic intermittent diarrhea
3. Electrolyte abnormalities
4. Type 2 DM
5. Lorazepam PRN agitation

▶ Questions

Problem Identification

1. a. Create a list of the patient's drug-related problems.
   b. What information (signs, symptoms, laboratory values) indicates the presence or severity of hypokalemia, hypomagnesemia, and hypocalcemia?
   c. What are the potential causes of the electrolyte disorders in this patient?
   d. What additional information is needed to satisfactorily assess this patient?

Desired Outcome

2. What are the goals of pharmacotherapy in this patient?

Therapeutic Alternatives

3. What feasible pharmacotherapeutic alternatives are available for treatment of dehydration, hypokalemia, hypomagnesemia, and hypocalcemia?

Optimal Plan

4. Given the above therapeutic alternatives, what therapy would be the most appropriate?

Outcome Evaluation

5. What clinical and laboratory parameters are necessary to evaluate the therapy for the desired therapeutic outcome and prevention of adverse effects?

Patient Counseling

6. When the patient is to be discharged on oral potassium and magnesium supplementation, what information should be provided to her to ensure successful therapy and minimize adverse effects?

▶ Follow-up Questions

1. What medical options are available for the treatment of this patient's chronic pancreatitis?
2. What changes should be made in the therapy for the patient's other medical conditions?

▶ Self-study Assignments

1. Outline a therapeutic plan for the treatment of chronic pain in this patient.
2. Search the literature for information on the treatment or prevention of withdrawal symptoms in hospitalized alcoholics. What drug therapy would you recommend? Defend your choice.
3. Describe how a patient's acid–base status can affect serum electrolyte concentrations.

▶ Clinical Pearl

The addition of small amounts of potassium (20 to 30 mEq/L) to dextrose solutions for replacement may lead to a transient decrease in serum potassium. The glucose solution may stimulate insulin secretion causing an intracellular shift of potassium.

References

1. Dyckner T, Wester PO. Ventricular extrasystoles and intracellular electrolytes in hypokalemic patients before and after correction of the hypokalemia. Acta Med Scand 1978;204:375–379.
2. Kruse JA, Carlson RW. Rapid correction of hypokalemia using concentrated intravenous potassium chloride infusions. Arch Intern Med 1990;150:613–617.
3. Hamill RJ, Robinson LM, Wexler HR, et al. Efficacy and safety of potassium infusion therapy in hypokalemic critically ill patients. Crit Care Med 1991;19: 694–699.

43 HYPERKALEMIA, HYPERPHOSPHATEMIA, AND HYPOCALCEMIA

▶ A Lesson in Homeostasis (Level II)

Brian K. Bond, PharmD
Mary K. Stamatakis, PharmD

▶ After completing this case study, students should be able to:

- Recognize clinical and laboratory findings that support the diagnosis of hyperkalemia and hyperphosphatemia.
- Recommend patient-specific therapeutic plans for the treatment of hyperkalemia and hyperphosphatemia.
- Outline appropriate monitoring parameters to assess the recommended pharmacotherapeutic plans.
- Counsel patients with renal disease on the over-the-counter medications that can worsen hyperkalemia and hyperphosphatemia.

☀ PATIENT PRESENTATION

Chief Complaint
"I'm not feeling too good."

HPI
Terry James is a 34 yo man with IDDM, HTN, and ESRD. He receives hemodialysis three times a week. Two days prior to admission, he developed fever, chills, general malaise, midsternal chest pain, and SOB. On the day of admission, he complained of nausea and vomiting. He admits to missing his HD session yesterday.

PMH

IDDM since age 18
HTN × 12 years
ESRD on HD for the past 6 months
Left arm AV graft thrombus formation with thrombectomy last month
AV graft infected with MRSA 2 months ago

FH

Father with CAD; no family history of DM, HTN, CA

SH

Retired from a glass factory; on disability; past history of smoking, quit 3 years ago; (−) EtOH for the past 7 years; H/O IVDA, quit 7 years ago

ROS

Complaints of decreased appetite, intermittent headache, and left arm pain

Meds

Warfarin 2.5 mg po QD
Ranitidine 150 mg po QD
Calcium acetate 667 mg po TID
Clonidine patch, TTS-2, 1 patch Q week
Procardia XL 60 mg po QD
NPH insulin 30 units SC Q AM and 15 units SC Q PM
Epogen 6000 IU IV 3 times a week with hemodialysis
Metamucil effervescent powder, 1 packet dissolved in water, po TID

All

NKDA

PE

Gen

Patient appears to be in mild to moderate distress

VS

BP 172/86, P 122, RR 18, T 39.0°C; Wt 62 kg, Ht 5'11"

Skin

Erythematous left arm AV graft site with marked tenderness, warm to the touch

HEENT

NC/AT, PERRLA, EOMI, funduscopy WNL, oral pharyngeal mucosa clear

Neck/LN

No JVD or lymphadenopathy, normal thyroid

Lungs

CTA bilaterally

CV

Tachycardia; normal S_1 and S_2; no S_3 or S_4; II/VI SEM at apex radiating to LSB

Abd

Soft, NT/ND, no HSM

Genit/Rect

Normal prostate, guaiac negative stool

MS/Ext

Trace bilateral pedal edema, no clubbing or cyanosis

Neuro

A & O × 3, CN II–XII intact, normal DTRs bilaterally

Labs

Na 135 mEq/L	Hgb 7.3 g/dL	Ca 7.3 mg/dL
K 6.0 mEq/L	Hct 21.5%	Mg 1.9 mg/dL
Cl 97 mEq/L	Plt $192 \times 10^3/mm^3$	Phos 7.4 mg/dL
CO_2 22 mEq/L	WBC $14.4 \times 10^3/mm^3$	Alb 3.2 g/dL
BUN 71 mg/dL		Intact PTH 110 pg/mL
SCr 8.8 mg/dL		
Glu 200 mg/dL		

Chest X-ray

No infiltrates or effusions

ECG

Sinus tachycardia

Bacteriology

Blood culture from AV graft positive for coagulase-positive cocci

Assessment

34 yo man with IDDM, ESRD on HD with infected AV graft site, hyperkalemia, hyperphosphatemia, and hypocalcemia

Plan

Start vancomycin for probable MRSA-infected dialysis graft
Patient missed HD session yesterday. Will dialyze now and correct electrolyte abnormalities

---

▶ Questions

Problem Identification

1. a. Create a list of the patient's drug-related problems.

Problem 1: Hyperkalemia

b. What information (signs, symptoms, laboratory values) indicates the presence or severity of hyperkalemia?

c. Could any of the patient's medications be contributing to his hyperkalemia?

d. *What is the pathophysiology of the patient's hyperkalemia?*

e. *What are the clinical consequences of hyperkalemia?*

Desired Outcome

2. *What are the goals for treating this patient's hyperkalemia?*

Therapeutic Alternatives

3. a. *What non-drug therapies are available for the treatment of hyperkalemia?*

   b. *What feasible pharmacotherapeutic alternatives are available for treatment of hyperkalemia?*

Optimal Plan

4. *What pharmacotherapeutic recommendations are optimal for treatment of this patient's hyperkalemia?*

Outcome Evaluation

5. *What clinical and laboratory parameters are necessary to evaluate the therapy for achievement of the desired therapeutic outcomes and to detect or prevent adverse effects?*

Patient Counseling

6. *What information should be provided to the patient regarding OTC medications that should be avoided to reduce the risk of hyperkalemia?*

Problem 2: Hyperphosphatemia and Hypocalcemia

1. b. *What information (signs, symptoms, laboratory values) indicates the presence or severity of hyperphosphatemia and hypocalcemia?*

   c. *Could any of the patient's medications be contributing to his hyperphosphatemia and hypocalcemia?*

   d. *What is the pathophysiology of the patient's hyperphosphatemia and hypocalcemia?*

   e. *What are the clinical consequences of hyperphosphatemia and hypocalcemia?*

   f. *What is the patient's corrected calcium concentration based on his albumin concentration?*

Desired Outcome

2. *What are the goals of pharmacotherapy for treating this patient's hyperphosphatemia and hypocalcemia?*

Therapeutic Alternatives

3. a. *What non-drug therapies are available for the treatment of hyperphosphatemia?*

   b. *What feasible pharmacotherapeutic alternatives are available for the treatment of hyperphosphatemia?*

   c. *What pharmacotherapeutic alternatives are available for the treatment of hypocalcemia?*

Optimal Plan

4. *What drug recommendations are optimal for treatment of this patient's hyperphosphatemia and hypocalcemia?*

Outcome Evaluation

5. *How should laboratory parameters be monitored to assess the effectiveness of the therapy for hyperphosphatemia and hypocalcemia?*

Patient Counseling

6. *What information should be provided to the patient to help ensure successful therapy and prevent future complications?*

▶ Follow-up Questions

1. *What is an appropriate dosage of vancomycin for treatment of presumed MRSA bacteremia in this patient who receives dialysis with a cellulose acetate (low-flux) dialyzer?*

2. *What additional information would you need to assess this patient's anemia of chronic renal disease?*

▶ Clinical Pearl

Electrolyte disorders such as hyperkalemia and hypercalcemia can be prevented in dialysis patients by lowering dialysate potassium and calcium concentrations.

▶ Self-study Assignments

1. The following laboratory values and erythropoietin dosages were available from the outpatient hemodialysis unit. Formulate a treatment plan to improve the patient's anemia.

Time	Hct %	Ferritin (ng/mL)	% Transferrin Saturation	Erythropoietin Dosage
2 weeks ago	25	85	16	6000 IU 3 ×/week
1 month ago	28			6000 IU 3 ×/week

2. Compare the cost of a one-month supply of the available phosphate binders using usual dosages.

References

1. Allon M. Hyperkalemia in end-stage renal disease: Mechanisms and management. J Am Soc Nephrol 1995;6:1134–1142.

2. Mandal AK. Hypokalemia and hyperkalemia. Med Clin North Am 1997;81:611–639.

3. Delmez JA, Slatopolsky E. Hyperphosphatemia: Its consequences and treatment in patients with chronic renal disease. Am J Kidney Dis 1992;19:303–317.

4. Ben Hamida F, el Esper I, Compagnon M, et al. Long-term (6 months) cross-over comparison of calcium acetate with calcium carbonate as phosphate binder. Nephron 1993;63:258–262.

44 HYPERCALCEMIA

▶ **Crazy From the Calcium**   (Level I)

James S. Lewis II, PharmD
Daniel Sageser, PharmD

▶ After completing this case study, students should be able to:
- Systematically evaluate the treatment options for hypercalcemia.
- Describe the clinical signs and symptoms of hypercalcemia.
- Devise rational treatment strategies for patients with hypercalcemia.
- Develop monitoring strategies to assess the response to treatment of hypercalcemia.
- Present necessary drug and disease state information to patients and their families.

PATIENT PRESENTATION

Chief Complaint
"My husband isn't acting normal."

HPI
Michael Prince is an 80 yo man with a 6-month history of multiple myeloma and pancytopenia lasting for 6 weeks after chemotherapy. He presents to the ED this morning with his wife who states, "He's just so confused, and I don't know what to do to help him. He's been talking to walls and is just not himself." His wife also reports that this morning at 0700 the patient experienced a bout of coffee-ground emesis. The patient also had 2 bouts of emesis yesterday, which were negative for gross blood. The patient's wife reports that he has been increasingly weak, fatigued, and confused over the last 4 days.

PMH
Discharged 7 days ago after treatment for a UTI; receiving cephalexin 500 mg po QID × 4 more days
Multiple myeloma diagnosed 6 months ago; received one cycle of vincristine, doxorubicin, and dexamethasone 5 months ago with prolonged and profound bone marrow suppression. Despite the physician's recommendation, the patient and family then jointly decided that no further chemotherapy would be used.
UGI bleed 13 years ago
Spontaneous subdural hematoma with seizure disorder and sequelae 3 years ago
HTN × 20 years
BPH with recurrent UTIs × 10 years
CRI secondary to multiple myeloma
Dyspepsia × 5 years

FH
Father died at age 65 of an MI; mother had colon cancer and died at age 84 of a CVA. Patient has one younger brother who is 62 and has HTN. The patient has one daughter who is healthy except for allergic rhinitis.

SH
Patient is a retired shipyard worker who moved to this area 10 years ago. He was an avid tennis player and was very active in his church until the diagnosis of his malignancy. According to his wife, the patient continues to consume 2 martinis nightly and has done so for at least 30 years. He has never used tobacco and to her knowledge has never used any illicit drugs.

ROS
Per spouse: Patient is reported to be weak, easily fatigued, and confused; has had nausea with vomiting × 3; frequent urination; constipated for the last several days. No recent headache, sore throat, ear pain, eye problems, SOB, or pain with breathing

Meds
Percocet 1 to 2 tablets po Q 4–6 H PRN pain
Sorbitol 15 to 30 mL po BID
Cephalexin 500 mg po QID × 10 days (4 days remaining)
Duragesic Transdermal System 100 μg/hr patch + 50 μg/hr patch (total 150 μg/hr) Q 3 days
Phenytoin 200 mg po BID
Pepcid 20 mg po QD
Promethazine 25 mg po Q 4 H PRN nausea

All
Sulfa (mild rash)

PE

Gen
Patient is a well-developed, elderly man who is obviously confused but in NAD.

VS
BP 124/58, P 58, RR 18, T 36.1°C; Wt 81 kg

Skin
Cool, dry skin with normal color and turgor

HEENT
PERRL; pupils constricted to 3 mm with no nystagmus present; TMs normal; oropharynx with 2 abrasions on the anterior right side of the tongue that are not oozing; ecchymotic lesion on the left cheek that is not oozing

Neck
Supple; no lymphadenopathy or thyromegaly

Chest
CTA

Cardiac
RRR with no murmurs

Abd
Soft, nontender without masses; no HSM

Genit/Rect
No obvious blood per rectum and no melena; stool guaiac (−)

Ext
Warm and dry with capillary refill <2 seconds

Neuro
Hyporeflexive with pronounced muscle weakness in upper and lower extremities

Labs

Na 136 mEq/L	Hgb 10.0 g/dL	Ca 13.4 mg/dL	AST 84 IU/L
K 4.2 mEq/L	Hct 30.1%	Mg 1.9 mg/dL	ALT 100 IU/L
Cl 99 mEq/L	Plt $30 \times 10^3/mm^3$	Phos 4.5 mg/dL	LDH 1249 IU/L
CO_2 25 mEq/L	WBC $2.3 \times 10^3/mm^3$	Uric acid 6.6 mg/dL	Alb 3.5 g/dL
BUN 67 mg/dL			Phenytoin 12.6 µg/mL
SCr 2.5 mg/dL			
Glu 137 mg/dL			

Blood and Urine Cultures
Pending

ECG
Sinus bradycardia with QT interval of 0.26 seconds, PR interval of 0.24 seconds.

Assessment
A 70 year old well developed male in NAD with a history of increasing fatigue, weakness, confusion, and evidence of an isolated bout of coffee ground emesis. Will transfuse with 2 units of PRBCs and observe for signs of active bleeding. Most likely patient is confused due to elevated calcium, but medications may also be playing a role. Patient has a history of rapid consumption of platelet infusions so will hold off until evidence of active bleeding is present.

▶ Questions

Problem Identification

1. a. Create a drug-related problem list for this patient.
   b. What signs and symptoms in this patient are consistent with the diagnosis of hypercalcemia?

Desired Outcome

2. What are the goals of pharmacotherapy for hypercalcemia in this case?

Therapeutic Alternatives

3. What pharmacotherapeutic options are available for the treatment of this patient's hypercalcemia?

Optimal Plan

4. What drug, dosage form, dose, schedule, and duration of therapy are best for reversing this patient's hypercalcemia?

Outcome Evaluation

5. What clinical and laboratory parameters are necessary to evaluate the therapy for achievement of the desired therapeutic outcome and to detect or prevent adverse events?

Patient Counseling

6. What information should be provided to the patient to enhance compliance, ensure successful therapy, and minimize adverse effects?

▶ Self-study Assignments

1. Organize a debate on the use of alendronate for hypercalcemia of malignancy.
2. Create a one-page table outlining the various treatment options for hypercalcemia with their advantages and disadvantages.

▶ Clinical Pearl

Oncology patients are often confused due to pain medications or the underlying malignancy. However, hypercalcemia is a life threatening complication associated with many malignancies that must always be considered in a confused oncology patient.

References

1. Mundy GR, Guise TA. Hypercalcemia of malignancy. Am J Med 1997; 103:134–145.
2. Chisholm MA, Mulloy AL, Taylor AT. Acute management of cancer-related hypercalcemia. Ann Pharmacother 1996;30:507–513.

45 METABOLIC ACIDOSIS

▶ **Of Proximal Tubules, Normal Anion Gaps, and RTA**   (Level II)

Melanie S. Joy, PharmD

▶ After completing this case study, students should be able to:

- Recognize the clinical and laboratory manifestations of metabolic acidosis.
- Differentiate between the types of renal tubular acidosis.
- Develop a patient-specific pharmacotherapeutic plan for the treatment of chronic metabolic acidosis.
- Provide medication counseling for patients with chronic metabolic acidosis.

☼ PATIENT PRESENTATION

Chief Complaint
"I just feel so weak all the time."

HPI
Carla Snyder is a 27 yo woman who was referred to the nephrology clinic for the management of fatigue, dyspnea, somnolence, lethargy, and increased proximal muscle weakness, particularly with hip extension. She has required the use of her upper extremities to arise from a seated position. In addition, she also notes increasing pain in the left shoulder and hips, as well as discomfort in the quadriceps region. There is no history of diarrhea.

PMH
Four pregnancies with normal uncomplicated vaginal deliveries

SH
She has been divorced from her husband for 8 years and currently lives with her 4 children. There is no history of tobacco habituation or recreational drug use.

FH
History of unspecified arthritis and cancer, and a questionable history of renal disease in the patient's mother

ROS
As per HPI

Meds
None

All
NKDA

PE

Gen
Pleasant African-American woman in NAD

VS
BP 124/80, P 80, RR 22, T 37.2°C; Wt 75 kg, Ht 5'7"

HEENT
No hemorrhages or exudates on funduscopic examination

Neck/LN
JVP was 5 cm; carotid pulses were 2+ bilaterally; no thyromegaly or lymphadenopathy

Lungs
CTA & P

CV
Unable to palpate PMI; regular rate and rhythm; normal S_1 and S_2; no murmurs

Abd
Obese, soft, non-tender, normoactive bowel sounds, no organomegaly

MS/Ext
Minimal sternal and quadriceps tenderness

Neuro
No focal cranial nerve deficits, weakness in hip flexion and extension with strength graded at 3/5. DTRs are 1+ brachioradialis, 2+ biceps, 2+ quadriceps, 1+ ankle jerks, toes downgoing bilaterally

Labs

Na 143 mEq/L	Hgb 15 g/dL	AST 13 IU/L	1, 25-OH-D_3 32 pg/mL
K 3.2 mEq/L	Hct 45%	ALT 7 IU/L	25-OH D_3 10 ng/mL
Cl 119 mEq/L	Plt 225 × 10³/mm³	Alk phos 113 IU/L	T4 5.8 μg/dL
CO_2 12 mEq/L	WBC 7.6 × 10³/mm³	GGT 14 IU/L	TSH 4.5 μIU/mL
BUN 15 mg/dL	Ca 7.4 mg/dL	T. bili 0.4 mg/dL	
SCr 1.2 mg/dL	Mg 2.2 mg/dL	Alb 4.6 g/dL	
Glu 75 mg/dL	Phos 1.0 mg/dL		

ABG on RA
pH 7.27, pco₂ 27 mm Hg, po₂ 106 mm Hg, bicarbonate 12.1 mEq/L

UA
SG 1.010; pH 5.0. Fractional excretion of bicarbonate following bicarbonate infusion to increase serum level to 25 mEq/L >25%

KUB
No nephrocalcinosis

Radiology
Bilateral femur and tibia films demonstrated pseudofracture or stress response to the right proximal femur; cortical reabsorption in the left proximal femur

Assessment
1. Acidosis
2. Hypocalcemia
3. Hypophosphatemia
4. Osteomalacia

▶ Questions

Problem Identification

1. a. Identify the type of acidosis (metabolic versus respiratory) this patient exhibits, calculate the anion gap, and identify the potential causes.

   b. What medical conditions present in this patient are either untreated or inadequately treated?

   c. What information obtained from the patient's symptoms, physical examination, and laboratory analysis indicates the presence of a chronic metabolic acidosis with a renal tubular acidosis component or one of its complications?

   d. What are the different types of renal tubular acidosis (RTA), *and how do they differ with respect to etiology, mechanisms, and clinical/laboratory findings?*

   e. *Which type of RTA is most likely present in this patient?*

Desired Outcome

2. *What are the pharmacotherapy goals for this patient?*

Therapeutic Alternatives

3. *What treatment alternatives are available to achieve the desired therapeutic outcomes?*

Optimal Plan

4. *Design a pharmacotherapeutic plan for the management of metabolic acidosis and its complications in this patient.*

Outcome Evaluation

5. *Outline a clinical and laboratory monitoring plan to assess the patient's response to the pharmacotherapeutic regimen you recommended.*

Patient Counseling

6. *How should the patient be counseled about the drug therapy to treat chronic metabolic acidosis and renal tubular acidosis?*

▶ ## Clinical Course

At the patient's 6-month clinic visit, 2+ pedal edema and symptoms of depression are noted. During the patient interview, she suggests that she has not been compliant with medications due to depressive symptoms. Labs:

Na 139 mEq/L	Ca 7.1 mg/dL
K 3.3 mEq/L	Mg 1.9 mg/dL
Cl 114 mEq/L	Phos 0.9 mg/dL
CO_2 14 mEq/L	Alb 4.6 g/dL
BUN 12 mg/dL	UA: Trace glucose
SCr 0.9 mg/dL	
Glu 99 mg/dL	

Furosemide 40 mg po QD, Neutra-Phos 3 packets po TID, and amitriptyline 25 mg po HS were added to the medication regimen. In addition, the patient was advised to take an extra 80 mEq potassium over the ensuing 24 hours.

▶ ## Self-study Assignments

1. Differentiate the bone disease of metabolic acidosis versus those associated with chronic renal failure and osteoporosis.
2. Discuss the basis for the diagnosis of the various forms of RTA by evaluating the urinalysis and serum chemistries.

▶ ## Clinical Pearl

When differentiating between types I and II RTA, consider the urine pH, fractional excretion of bicarbonate, serum potassium, presence or absence

	Type I RTA	Type II RTA
Urine pH (serum <7.4)	>5.3	<5.3
F.E. HCO_3[a]	<3%	>15–20%
Serum K	Normal, reduced, elevated	Normal or reduced
Complications	Nephrocalcinosis	Osteomalacia
Bicarbonate dose	1–2 mEq/kg	10–15 mEq/kg

[a] Denotes the fractional excretion of bicarbonate after the administration of a bicarbonate infusion to increase the plasma bicarbonate concentration to 25 mEq/L.

of nephrocalcinosis and bone disease, and dose of bicarbonate needed to normalize plasma bicarbonate.

References

1. Eiam-ong S, Kurtzman NA. Metabolic acidosis and bone disease. Miner Electrolyte Metab 1994;20:72–80.
2. Oh MS. Irrelevance of bone buffering to acid–base homeostasis in chronic metabolic acidosis. Nephron 1991;59:7–10.
3. Smulders YM, Frissen PH, Slaats EH, et al. Renal tubular acidosis. Pathophysiology and diagnosis. Arch Intern Med 1996;156:1629–1636.
4. Metabolic Acidosis. In: Rose BD, ed. Clinical Physiology of Acid–Base and Electrolyte Disorders, 3rd ed. New York, McGraw-Hill, 1994:540–603.

46 · METABOLIC ALKALOSIS

▶ ## The ABCs of Acid–Base Chemistry (Level I)

Jennifer Stoffel, PharmD, BCPS

▶ After completing this case study, students should be able to:

- Determine the type of acid–base disorder a patient is experiencing when given patient history and pertinent laboratory values.
- Describe patient-specific factors that contribute to the development of metabolic disorders.
- Recommend appropriate therapeutic alternatives for the treatment of metabolic alkalosis.
- Formulate a patient-specific pharmacotherapeutic plan for the treatment and monitoring of metabolic alkalosis.

☼ PATIENT PRESENTATION

Chief Complaint

"I seem to be so short of breath lately."

HPI

Henry Alstoff is a 72 yo man who presents to the ED with complaints of shortness of breath and generalized pain. He was discharged yesterday from a hospital near his home where he had been admitted with symptoms consistent with CHF. During that hospitalization he was treated with furosemide and supplemental oxygen. He was breathing comfortably on discharge. The patient also reports worsening shortness of breath, increased weakness, and "shakiness" over the past 24 hours.

PMH

Hx CHF
CABG 14 years ago
Orthotopic liver transplantation 7 years ago for end-stage liver disease secondary to alcoholic cirrhosis
Chronic renal insufficiency (SCr 2.0 mg/dL 1 month ago)
Insulin-dependent diabetes mellitus

FH

Not Available

SH

Significant history of alcohol consumption but has not had an alcoholic beverage for 8 years. There is no history of tobacco or illicit drug use. He is a retired carpenter and lives at home with his wife.

ROS

The patient denies recent weight gain or loss, loss of appetite, nausea, or vomiting. Also denies fever, chills, or night sweats. Does admit to a non-productive cough. No reported chest pain, palpitations, or diaphoresis. Denies diarrhea, constipation, change in bowel habits, or color of stool. Urine output has decreased over the past 24 hours.

Meds

Prograf 1 mg po BID × 7 years; last dosage change 6 months ago
Prednisone 5 mg po QD × 7 years
Furosemide 80 mg po QD; increased from 40 mg po QD 5 days ago
Dapsone 100 mg po QD × 4 years
Florinef 0.1 mg po QD × 8 months
Magnesium oxide 400 mg po BID × 8 months
Calcium carbonate 500 mg po BID × 8 months
Questran 4 grams po BID × 8 years
Humulin-N insulin 24 units SC Q AM, 18 units SC Q PM; has required insulin × 7 years; last dosage change 1 month ago
Captopril 12.5 mg po BID × 1 year

All

NKDA

PE

Gen

The patient is shaking and looks uncomfortable. Breathing is labored.

VS

BP 132/78, HR 96, RR 26, T 38.2°C; Wt 111 kg; Ht 5′10″; O$_2$ sat 89% on RA

Skin

Decreased skin turgor

HEENT

NC/AT, EOMI, PERRLA, sclerae anicteric. Funduscopic exam is normal.

No sinus tenderness. Dry tongue and mucous membranes. No oral lesions or exudates

Neck/LN

No JVD or bruits. No lymphadenopathy or thyromegaly

Chest

Scattered rhonchi at bases

CV

RRR, normal S$_1$, S$_2$, no S$_3$ or S$_4$, no murmurs

Abd

Soft, NT/ND; old surgical scars evident; (+) bowel sounds

GU

Noncontributory

Ext

Distal pulses trace bilaterally. Femoral pulses 1+ bilaterally

Neuro

A & O × 3. DTR 1+ and symmetrical bilaterally. UE/LE strength 4/5. Fine tremor in upper extremities and trunk. CN II–XII intact. Babinski negative bilaterally.

Labs

Na 137 mEq/L	Hgb 12.0 g/dL	AST 13 IU/L
K 5.5 mEq/L	Hct 37.1%	ALT 23 IU/L
Cl 90 mEq/L	Plt 361 × 10^3/mm^3	GGT 60 IU/L
CO$_2$ 35 mEq/L	WBC 17.4 × 10^3/mm^3	T. bili 0.4 mg/dL
BUN 99 mg/dL	Mg 2.5 mEq/L	PT 12.1 sec
SCr 2.9 mg/dL	Phos 2.7 mg/dL	PTT 21.9 sec
Glu 305 mg/dL		Tacrolimus 6.5 ng/mL[a]

[a] Tacrolimus 2 (whole blood, MEIA), therapeutic range 5 to 20 ng/mL

ABG

pH 7.42, pco$_2$ 55 mm Hg, po$_2$ 83 mm Hg

UA

Urine sodium 14 mEq/L, potassium 10 mEq/L, chloride 18 mEq/L

Blood and Sputum Cultures

Pending

Chest X-ray

RLL infiltrate

ECG

Normal

Assessment

Admit patient for a presumed respiratory tract infection, worsening renal function, and electrolyte abnormalities

Follow-Up

Shortly after admission, the patient is intubated and empiric IV antibiotics are initiated.

► Questions

Problem Identification

1. a. Create a list of this patient's drug-related problems.
   b. Describe the clinical findings that are consistent with metabolic alkalosis and those that are not consistent with this acid–base disorder.
   c. Explain how diuretics such as furosemide can result in a metabolic alkalosis.

Desired Outcome

2. What are the desired therapeutic outcomes for this patient?

Therapeutic Alternatives

3. What pharmacologic and non-pharmacologic alternatives should be considered for the treatment of metabolic alkalosis in this patient?

Optimal Plan

4. a. What drug, dosage form, dose, schedule, and duration of therapy are best for this patient?
   b. What other modifications to the patient's current drug regimen are warranted? Include your rationale.

Outcome Evaluation

5. a. What clinical and laboratory parameters are necessary to evaluate the therapy for achievement of the desired outcome and prevention of adverse effects?

► Clinical Course

The patient was started on the therapy for metabolic alkalosis that you recommended. Physician and nursing assessments note improvement in skin turgor and the moistness of oral mucous membranes. Urine output improved from 15 mL/hr during the first 2 hours after admission to 40 mL/hr. Total fluid intake was 4.2 L and urine output was 1.2 L for the first 24 hours. The next morning, a chest x-ray shows no change in the RLL infiltrate and no pulmonary edema. Laboratory values 24 hours after the initiation of therapy are as follows:

Na 142 mEq/L	BUN 80 mg/dL	ABG
K 4.8 mEq/L	SCr 2.6 mg/dL	pH 7.45
Cl 99 mEq/L	Mg 2.3 mEq/L	Pco_2 45 mm Hg
CO_2 30 mEq/L		po_2 95 mm Hg

After the completion of BAL for culture specimens, ticarcillin/clavulanate 3.1 g IV Q 12 H and erythromycin 1 g IV Q 6 H were started as empiric therapy for presumed hospital-acquired pneumonia. After 48 hours, cultures from the BAL were positive for beta-lactamase producing *Haemophilus influenzae*. At this time the patient had been afebrile for 24 hours and the white count had decreased to $12.1 \times 10^3/mm^3$. The patient was extubated on the third day after admission. For the treatment of congestive heart failure, the patient's captopril was discontinued and isosorbide dinitrate 20 mg po TID and hydralazine 25 mg QID were initiated.

b. What is your assessment of the patient's response to the therapy initiated for treatment of metabolic alkalosis?

Patient Counseling

6. What information should be provided to the patient regarding the isosorbide dinitrate and hydralazine started for the treatment of CHF?

► Self-study Assignments

1. Calculate the expected respiratory compensation for this patient's metabolic alkalosis. Discuss how various respiratory disease states would affect compensation.
2. Discuss how urine electrolytes play a role in the diagnosis and treatment of metabolic alkalosis.

► Clinical Pearl

It is important to identify the cause of metabolic alkalosis and correct it. However, correcting the underlying cause does not always reverse the alkalosis, and additional therapy will be required.

References

1. Martin WJ, Matzke GR. Treating severe metabolic alkalosis. Clin Pharm 1982;1:42–48.
2. Marik PE, Kusman BD, Lipman J, et al. Acetazolamide in the treatment of metabolic alkalosis in critically ill patients. Heart Lung 1991;20(5 Pt 1):455–459.
3. Brimioulle S, Berre J, Dufaye P, et al. Hydrochloric acid infusion for treatment of metabolic alkalosis associated with respiratory acidosis. Crit Care Med 1989;17:232–236.
4. Cochran EB, Kamper CA, Phelps SJ, et al. Parenteral nutrition in the critically ill patient. Clin Pharm 1989;8:783–799.
5. Anderson PO, Knoben JE. Handbook of Clinical Drug Data, 8th ed. Stamford, CT, Appleton & Lange, 1997:908.

47 BENIGN PROSTATIC HYPERPLASIA

► Get Me to the Bathroom on Time (Level II)

Catherine A. Heyneman, PharmD, MS
Richard S. Rhodes, PharmD

► After completing this case study, students should be able to:

- Recognize the clinical manifestations of BPH.
- Differentiate between obstructive and irritative symptoms.
- Recommend appropriate pharmacotherapeutic treatment for BPH.
- Recognize when surgical therapies should be considered.
- Understand how some drugs can exacerbate BPH symptoms.

PATIENT PRESENTATION

Chief Complaint
"I can't sleep at night. I'm up 4 or 5 times feeling that I have to urinate, and then when I get to the bathroom all I can do is dribble. Sometimes I don't even make it to the bathroom in time. I've been really depressed lately."

HPI
Hugh Rowlett is a 79 yo man with a long-standing history of UTIs. He has been hospitalized twice in the past 3 years for urosepsis. He is currently being evaluated because of a guaiac-positive stool detected last week and complaints of the recent-onset of urinary hesitancy, nocturia, and dribbling.

PMH
Severe OA with L total hip replacement 9 years ago and R total hip replacement 3 years ago
Laminectomy 10 years ago
BPH with urge incontinence
Chronic UTIs
Type 2 DM (well-controlled with tolbutamide)
UGI bleed 2 months ago
Obesity
Hx Headaches
CHD
Lipoma—lower back
Chronic major depression diagnosed 15 years ago

FH
Caucasian male educated through the 6th grade. Father died of massive MI at age 72; mother still alive at age 94

SH
Worked for 35 years as a railroad diesel refrigeration mechanic; retired 17 years ago. Married twice. Second wife deceased 5 years ago (stroke); one daughter, two granddaughters. Admitted to a long-term care facility 3 years ago; was living with one granddaughter who could no longer care for him because of his fading memory and walking/hearing limitations. He has a strained relationship with that granddaughter; he recently changed his power of attorney to his other granddaughter. Used smokeless tobacco × 55 years; heavy EtOH in the past, none now. He is socially active; is chairman of the resident council at the nursing home

ROS
In conversation, he seems alert, friendly, and courteous but complains that his depression is getting significantly worse. He has no c/o dyspepsia, dysphagia, abdominal pain, hematemesis, or visible blood in the stool.

Meds
Tagamet 400 mg po BID for PUD
Tolbutamide 500 mg po TID for DM
Amitriptyline 50 mg po Q HS for HA prophylaxis
Ibuprofen 800 mg po BID for OA
Trazodone 50 mg 4 1/2 tabs po Q HS for depression
Capoten 25 po TID for prevention of diabetic nephropathy

All
NKDA

PE

Gen
Elderly Caucasian man in NAD; well-kept appearance; A & O × 3; poor historian

VS
BP 132/80, P 72, RR 24, T 98.6°F; Wt 254 lbs., Ht 5'6"

Skin
Vertical scars on neck and lower back from laminectomies

HEENT
PERRLA, EOMI, TMs WNL, nose and throat clear w/o exudate or lesions

Neck/LN
Supple w/o LAD or masses; thyroid in midline

Lungs/Thorax
CTA, distant sounds

CV
RRR w/o murmurs

Abd
Soft, NT/ND w/o masses or scars; (+) BS

Genit/Rect
Testes ↓↓, penis circumcised w/o DC

MS/Ext
Neurovascular intact, distal pulses 1-2+

Neuro
DTRs 2+; CN II–XII grossly intact

Labs

Na 136 mEq/L	Hgb 12.6 g/dL	WBC 5.6 × 10³/mm³	AST 12 IU/L	Ca 8.5 mg/dL
K 4.1 mEq/L	Hct 37.9%	Neutros 75%	ALT 16 IU/L	Phos 3.5 mg/dL
Cl 103 mEq/L	MCV 92.5 μm³	Lymph 16%	Alk Phos 55 IU/L	Uric Acid 3.5 mg/dL
CO_2 41 mEq/L	MCH 30.8 pg	Monos 5%	LDH 121 U/L	T_4 7.3 μg/dL
BUN 9 mg/dL	MCHC 33.3 g/dL	Eos 3%	T. bili 0.6 mg/dL	TSH 1.04 μIU/mL
SCr 0.7 mg/dL	Plt 191 × 10³/mm³	Basos 1%	T. prot 6.1 g/dL	
Glu 165 mg/dL			T. chol 146 mg/dL	

UA

Color straw; appearance clear; SG 1.010; pH 6.5; glucose (–), bilirubin (–), ketones (–), blood (–), urobilinogen 0.2 mg/dL, nitrite (–), leukocyte esterases (–), epithelial cells–occasional per hpf; WBC–occasional per hpf, RBC–none seen; bacteria–trace; amorphous–none seen; crystals–1+ calcium oxalate; mucous–none seen. Culture not indicated

GU Consult

Patient treated for UTI 2 weeks ago with Cipro. Urine clear, negative for glucose. Bladder exam with ultrasound revealed post-void residual estimate of 20 mL. Prostate approximately 25 g, small, benign

Assessment

BPH with urge incontinence
Normocytic anemia possibly secondary to UGI bleed
Chronic major depression

▶ Questions

Problem Identification

1. a. Create a list of the patient's drug-related problems.
   b. Describe the natural history and epidemiologic characteristics of BPH.
   c. Which of this patient's complaints are consistent with obstructive symptoms of BPH? Which are consistent with irritative symptoms?
   d. What steps are recommended in the initial evaluation of all patients presenting with BPH?
   e. What other medical conditions should be ruled out before treating this patient for BPH?
   f. Could any of this patient's problems have been exacerbated by drug therapy?
   g. Are any of this patient's problems amenable to pharmacotherapy?

Desired Outcome

2. What are the goals of pharmacotherapy in this case?

Therapeutic Alternatives

3. What are the treatment alternatives for BPH?

Optimal Plan

4. What drug, dosage form, dose, schedule, and duration of therapy are best for this patient?

Outcome Evaluation

5. What clinical and laboratory parameters are necessary to evaluate the therapy for achievement of the desired therapeutic outcome and to detect or prevent adverse effects?

Patient Counseling

6. What information should be provided to the patient to enhance compliance, ensure successful therapy, and minimize adverse effects?

▶ Clinical Course

Mr. Rowlett's BPH symptoms improved within days after discontinuation of two of his medications. He required no further drug therapy for BPH. Six months later, however, his symptoms returned and he opted for laser prostatectomy. This procedure was successful in alleviating his symptoms, but left him impotent. The resolution of urge incontinence was such a relief to him that he considered his situation greatly improved.

▶ Self-study Assignments

1. Compare the efficacy of saw palmetto (Serenoa repens) to finasteride and α_1-antagonists for the treatment of BPH.
2. Perform a literature search for evidence that supports the use of finasteride and α_1-antagonists as combination therapy for BPH.

▶ Clinical Pearl

Physiologic measurements such as post-void residuals, uroflowmetry, and pressure-flow studies often do not correlate well with the patient's perception of symptom severity.

References

1. Lee M, Sharifi R. Benign prostatic hyperplasia: Diagnosis and treatment guideline. Ann Pharmacother 1997;31:481–486.
2. McConnell JD, Barry MJ, Bruskewitz RC, et al. Benign prostatic hyperplasia: Diagnosis and treatment. Clinical Practice Guideline, number 8. AHCPR publication no. 94-0582. Rockville, MD, Agency for Health Care Policy and Research, Public Health Service, U.S. Department of Health and Human Services, February 1994.
3. Wilde MI, McTavish D. Tamsulosin: A review of its pharmacological properties and therapeutic potential in the management of symptomatic benign prostatic hyperplasia. Drugs 1996;52:883–898.
4. Lepor H, Williford WO, Barry MJ, et al. The efficacy of terazosin, finasteride, or both in benign prostatic hyperplasia. N Engl J Med 1996;335:533–539.
5. McConnell JD, Bruskewitz R, Walsh P, et al. The effect of finasteride on the risk of acute urinary retention and the need for surgical treatment among men with benign prostatic hyperplasia. N Engl J Med 1998;338:557–563.

6. Wasson JH. Finasteride to prevent morbidity from benign prostatic hyperplasia. N Engl J Med 1998;338:612–613.
7. Tammela T. Benign prostatic hyperplasia. Practical treatment guidelines. Drugs Aging 1997;10:349–366.

48 NEUROGENIC BLADDER AND URINARY INCONTINENCE

▶ **Bladder Matters**   (Level III)

Mary Lee, PharmD, BCPS, FCCP

▶ After completing this case study, students should be able to:

- Distinguish among four types of urinary incontinence: urge, stress, overflow, and functional incontinence.
- Determine when anticholinergic and muscle relaxant drugs should be recommended for the management of urge incontinence based on their mechanism of action and adverse effects.
- Recognize concomitant drug therapy that may exacerbate urge incontinence.
- Recommend appropriate non-drug therapy for the management of urge incontinence.
- Explain why anticholinergic and muscle relaxant drugs should be used cautiously in patients with bladder outlet obstruction.

☀ PATIENT PRESENTATION

Chief Complaint
"I can't seem to get to the bathroom on time because I can't control my urinary stream."

HPI
John Brown is a 74 yo man with urinary urgency and frequency for 6 weeks following a CVA. He reports soiling his underwear at least four times during the day and several times during the night and has resorted to wearing adult diapers. The patient has curtailed much of his volunteer work and social activities because of this problem.

PMH
HTN for many years, treated with medications for 20 years
CVA 6 weeks ago, appears to have no residual neurological deficits except for urinary incontinence

FH
Non-contributory

SH
Non-smoker, social drinker, married

Meds
Hydrochlorothiazide 25 mg po QD with supper
Terazosin 10 mg po QD
Aspirin 325 mg po Q AM

All
NKDA

ROS
WDWN man who looks healthy but smells of urine. Patient complains that he can't control his urinary stream and leaks urine repeatedly throughout the day. Patient reports good control of his blood pressure and has no complaints of weakness, fatigue, dizziness, or headaches.

PE

VS
BP 150/90, P 90, RR 16, T 37°C; Wt 80 kg, Ht 5'6"

Skin
No rashes, wounds, or open sores

HEENT
PERRLA, EOMI; no AV nicking or hemorrhages

Neck/LN
No palpable thyroid masses; no lymphadenopathy

CV
Regular S_1, S_2; (+) S_4; (−) S_3, murmurs, or rubs

Pulm
Clear to A & P

Abd
Soft, NT/ND, (+) bowel sounds

Rect
External hemorrhoids; heme (−) stool; prostate mildly enlarged; external genitalia normal

Ext
Normal; equal motor strength in both arms and legs

Neuro
A & O × 3, CN II–XII grossly intact; DTRs 3/5 bilaterally; negative Babinski

Labs
Na 137 mEq/L	Hgb 13 g/dL
K 3.7 mEq/L	Hct 40%
Cl 102 mEq/L	Plt 400×10^3/mm³
CO_2 28 mEq/L	WBC 5.6×10^3/mm³
BUN 30 mg/dL	
SCr 1.4 mg/dL	
Glu 139 mg/dL	

UA
No bacteria, no WBC

Cystoscopy

No urethral or bladder abnormalities noted, prostate does not appear to cause bladder outlet obstruction. Urinary flow rate 16 mL/second

Cystometrogram (CMG)

Bladder capacity 130 mL with maximal detrusor pressure of 75 cm Hg at time of bladder emptying. During the CMG, uninhibited detrusor muscle contractions documented at lower detrusor muscle pressures of 40–60 cm Hg. Bladder sensation is intact.

Assessment

Urge incontinence secondary to CVA, and possibly exacerbated by drug therapy

► Questions

Problem Identification

1. a. Create a list of the patient's drug-related problems.
   b. What information (signs, symptoms, medical history, laboratory values, other test results) indicates the presence or severity of urge incontinence?
   c. Differentiate urge incontinence from stress incontinence, overflow incontinence, and functional incontinence.
   d. In addition to the medications the patient is currently taking, what other drugs could exacerbate urge incontinence?

Desired Outcome

2. What are the goals of pharmacotherapy in this case?

Therapeutic Alternatives

3. a. What non-drug therapies might be useful for this patient?
   b. What feasible pharmacotherapeutic alternatives are available for treatment of urge incontinence?

Optimal Plan

4. What drug, dosage form, dose, schedule, and duration of therapy are best for this patient?

Outcome Evaluation

5. What clinical and laboratory parameters are necessary to evaluate the therapy for achievement of the desired therapeutic outcome and to detect or prevent adverse effects?

Patient Counseling

6. What information should be provided to the patient to enhance compliance, ensure successful therapy, and minimize adverse effects?

► Clinical Course

The patient was started on the medication regimen you recommended but experienced severe constipation and excessive sedation. Adverse effects did not abate despite continuation of therapy for 1 week. For this reason, the drug was changed to a drug with a different mechanism of action. The patient had complete relief of symptoms of urinary leakage with this regimen and continued to take it for 1.5 years. During the last 6 months of treatment, the patient noted that he was developing a slower urinary stream. He seemed to have greater difficulty emptying his bladder completely and always felt that his bladder was still full despite having just voided. He has required antibiotic treatment regularly for relapsing urinary tract infections. He sought medical attention and was referred to a urologist. Rectal examination revealed a significantly enlarged 30-g smooth prostate (normal, 15 to 20 g). A PSA was 1.0 ng/dL; BUN and serum creatinine were unchanged from the last visit. Repeat cystoscopy showed a large obstructing prostate at the bladder neck and a hypertrophied, noncontractile detrusor muscle. Peak urinary flow rate was 3 mL/second. Post void residual bladder volume is 1200 mL.

► Follow-up Questions

1. Why has the patient developed new and different voiding symptoms?
2. How should this patient's voiding problem now be managed?

► Self-study Assignments

1. Conduct a literature search to identify current studies that compare the efficacy and safety of terodiline for treatment of urge incontinence. This investigational drug may soon be available on the U.S. market.
2. Tricyclic antidepressants have been used to treat stress incontinence. Explain the rationale for the use of this class of drugs for this disorder.

► Clinical Pearl

Proper classification of the type of urinary incontinence is key to selecting appropriate drug therapy. Urge incontinence responds to anticholinergics or muscle relaxants. Overflow urinary incontinence may respond to α-adrenergic blocking agents or cholinergic stimulants. Stress incontinence responds to α-adrenergic stimulants.

ACKNOWLEDGMENT

The author would like to acknowledge the assistance and kind help of Dr. Roohollah Sharifi, Professor of Urology, University of Illinois at Chicago College of Medicine.

References

1. Wein AJ. Pharmacologic treatment of incontinence. J Am Geriatr Soc 1990;38: 317–325.
2. Resnick NM. Geriatric incontinence. Urol Clin North Am 1996; 23:55–74.
3. Ouslander JG, Schnelle JF, Uman G, et al. Does oxybutynin add to the effectiveness of prompted voiding for urinary incontinence among nursing home residents? A placebo-controlled trial. J Am Geriatr Soc 1995;43:610–617.
4. Jonas U, Hofner K, Madersbacher H, et al. Efficacy and safety of two doses of tolterodine versus placebo in patients with detrusor overactivity and symptoms of frequency, urge incontinence, and urgency: Urodynamic evaluation. World J Urol 1997;15:144–151.

49   ERECTILE DYSFUNCTION

▶   A Sensitive Issue   (Level III)

Cara Lawless-Liday, PharmD
Rex W. Force, PharmD, BCPS

▶   After completing this case study, students should be able to:

- Identify the different etiologies of erectile dysfunction (ED).
- Recognize risk factors for the development of ED.
- Provide brief descriptions of the advantages and disadvantages of the common methods available for the treatment of ED.
- Recommend appropriate therapy and alternative treatments for ED.
- Counsel patients on treatment options, proper administration of selected treatments, and possible side effects.

☀ PATIENT PRESENTATION

Chief Complaint
"I've been having some problems with my sex life."

HPI
Roy Johnson is a 39 yo man who presents to his PCP with the above complaint. Upon questioning, he states that for the last 10 months he has only been able to achieve partial erections that are not sufficient for intercourse. He notices occasional nocturnal penile tumescence, but these are also only partial erections.

PMH
Type 2 DM × 6 years
HTN × 27 years
COPD × 4 years
GERD × 2 years
Carpal tunnel release surgery in both wrists 2 years ago
No history of STDs

FH
Strong for polyps of the colon. Brother had colitis. Father recently died at age 64 of COPD and cardiac arrest

SH
Patient is single and lives alone. Currently has a girlfriend and desires a monogamous sexual relationship. Has a 25 pack-year smoking history but quit smoking 2 years ago. Drinks alcohol only around holidays

ROS
Denies significant life stressors, nausea, vomiting, sweating, blurry vision, dizziness, nocturia, urgency, or symptoms of prostatitis. Complains of slight SOB, cold and hypersensitive feet, impotence (difficulty achieving and maintaining erections), seasonal allergies, diarrhea for the last 2 months (1 or 2 loose stools/day; normal to small amounts of stool), and dental caries

Meds
Lotensin 40 mg po BID
Cardura 8 mg po Q HS
HCTZ 12.5 mg po QD
Glucophage 850 mg po TID
Glyburide 1.25 mg po Q AM
Prilosec 20 mg po QD
Albuterol MDI PRN

All
NKDA

PE

Gen
Alert, cooperative, anxious, obese man in NAD

VS
BP 138/78, P 100, RR 20, T 99°F; Wt 128 kg, Ht 5'10"

Skin
Warm, dry; no lesions

HEENT
NC/AT; EOMI; PERRLA; funduscopic exam shows no arteriolar narrowing, hemorrhages, or exudates; TMs WNL bilaterally

Neck/LN
Supple without lymphadenopathy, masses, or goiter

Lungs/Chest
Clear to A & P bilaterally

CV
RRR; normal S_1 and S_2; no m/r/g

Abd
Soft, obese; NT/ND; normal bowel sounds; no masses or organomegaly

Genit/Rect
Normal scrotum, testes descended; NT w/o masses. Penis without discharge

MS/Ext
Muscle strength 5/5 throughout; full ROM in all extremities; pulses 2+ throughout; ingrown toenail on left great toe

Neuro

CN II–XII intact; DTRs 2+ and equal bilaterally. No sensory/motor deficits; some hypersensitivity in lower extremities

Labs

Na 137 mEq/L Hcg 15.0 g/dL Ca 9.4 mg/dL
K 4.0 mEq/L Hct 48% Mg 1.6 mEq/L
Cl 100 mEq/L WBC 7.6 × 10³/mm³ Phos 4.0 mg/dL
CO_2 27 mEq/L   T. chol 179 mg/dL
BUN 9 mg/dL   Non-fasting finger stick glu 223 mg/dL
SCr 0.6 mg/dL HbA_{1c} 11.8%

UA

SG 1.015, pH 5.0, leukocyte estrase (−), nitrite (−), protein 100 mg/dL, ketones (−), urobilinogen normal, bilirubin (−), blood 10 RBC/μL.

Assessment

1. Erectile dysfunction
2. Poor long-term control of type 2 DM

► Questions

Problem Identification

1. a. Create a list of the patient's drug-related problems.
   b. What risk factors for ED are present in this patient?
   c. What are the etiologies of ED, and what is this patient's most likely etiology?
   d. Could any of the patient's problems have been caused by drug therapy?

Desired Outcome

2. What are the goals of therapy in this case?

Therapeutic Alternatives

3. a. What non-pharmacologic alternatives are available for the treatment of ED?
   b. What pharmacologic alternatives are available for the treatment of ED?

Optimal Plan

4. What therapy is most appropriate and effective for initial treatment of this patient? If drug therapy is indicated, list the drug, dosage form, dose, schedule, and duration of therapy.

Outcome Evaluation

5. What clinical parameters are necessary to evaluate the therapy for achievement of the desired therapeutic outcome and to detect or prevent adverse effects?

Patient Counseling

6. What information should be provided to the patient to enhance compliance, ensure successful therapy, and minimize adverse effects?

► Self-study Assignments

1. Investigate the treatments for priapism and write a two-page report that includes your conclusion about the most effective treatment.
2. Prepare a list of the medications that have been associated with ED. Provide literature evidence on the strength of the association with each medication.
3. Perform a literature search to identify new oral therapies for ED. Compare the potential advantages and disadvantages of each treatment.

► Clinical Pearl

Some degree of erectile dysfunction is experienced by 20 to 30 million American men, but many do not receive effective treatment because they are hesitant to discuss the issue with their physicians. The advent of oral therapies has revolutionized the treatment of erectile dysfunction.

References

1. Greiner KA, Weigel JW. Erectile dysfunction. Am Fam Physician 1996;54:1675–1682.
2. Saulie BA, Campbell RK. Treating erectile dysfunction in diabetes patients. Diabetes Educ 1997;23:29–33.
3. Khedun SM, Naicker T, Maharaj B. Zinc, hydrochlorothiazide and sexual dysfunction. Centr Afr J Med 1995;41:312–315.
4. Carvajal A, Martin Arias LH. Gynecomastia and sexual disorders after the administration of omeprazole. Am J Gastroenterol 1995;90:1028–1029. Letter.
5. Padma-Nathan H, Hellstrom WJ, Kaiser FE, et al. Treatment of men with erectile dysfunction with transurethral alprostadil. Medicated Urethral System for Erection (MUSE) Study Group. N Engl J Med 1997;336:1–7.

SECTION 5

Neurologic Disorders

Barbara G. Wells, PharmD, FASHP, FCCP, BCPP, Section Editor

50   MULTIPLE SCLEROSIS

▶ **Relapses and Remissions**   **(Level I)**

Barry E. Gidal, PharmD
John O. Fleming, MD

▶ After completing this case study, students should be able to:

- Understand that the signs and symptoms of multiple sclerosis often mimic those of other neurologic diseases.

- Design a pharmacotherapeutic regimen for treatment of an acute exacerbation of multiple sclerosis.

- Identify patients for whom disease-modifying therapy would be appropriate and recommend the most appropriate alternative for an individual patient.

- Provide patient counseling on the proper dosing, self-administration, adverse effects, and storage of interferon beta-1a, interferon beta-1b, and glatiramer acetate.

☀ PATIENT PRESENTATION

Chief Complaint
"My left foot is numb, and I'm having trouble walking."

HPI
Cathy Olson is a 24 yo woman who was in excellent health until 10 months ago when she developed progressive sensory loss on her right face, "distorted" hearing in the right ear, and intense vertigo. These symptoms intensified over 10 days at which time she was hospitalized. A head MRI showed a probable demyelinating lesion in her right pons, and CSF evaluation revealed elevated protein and cell counts. She presents to clinic today indicating that she has had progressive left-sided sensory loss resulting in difficulty ambulating that began about a week ago when she had a mild URI and was experiencing increased stress at work.

PMH
Frequent migraine headaches since adolescence that have been difficult to control despite therapy with ibuprofen and sumatriptan.
Mild to moderate, recurrent bouts of depression that have not been treated pharmacologically.

FH
The patient is of Norwegian descent. She was born and raised in Wisconsin. She has no siblings, and both parents are alive and well. There is no family history of neurological disease.

SH
The patient is single and is employed as an accountant. She has not smoked for 3 years; prior to that she smoked 1 ppd. Her use of alcohol is limited to an occasional glass of wine or beer on weekends.

Meds
Ibuprofen 400 mg po PRN headache

All
NKDA

ROS
Unremarkable except that she reports feeling run down and tired. Also reports past difficulty with urinary control (incontinence) and a subjective feeling of weakness in hot weather. No previous history of visual disturbance (e.g., pain, blurred or double vision), or motor disturbance.

PE

Gen

The patient is a Caucasian woman who appears to be slightly anxious but is otherwise in NAD.

VS

BP 106/60, P 72 and regular, RR 12, T 97.1°C; Wt 55 kg, Ht 5′5″

Skin

Normal turgor; no obvious lesions, tumors, or moles

HEENT

PERRLA; visual acuity is 20/20 OU. Funduscopic exam is normal. EOMs are full in extent. Slight nystagmus present

Neck/LN

Supple, without lymphadenopathy or thyromegaly

Cor

RRR; S_1, S_2 normal; no m/r/g

Lungs

Clear to A&P

Abd

NT/ND

Genit/Rect

Deferred

MS/Ext

Normal ROM; pulses 2+ throughout

Neuro

The patient is alert, oriented, and cooperative. Mild subjective sense of auditory distortion and tinnitus AD despite intact auditory acuity. CN II through XII are intact. Motor tone and strength are normal throughout. DTRs are hyperactive throughout. Sensory exam reveals moderate diminution in the subjective intensity of light touch and pinprick on the left, with maximal deficits noted in the left foot. Coordination testing is normal except for modest unsteadiness on performing tandem walking. Romberg maneuver is positive.

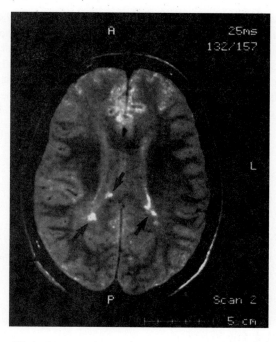

Figure 50–1. Head MRI scan. Arrows highlight typical periventricular white matter lesions seen in multiple sclerosis.

Labs

Na 140 mEq/L	AST 12 IU/L
K 4.1 mEq/L	ALT 40 IU/L
Cl 99 mEq/L	GGT 33 IU/L
CO_2 23 mEq/L	Wintrobe ESR 20 mm/hr
BUN 11 mg/dL	TSH 2.0 μIU/mL
SCr 0.9 mg/dL	ANA negative
Glu 109 mg/dL	VDRL negative
	Lyme serology negative

Head MRI

Multiple areas of increased periventricular white matter signal (plaque); see Figure 50–1.

▶ Questions

Problem Identification

1. a. What information (patient demographics, signs, symptoms, lab values) indicates the presence or severity of multiple sclerosis in this patient?
    b. What additional information (laboratory tests, diagnostic procedures) may be useful in assessing this patient?

Desired Outcome

2. What are the goals of therapy for this patient?

Therapeutic Alternatives

3. a. What pharmacotherapeutic options are available to treat this patient's acute exacerbation, and which one would you recommend?
    b. What adjunctive treatments may be indicated for this patient?
    c. What adverse effects might be anticipated for both first-line and adjunctive treatments?

▶ Clinical Course

The patient was treated with the regimen you recommended with gradual resolution of her symptoms. Six months after the initial presentation, she returns to clinic with complaints of increased difficulty walking and some blurring of her vision. Her muscle strength is intact in the upper extremities, but there is marked weakness in the lower extremities, especially the left side. DTRs are hyperactive in the lower extremities, and tone is slightly spastic. The patient's gait is slow, but she is able to walk without assistance. Her affect is sad, and she is tearful during the examination. She states that she is concerned about the progression of her disease.

> *d. What therapeutic options are available to modify this patient's disease course?*

Optimal Plan

> *4. Design an optimal pharmacotherapeutic plan for reducing the frequency of MS exacerbations in this patient.*

Outcome Evaluation

> *5. What clinical and laboratory parameters are necessary for assessment of both efficacy and toxicity?*

Patient Counseling

> *6. What information would you provide to this patient about her long-term MS therapy?*

▶ Self-study Assignments

1. Identify recent clinical trials assessing the efficacy and toxicity of cyclosporine or IV immune globulin (IVIG) for MS. Considering the data available, define the potential role(s) of these agents for patients with MS.
2. Review the clinical studies evaluating glatiramer for MS. How does this agent compare to interferon beta-1b and interferon beta-1a in terms of both efficacy and toxicity?
3. Outline a plan for providing patient counseling on the dosing, administration, and storage of interferon beta-1b, interferon beta-1a, and glatiramer.
4. Obtain relevant information and formulate an opinion on the role of plasmapheresis in the treatment of MS.

▶ Clinical Pearl

Many patients do not feel better with interferon therapy and may experience unpleasant adverse effects. Adequate counseling about the potential benefits and expected side effects is essential to ensuring adherence to the therapy.

References

1. Schapiro RT. Symptom management in multiple sclerosis. Ann Neurol 1994;36(suppl):S123–S129.
2. The IFNB Multiple Sclerosis Study Group. Interferon beta-1b is effective in relapsing-remitting multiple sclerosis. I. Clinical results of a multicenter, randomized, double-blind, placebo-controlled trial. Neurology 1993;43:655–661.
3. Paty DW, Li DK. Interferon beta-1b is effective in relapsing-remitting multiple sclerosis. II. MRI analysis results of a multicenter, randomized, double-blind, placebo-controlled trial. Neurology 1993;43:662–667.
4. The INFB Multiple Sclerosis Study Group and the British Columbia MS/MRI Analysis Group. Interferon beta-1b in the treatment of multiple sclerosis: Final outcome of the randomized controlled trial. Neurology 1995;45:1277–1285.
5. Jacobs LD, Cookfair DL, Rudick RA, et al. Intramuscular interferon beta-1a for disease progression in relapsing multiple sclerosis. The Multiple Sclerosis Collaborative Research Group. Ann Neurol 1996;39:285–294.
6. Johnson KP, Brooks BR, Cohen JA, et al. Copolymer 1 reduces relapse rate and improves disability in relapsing-remitting multiple sclerosis: Results of a phase III multicenter, double-blind, placebo-controlled trial. The Copolymer 1 Multiple Sclerosis Study Group. Neurology 1995;45: 1268–1276.
7. Hunter SF, Weinshenker BG, Carter JL, et al. Rational clinical immunotherapy for multiple sclerosis. Mayo Clin Proc 1997;72:765–780.

51 COMPLEX PARTIAL SEIZURES

▶ A Lifelong Pattern   (Level I)

James W. McAuley, RPh, PhD

▶ After completing this case study, students should be able to:

- Identify necessary patient- and disease-specific data to collect for patients with complex partial seizures.
- Define potential drug-related problems for established and new antiepileptic drugs.
- List desired therapeutic outcomes for patients with complex partial seizures.
- Based on patient characteristics, choose appropriate pharmacotherapy for treatment of partial seizures and develop a suitable care plan.

☀ PATIENT PRESENTATION

Chief Complaint
"My regular doctor told me I should see a neurologist about my seizures."

HPI
Peggy Livingston is a 60 yo woman referred to the epilepsy clinic by her PCP for evaluation of anticonvulsant therapy. She continues to have seizures, with the last one being 1 week ago that resulted in a fall down a flight of stairs. Her seizures started at a very early age. She remembers first having them in first grade and being confused a lot throughout her schooling. She was briefly tried on phenobarbital but has been on phenytoin most of her life. She has poor seizure control with no extended seizure-free periods. She has not seen a neurologist for years, if ever. She has not had any neuroimaging studies and provides no previous EEG results.

Most of her seizures are complex partial seizures where she "blacks out" and loses sense of time. Occasionally, she has secondarily generalized tonic–clonic convulsions. She is more likely to have a seizure if she gets "over tired" or stressed. She has no significant risk factors for seizures. She states that at some time in her past, she "felt terrible" on higher doses of phenytoin. She confirms that she is very compliant, although she has run out of her medications more than once. Because she is having seizures, she does not drive and therefore must rely on others for transportation.

Data gathered from reviewing her seizure calendar with her and her husband suggest that she is experiencing approximately 2 "small" seizures per week (complex partial seizures with no secondary generalization) and 1 "big" seizure per month (a secondarily generalized tonic–clonic seizure). Her interview details and her overall score on her responses to the Quality of Life in Epilepsy questionnaire (QOLIE-89) show a significant impact of her seizures on her quality of life. Her scores on the energy/fatigue, pain, and social support domains are especially low in comparison to a cohort of other patients with epilepsy.

PMH
s/p hysterectomy at age 44

FH
Both parents deceased, 1 younger brother in good health. No seizure disorder, cancer, or cardiovascular disease.

SH
Married; retired from a local seamstress shop; denies tobacco and alcohol use; finished high school.

ROS
Tires easily, but no problem with balance

Meds
Phenytoin 100 mg po TID

All
NKDA

PE

Gen
Pleasant Caucasian woman in NAD

VS
BP 126/73, P 63, RR 17, T 97.1°F; Ht 5'1", Wt 50.8 kg

Skin
Normal color, hydration, and temperature

HEENT
Mild hirsutism, (−) gingival hyperplasia, (+) cataract OS

Neck/LN
(−) JVD, (−) lymphadenopathy

Lungs/Thorax
CTA

Breasts
Deferred

CV
Normal S_1 & S_2, RRR, NSR, normal peripheral pulses

Abd
NTND, (+) BS, no HSM

Genit/Rect
Deferred

MS/Ext
Significant burn on right hand from seizure while cooking

Neuro
CN II–XII intact, slight lateral gaze nystagmus noted. Motor: 4/5 muscle strength on left side, 5/5 on right side. DTRs: 2+ RUE, 1+ LUE, 0 RLE, 0 LLE. Sensory: normal light touch and pin prick. Station: NL.

Labs

Na 137 mEq/L	Hgb 14.5 g/dL	AST 31 IU/L
K 4.1 mEq/L	Hct 41.7%	ALT 22 IU/L
Cl 100 mEq/L	RBC $4.71 \times 10^6/mm^3$	Alk phos 187 IU/L
CO_2 29 mEq/L	MCV 88.6 μm^3	GGT 45 IU/L
BUN 9 mg/dL	MCHC 34.7 g/dL	Ca 7.3 mg/dL
SCr 0.6 mg/dL	Plt $212 \times 10^3/mm^3$	Alb 3.9 g/dL
Glu 107 mg/dL	WBC $5.4 \times 10^3/mm^3$	

EEG
Abnormal for bitemporal slowing, which is more significant in the left temporal region as characterized with polymorphic and epileptiform discharges consistent with a history of seizure disorder

Assessment
Uncontrolled complex partial seizures, with occasional secondary generalization

---

▶ Questions

Problem Identification

1. a. Create a list of the patient's drug-related problems.

   b. What information (signs, symptoms, laboratory values) indicates the presence or severity of complex partial seizures?

Desired Outcome

2. What are the goals of pharmacotherapy in this case?

Therapeutic Alternatives

3. a. What non-drug therapies might be useful for this patient?

   b. What feasible pharmacotherapeutic alternatives are available for treatment of complex partial seizures in this patient?

Optimal Plan

4. What drug, dosage form, dose, schedule, and duration of therapy are best for this patient?

Outcome Evaluation

5. *What clinical and laboratory parameters are necessary to evaluate the therapy for achievement of the desired therapeutic outcome and to detect or prevent adverse effects?*

Patient Counseling

6. *What information should be provided to the patient to enhance compliance, ensure successful therapy, and minimize adverse effects?*

▶ Clinical Course

A collective decision was made among the health care practitioners, the patient, and her husband to add one of the new antiepileptic drugs to her current drug regimen and to see her back in 3 months. She was given written and verbal information on this new drug and instructed to call with any questions, problems or concerns. At her next visit, the patient reported that there had been an initial response to the addition of the new antiepileptic drug (i.e., fewer seizures), but then a return to 2 "small" seizures per week and 1 "big" seizure per month. There are no recent laboratory data. Her neurologic exam is unchanged.

▶ Follow-up Question

1. *Other than non-compliance, what are the potential explanations for this situation?*

▶ Clinical Course

Upon further questioning about compliance, the patient reports that she has not been taking her new antiepileptic drug for the last 2 months. This was due to having no prescription insurance coverage and financial problems at home. She was able to continue her phenytoin as directed. She is offered enrollment forms for a patient assistance program in order to obtain her medications at a reduced cost, and the need to be compliant with her medications was reemphasized. She then stated that 2 months ago she fell and broke her hip. It has healed well, but she is now more concerned about her "brittle bones."

▶ Self-study Assignments

1. Outline a plan for assessing this patient's compliance with her medication regimen.
2. What risk factors does this patient have for osteoporosis? What interventions should be made?
3. Would switching this patient from phenytoin to carbamazepine be an appropriate alternative? If so, would Tegretol XR be an appropriate dosage form?

▶ Clinical Pearl

Although epilepsy affects men and women equally, there are many women's health issues in epilepsy, including menstrual cycle influences on seizure activity, contraceptive-antiepileptic drug interactions, teratogenicity of antiepileptic drugs, and influence of hormone replacement on seizure activity.

References

1. Vickrey BG, Perrine KR, Hays RD, et al. Quality of life in epilepsy QOLIE-89: Scoring manual and patient inventory. Santa Monica, RAND, 1993:1–16.
2. Marson AG, Kadir ZA, Chadwick DW. New antiepileptic drugs: A systematic review of their efficacy and tolerability. BMJ 1996;313:1169–1174.
3. Dichter MA, Brodie MJ. New antiepileptic drugs. N Engl J Med 1996;334:1583–1590.
4. Hahn TJ. Bone complications of anticonvulsants. Drugs 1976;12:201–211.

52 STATUS EPILEPTICUS

▶ Not Just Another Seizure　　　(Level I)

Sharon M. Tramonte, PharmD

▶　After completing this case study, students should be able to:
- Define status epilepticus and its precipitating causes.
- Identify measures that should be taken in the ED for a patient in status epilepticus.
- Recommend appropriate drug treatment for status epilepticus.
- Recommend an appropriate pharmaceutical care plan for a patient with status epilepticus.

☀ PATIENT PRESENTATION

Chief Complaint
As given by a friend of the patient: "We were out playing basketball and he fell to the ground and started having seizures. We couldn't wake him up so we brought him here."

HPI
Michael Stillman is a 29 yo man brought to the ED by his wife and three friends. His wife reports that she thinks he stopped taking his medications a few weeks ago because he hasn't had seizures in years and doesn't think he needs them anymore.

PMH
Medical records revealed that the patient developed generalized tonic–clonic seizures in childhood. Phenobarbital was initiated and controlled the seizures for many years. Withdrawal of phenobarbital was attempted 15 years ago after several years of being seizure free. The drug was restarted when seizures occurred during the attempted taper. Phenobarbital was replaced with carbamazepine because of sedation and lethargy. Phenytoin was added 8 years ago because of frequent and prolonged breakthrough seizures. He has not had a seizure since that time.

FH

Negative for epilepsy; the patient has 5 siblings, all alive and well. No other information on family history was obtained.

SH

Married with no children; no tobacco use; reports drinking up to 3 beers per month

Meds

Carbamazepine 500 mg po TID
Phenytoin 100 mg po BID

All

NKDA

Adverse Drug Effect History

Phenobarbital (sedation, lethargy), phenytoin (gingival hyperplasia)

PE

Gen

WDWN Caucasian man who is unarousable; clothes are wet from urinary incontinence

VS

BP 150/90, P 150, RR 25, T 37.5°C; Ht 5'7", Wt 79.4 kg

Skin

Warm, dry and pale; nail beds are pale

HEENT

Mild gingival hyperplasia; mucous membranes are dry

Neck/LN

Supple; no thyromegaly or lymphadenopathy

Chest/Lungs

Symmetric, lungs CTA

CV

RRR, no m/r/g

Abd

Soft, no HSM, (+) BS

MS/Ext

Muscle mass normal, full ROM

Neuro

Unarousable; reflexes 3+ bilaterally

Labs

Na 136 mEq/L	Hgb 12.8 g/dL	Drug Screen: pending
K 4.5 mEq/L	Hct 41%	Carbamazepine: pending
Cl 97 mEq/L	Plt $320 \times 10^3/mm^3$	Phenytoin: pending
CO_2 28 mEq/L	WBC $9.0 \times 10^3/mm^3$	
BUN 16 mg/dL	Diff WNL	
SCr 1.0 mg/dL		
Glu 60 mg/dL		

EEG

Baseline from medical record: Diffuse background slowing; no focal changes or epileptiform activity present; photic stimulation failed to produce other changes

Assessment

29 yo man with a history of tonic–clonic seizures now in status epilepticus

---

▶ Questions

Problem Identification

1. a. What are this patient's drug-related problems?
   b. What steps should be taken when the patient is first seen in the ED?

Desired Outcome

2. What are the goals of pharmacotherapy in this case?

Therapeutic Alternatives

3. What pharmacotherapeutic options are available to treat status epilepticus?

Optimal Plan

4. What is the best pharmacotherapeutic plan for this patient?

Outcome Evaluation

5. What clinical and laboratory parameters are needed to evaluate the therapy to ensure the best possible outcome?

Patient Counseling

6. What information should the patient receive to ensure successful therapy and to minimize adverse effects?

▶ Self-study Assignments

1. There are several drug interactions with phenytoin and carbamazepine. Describe the effects that these drugs have on one another. What, if anything, should be done to compensate for these drug interactions?
2. There are several sports that patients with epilepsy should not participate in. What are some of these sports, and why should they not participate in them?

3. Finger-stick assays are available for phenytoin, carbamazepine, and phenobarbital. What role might they play in the emergent therapy of status epilepticus? Characterize the accuracy of these tests.
4. Prepare a two-page paper summarizing the hematologic adverse effects of all of the anticonvulsants.

▶ Clinical Pearl

In non-convulsive status epilepticus, it is often impossible to determine if seizures have stopped without obtaining an EEG.

References

1. Weise KL, Bleck TP. Status epilepticus in children and adults. Crit Care Clin 1997;13:629–646.
2. Lowenstein DH, Aminoff MJ, Simon RP. Barbiturate anesthesia in the treatment of status epilepticus: Clinical experience with 14 patients. Neurology 1988;38:395–400.
3. Kumar A, Bleck TP. Intravenous midazolam for the treatment of refractory status epilepticus. Crit Care Med 1992;20:483–488.

53 ACUTE MANAGEMENT OF THE HEAD INJURY PATIENT

▶ Bowled Over   (Level III)

Denise H. Rhoney, PharmD
Mark S. Luer, PharmD

▶ After completing this case study, students should be able to:

- Discuss the goals of cerebral resuscitation.
- Identify parameters beneficial in assessing the severity of the head injury.
- Discuss the therapeutic management of increased intracranial pressure.
- Recommend appropriate therapy to prevent medical complications after head injury.

☀ PATIENT PRESENTATION

Chief Complaint
Not available—the patient was brought in by EMS as a trauma code.

HPI
Jonathan Bowle is a 25 yo, 80 kg man involved in an MVA in which his car veered off the road into a tree about 45 minutes PTA. He was not wearing a seat belt at the time of the collision. Witnesses report that he was initially lucid at the scene but has become progressively less responsive since then.

PMH
Unknown

FH
Unknown

SH
Unknown, but possible alcohol abuse

ROS
Unobtainable

Meds
Unknown

All
Unknown

PE

Gen
Well-developed male who is unresponsive with extensor posturing; heavy smell of alcohol. Mood and affect are not assessable.

VS
BP 175/85, P 140, RR 40, T 101.2°F; Wt 80 kg, Ht 6'2"

Skin
Several abrasions noted

HEENT
Inspection of conjunctivae and lids reveal bilateral periorbital ecchymoses. The left pupil is 6 mm and nonreactive and the right pupil is 3 mm and nonreactive. EOMs are not reactive and not moving. External inspection of ears and nose reveals no acute abnormalities. There is some dried blood in both nares and mouth. Internal inspection of the ears reveals evidence of hemotympanum. Battle's sign and raccoon eyes are present. The head has a 4-cm scalp laceration over the left frontal region of the skull with some swelling. Neck is in a cervical collar, therefore movement was not attempted. There is no bony step-off noted and no gross masses in the neck.

Lungs
Increased respiratory effort with retractions and rhonchi noted diffusely

Heart
Auscultation reveals a tachycardic rhythm with no abnormal sounds

Abd
Soft with no masses or tenderness but decreased bowel sounds. There is no gross HSM

Ext
No non-traumatic edema is noted

Neuro
There is no response other than extensor posturing to pain

Labs

Na 145 mEq/L	Hgb 13.4 g/dL	Ca 8.7 mg/dL	ABG
K 3.8 mEq/L	Hct 40.7%	Mg 1.2 mg/dL	pH 7.5
Cl 109 mEq/L	Plt 101 × 10³/mm³	Phos 1.4 mEq/L	HCO_3 18 mEq/L
CO_2 21 mEq/L	WBC 16.0 × 10³/mm³	Alb 2.4 g/dL	pco_2 28 mm Hg
BUN 15 mg/dL	Diff N/A	Ethanol 312 mg/dL	po_2 71 mm Hg
SCr 1.2 mg/dL			O_2 sat 80% on RA
Glu 235 mg/dL			

Portable Chest X-ray

No evidence of pneumothorax, hemothorax, or rib fractures; the ET tube is above the carina

Head CT

Small, left frontal-parietal acute subdural hematoma with subarachnoid blood and a nondepressed linear skull fracture

Assessment

1. Status post MVA
2. Intracranial bleed
3. Coma
4. Respiratory distress

► Clinical Course

Upon arrival in the ED, IV access was initiated, and the patient was intubated orally using a rapid sequence intubation technique (10 mg IV vecuronium followed by 100 mg IV lidocaine, 2 mg IV midazolam, and 100 mg IV succinylcholine). The patient was taken to the operating room immediately for evacuation of the hematoma and ventriculostomy placement for monitoring of ICP. The patient will then be transferred to the neurotrauma unit for monitoring.

► Questions

Problem Identification

1. a. What information (signs, symptoms, laboratory values) indicates the severity of this patient's head injury?
   b. What is the Glasgow coma score for this patient?
   c. Does this patient have any factors that may complicate assessment of the neurologic examination?

Desired Outcome

2. a. What are the goals of therapy for this patient?
   b. What are the goals of fluid resuscitation and hemodynamic monitoring for this patient?

Therapeutic Alternatives

3. a. What therapeutic alternatives are available for fluid resuscitation, and which would be the most appropriate for this patient?
   b. What non-drug therapies may be useful in preventing or treating increased ICP?
   c. What pharmacotherapeutic alternatives are available for the treatment of increased ICP?

Optimal Plan

4. a. Develop an optimal pharmacotherapeutic plan to treat the patient's increased ICP.
   b. Outline a pharmacotherapeutic plan for prevention of medical complications that may occur in this patient.

Outcome Evaluation

5. What monitoring parameters should be instituted to ensure efficacy and prevent toxicity for the therapy recommended for treating increased ICP?

Patient Counseling

6. What medication counseling should this patient receive if he is discharged on phenytoin?

► Self-study Assignments

1. Review the different types of neurologic monitoring devices that are available and how drug therapy might influence these monitoring parameters.
2. Review cerebral autoregulation in the normal brain and injured brain and discuss the potential use of hypertensive cerebral perfusion pressure as a treatment modality for increased ICP.

► Clinical Pearl

There are only three standards of care for severe head injury patients: (1) use of corticosteroids is not recommended for improving outcome or reducing ICP; (2) in the absence of increased ICP, chronic prolonged hyperventilation ($Paco_2$ ≤25 mm Hg) should be avoided; and (3) prophylactic use of antiepileptic drugs is not recommended for preventing late posttraumatic seizures (>7 days).

References

1. Chesnut RM, Marshall LF, Klauber MR, et al. The role of secondary brain injury in determining outcome from severe head injury. J Trauma 1993;34:216–222.
2. Muizelaar JP, Marmarou A, Ward JD, et al. Adverse effects of prolonged hyperventilation in patients with severe head injury: A randomized clinical trial. J Neurosurg 1991;75:731–739.
3. Hsiang JK, Chesnut RM, Crisp CB, et al. Early, routine paralysis for intracranial pressure control in severe head injury: Is it necessary? Crit Care Med 1994;22:1471–1476.

4. Temkin NR, Dikmen SS, Wilensky AJ, et al. A randomized, double-blind study of phenytoin for the prevention of post-traumatic seizures. N Engl J Med 1990;323:497–502.

5. Reusser P, Gyr K, Scheidegger D, et al. Prospective endoscopic study of stress erosions and ulcers in critically ill neurosurgical patients: Current incidence and effect of acid-reducing prophylaxis. Crit Care Med 1990;18:270–274.

6. Black PM, Baker MF, Snook CP. Experience with external pneumatic calf compression in neurology and neurosurgery. Neurosurgery 1986;18:440–444.

54　PARKINSON'S DISEASE

▶ On Shaky Ground　　　　　　　　(Level II)

Mary Louise Wagner, MS, PharmD

▶　After completing this case study, students should be able to:

- Recognize motor and non-motor symptoms of Parkinson's Disease (PD).

- Develop an optimal pharmacotherapeutic plan for a patient with PD.

- Recommend alterations in therapy for a patient experiencing adverse drug effects.

- Counsel patients with PD about the disease and its drug therapy.

☀ PATIENT PRESENTATION

Chief Complaint
"I just can't sleep anymore."

HPI
Ron Vaser is a 73 yo man who presents to the neurology clinic for his routine 3-month evaluation. He feels he has good and bad days, but overall his Sinemet doses are not lasting as long as they used to. He complains that it takes him a long time to go to sleep and that he often awakens in the morning with a painful cramp in his foot. Many afternoons he refuses to leave the house because he feels unsteady when walking. He also complains of decreased appetite; he states that he is "just not interested in food." He eats 3 small meals daily (i.e., 1/2 bowl of cereal in the morning, 1/2 sandwich at noon, and he "never finishes supper"). His wife states that he is sleeping more during the day and that he appears depressed during many afternoons.

PMH
PD × 6 years
BPH × 4 years
Hypothyroidism × 8 years

FH
Mother died at age 64 of ovarian CA; father died of "old age"; 2 daughters are alive and in good health.

SH
(−) Alcohol, (−) tobacco, married for 52 years.

ROS
The patient has no complaints other than those noted in the HPI. He denies constipation, sweating, and dizziness. He also reports no problems with swallowing, writing, or urination.

Meds
Eldepryl 5 mg at breakfast and at bedtime (started 3 months ago)
Sinemet 25/100, 1 tablet @ 8:00 A.M., 12:00 P.M., 4:00 P.M., and 8:00 P.M. (started 6 years ago with many dose changes since that time)
Synthroid 0.075 mg po QD (started 8 years ago)
Hytrin 1 mg po QD (started 4 years ago)

All
Shellfish (shortness of breath and rash)

PE

Gen
The patient is an elderly Caucasian man who appears his stated age

VS
BP 114/70 sitting, 110/68 standing; P 60; RR 13; T 98.2°F; Wt 75 kg, Ht 69″

Skin
Small amount of dry yellow scales on forehead

HEENT
Decreased volume of speech, facial masking, decreased eye blinking; PERRLA; EOMI

Neck/LN
Supple, no masses, normal thyroid, no bruits

Lungs/Thorax
Normal breath sounds

CV
Regular pulse, no murmurs

Abd
Soft, non-tender

Genit/Rect
Enlarged prostate, but no nodules palpated; no rectal polyps

MS/Ext
Resting tremor (L > R), cogwheel rigidity, and poor postural stability. Normal peripheral pulses

Neuro
CNs intact. UPDRS exam (Unified Parkinson's Disease Rating Scale) during an on-period: motor score 25, ADL score 9, mentation behavior and mood score 2 (indicating no problem with memory or behavior, but he has depression and apathy mostly during off-periods). His daily off time is 4 to 5 hours per day. (Note that scores will be higher during his off-periods.)

Labs
Hgb 15 g/dL
Hct 44%
WBC $7.0 \times 10^3/mm^3$
SCr 1.0 mg/dL
TSH 2.0 µIU/mL
T_4 total 1.0 µg/dL

Activities of Daily Living

No difficulties in swallowing, salivation, or cutting food. No episodes of falling or freezing. Able to maintain good hygiene. Micrographic handwriting but legible. Dressing time in the morning increased since last visit. Increased difficulty turning in bed and adjusting the sheets.

Assessment

Based on the HPI and UPDRS, the patient's resting tremor, rigidity, and bradykinesia are about the same, but his gait and postural imbalance are worse than at the last visit. He has increased off-periods. His PD is worsening, but his other medical conditions are stable.

► Questions

Problem Identification

1. a. Create a list of the patient's drug-related problems.
   b. What signs and symptoms of PD are present in this patient?
   c. According to the Hoehn–Yahr Scale, what stage is his disease?

Desired Outcome

2. What are the goals of therapy for PD?

Therapeutic Alternatives

3. a. What non-pharmacologic alternatives may be beneficial for the treatment of PD in this patient?
   b. Based upon the patient's signs and symptoms, which pharmacotherapeutic alternatives are viable alternatives for him at this time?

Optimal Plan

4. What drug, dosage form, dose, schedule, and duration of therapy are best for this patient?

Outcome Evaluation

5. What monitoring parameters should be used to evaluate the patient's response to medications and to detect adverse effects?

Patient Counseling

6. How would you counsel this patient to ensure successful therapy, enhance compliance, and minimize adverse effects?

► Clinical Course

The pharmacotherapeutic plan that was recommended is as follows: Discontinue selegiline and add pergolide 0.25 mg po TID. A week later the patient's wife calls the neurologist complaining that her husband is very nauseated, vomiting, and claims to be seeing Bugs Bunny leaving carrots around the house. He is sleeping better through the night and less during the daytime since discontinuing the selegiline. He is experiencing less wearing-off periods and is able to get out of the house more often. He no longer complains of unsteadiness, trouble walking, or cramps. His wife reports that he is eating better and that he is more pleasant. He is less apathetic and moody.

► Follow-up Questions

1. What side effects of therapy does the patient now manifest?
2. What adjustments in drug therapy do you recommend at this time?
3. What new patient education should be provided to the patient?

► Self-study Assignments

1. Evaluate the use of apomorphine in the treatment of PD.[5]
2. Evaluate the use of liquid Sinemet in the treatment of PD.[6]

► Clinical Pearl

As Parkinson's disease progresses, the timing of medications needs to coincide with symptoms. Patient symptoms may worsen when they are forced to receive their medications at predetermined dosing times such as those used in hospitals and nursing homes.

ACKNOWLEDGMENT

The author would like to thank Jacob Sage, MD, and Margery Mark, MD, for providing the patient case and for their editorial comments.

References

1. Lees AJ. Comparison of therapeutic effects and mortality data of levodopa and levodopa combined with selegiline in patients with early, mild Parkinson's disease. Parkinson's Disease Research Group of the United Kingdom. BMJ 1995;311:1602–1607.
2. Lang EA. Clinical rating scales and videotape analysis. In: Koller WC, Paulson G. eds. Therapy of Parkinson's Disease, 2nd ed. New York, Marcel Dekker, 1995;21–46.
3. Olanow CW, Koller WC. An algorithm (decision tree) for the management of Parkinson's disease: Treatment guidelines. American Academy of Neurology. Neurology 1998;50(suppl 3):S1–S57.

4. Corboy D, Wagner ML, Sage JI. Apomorphine for motor fluctuations and freezing in Parkinson's disease. Ann Pharmacother 1995;29:282–288.
5. Zoldan J, Friedberg G, Livneh M, et al. Psychosis in advanced Parkinson's disease: Treatment with ondansetron, a 5-HT3 receptor antagonist. Neurology 1995;45:1305–1308.
6. Pappert EJ, Goetz CG, Niederman F, et al. Liquid levodopa/carbidopa produces significant improvement in motor function without dyskinesia exacerbation. Neurology 1996;47:1493–1495.

55 PAIN MANAGEMENT

▶ A Pain in the Iliac   (Level II)

Karen Beauchamp, BPharm, RPh
Daniel Sageser, PharmD

▶ After completing this case study, students should be able to:

- Define the goals for pain management in a patient with multiple debilitating disease states.
- Design a pharmacotherapeutic pain management plan.
- Understand the use of NSAIDs and other non-opioids in the treatment of pain.
- Determine the monitoring parameters for safety and efficacy in pain treatment for immobilized patients.

☼ PATIENT PRESENTATION

Chief Complaint
"It hurts when I move or walk. I especially feel the pain when I try to reach up in my kitchen cupboards for things. About the only time I'm not in pain is when I'm lying flat in bed."

HPI
Olivia Conner is a 68 yo woman who developed significant low back pain 1 month ago without precipitating injury or incident. She was diagnosed with multiple myeloma 5 years ago. She received a course of melphalan 8 mg/m^2 and prednisone 40 mg/m^2 1 year ago that had to be discontinued after 3 sessions due to pancytopenia. Her myeloma is currently being treated with intermittent doses of Decadron. Her back pain has generally been getting worse over the last month. Within the last week the patient has had an extensive work-up, including MRI scans, DEXA scans, bone scans, and x-ray studies. A recent MRI shows compression fractures at T12, L3, and L5. Total body bone scan reveals intense uptake at T12. Plain x-rays of the lumbar spine demonstrate severe osteopenia.

PMH
Multiple myeloma × 5 years
Cholelithiasis, resolved with surgery 12 years ago
Type 2 DM × 5 years

SH
Lives at home with her husband. Patient is a retired secretary. She is a life-long non-smoker. She rarely drinks alcohol.

FH
Two brothers who were smokers died of emphysema. She has 5 children in good health.

Meds
Dexamethasone 40 mg po QD × 4 days, then off 5 days for 3 cycles (4 days on, 5 days off) ending with a 14-day rest period, then restart.
Medroxyprogesterone 2.5 mg po QD
Conjugated estrogens 0.625 mg po QD
Glyburide 5 mg po BID

All
NKDA

ROS
Positive for pain radiating from the thoracic/lumbar area, exacerbated by movement. Occasional heartburn after large meals.

PE

Gen
Patient is a 68 yo woman in obvious pain and discomfort related to her spine. She presents using a walker.

VS
BP 164/94, P 72, RR 15, T 37.4°C; Wt 65.4 kg, Ht 5'7"

HEENT
PERRLA, EOMI, TMs intact; dry buccal mucosa

Neck
Supple, no JVD, no lymphadenopathy

Resp
CTA & P. No crackles or wheezes

Thorax
Patient stands with a forward list and moves in a very slow and guarded fashion. The thoracolumbar range of motion is markedly limited with pain.

CV
NSR without murmurs, rubs, or gallops

Breasts
Negative

Abd
Soft, NT, liver and spleen not palpable, (+) BS

Genit/Rect
Deferred

Ext
There is some mild edema of the left ankle, without pitting. There is no tenderness farther up and no pitting edema in the pretibial areas.

Homan's sign is negative. Distal pulses are 2+ and symmetrical. Gait is very slow and painful. She is able to walk on the heels and toes with some encouragement. Squat and rise are normal.

Neuro

A & O × 3; DTRs are 2+ and symmetrical in the knees and ankles. Great toes are downgoing bilaterally to plantar stimulation. There is no fasciculation or clonus noted in the lower extremities. Manual muscle testing shows normal strength in all muscle groups of the lower extremities.

Labs

Na 140 mEq/L	Ca 8.7 mg/dL	AST 78 IU/L
K 3.8 mEq/L	Phos 4.1 mg/dL	ALT 70 IU/L
Cl 110 mEq/L	U.A. 6.8 mg/dL	Alk Phos 93 IU/L
CO_2 22 mEq/L	T. Prot 11.2 g/dL	GGT 121 IU/L
BUN 13 mg/dL	Alb 3.2 g/dL	LDH 391 IU/L
SCr 0.8 mg/dL	T. Chol 100 mg/dL	T. bili 0.7 mg/dL
Glu 140 mg/dL	Trig 270 mg/dL	

Assessment

Multiple myeloma with compression fractures

▶ Questions

Problem Identification

1. a. Create a list of all of the patient's drug-related problems.
   b. What are the possible causes of spinal fracture in this patient, and what additional diagnostic tests might be helpful in determining their etiology?
   c. List appropriate questions and the tools you would use in assessing pain severity and foci in this patient.

Desired Outcome

2. What are the goals for pain management in this patient?

Therapeutic Alternatives

3. Compare the pharmacotherapeutic alternatives available for treatment of this patient's pain.

Optimal Plan

4. Design a pharmacotherapeutic pain management plan specific for this patient.

Outcome Evaluation

5. Identify monitoring parameters both for efficacy and adverse effects of your pain management plan.

Patient Counseling

6. Outline pertinent medication information you would provide to this patient and her family regarding her pharmaceutical care plan.

▶ Clinical Course

The patient's physician accepted your care plan and prescribed what you recommended to treat her pain. The patient gained some initial relief from your regimen. Four weeks later, she returns to the clinic complaining of dramatically increased pain and frequent nausea. She has not had a bowel movement in 5 days. The patient's primary cancer state is also progressing, and laboratory testing reveals SCr 3.0 mg/dL and BUN 45 mg/dL. Her physician places her in a body-jacket type brace and wheelchair to restrict her movement to promote healing.

▶ Follow-up Questions

1. How would you alter your care plan for this patient?
2. What additional monitoring parameters should you consider in an immobilized patient?

▶ Self-study Assignments

1. Construct a chart of opioid and analgesic medications categorized by sites of metabolism and excretion.
2. Develop a 15-minute presentation on the use and efficacy of calcitonin in bone pain management.

▶ Clinical Pearl

Nonsteroidal anti-inflammatory drugs are often overlooked but effective first-line agents in the treatment of bone pain.

References

1. Agency for Health Care Policy and Research. Management of cancer pain: Adults. Am J Hosp Pharm 1994;51:1643–1656.
2. Portenoy RK, Ingham J. The measurement of pain and other symptoms. In: Doyle D, Hanks GWC, MacDonald N. Oxford Textbook of Palliative Medicine, 2nd ed. New York, Oxford University Press, 1993:203–219.
3. Daut RL, Cleeland CS, Flanery RC. Development of the Wisconsin Brief Pain Questionnaire to assess pain in cancer and other diseases. Pain 1983;17:197–210.
4. Ferrell BR. The impact of pain on quality of life: A decade of research. Nursing Clin North Am 1995;30:609–624.

56 HEADACHE DISORDERS

▶ **Streaks of Light**   (Level II)

Mark S. Luer, PharmD
Susan R. Winkler, PharmD, BCPS

▶ After completing this case study, students should be able to:

- Develop both short-term and long-range goals for the treatment and prevention of migraine headaches.

- Make recommendations regarding pharmacotherapeutic regimens for an individual patient based on information concerning the patient's headache type and severity, medical history, previous drug therapy, concomitant problems, and pertinent laboratory data.

- Provide counseling to patients on the use of transnasal abortive agents for the treatment of migraine headaches.

- Describe the appropriate use of a headache diary and how it may be used to refine headache treatment.

☼ PATIENT PRESENTATION

Chief Complaint
"I am queasy and seeing streaks of light."

HPI
Caroline Parker is a 28 yo woman who is well known to the medical staff. She presents to the walk-in clinic today for treatment of an impending migraine headache. She began experiencing an aura about 30 minutes ago. Her aura consists of nausea and streaks of pastel lights flashing throughout all visual fields. She admits to not taking her carbamazepine for the past 2 days. Her typical headache usually evolves quickly (within 1 hour) and involves severe throbbing pain, which is unilateral and temporal in distribution and preceded by an aura. It frequently involves photophobia and nausea. Vomiting may occur with an extreme headache. She describes her headaches as "almost crippling," necessitating a return to her residence, covering her windows, and placing her head under a pillow until the headache abates. Without treatment, headaches can last for up to 72 hours. She rates a typical headache as 7 to $7^{1}/_{2}$ on a scale of 0 to 10, with 10 being the worst possible headache. The frequency of her headaches has decreased since she started carbamazepine, but the intensity remains the same. Currently, headaches are sporadic (1 or 2 per month). There is no identifiable relationship between her headaches and the timing of her menses.

PMH
Migraine with aura since age 13; previous medical work-up, including an EEG and a head MRI, demonstrated no PVD, CVA, brain tumor, infection, cerebral aneurysm, or epileptic component. Previously, it was thought that she may have epilepsy, and she was started on valproic acid empirically. While epileptic events were subsequently ruled out, she did experience some improvement in her headaches with daily antiepileptic therapy. Drug therapies have included the following.

Abortive therapies
   Simple analgesics, NSAIDs, and Midrin (no efficacy)
   Ergotamine tartrate suppository, which caused severe vomiting with no headache relief
   Narcotics (good efficacy, but puts her "out of commission for days")
   Oral sumatriptan (Imitrex po worked well for 3 to 4 months, but no longer has efficacy)
   SC sumatriptan (Imitrex SC had good efficacy; occasionally has a return of the headache 24 to 48 hours later; she requires medical assistance for drug administration because she refuses to self-administer)
Prophylactic therapies
   Valproic acid (good efficacy, caused an increase in appetite and a 15 lb. weight gain in 2 weeks)
   Carbamazepine (good efficacy with no apparent adverse effects)
Other medical problems include endometriosis and chronic mild depression for 18 months

FH
Positive for migraines (both parents).

SH
Pre-med student. Denies tobacco or alcohol use. Occasional caffeine intake.

ROS
Complains of diminished sight in all visual fields, streaking lights of pastel colors; (+) nausea but no vomiting or diarrhea; regular menses with oral contraceptive.

Meds
   Loestrin 21, 1 tablet po QD (for endometriosis)
   Carbamazepine 200 mg po Q HS, started 6 months ago
   Sertraline 50 mg po Q HS
   Imitrex 6 mg SC STATdose System PRN headache (administered in physician's office only)

All
None

PE

Gen
WDWN woman in moderate distress

VS
BP 132/86, HR 76, RR 18, T 37.2°C; Ht 5'6", Wt 56.7 kg

Skin
Normal skin turgor; no diaphoresis

HEENT
PERRLA; EOMI; funduscopic exam shows sharp discs, normal vessel number and size, (−) hemorrhages or papilledema

Neck
Supple; no masses, thyroid enlargement, adenopathy, bruits, or JVD

Chest
Good breath sounds bilaterally; clear to A & P

CV
RRR, S_1, S_2 normal, no m/r/g

Abd
Soft, NT/ND, no hepatosplenomegaly, (+) BS

Genit/Rect
Deferred

MS/Ext
UE/LE strength 5/5 with normal tone; radial and femoral pulses 3+ bilaterally; no edema; no evidence of thrombophlebitis; full ROM

Neuro
A&O × 3; no dysarthria or aphasia; memory intact; no nystagmus; no fasciculations, tremor, or ataxia; (−) Romberg; CN II–XII intact; sensory intact; DTRs: 2+; Babinski ↓ bilaterally

Labs
None obtained; urine pregnancy test (−)

Assessment
Aura, with impending migraine headache

► Questions

Problem Identification

1. a. Create a list of the patient's drug-related problems related to this clinic visit.

b. What information indicates the presence or severity of the migraine headache?

c. Could any of the patient's problems have been caused or exacerbated by her drug therapy?

Desired Outcome

2. What are the initial and long-term goals of therapy for this patient?

Therapeutic Alternatives

3. a. What pharmacotherapeutic alternatives are available for treatment of the patient's nausea, and how will they impact potential abortive therapies?

b. What pharmacotherapeutic alternatives are available for aborting her current migraine attack?

Optimal Plan

4. Considering this patient's past successes and failures in treating her migraine attacks, design an optimal pharmacotherapeutic plan for aborting her headaches now and in the future.

Outcome Evaluation

5. What clinical and/or laboratory parameters should be assessed regularly to evaluate the therapy for achievement of the desired therapeutic outcome and to detect or prevent adverse effects?

Patient Counseling

6. What information should be provided to the patient regarding her new abortive therapy?

► Follow-up Question

1. Describe how a headache diary could help the treatment of this patient's migraine headaches (see Figure 56–1).

► Self-study Assignments

1. Review the literature regarding other intranasal agents (including butorphanol and lidocaine) that are also used for aborting migraines.
2. Familiarize yourself with common medications implicated as trigger factors for migraines.
3. Prepare a report highlighting antiepileptic drugs that are used in the prophylaxis of migraines.

► Clinical Pearl

Headaches that occur every day or almost every day are sometimes caused by the overuse of the medicines used to abort migraines (i.e., simple analgesics) and are called rebound headaches.

References

1. Silberstein SD. The role of sex hormones in headache. Neurology 1992;42(3 suppl 2):37–42.
2. Moore KL, Noble SL. Drug treatment of migraine: Part I. Acute therapy and drug-rebound headache. Am Fam Physician 1997;565:2039–2048.
3. Ryan R, Elkind A, Baker CC, et al. Sumatriptan nasal spray for the acute treatment of migraine. Results of two clinical studies. Neurology 1997;49:1225–1230.
4. Mathew NT, Asgharnejad M, Peykamian M, et al. Naratriptan is effective and well tolerated in the acute treatment of migraine. Results of a double-blind, placebo-controlled, crossover study. Neurology 1997;49:1485–1490.
5. Edmeads JG, Millson DS. Tolerability profile of zolmitriptan (Zomig; 311C90), a novel dual central and peripherally acting 5HT1B/1D agonist. International clinical experience based on >3000 subjects treated with zolmitriptan. Cephalalgia 1997;17(suppl 18):41–52.
6. Visser WH, Terwindt GW, Reines SA, et al. Rizatriptan vs sumatriptan in the acute treatment of migraine. A placebo-controlled, dose-ranging study. Arch Neurol 1996;53:1132–1137.

Name: _____   Month: _____   Year: _____

Date of Headache													
Headache Intensity													
Excruciating pain	10	10	10	10	10	10	10	10	10	10	10	10	10
	9	9	9	9	9	9	9	9	9	9	9	9	9
Severe pain	8	8	8	8	8	8	8	8	8	8	8	8	8
	7	7	7	7	7	7	7	7	7	7	7	7	7
Severe pain	6	6	6	6	6	6	6	6	6	6	6	6	6
	5	5	5	5	5	5	5	5	5	5	5	5	5
Moderate pain	4	4	4	4	4	4	4	4	4	4	4	4	4
	3	3	3	3	3	3	3	3	3	3	3	3	3
Mild pain	2	2	2	2	2	2	2	2	2	2	2	2	2
Aura only	1	1	1	1	1	1	1	1	1	1	1	1	1
Headache Duration (hours)													
Level of Disability													
Hospitalized													
Treatment by healthcare professional													
Bedrest required													
Decrease in activity by 50%													
Decrease in activity by 25%													
Normal activity													
Other (comment below)													
Associated Symptoms													
Nausea													
Vomiting													
Visual disturbances													
Menstrual period													
Neurological													
Other (comment below)													
Medications Taken													
1.													
2.													
3.													
4.													
5.													
Treatment Results													
Complete relief													
75% relief													
50% relief													
25% relief													
No relief													
Other (comment below)													
General Comments													

Note: A normal diary includes space to record a full month of headache activity. This form has been truncated for space purposes.

Figure 56-1 A headache diary.

SECTION 6

Psychiatric Disorders

Barbara G. Wells, PharmD, FASHP, FCCP, BCPP, Section Editor

57 ATTENTION-DEFICIT HYPERACTIVITY DISORDER

▶ **The Keys to My Success** (Level I)

William H. Benefield, Jr, PharmD, BCPP, FASCP
Donna M. Jermain, PharmD, BCPP

▶ After completing this case study, students should be able to:

- Identify the target symptoms of attention-deficit hyperactivity disorder (ADHD).

- Recommend appropriate therapeutic options for treating ADHD.

- Describe the presentation of adult-onset ADHD.

- Perform patient assessment to determine the presence of the major side effects of pharmacotherapy for ADHD.

☀ PATIENT PRESENTATION

Chief Complaint
"Sorry I'm late. . . . I couldn't find my keys."

HPI
Annie Mitchell is a 33 yo woman who presents 40 minutes late to her appointment at a psychiatrist's office. She is seeking an evaluation after realizing that she may have symptoms of ADHD. These symptoms were brought to her attention by a preceptor during her pharmacy practice residency. She states that her symptoms began in about the third grade; she

felt bored all the time, failed to pay attention in class, and daydreamed constantly. She also did not complete assignments and lost important papers. She managed to receive good grades throughout school despite these symptoms.

She recounts a particular episode that occurred while baby-sitting her two-year-old sister when she was a teenager. She was distracted by a rainstorm and left the house to unclog drains throughout the neighborhood with a friend. She left the door wide open with her younger sister upstairs alone until her parents got home. Her parents were not pleased.

Other symptoms that continued into adulthood include lack of organization, losing important documents and papers, locking her keys in her car, failing to meet deadlines, and forgetting appointments. Recently, on a trip to speak at a national meeting, she could not find her airline ticket. She purchased another one at the airport and left that one on the plane while making her connection. Upon arrival, her handout was not complete and she stayed up most of the night in order to complete it for the next morning's talk. Similar engagements and writing projects have also ended with completion of the project several months after the deadline.

PMH
No previous psychiatric history or major medical problems.

FH
Both a paternal and maternal uncle have a history of hyperactivity, and a cousin has a diagnosis of ADHD. Her mother has diabetes that is diet-controlled, and her sister has migraine headaches.

SH
Dr. Mitchell plans to practice in an institutional setting after completing her residency. She is single but is currently dating one man. She enjoys snow skiing. She drinks alcohol socially and denies tobacco or other substance use.

ROS

She has no menstrual difficulties; no recent change in weight, appetite, or cramping with menses. She denies having heavy bleeding, breast tenderness, acne, or mood swings related to menses.

Meds

Lo-Ovral 28, 1 po QD

All

Cats and dust mites cause sneezing and rhinorrhea. Sulfa drugs resulted in a rash.

PE

Gen

She is a healthy-appearing, slender woman in NAD.

VS

BP 110/60, P 62, RR 20, T 98.8°F; Wt 59 kg, Ht 64″

Skin

Warm and dry

HEENT

PERRLA

Neck/LN

No palpable nodes or thyromegaly

Lungs

CTA

Breasts

Mild fibrocystic changes

CV

No m/r/g

Abd

No obesity, non-tender

Genit/Rectal

Deferred

MS/Ext

Normal ROM; pulses 2+ throughout; no CCE

Neuro

A & O × 3; CN II–XII intact; DTRs 2+; Babinski negative

Labs

Hgb 141.1 g/dL	WBC 7.6×10^3/mm^3	*Fasting Lipid Profile*
Hct 39.3%	Neutros 81%	T. chol 130 mg/dL
RBC 4.8×10^6/mm^3	Lymphs 15%	HDL 64 mg/dL
Plt 183×10^3/mm^3	Monos 4%	LDL 51 mg/dL
MCV 98.8 μm^3	Eos 0%	Trig 75 mg/dL
MCH 34 pg	Basos 0%	
MCHC 33.5 g/dL	TSH 1.7 μIU/mL	

Assessment

ADHD

▶ Questions

Problem Identification

1. a. *Create a list of the patient's drug-related problems.*
   b. *What information (signs, symptoms, laboratory values) indicates the presence or severity of ADHD?*

Desired Outcome

2. *What are the goals of pharmacotherapy in this case?*

Therapeutic Alternatives

3. a. *What non-drug therapies might be useful for this patient?*
   b. *What feasible pharmacotherapeutic approaches are available for treatment of ADHD in this patient?*

Optimal Plan

4. a. *What drug, dosage form, dose, schedule, and duration of therapy are best for this patient?*
   b. *What alternatives would be appropriate if the initial therapy fails or cannot be used?*

Outcome Evaluation

5. *What clinical and laboratory parameters are necessary to evaluate the therapy for achievement of the desired therapeutic outcome and to detect or prevent adverse effects?*

Patient Counseling

6. *What information should be provided to the patient to enhance compliance, ensure successful therapy and minimize adverse effects?*

▶ Clinical Course

Dr. Mitchell returns to the clinic 2 weeks later and is taking methylphenidate 10 mg po Q AM and 10 mg at noon with minimal response. She also complains of tachycardia with all the coffee she drinks throughout the day.

▶ Follow-up Question

1. *Given this new information, what interventions, if any, would you recommend at this time?*

► Self-study Assignments

1. Perform a literature search to acquire recent data on the concern about growth suppression in children taking stimulants.
2. Which herbal therapies have been studied in ADHD, and what have the results shown?
3. What is the role of pemoline in the treatment of ADHD?

► Clinical Pearl

If significant comorbidity symptoms exist (i.e., a significant depression), antidepressant therapy may be considered first-line treatment for ADHD in children and perhaps in adults.

References

1. Spencer T, Biederman J, Wilens T, et al. Pharmacotherapy of attention-deficit hyperactivity disorder across the life cycle. J Am Acad Child Adolesc Psychiatry 1996; 35:409–432.
2. Popper CW. Antidepressants in the treatment of attention-deficit/hyperactivity disorder. J Clin Psychiatry 1997;58(suppl 14):14–29.
3. Spencer T, Wilens T, Biederman J, et al. A double-blind, crossover comparison of methylphenidate and placebo in adults with childhood-onset attention-deficit hyperactivity disorder. Arch Gen Psychiatry 1995;52:434–443.

58 ANOREXIA NERVOSA

► Sweet Sixteen   (Level I)

Rae Ann Maxwell, RPh, PhD

► After completing this case study, students should be able to:

- Identify specific factors that differentiate anorexia nervosa from bulimia nervosa.
- Describe physiologic symptoms that may be associated with anorexia nervosa.
- Describe secondary medical complications that may occur due to the starvation activities associated with anorexia nervosa.
- Develop a treatment plan that addresses selection of psychotherapy and pharmacotherapy, defining patient goals, and monitoring for achievement of the desired outcome.

☼ PATIENT PRESENTATION

Chief Complaint
"I have no energy and I need to lose weight."

HPI

Jennifer Carter is a 16 yo young woman who is in 11th grade at Epperson High School. This is her first visit to the Eating Disorder Clinic (EDC). She was referred to the EDC by physicians at a local ED. She had fainted in school while walking to class. She sustained no injuries.

When she was younger she was of normal height and weight and ate freely from all food groups. Her parents divorced when she was 12 yo, and she began living with her mother and brother. At the age of 13 she was 5 ft 5 inches tall, weighed between 125 and 130 lbs., and entered menarche. She felt that she could lose some weight but did not feel that she was overweight—"just a little pudgy." She began to exercise by walking 10 to 15 minutes 3 times a week and tried out for the basketball and volleyball teams at school (she played both sports). At the age of 14 she weighed 138 pounds (her highest weight) and began to run track. She still participated in volleyball, but team sports did not bring her the satisfaction of accomplishment on her own. In September 2 years ago she read a magazine article on the health benefits of low-fat meals. She began to prepare the family meals and involve them in "eating healthier" with the low-fat diets she collected. By December, her weight had dropped to 125 lbs.

The following May, she began to restrict her food intake (started eating only half-portions of any food) and felt that she needed to lose several more pounds but would not define the exact number. She moved in with her father at this time because she could not deal with her brother's "problem" anymore. Her brother has ADHD, and she states that he would hit her. Her mother is also dating a gentleman whom Jennifer does not like. While living with her father, she was able to skip breakfast and lunch (he left for work before she would go to school) and for dinner have a bowl of soup or cereal and would feel full. She does like cooking for her dad since "he is too busy to do it himself." The apartment building has a weight room, so she would lift weights for an hour a day, jog for an hour, and then do as many sit-ups as she could (usually over 300). This was in addition to the conditioning she does at school as part of track and volleyball.

She did experiment with taking Lasix (which she had taken from her mother) for 2 weeks 5 months ago but decided it did not help her lose the weight she desired to. Four months ago, she began taking Dexatrim 2 or 3 times a week (up to 4 capsules a day); the last time she took any was 1 week ago. She denies using any laxatives or ipecac. She denies any forced vomiting. Both parents state that they have noticed that she has been irritable and has been crying for no apparent reason, which is not like her since she is a "good girl" with school work and her other activities and doing what is expected of her (e.g., looking out for her little brother). Jennifer never refers to any particular friends at school. She does admit to having suicidal ideation but no plan and would probably "not have the guts" to follow through with it.

PMH
Negative for surgeries or hospitalizations
Negative for serious injuries or bone fractures
Chicken pox at the age of 6

FH
Oldest of two siblings; has an 11 yo brother diagnosed with ADHD and depression. Parents have been divorced for 4 years; father is a financial consultant, mother is a teacher. Mother was treated for depression with nortriptyline for one year 3 years ago. A maternal uncle has been diagnosed with depression; her maternal grandfather is an alcoholic.

SH

Straight "A" student, would like to go to Princeton. Enjoys reading. Very active in various student activities, including track and volleyball; is on the student council and is a class officer. Denies use of tobacco, alcohol, or illicit substances.

ROS

She complains of dizziness and states that she feels her heart "flutter" from time to time but denies chest pain. No history of seizures. She reports a decrease in appetite and energy and has felt fatigued over the last 2 to 3 weeks. She has no c/o epigastric or abdominal pain. She usually has a bowel movement every other day, but admits that she has not had one in a week. She has intolerance to cold. Her last menses was 1 year ago.

Meds

No prescribed medications, but she has been taking Dexatrim (phenylpropanolamine 75 mg) and furosemide 20 mg (taken from her mother's medicine cabinet) on her own.

All

NKDA

PE

Gen

The patient is a pleasant, young female. Appropriately dressed with regard to clothing size. Appears to be low weight. Easily engaged in conversation. Cooperative to answering questions, not guarded in responses, and makes eye contact with interviewer. No odd or inappropriate motor behavior.

VS

BP 104/78, P 70, RR 16, T 36.6°C; Ht 66″, Wt 101.5 lb (lowest to date)

Skin

Dry, some scaling, negative for rashes, skin tone normal in color, acne on forehead

HEENT

PERRLA; EOMI; TMs intact; teeth show no signs of erosion; throat without erythema or soreness. Hair is thin and dry, "downy-like" in appearance

Neck/LN

Neck supple without lymphadenopathy or thyromegaly

Breasts

Normal without masses

CV

Heart RRR, no m/r/g

Abd

Soft, NT, hypoactive bowel sounds, no organomegaly

Genit/Rect

Refused exam

MS/Ext

No CCE; range of motion intact; good peripheral pulses bilaterally

Neuro

A & O × 3; CN II–XII intact; DTRs 2+ throughout; Babinski (−)

Labs

Na 144 mEq/L	Hgb 13.0 g/dL	AST 17 IU/L
K 4.8 mEq/L	Hct 39%	ALT 23 IU/L
Cl 104 mEq/L	Plt $200 \times 10^3/mm^3$	Alk phos 51 IU/L
CO_2 24 mEq/L	WBC $5.0 \times 10^3/mm^3$	GGT 20 IU/L
BUN 7 mg/dL	Ca 10.5 mg/dL	TSH 1.834 μIU/mL
SCr 0.9 mg/dL	Mg 1.4 mg/dL	
Glu 83 mg/dL	Phos 2.6 mg/dL	

Assessment

Anorexia nervosa, malnutrition, depressive symptoms

► Questions

Problem Identification

1. a. Create a list of this patient's drug-related problems.
   b. What information from the history and physical exam is consistent with a diagnosis of anorexia nervosa?
   c. What signs and symptoms of malnutrition often seen in anorexia nervosa are not exhibited by this patient?
   d. Classify the subtype of anorexia that this patient has. How severe is the disorder at this point?

Desired Outcome

2. a. What are the goals of treatment for this patient?
   b. What secondary complications do you want to avoid in this patient?

Therapeutic Alternatives

3. a. What non-pharmacologic interventions must be considered for this patient?
   b. What pharmacologic interventions may be considered for this patient?

Optimal Plan

4. Design an optimal therapeutic regimen for this patient.

Outcome Evaluation

5. How should the therapy you recommended be monitored for efficacy and side effects?

Patient Counseling

6. What information should be provided to the patient about her non-drug and drug therapies?

▶ Follow-up Question

   1. *What is the likelihood of relapse or resistance to therapy?*

▶ Self-study Assignments

   1. Regulation of hunger and feeding involve the interregulation of several neurotransmitters (norepinephrine, serotonin, dopamine) and neuropeptides (CCK and pancreatic polypeptides). Review how these interrelate with each other and the proposed mechanism of action. How would this aid in the future development of medications to target these systems?
   2. Compare and contrast the symptoms and signs of anorexia nervosa to bulimia nervosa. Does pharmacotherapy improve outcome any better with bulimia nervosa?

▶ Clinical Pearl

The primary treatment modalities for anorexia nervosa are weight restoration, behavior modification, and psychotherapy. Pharmacotherapy is adjunctive and has had limited success in treatment.

References

1. Jarry JL, Vaccarino FJ. Eating disorder and obsessive-compulsive disorder: Neurochemical and phenomenological commonalties. J Psychiatry Neurosci 1996;21: 36–48.
2. Rock CL, Curran-Celentano J. Nutritional management of eating disorders. Psychiatr Clin North Am 1996;19:701–713.
3. Walsh BT, Devlin MJ. Psychopharmacology of anorexia nervosa and bulimia nervosa and binge eating. In: Bloom FE, Kupfer D, eds. Psychopharmacology: The Fourth Generation of Progress. New York, Raven Press, 1995:1581–1589.
4. Jimerson DC, Wolfe BE, Brotman AW, et al. Medications in the treatment of eating disorders. Psychiatr Clin North Am 1996;19:739–754.

59 ALZHEIMER'S DISEASE

▶ **Irreversible, But Not Untreatable** (Level I)

Cynthia P. Koh-Knox, PharmD
Virginia L. Stauffer, PharmD, BCPS

▶ After completing this case study, students should be able to:

   • State cognitive deficits and noncognitive/behavioral symptoms of Alzheimer's disease (AD).

   • Recommend pharmacotherapy to manage the cognitive and behavioral symptoms of AD.

   • Provide education and counseling to the patient and caregivers about AD, the possible benefits and adverse effects of donepezil therapy, and the importance of adherence to therapy.

   • List at least three theories of AD etiologies and agents under investigation based on those theories.

☼ PATIENT PRESENTATION

Chief Complaint
"My memory seems to be slipping."

HPI
Thelma Day is a 67 yo woman who presents to the clinic for the first time accompanied by 2 of her children. The children report that short-term memory loss began approximately 1 year ago. Cognitive symptoms have since progressed and include forgetting times and dates easily, misplacing and losing items, repeating questions and current events, inability to answer questions, and increasing difficulty with managing finances. Her family is concerned about her lack of interest in family conversations, which require urging her to participate. Mrs. Day also reports tearful periods and difficulty sleeping.

PMH
   Glaucoma in both eyes diagnosed 3 years ago
   Osteoarthritis in both knees × 5 years
   No previous history of psychological or psychiatric problems

FH
Noncontributory, both parents deceased. Ten children, 7 who live nearby.

SH
Lives alone and has been widowed for 1 year (husband died of cancer).

Meds
None

All
NKA

ROS
Complains of occasional knee pain; no complaints of vision problems due to glaucoma.

PE

Gen
WD woman who appears her stated age

VS
BP 142/80 sitting, 136/90 standing; P 76; RR 20; T 37°C; Wt 114 lb., Ht 5′6″

Skin
Normal texture and color

HEENT
WNL, TMs intact

Neck/LN
Neck supple without thyromegaly or lymphadenopathy

Lungs/Thorax
Clear, normal breath sounds

Breasts
No masses or tenderness

CV
RRR, no murmurs or bruits

Abd
Soft, NTND

Genit/Rect
Normal external female genitalia

MS/Ext
No CCE, normal ROM

Neuro
Motor, sensory, CNs, cerebellar, and gait normal. Folstein MMSE score 19/30. Disoriented to season, month, date, and day of week. Disoriented to country. Good registration but impaired attention and very poor short-term memory. Unable to remember any of 3 items after 3 minutes.

Labs

Na 139 mEq/L	Hgb 13.7 g/dL	AST 32 IU/L	T. prot 7.5 g/dL	UA 5.8 mg/dL
K 4.1 mEq/L	Hct 41.0 %	ALT 28 IU/L	Alb 4.5 g/dL	B_{12} 330 pg/mL
Cl 101 mEq/L	RBC 4.42×10^6/mm³	Alk phos 81 IU/L	Chol 232 mg/dL	
CO_2 28 mEq/L	Plts 395×10^3/mm³	GGT 26 IU/L	Trig 181 mg/dL	
BUN 8 mg/dL	WBC 7.4×10^3/mm³	LDH 95 IU/L	Ca 9.7 mg/dL	
SCr 0.7 mg/dL	Neutros 65 %	T. bili 0.9 mg/dL	Phos 4.5 mg/dL	
Glu 102 mg/dL	Lymphs 29%	D. bili 0.4 mg/dL	TSH 3.7 µIU/mL	
	Monos 6%		T_4 6.9 ng/dL	

CT Scan
Mild to moderate generalized cerebral atrophy

Assessment
1. Probable Alzheimer's disease, stage 4 on the global deterioration scale (borderline moderate in severity)
2. Mild depressive symptoms

▶ Clinical Course

Mrs. Day and 7 of her children met with the geriatric care team and discussed the diagnosis of probable Alzheimer's disease. It was explained that Mrs. Day was in the early moderate stage and it was to be expected that she would have waxing and waning of symptoms that would result in good and bad days. The family expressed the desire to try to manage their mother at home, and responsibilities would be divided among the children. Tacrine was initiated for cognitive symptoms and sertraline was started for depression.

One year later, Mrs. Day and 2 of her children return to clinic for a follow-up visit. The patient reports that she has missed taking some of her medication because she is confused about how to take it. Since being started on tacrine, she has developed GERD and has experienced nausea and vomiting. She has lost 8 pounds in the past 5 months. However, her children report that she has been participating more actively in family and social functions. Mrs. Day states that she has had fewer tearful periods and feels happy most of the time. She reports no GERD symptoms. She exhibits impaired cognitive function as displayed on the Folstein MMSE score of 20/30. Upon neurologic assessment, the patient's Alzheimer's disease is at Stage 4 on the global deterioration scale. Medications include tacrine 10 mg po alternating with 20 mg po QID (10-20-10-20 mg), sertraline 50 mg po QD, Pepcid AC 20 mg po Q HS PRN, and Ensure drinks PRN. Laboratory results include AST 72 IU/L, ALT 70 IU/L, and LDH 472 IU/L. The geriatric care team is considering a change in the patient's therapy because of the complexity of tacrine administration, the difficulty in adhering to the regimen, and the elevated liver enzymes.

▶ Questions

Problem Identification

1. a. *Create a list of the patient's drug-related problems.*
   b. *What information (signs, symptoms, laboratory values) indicates the presence or severity of Alzheimer's disease?*
   c. *Could any of the patient's problems have been caused by drug therapy?*

Desired Outcome

2. *What are the goals of pharmacotherapy in this case?*

Therapeutic Alternatives

3. a. *What non-drug therapies might be useful for this patient?*
   b. *What feasible pharmacotherapeutic alternatives are available for the treatment of Alzheimer's disease?*
   c. *What economic, psychosocial, racial, and ethical considerations are applicable to this patient?*

Optimal Plan

4. a. *What drug, dosage form, dose, schedule, and duration of therapy are best for this patient?*
   b. *What alternatives would be appropriate if the initial therapy fails or cannot be used?*

Outcome Evaluation

5. *What clinical and laboratory parameters are necessary to evaluate the therapy for achievement of the desired therapeutic outcome and to detect or prevent adverse effects?*

Patient Counseling

6. *What information should be provided to the patient to enhance compliance, ensure successful therapy, and minimize adverse effects?*

► Self-study Assignments

1. What are the stages of cognitive decline as defined by the global deterioration scale? At what stage is AD identified?
2. List at least three theories of the etiology of AD. What therapies are under investigation to support these theories?
3. Describe neurofibrillary tangles and neuritic plaques and their roles in AD development.
4. Differentiate cognitive deficits and noncognitive/psychiatric symptoms and behaviors.

► Clinical Pearl

Depressive symptoms occur commonly in the early stages of Alzheimer's disease and may warrant antidepressant treatment. If symptoms improve over 9 to 12 months, antidepressant therapy should be tapered. Patients often remain on antidepressants longer than necessary.

References

1. Filley CM. Alzheimer's disease: It's irreversible but not untreatable. Geriatrics 1995;50:18–23.
2. Rogers SL, Friedhoff LT, and the Donepezil Study Group. The efficacy and safety of donepezil in patients with Alzheimer's Disease: Results of a US multicentre, randomized, double-blind, placebo-controlled trial. Dementia 1996;7:293–303.
3. Paganini-Hill A, Henderson VW. Estrogen in the treatment and prevention of Alzheimer's disease. Int J Pharmaceutical Compounding 1998;2:24–29.
4. Le Bars PL, Katz MM, Berman N, et al. A placebo-controlled, double-blind, randomized trial of an extract of Gingko biloba for dementia. North American EGb Study Group. JAMA 1997;278:1327–1332.
5. Sano M, Ernesto C, Thomas RG, et al. A controlled trial of selegiline, alpha-tocopherol, or both as treatment for Alzheimer's disease. The Alzheimer's Disease Cooperative Study. N Engl J Med 1997;336:1216–1222.

60 ALCOHOL WITHDRAWAL

► No More Drinking and Driving (Level I)

Jill Slimick-Ponzetto, PharmD, BCPS

► After completing this case study, students should be able to:

- Identify the signs and symptoms of alcohol dependence.
- Recognize the common signs and symptoms of alcohol withdrawal.
- Recognize the common laboratory abnormalities seen in an alcohol dependent patient.
- Develop a treatment plan for alcohol withdrawal.

☀ PATIENT PRESENTATION

Chief Complaint
"I have been sweating, shaking, vomiting, and running a fever for 2 days."

HPI
Aaron Jackson is a 69 yo man who presents to the ED stating that he drinks too much and needs alcohol rehabilitation. He states that he was released yesterday after spending 2 days in jail for driving while intoxicated. The patient states that he has been drinking one 750-mL bottle of vodka per day for 7 to 8 years. He had become increasingly depressed over the time prior to his arrest because his wife had left him. He states that he was on a drinking binge for 7 days prior to being arrested. The patient has not had any alcohol since the arrest.

PMH
Alcohol dependence
Hx Depression (unknown history and duration)
Post-traumatic stress disorder (PTSD) s/p Korean War veteran
HTN × 10 years
BPH × 5 years

FH
Patient has 3 brothers and a sister; medical histories unknown. Parents are deceased; patient is unable to give medical histories.

SH
Currently unemployed and has had sporadic employment (frequently fired due to call-offs) over the last 9 years. The patient has attended the PTSD group therapy on a monthly basis for several years. Divorced × 2; current wife moved out 2 weeks ago; drinks 750 mL vodka/day × 7 to 8 years; (+) tobacco 1½ ppd × 20 years; denies any illicit drug use.

ROS
Normal except for sweating, tremors in both hands, and fever. Patient states that he is feeling nervous and anxious.

Meds
Minipress 1 mg po Q HS
Plendil 5 mg po QD
Colace 100 mg po BID
Ibuprofen 400 mg po Q 6 H PRN headaches
Gaviscon 1 to 2 tablets po QID PRN GI upset

All
NKDA

PE

Gen

Patient is a WDWN African-American man lying comfortably on a gurney; there is an odor of alcohol, sweat, and urine in the room. Patient's clothes are soiled with urine. Upon interview, the patient's mental status fluctuated from confusion to coherence. Patient also stated that he heard "female voices" talk to him last night, even though he now lives alone.

VS

BP 151/115, P 115, RR 22, T 100°F

Skin

Moist secondary to diaphoresis

HEENT

NC/AT; PERRLA

Neck/LN

No lymphadenopathy, JVD, or carotid bruits

Lungs

Clear bilaterally, no crackles

CV

Normal S_1 and S_2; no m/r/g; occasional premature beats

Abd

Soft, obese; NT; (+) bowel sounds; (+) hepatomegaly; (−) splenomegaly

Genit/Rect

(+) Enlarged prostate, (−) occult blood in stool

MS/Ext

Tremor in both hands (R > L), pulses 1+ dorsalis pedis, none in posterior tibial

Neuro

A & O × 3, (+) tremors in both hands, CN II–XII intact; DTRs are exaggerated

Labs

Na 139 mEq/L	AST 254 IU/L	Ca 9.8 mg/dL
K 3.7 mEq/L	ALT 113 IU/L	Mg 1.2 mg/dL
Cl 108 mEq/L	Alk phos 41 IU/L	Phos 2.5 mg/dL
CO_2 25.5 mEq/L	GGT 265 IU/L	UA 10.8 mg/dL
BUN 9 mg/dL	LDH 321 IU/L	Alb 4.3 g/dL
SCr 1.4 mg/dL	T. bili 1.1 mg/dL	PT 12.2 sec
Glu 136 mg/dL	D. bili 0.4 mg/dL	INR 1.03

Other

The patient became very agitated and started having auditory hallucinations; he had to be physically restrained in the ED after his physical exam.

Toxicology Screen

(−) For illicit drugs, (−) alcohol

Assessment

The patient appears to be going through alcohol withdrawal with delirium tremens.

▶ Questions

Problem Identification

1. a. Create a list of the patient's drug-related problems.
   b. What information (signs, symptoms, laboratory values) indicates that the patient is going through alcohol withdrawal?
   c. What signs and symptoms are consistent with delirium tremens?
   d. What signs, symptoms, and history are consistent with alcohol dependence in this patient?
   e. What laboratory abnormalities may be expected in a patient with a history of alcohol abuse?

Desired Outcome

2. What are the short-term and long-term goals of pharmacotherapy in this case?

Therapeutic Alternatives

3. What pharmacotherapeutic alternatives are available for the treatment of alcohol withdrawal and to prevent further alcohol withdrawal complications?

Optimal Plan

4. Design an optimal pharmacotherapeutic plan to rapidly control withdrawal symptoms in this patient and to prevent further withdrawal complications. Explain the rationale for your selections.

Outcome Evaluation

5. What clinical and laboratory parameters are necessary to evaluate your chosen therapy for the achievement of desired outcome and to detect or prevent adverse effects?

Patient Counseling

6. What information should be provided to the patient to enhance compliance, ensure successful therapy, and to minimize adverse effects?

▶ Clinical Course

After 1 week of detoxification and taper, Mr. Jackson's tremor has disappeared, vital signs are within normal limits, and his auditory hallucinations have disappeared. He is calm and able to think clearly. He still craves alcohol but has entered into Alcoholics Anonymous and has agreed to increase his visits at the PTSD discussion group as well as enroll in individual psychiatric therapy for his depression. The patient vows to try to maintain sobriety in the future.

▶ Self-study Assignments

1. Design an outpatient pharmacotherapeutic plan for this patient after discharge.
2. Describe the Alcoholics Anonymous 12-step approach to staying sober.
3. Discuss the pharmacologic options that are currently marketed in the United States (FDA-approved drugs) for the treatment of alcohol dependence.

▶ Clinical Pearl

In a patient with chronic alcoholism, parenteral thiamine should be administered before or concurrently with dextrose-containing intravenous fluids to prevent Wernicke's encephalopathy, a neurologic disorder common in alcoholics caused by thiamine deficiency.

References

1. Mayo-Smith MF. Pharmacological management of alcohol withdrawal: a meta-analysis and evidence-based practice guideline. The American Society of Addiction Medicine Working Group on Pharmacological Management of Alcohol Withdrawal. JAMA 1997;278:144–151.
2. Saitz R, O'Malley SS. Pharmacotherapies for alcohol abuse: Withdrawal and treatment. Med Clin North Am 1997;81;881–907.
3. Moskowitz G, Chalmers TC, Sacks HS, et al. Deficiencies of clinical trials of alcohol withdrawal. Alcohol Clin Exp Res 1983;7:42–46.
4. Sullivan JT, Sykora K, Schneiderman J, et al. Assessment of alcohol withdrawal: The revised clinical institute withdrawal assessment for alcohol scale (CIWA-Ar). Br J Addict 1989; 84:1353–1357.

61 NICOTINE ADDICTION

▶ Kicking Mr. Butts   (Level I)

Julie A. Cold, PharmD, BCPP

▶ After completing this case study, students should be able to:

- Identify the pharmacist's role in promoting smoking cessation and nicotine abstinence.
- Provide recommendations for initiating life-style modifications and pharmacological treatments, based upon patient characteristics and disease states, using the Agency for Health Care Policy and Research (AHCPR) smoking cessation clinical guideline[1] to help the nicotine-addicted individual stop using tobacco.
- Recommend alternative treatments and monitoring plans for nicotine addiction if the initial plan fails.
- Provide patient counseling on the use of pharmacotherapeutic agents used to treat nicotine addiction.

☼ PATIENT PRESENTATION

Chief Complaint
"It's getting harder and harder to breathe each day. Do you think cigarette smoking is a factor in this problem?"

HPI
Sue Tried is a 55 yo woman who presents to the community pharmacy with complaints of breathing difficulties that have become increasingly worse during the past week. She states that she has not used her inhaler during the past 2 weeks and needs to have her prescription refilled.

PMH
Hypothyroidism diagnosed at age 39
Menopausal hot flushes diagnosed at age 42
Emphysema diagnosed at age 45
Osteoporosis diagnosed at age 53

FH
Mother died at age 38 of a heart attack. Father is alive and suffers from diabetes and arthritis. Consumer is the second child of four siblings. All close family members are cigarette smokers.

SH
Lives alone since her husband's death 3 years ago; she is a retired homemaker; smokes 2 ppd (has smoked for the past 40 years); drinks 1 to 2 glasses of wine each night; does not exercise on a regular basis. Three adult children and 7 grandchildren live in the local area.

ROS
Negative except for the problem described above.

Meds
Atrovent inhaler 2 inhalations QID
Premarin 0.3 mg/day for 3 weeks out of the month
Synthroid 75 μg po QD
Fosamax 10 mg po QD

All
NKDA

PE

Gen
Well groomed, thin woman who looks her stated age with a flushed face and obvious respiratory distress. Sitting during the interview with chest forward and hands resting on her knees

VS
BP 128/75, P 102 obtained at the pharmacy

Skin
Marked "crow's feet" wrinkling around the eyes

HEENT
Wears dentures

Lungs
Breathing through pursed lips

No other PE information is available.

Labs
None available

Assessment
Consumer's quality of life is greatly compromised by untreated emphysema exacerbated by cigarette smoking

---

▶ Questions

Problem Identification

1. a. *Create a list of this patient's drug-related problems.*
   b. *What information in the patient's history can be identified as disease or symptomatology that is probably directly related to the consumer's smoking history?*
   c. *What stage of change for smoking cessation is the consumer in at this time?*
   d. *What signs or symptoms in this consumer's presentation indicate the severity of this consumer's nicotine addiction?*
   e. *List other questions that you can ask the consumer to determine her dependence upon nicotine.*

Desired Outcome

2. *What are the goals of smoking cessation pharmacotherapy in this case?*

Therapeutic Alternatives

3. a. *Describe non-drug therapies that may help this consumer quit smoking.*
   b. *What feasible pharmacotherapeutic alternatives are available for the treatment of the nicotine dependence?*
   c. *What economic, psychosocial, racial, and ethical considerations are applicable to this consumer?*

Optimal Plan

4. *What drug, dosage form, dose, schedule, and duration of therapy are best for this patient?*

Outcome Evaluation

5. *What clinical and laboratory parameters are necessary to evaluate the therapy for achievement of the desired therapeutic outcome and to detect or prevent adverse effects?*

Patient Counseling

6. *What information should be provided to the patient to enhance compliance, ensure successful therapy, and minimize adverse effects?*

▶ Clinical Course

The patient complains of a rash at the patch site 3 days after starting on the nicotine transdermal patch you recommended. She informs you that she can't stand the itching and would rather quit using the patch than continue if it is going to mean this much misery. In addition, she states that she can't sleep at night and has noticed a large increase in her appetite and fears gaining a lot of weight.

▶ Follow-up Questions

1. *What is the risk of smoking relapse at this point?*
2. *Has the treatment goal changed at this point?*
3. *Evaluate the consumer's complaints and recommend alternative treatments that should be reinforced at this point.*
4. *Design an alternative pharmacotherapeutic plan to address the consumer's nicotine addiction.*
5. *Describe clinical monitoring parameters for the consumer at this point in treatment.*

▶ Clinical Course

The consumer was successful in smoking cessation for the 8 weeks that she wore the nicotine transdermal patch. Five months later, she returns to your pharmacy to have her prescriptions filled. She has been hospitalized 2 times in the past 6 weeks to treat respiratory infections, and she is feeling very down about her ill health and because she has relapsed to smoking again. She would like to know if there are any new medications available to help her quit smoking. She states that when she was not smoking she had a strong craving to smoke.

▶ Follow-up Questions

1. *To determine what pharmacotherapy may be beneficial at this point, list the positive and negative factors that are important in determining whether the patient is ultimately able to become smoking abstinent.*
2. *Evaluate the consumer's complaints and recommend alternative treatments that should be reinforced at this point.*
3. *Design an alternative pharmacotherapeutic plan to address her nicotine addiction.*
4. *What information should be provided to the patient to enhance compliance, ensure successful therapy, and minimize adverse effects?*

▶ Self-study Assignments

1. Perform a literature search to determine if an alcoholic patient in recovery will need different smoking cessation intervention than a

person who is not alcoholic. Write a two-page paper outlining the differences that might be required.

2. Devise a plan to encourage administrators in health care systems to actively promote smoking cessation in each of their systems.

3. Review the literature concerning the use of combination pharmacotherapy to treat nicotine addiction. Write a paper that describes the potential benefits and drawbacks of combination therapy and suggest the type of patient for whom combination therapy might be beneficial.

▶ Clinical Pearl

Smoking cessation is achieved through a dynamic process; the smoker's stage of change must be identified so that effective smoking cessation intervention can be implemented for the smoker at their stage of change.

References

1. Nunn-Thompson C, Barr CC, Tommasello AC, et al. APhA Special Report: A Review of the New Smoking Cessation Strategies for the Agency for Health Care Policy and Research. Washington, DC, American Pharmaceutical Association, 1996.
2. Hudmon KS, Berger BA. Pharmacy applications of the transtheoretical model in smoking cessation. Am J Health-Syst Pharm 1995;52:282–287.
3. Wongwiwatthananukit S, Jack HM, Popovich NG. Smoking cessation: Part 1—an overview. J Am Pharm Assoc 1998;38:58–70.
4. Setter SM, Johnson MD. Smoking cessation and drug therapy. US Pharmacist January 1997:91–102.

62 SCHIZOPHRENIA

▶ !Yo Quiero Taco (I Want a Taco) (Level I)

William H. Benefield, Jr., PharmD, BCPP, FASCP
Lawrence J. Cohen, PharmD, BCPP, FASHP, FCCP

▶ After completing this case study, students should be able to:

- Identify the target symptoms of schizophrenia.
- Manage an acutely psychotic patient with appropriate pharmacotherapy.
- Manage adverse effects of the antipsychotics.
- Discuss the role of atypical antipsychotics in the treatment of schizophrenia.

☀ PATIENT PRESENTATION

Chief Complaint
"Police brought me in a patrol car."

HPI
This is the first admission for Thelma Baker, a 35 yo woman who was brought to the state hospital by the police. The patient apparently has been delusional and believes people sneak into her room at night when she is asleep and put worms inside her body. She also believes that she is being raped by passing men on the street. She is quite preoccupied about having massive wealth. She claims to have bought some gold and left it at the grocery store. She believes that her ideas have been given to a communist who has had plastic surgery to look like her and is using her ID to take possession of all of her property. She states that she is having difficulty getting her property back.

Apparently, the precipitating event causing her hospitalization was that she created a disturbance at a Mexican fast-food restaurant, claiming that she owned it. Because of the disturbance, police were called and she subsequently was sent here on an order of protective custody. According to the patient, she bought a taco and sat down to eat it, and for some reason somebody called the police and charged her with illegal trespassing. She claims that 6 years ago she was raped by a relative of a sister and broke her hip in the process. She states that her feet were cut off because she would not do what her impostors wanted her to do, and her feet were subsequently sent back to her from India and were reattached.

Her speech is quite rambling, and she speaks of having been part of an experiment in Alabama where 38 eggs were taken from her body, and children were produced from them and killed by the government. She also reports that she took part in signing the treaty in 1945 when Germany surrendered. She claims that she has worms in her that are the type that kill dogs and horses, and says that they have been put there by the government. She also claims that at one time she had transmitters in her backbone and that it took three years to have them taken out by the government. She claims to have had surgery in the past, and the surgeon didn't know what he was doing and took out her gallbladder and put it in the intestines where it exploded. The patient also states that on one occasion a physician was removing the snakes from her abdominal cavity, and the snakes killed the doctor and a nurse. She also claims that she worked as a surgeon herself before 1963.

Past Psychiatric History
The patient denies any prior hospitalization for mental problems, denies any street drugs or significant substance use. There is some history of her having frequent visits to the local hospital. She denies any drug or alcohol use and denies using any tobacco products.

PMH
The patient's past records indicate that she did have gallbladder surgery (cholecystectomy) 2 months ago. There is no record of her ever being raped or having a broken hip. No further medical history is known.

Family Psychiatric History
The patient claims that her alleged family is not really her family and that she is not sure who is her family.

Meds
None noted

All
Penicillin → rash

Legal/Social Status

Divorced, heterosexual; lives in an apartment alone; employment history unknown.

Mental Status Exam

The patient is a Caucasian female, modestly dressed with some disarray. Her hair is brown and unwashed. She is alert, oriented and in no acute distress. Her speech is clear, constant, pressured, with many grandiose delusions and illogical thoughts. She is quite rambling, going from one subject to the other without interruption. Her affect is mood congruent, her mood is euphoric, and there is a marked degree of grandiosity. Her thought processes are quite illogical with marked delusional thinking. There is no evidence of auditory hallucinations, and she denies visual hallucinations. She denies any suicidal or homicidal ideation, but she is quite verbal and pressured in her thought content, verbalizing a great deal about the things that have been taken away from her illegally by people impersonating her. She has marked delusional symptoms with paranoid ideation prominent. Her memory (immediate, recent, and remote) is fair. Her cognition and concentration are adequate. Her intellectual functioning is within the average range. Insight and judgment are markedly impaired.

ROS

Reports occasional GI upset; complains that worms are inside her stomach. Otherwise negative.

PE

VS

BP 132/79, P 80, RR 17, T 37.1°C; Wt 80 kg; Ht 63″

HEENT

PERRLA; EOMI; fundi benign; throat and ears clear; TMs intact

Skin

Scratches on both hands

Neck

Supple, no nodes; normal thyroid

CV

RRR, normal S_1 and S_2

Lungs

CTA & P

Abd

(+) BS, non-tender

Ext

Full ROM, pulses 2+ bilaterally

Neuro

A & O × 3; reflexes symmetric; toes downgoing; normal gait; normal strength; sensation intact; CN II–XII intact

Labs

Na 140 mEq/L	Hgb 14.6 g/dL	WBC 11.0×10^3/mm³	AST 34 IU/L	Ca 9.6 mg/dL
K 3.9 mEq/L	Hct 45.7%	Neutros 66%	ALT 22 IU/L	Phos 5.1 mg/dL
Cl 104 mEq/L	RBC 4.7×10^6/mm³	Lymphs 24%	Alk phos 89 IU/L	TSH 4.5 μIU/mL
CO_2 22 mEq/L	MCV 90.2 μm³	Monos 8%	GGT 38 IU/L	RPR negative
BUN 19 mg/dL	MCH 31 pg	Eos 1%	T. bili 0.9 mg/dL	Urine pregnancy (−)
SCr 1.1 mg/dL	MCHC 34.5 g/dL	Basos 1%	Alb 3.6 g/dL	
Glu 91 mg/dL	Plt 232×10^3/mm³		T. chol 190 mg/dL	

UA

Color, yellow; appearance, slightly cloudy; glucose (−); bili (−); ketones, trace; SG 1.025; blood (+); pH 6.0; protein (−); nitrites (−); leukocyte esterase (−)

Assessment

Axis I: Schizophrenia, paranoid type, acute exacerbation

Axis II: None

Axis III: Patient allergic to penicillin by history, S/P gallbladder surgery 2 months ago

Axis IV: Unemployment

Axis V: Global Assessment of Functioning (GAF) Scale = 32

▶ Questions

Problem Identification

1. a. Create a list of the patient's drug-related problems.
   b. What information (signs, symptoms, laboratory values) indicates the presence or severity of an acute exacerbation of schizophrenia, paranoid type?

Desired Outcome

2. What are the goals of pharmacotherapy in this case?

Therapeutic Alternatives

3. a. What non-drug therapies might be useful for this patient?
   b. What pharmacotherapeutic alternatives are available for the treatment of this patient?

Optimal Plan

4. a. *What drug, dosage form, dose, schedule, and duration of therapy are best for this patient?*
   b. *What alternatives would be appropriate if the initial therapy fails or cannot be used?*

Outcome Evaluation

5. *What clinical and laboratory parameters are necessary to evaluate the therapy for achievement of the desired therapeutic outcome and to detect or prevent adverse effects?*

Patient Counseling

6. *What information should be provided to the patient to enhance compliance, ensure successful therapy and minimize adverse effects?*

▶ Self-study Assignments

1. Develop a formulary for antipsychotic medications for your institution. Which ones should you include and why?
2. Review the pharmacoeconomic literature for the atypical antipsychotics. For your geographical area, compare costs for the average daily doses of haloperidol, olanzapine, risperidone, clozapine, and quetiapine.
3. Perform a literature search on the use of vitamin E for the treatment and prevention of tardive dyskinesia. What is the proposed mechanism of action? Would you recommend this therapy and, if so, what dose would you suggest?

▶ Clinical Pearl

A benzodiazepine (lorazepam) can be scheduled routinely during the initiation of an antipsychotic to minimize aggression and allow time for the antipsychotic to take effect. The addition of lorazepam may also allow lower initial dosages to be used initially and during the maintenance phase of treatment.

References

1. Marder SR. Facilitating compliance with antipsychotic medication. J Clin Psychiatry 1998;59(suppl 3):21–25.
2. Revicki DA. Methods of pharmacoeconomic evaluation of psychopharmacologic therapies for patients with schizophrenia. J Psychiatry Neurosci 1997;22:256–266.
3. Glazer WM. Olanzapine and the new generation of antipsychotic agents: Patterns of use. J Clin Psychiatry 1997;58(suppl 10):18–21.
4. Sharma T, Mockler D. The cognitive efficacy of atypical antipsychotics in schizophrenia. J Clin Psychopharmacol 1998;18(suppl 1):12S–19S.

63 MAJOR DEPRESSION

▶ A Life Worth Living   (Level I)

Brian L. Crabtree, PharmD, BCPP

▶ After completing this case study, students should be able to:
- Identify the signs and symptoms of depression.
- Develop a pharmacotherapy plan for a patient with depression.
- Compare side-effect profiles of various antidepressant drugs.
- Discuss pharmacoeconomic considerations in antidepressant therapy.

☼ PATIENT PRESENTATION

Chief Complaint
"I don't think I can go on like this. I can't sleep. I can't eat. I can't think straight. Sometimes I wonder if life is worth living."

HPI
Ella Mae is a 38 yo woman who presents to her family physician with the above complaint. She separated from her husband 3 months previously. She has felt down, sad, and worried for over a year, but her symptoms have become worse over the last couple of months.

Ella Mae left her husband, Robert, after 5 years of marriage. This was her second marriage. Violent arguments between them, during which Ella was beaten by her husband, had occurred for the last 4 years of their marriage. They had daily arguments during which Robert hit her hard enough to leave bruises on her face and arms. During their final argument, about Ella Mae buying a gift for a favorite niece, Robert threatened to take the gift away from the niece and destroy it if she didn't agree to return it to the store for a refund. Ella Mae has obtained a court order of protection that prevents Robert from having any contact with her. She has moved in with her parents.

In the 3 months since she left her husband, Ella Mae has become increasingly depressed. Her appetite has been poor, she has little interest in food, and she has lost 14 pounds. She cries frequently and wakes up around 3:00 AM, unable to get back to sleep. She lies awake at night when she goes to bed, crying and tossing and turning for hours before falling asleep. She experiences nightmares about the previous deaths of her sisters. In these nightmares, the sisters summon her to join them. She is unable to concentrate as well as before. She has tried to read the Bible to comfort herself, but she finds herself just reading the same lines over and over. Most recently, she has had thoughts that she wishes she could just go to sleep and not wake up.

PMH
Childhood illnesses—she has had all of the usual childhood illnesses.
Adult illnesses—no current nonpsychiatric adult illnesses; no previous psychiatric treatment, but reports a life-long history of occasional periods of intense sadness lasting several weeks. During these times, she would lose

interest in her usual activities, sometimes missing school or work as a result.

Trauma—fractured arm due to bicycle accident at age 9, otherwise unremarkable.

Surgeries—hx childbirth by CS; tonsillectomy at age 6.

Travel—no significant travel history.

Diet—no dietary restrictions; has recently had a poor appetite and eats only sporadically, skipping many meals.

Exercise—no regular exercise program.

Immunizations—no personal records of childhood vaccinations; had tetanus booster 9 years ago.

FH

Mother has history of anxiety and depression, takes antidepressant medication; Ella Mae doesn't know which. Father is in good health except for well-controlled HTN. Two sisters, both deceased. One committed suicide by stepping in front of a train.

SH

High school graduate with 2 years education at a community college; now unemployed but worked as a secretary before getting married. Married for 5 years, now separated for 3 months. Lives with her parents. Health insurance is through husband's employer (he services photocopiers for an office supply business). Attended church occasionally (Baptist) in the past, but not in the last year or so.

Drinks alcohol (wine and beer) once or twice a month; denies drinking to intoxication. Smokes about 1 ppd with about 14 pack-year history. Drinks 3–4 cups of caffeinated coffee per day; usually drinks iced tea with evening meal; drinks colas as leisure beverage. Used marijuana a few times after high school, denies any use in over 10 years; denies use of other illicit substances.

ROS

General Appearance—Pt c/o feeling tired much of the time.

HEENT—has frequent headaches for last several weeks; no c/o dizziness; wears contact lenses; no tinnitus, ear pain, or discharge; no c/o nasal congestion; hx of dental repair for caries

Chest—no hx of asthma or other lung disease

CV—reports occasional feelings of "racing heartbeat." No hx of heart disease.

GI—reports infrequent constipation, takes MOM PRN. Has lost 14 lb in last 3 months.

GU—has regular menses associated with some cramping

Neuromuscular—often feels stiff and tense in neck and shoulders

Skin—no complaints

PE

Performed by nurse practitioner.

Gen

Thin WF, slightly unkempt and no makeup

VS

BP 112/68, P 92, RR 22, T 36.9°C; Wt 50.3 kg, Ht 66″

Skin

Normal skin, hair, and nails

Neck/LN

Supple without thyromegaly or lymphadenopathy

HEENT

PERRLA; EOM intact, no nystagmus. Fundus—disks sharp, no retinopathy; no nasal discharge or nasal polyps; TMs gray and shiny bilaterally; minor accumulation of cerumen.

Chest/Lungs

Frequent sighing during examination, but no tachypnea or SOB; chest CTA

Heart

RRR without murmur

Breasts

No masses or tenderness

Abdomen

Soft, non-tender; (+) BS; no organomegaly

Genit/rect

Deferred

Ext

Unremarkable

Neuro

CN II–XII intact. Negative Romberg. Finger-to-nose normal. Motor—normal grip strength, bilaterally symmetric. DTRs 2+ and equal. Sensory—intact bilaterally.

Mental Status

The patient is pale and thin, dressed in worn-out jeans and dark blue sweater. Her hair looks unwashed, and she appears older than her stated age. She speaks slowly, describing her depressed mood and lack of energy. She says that she has no pleasure in her life. She has no social contacts other than with her parents. She feels worthless and blames herself for her marital discord. She is often anxious and worries about the future. Speech and thought are logical, coherent, and goal-oriented. No active suicidal ideas, but admits to wishing she could "just pass away." No homicidal ideas. She denies hallucinations. Paranoid delusions, flight of ideas, ideas of reference, and looseness of associations are absent.

Meds

Ortho-Novum 1/35-28, 1 po QD; hasn't taken for 2 months.

Took Tranxene (unknown dosage) for about 2 weeks while in college, Rx by family MD.

St. John's wort 300 mg po TID for the last month or so (purchased at health food store; someone told her it would "lift my spirits").

OTC ibuprofen 400 mg (2 × 200 mg tablets) PRN for headache pain or menstrual cramps, not daily.

Uses non-Rx antihistamines and decongestants for colds or allergies, none in recent months.

MOM 2 tbsp PRN for occasional constipation.

All

NKDA

Labs

Specimens collected 11:45 AM.

Na 139 mEq/L	Hgb 14.0 g/dL	AST 34 IU/L
K 4.2 mEq/L	Hct 46.2%	ALT 42 IU/L
Cl 102 mEq/L	MCV 92 μm^3	GGT 38 IU/L
CO_2 24 mEq/L	MCH 29 pg	T. bili 0.8 mg/dL
BUN 12 mg/dL	Plt 234 × $10^3/mm^3$	T. prot 7.0 g/dL
SCr 0.9 mg/dL	WBC 7.3 × $10^3/mm^3$	Alb 4.4 g/dL
Glu 98 mg/dL	Segs 49%	CK 57 IU/L
Ca 9.5 mg/dL	Bands 1%	T_4 8.6 μg/dL
Mg 1.7 mEq/L	Lymphs 42%	T_3 uptake 29%
Uric acid 4.0 mg/dL	Monos 2%	TSH 2.8 μIU/mL
	Eos 6%	

UA

Glucose neg; ketones neg; pH 5.8; SG 1.016; bilirubin neg; WBC 1/hpf, protein neg, amorphous—rare, epithelial cells 1/hpf; color yellow; blood neg, RBC 0/hpf; mucus—rare; bacteria—rare; casts 0/lpf; appearance clear

Assessment

Major depressive disorder, recurrent, with melancholic features

Plan

Refer for support group, psychotherapy; begin antidepressant medication

---

▶ Questions

Problem Identification

1. a. Create a list of this patient's drug-related problems.
   b. What signs, symptoms, and laboratory values indicate depression in this patient?
   c. What factors in the family history support a diagnosis of depression?
   d. Why is this patient's depression considered to be recurrent even though this is her first psychiatric treatment?
   e. Is there anything in the patient's medication history that could cause or worsen depression?

Desired Outcome

2. What are the goals of pharmacotherapy in this case?

Therapeutic Alternatives

3. a. What non-pharmacologic treatments are important in this case? Should non-pharmacologic treatments be tried before beginning medication?
   b. What pharmacotherapeutic options are available for the treatment of depression?

Optimal Plan

4. a. What drug regimen (drug, dosage, schedule, and duration) is best for this patient?
   b. How should the patient be advised about the herbal therapy, St. John's wort?
   c. What alternatives would be appropriate if the patient fails to respond to initial therapy?

Outcome Evaluation

5. What clinical and laboratory parameters are necessary to evaluate the therapy for efficacy and adverse effects?

Patient Counseling

6. What information should be provided to the patient to enhance compliance, ensure successful therapy, and minimize adverse effects?

▶ Self-study Assignments

1. Since the SSRI antidepressants are commonly used and have the same reuptake pharmacology, contrast the agents in this class, considering relative side effects, dosing, and drug interactions.
2. Discuss pharmacoeconomic considerations in antidepressant therapy, including choice of agents for inclusion in the formulary of a hospital or health maintenance organization.
3. Review the medical literature and evaluate the scientific evidence for the efficacy of St. John's wort in the treatment of depression.

▶ Clinical Pearl

Although the newer antidepressants are more expensive than older antidepressants such as the tricyclic antidepressants, cost of therapy may be the same or less because of fewer adverse effects, fewer follow-up office visits, improved compliance, and less need for other concurrent medications.

References

1. Perry PJ. Pharmacotherapy for major depression with melancholic features: Relative efficacy of tricyclic versus selective serotonin reuptake inhibitor antidepressants. J Affect Disord 1996;39:1–6.
2. Preskorn SH. Comparison of the tolerability of bupropion, fluoxetine, imipramine, nefazodone, paroxetine, sertraline, and venlafaxine. J Clin Psychiatry 1995;56(suppl 6):12–21.
3. Frank E, Kupfer DJ, Perel JM, et al. Three-year outcomes for maintenance therapies in recurrent depression. Arch Gen Psychiatry 1990;47:1093–1099.
4. Linde K, Ramirez G, Mulrow CD, et al. St. John's wort for depression—an overview and meta-analysis of randomised clinical trials. Br Med J 1996;313:253–258.

64 BIPOLAR DISORDER

▶ **Love at First Bite** (Level II)

Andrea Eggert, PharmD, BCPP
William H. Benefield, Jr., PharmD, BCPP, FASCP

▶ After completing this case study, students should be able to:

- Outline a mental status examination and identify target symptoms of bipolar disorder when given patient interview information.

- Recommend appropriate pharmacotherapy for patients with acute mania.

- Generate parameters for monitoring anticonvulsant therapy for bipolar disorder.

- Identify the pharmacotherapeutic options for treating the subtypes of bipolar disorder.

☀ PATIENT PRESENTATION

Chief Complaint
"There are vampires in this city, and I have the documents to prove it."

HPI
Don Love is a 25 yo man brought to the hospital by police. This is his third psychiatric admission. According to neighbors who called the police, the patient has been acting increasingly strange. The lights in the house are left on all night, and spiritual music is played at all hours. Last evening, he dug a trench around his front yard with an electric lawn edger and filled it with garlic cloves. This evening, he painted crosses on the front of the house and threw furniture into his yard and the street. When approached by neighbors, he apparently began screaming and preaching at them. When the police arrived, they found the patient standing naked on the dining room table in his front yard preaching. When the police approached he began throwing garlic tablets at them and screaming, "become naked in the eyes of the Lord and you will be saved." He became increasingly hostile during the arrest shouting, "Don't hate me because I'm beautiful." He then tried to bite one of the officers.

PMH
Manic episodes first occurred while he was in college, leading to psychiatric admissions at ages 21 and 23 for acute mania. Patient was treated with haloperidol 5 mg po QD and lithium 600 mg po Q AM and 900 mg po Q HS, with adequate response and discharged on both occasions after about a month. Medical problems include migraine headaches.

Patient Interview
Patient is disheveled with pungent body odor. He is pacing the room, waving his hands in the air and preaching in an elated, loud, sing-songy voice. He is dressed flamboyantly in a brightly colored bathrobe and appears to be wearing a garlic necklace. He is carrying a Bible. When asked how he felt, he stated, "Playful, with intense clarity, sharp, spiffy, and clean." He then

became angry, insisting that he be discharged before sunrise or he would "face the light of the right and mighty and burn in 'demonocratic' hell." He then asked for a priest to exorcise the homosexual demons from his body. He believes that vampires live in the city. He stated he has the documents to prove it, and that the vampires are pursuing him to keep him from exposing their existence to Christians everywhere. He spoke in long run-on sentences with many political, religious, and sexual references. He was very difficult to interrupt. For example, at one point he stated, "Can't you see, or are you an idiot?! I am being persecuted by the right, 100 points of light, Republicans, redeeming the public, for the republic, under which I stand because I have no one to lean on, one gay man, bitten by the democrat, the demoncrat, doomed and miserable for loving the company I keep, and that's why misery loves company, and if you don't get that you're an idiot."

When asked about his sleep, he angrily replied, "Would you sleep at a time like this? If I sleep, America will fall, and it will all be on my shoulders." The patient stated that he has not been eating and has not taken his lithium in several days because, "Lithium is of the ground, the underworld. The Lord will sustain me."

Through his verbose conversation, it becomes apparent that he was bitten on the neck by a man he picked up in a gay bar last week. He also seems to believe that he has been given a mission from God as penance for visiting this bar. Several times during the interview, he began crying and wailing loudly begging to be saved, and shouting, "I'm sorry." He said something about the trials of Job and that he would be the next to die. He sang "Swing Low Sweet Chariot" in a very loud voice. When told that he might need to stay at the hospital so we could help him with his problems, he screamed, "You can't help me! Only the Lord can help me! They have drunk from the fruit of the vine. I am that fruit."

Abnormal Involuntary Movement Scale (AIMS)
Excessive eye-blinking and mild grimacing; unclear if abnormal (patient states this is the "demon blood" trying to take over his body). He is bothered by it in that to him it represents "his sinful nature."

FH
Father has a history of depression, paternal grandmother was placed in an "asylum" for hysteria secondary to childbirth. Mother and brother have type 2 diabetes.

SH
Recently fired from his job as a nurse at a local hospital. Patient is a single homosexual. Religious upbringing as a Southern Baptist. Smokes 1 ppd × 5 years. Patient states that he drinks "only occasionally," but he was noted to be intoxicated with a BAC 0.14% on a previous admission.

Meds
Ergotamine and ibuprofen PRN for migraines

All
NKA

ROS
Migraine headaches about 2 times a month, no aura, (+) nausea and photophobia. Occasional GI upset with no clear relationship to meals or time of day; frequent loose stools.

PE

VS

BP 118/73, P 83, RR 16, T 37.1°C; Wt 94 kg, Ht 6'2"

HEENT

PERRLA, EOMI, fundi benign, throat and ears clear, TMs intact; rapid eye-blinking and facial grimacing (may indicate early tardive dyskinesia)

Skin

Psoriasis evident on both elbows

Neck

Supple, bite mark, no nodes

Cor

RRR; S_1, S_2 normal; no m/r/g

Lungs

CTA & P

ABD

(+) BS, non-tender

Ext

Full ROM, pulses 2+ bilaterally

Neuro

A & O × 3, reflexes symmetric, toes downgoing, normal gait, normal strength, sensation intact, CN II–XII intact

Labs

Na 141 mEq/L	Hgb 14.6 g/dL	WBC 11.0×10^3/mm^3	AST 32 IU/L	Ca 9.7 mg/dL
K 3.8 mEq/L	Hct 45.7%	Neutros 67%	ALT 20 IU/L	Phos 5.3 mg/dL
Cl 103 mEq/L	RBC 4.73×10^6/mm^3	Lymphs 23%	Alk Phos 87 IU/L	TSH 4.1 μIU/mL
CO_2 24 mEq/L	MCV 90.2 μm^3	Monos 7%	GGT 36 IU/L	RPR: Neg
BUN 19 mg/dL	MCH 31 pg	Eos 2%	T. bili 0.9 mg/dL	Lithium 0.1 mEq/L
SCr 1.1 mg/dL	MCHC 34.4 g/dL	Basos 1%	Alb 3.7 g/dL	
Glu 89 mg/dL	Plt 256×10^3/mm^3		T. chol 218 mg/dL	

UA

Color yellow; appearance slightly cloudy; glucose (−), bili (−), ketones trace; SG 1.025, blood (−), pH 6.0, protein (−), nitrites (−), leukocyte esterase (−)

Assessment

Axis I: Bipolar disorder, current episode mixed
Axis II: Deferred
Axis III: Migraine headache by history

▶ Questions

Problem Identification

1. a. From the case information and patient interview, write a mental status examination for this patient.
   b. Create a list of this patient's drug-related problems.
   c. What information (target symptoms, laboratory values) indicates the presence and severity of bipolar disorder, mixed episode?

Desired Outcome

2. What are the goals of pharmacotherapy in this patient?

Therapeutic Alternatives

3. a. What non-drug therapies might be useful for this patient?
   b. What feasible pharmacotherapeutic alternatives are available for treatment of bipolar disorder?

Optimal Plan

4. a. What drug, dosage form, dose, schedule, and duration of therapy are best for this patient?
   b. What alternatives would be appropriate if the initial therapy fails or cannot be used?

Outcome Evaluation

5. What clinical and laboratory parameters are necessary to evaluate response to therapy and to detect or prevent adverse effects?

Patient Counseling

6. What information should be provided to the patient to enhance compliance, ensure successful therapy, and minimize adverse effects?

▶ Self-study Assignments

1. Perform a literature search and explore the role of the newer anticonvulsants (lamotrigine, gabapentin, and topiramate) in the treatment of bipolar disorder.
2. Perform a literature search on once-daily dosing of antimanic agents. How would you go about changing a patient's dosing regimen to increase compliance? Based on the literature, which patients are most suitable for conversion to once- or twice-daily dosing with lithium, carbamazepine, or valproate? Can regular-release products be used, or must the patient be converted to extended-release products?
3. Design an algorithm for the treatment of bipolar disorder. Include treatment strategies for acute mania, rapid cycling, depression, and mixed states.

► Clinical Pearl

When a patient admitted with acute mania is taking an antidepressant, the antidepressant should be tapered and withdrawn. In some patients, antidepressants may activate mania or increase the rate of cycling, and potentially prolong response to antimanic medication.

References

1. Swann AC, Bowden CL, Morris D, et al. Depression during mania: Treatment response to lithium or divalproex. Arch Gen Psychiatry 1997;54:37–42.
2. Freeman TW, Clothier JL, Pazzaglia P, et al. A double-blind comparison of valproate and lithium in the treatment of acute mania. Am J Psychiatry 1992;149:108–111.
3. Goldberg JF, Garno JL, Leon AC, et al. Rapid titration of mood stabilizers predicts remission from mixed or pure mania in bipolar patients. J Clin Psychiatry 1998;59:151–158.
4. Algorithm for patient management of acute manic states: Lithium, valproate, or carbamazepine? J Clin Psychopharmacol 1992;12:57S–63S.
5. McElroy SL, Keck PE, Tugrul KC, et al. Valproate as a loading treatment in acute mania. Neuropsychobiology 1993;27:146–149.

65 GENERALIZED ANXIETY DISORDER

► The Worrywart (Level I)

Chad M. VanDenBerg, PharmD
Michael W. Jann, PharmD, FCP, FCCP

► After completing this case study, students should be able to:

- Detect the target symptoms associated with generalized anxiety disorder (GAD).
- Outline non-pharmacologic therapeutic approaches to relieve anxiety.
- Recognize the role of pharmacologic agents in the treatment of anxiety.
- Devise a pharmaceutical care plan for a patient with GAD.

☼ PATIENT PRESENTATION

Chief Complaint
"I'm a worrier."

HPI
Karen Larson is a 23 yo woman who was evaluated by her family practitioner due to complaints of insomnia and restlessness despite feeling tired most of the day. In addition to being a full-time student, she works 24 hours/week as a cashier to make ends meet. She states that she has difficulty studying for her classes and concentrating at work. Furthermore, she constantly worries about school, grades, and her parents who are divorcing after 25 years of marriage. Car and school payments have always troubled her. These symptoms have been present for over 1 year but appear to have increased in frequency and intensity over the past 8 months. On more days than not, she complains of these symptoms and now she worries that these symptoms are not "normal" and that she is becoming mentally ill. Her family physician, upon consultation with the managed care consultant psychiatrist, agrees that she has generalized anxiety disorder (GAD).

PMH
Treated with alprazolam for anxiety 1 year ago by another physician; she discontinued this 6 months ago because she was afraid of becoming "addicted."
Alcohol abuse beginning 5 years ago; she was hospitalized for this problem 3 years ago and has not had an alcoholic drink since.
She has been evaluated by a gastroenterologist for her stomach problems and takes an occasional Tagamet HB for "heartburn."
Her current medical records note that over the past several years she has been a constantly anxious patient who worries continually about her life.

FH
Father had an episode of depression when his mother died 10 years ago but is otherwise well. Mother has traits of OCD but has not been diagnosed or treated. She has one sister who has no known psychological or medical problems.

SH
Student in dental hygiene school, smokes cigarettes 1–2 ppd, and drinks 4–5 cups of coffee per day; no alcohol use.

ROS
Only a mild dry mouth; negative for muscle aches, dizziness, diarrhea, palpitations, sweating, and shortness of breath.

Meds
Buspirone 10 mg po TID × 2 months; admits to having stopped this a few days ago due to perceived lack of efficacy.
Tagamet HB 200 mg po PRN heartburn

All
Sulfas (skin rash)

PE

Gen
Alert and well dressed, cooperative female patient, oriented × 3

VS
BP 136/88, P 72, RR 18, T 36.8°C; Wt 56.0 kg, Ht 65″

Skin
Warm and dry, no discoloration

HEENT
PERRLA; fundi benign; ear, nose, and throat clear; TMs intact

Neck/LN
Supple and without obvious nodes; no thyromegaly

Lungs
Clear to A & P

Breasts
Normal without masses

CV
NSR, S_1 and S_2 normal, no m/r/g

Abd
Soft to touch, non-tender, bowel sounds present

Neuro
Hyper-reflexive in both LE; Romberg (−); CN II–XII intact; normal gait; sensitive to light touch, pain, and vibration

Labs
Na 140 mEq/L
K 4.7 mEq/L
Cl 104 mEq/L
CO_2 27 mEq/L
BUN 17 mg/dL
SCr 1.1 mg/dL
Glu (fasting) 107 mg/dL

Hgb 13.2 g/dL
Hct 36%
TSH 1.9 μIU/mL
T_3 uptake 30%
T_4 5.6 mcg/dL

ECG
NSR, rate 76 bpm

Assessment
Psychiatric, generalized anxiety disorder

► Questions

Problem Identification

1. a. Create a list of the patient's drug-related problems.
   b. What information indicates the presence or severity of GAD?

Desired Outcome

2. What are the goals of pharmacotherapy in this case?

Therapeutic Alternatives

3. a. What non-drug therapies might be useful for the patient to consider?
   b. What feasible pharmacotherapeutic alternatives are available for the treatment of GAD?

► Clinical Course

Karen was referred to a cognitive and behavioral therapist for treatment of GAD. In addition, her physician restarted buspirone and increased the dose to 20 mg po TID. After 4 weeks of non-cognitive therapy (psychotherapy and behavioral therapy) and compliance with the new dose of buspirone, Karen feels that her anxiety has not been relieved although she feels more capable of coping with her feelings and wants to continue seeing the therapist.

Optimal Plan

4. a. What drug, dosage form, dose, schedule, and duration of therapy are best for this patient?
   b. What pharmacotherapeutic alternatives would be appropriate if the optimal plan fails?

Outcome Evaluation

5. What clinical and laboratory parameters are necessary to evaluate the therapy for achievement of the desired therapeutic outcome and to detect or prevent adverse effects?

Patient Counseling

6. What information should be provided to the patient to enhance compliance, ensure successful therapy, and minimize adverse events?

► Self-study Assignments

1. Perform a literature search to obtain recent information regarding the use of antidepressants in the treatment of GAD. Write a two-page critical review of your findings.
2. Familiarize yourself with the dose, duration of treatment, and adverse events of the various benzodiazepines used in treating GAD. Prepare a comprehensive table comparing benzodiazepines for future study and reference.
3. Discuss the pros and cons of using a placebo comparison in clinical trials for GAD. Write a one-page summary to support your view and refute the opposite view.

► Clinical Pearl

Benzodiazepines are not recommended for the treatment of anxiety in patients with a history of alcohol abuse.

References

1. Schweizer E, Rickels K. Strategies for treatment of generalized anxiety in the primary care setting. J Clin Psychiatry 1997;58(suppl 3):27–31.
2. Hoehn-Saric R. Generalised anxiety disorder: Guidelines for diagnosis and treatment. CNS Drugs 1998;9:85–98.
3. Rocca P, Fonzo V, Scotta M, et al. Paroxetine efficacy in the treatment of generalized anxiety disorder. Acta Psychiatr Scand 1997;95:444–450.
4. Nutt D. Management of patients with depression associated with anxiety symptoms. J Clin Psychiatry 1997;58(suppl 8):11–16.

66 PANIC DISORDER

▶ **Another Trip to the ER**   (Level I)

W. Alexander Morton, PharmD, BCPP

▶ After completing this case study, students should be able to:

- Describe the physical symptoms of a panic attack.
- Recognize the practice settings at which patients usually seek treatment.
- Discuss the likely consequences of patients not receiving adequate treatment.
- Recommend effective pharmacotherapy treatment plans for panic disorder.
- Discuss reasons why patients fail to receive adequate treatment of panic disorder.

☼ PATIENT PRESENTATION

Chief Complaint
"I get this tightness and squeezing in my chest."

HPI
Tina Brooks is a 33 yo woman who presents to your outpatient program in response to a television advertisement regarding a research program for anxiety. She describes experiencing sudden, spontaneous episodes of fearfulness accompanied by a crushing, tight sensation in her chest followed by shortness of breath. During this time she also has heart palpitations which feel like "my heart is about to jump out." She also reports vertigo, extreme nausea, diarrhea, shaking, sweating, and a fear that "I'm going to die."

She experiences 1 to 2 episodes a week, which "come out of nowhere" and can last from 3 to 10 minutes. She dates the onset of these attacks to 4 years ago when she was having trouble with her daughter in school. These episodes have been getting worse over the last year in both intensity and frequency. She has gone to the ER numerous times (twice in the last month) thinking she was having a heart attack but was told "it is all in your head." ECG and blood tests have all been normal. She has been seen by a cardiologist who performed 48-hour Holter monitor and a stress test, which were negative; she was told that she had a perfect heart.

She is currently fearful of driving her car because she experienced a bad panic attack on the highway. She is afraid she will "cause a pile-up." At times, she will not drive to work fearing she may lose control while driving. She relates one period of time when she did not leave her house for 3 months because she was fearful of having an attack. She avoids shopping, especially in large stores, because she feels like everything is closing in on her.

She states that she has received numerous medications in the past for these problems, but none have really helped. She is currently taking diazepam 2.5 mg po PRN, which was prescribed at the ER last night.

She also reports being on edge most of the time, expecting the worst in every situation. She excessively worries about finances and her husband's health. She is frequently tense, irritable, has difficulty getting a good night's rest, and feels fatigued all the time. She admits to a mildly depressed mood and a slight loss of interest in her activities, but she usually "snaps herself out of it." Her appetite and libido are normal, but concentration is "zero," and she frequently feels guilty about not being a good mother. She is afraid of high places, but this does not interfere with her life. She does not like to speak in front of others but has not been required to do so since high school, and she seldom thinks of doing this.

Past Psychiatric History
She reports one episode of depression in the past where she "lost interest in everything." She had difficulty sleeping, gained 30 pounds, had negative thoughts all the time, and frequently thought her "family would be better off if she was dead," but denied any specific suicide plan. She was treated with Elavil; after the first dose she had an anxiety attack and "wondered if the doctor knew what he was doing." She did not take it long because of the way it made her feel and did not return for follow-up.

PMH
Occasional dizziness/balance problem treated with Antivert with little relief of symptoms. Irritable bowel syndrome characterized by sudden cramping, abdominal pain, and diarrhea; medical evaluation was negative; was prescribed Librax but seldom takes it.

FH
No history of psychiatric problems. Her father died of an MI when he was 51 yo. Her mother is alive and in good health, "although she doesn't like to go out much." She has one younger brother who is healthy.

SH
She grew up in coastal North Carolina. Her parents were divorced when she was 5 yo, but they lived near to each other and she recalls mostly happy times. She graduated from high school and attended a university, graduating with a degree in journalism. She is happily married and has a 4 yo son and an 11 yo daughter who has ADHD. She has very few leisure activities ("I hardly do anything fun"). She tries to read to get her mind off her panic attacks. She will have a glass of wine to help relax her and help her fall asleep. She denies use of illegal substances. She does not use nicotine and avoids caffeine.

ROS
She reports frequent headaches, grinding of her teeth, and occasional muscle pain in her shoulders.

Meds
Diazepam 2.5 mg PRN for nervousness with no relief
Librax for irritable bowel syndrome
Antivert PRN for dizziness (not taken on a regular basis)
Ibuprofen 400 mg PRN headache
Recently started taking kava kava and St. John's wort because she heard they were recommended for anxiety

All
Avoids cold medicines because they make her anxious and feel "unreal."

MSE

A 33 yo cooperative, attractive, anxious female with mild psychomotor agitation. She is appropriately dressed for office work. She is mildly diaphoretic and her hands are cold. Speech is normal in rate and volume. There are no manic or psychotic symptoms present. There is no depressed affect and she doesn't appear to be delusional or hallucinating. She denies suicidal or homicidal ideation. She appears to have good attention and concentration. She reports her weight as 145 lb and height as 5'8".

PE

VS
BP 120/70, P 96, RR 18, T 37.1°C

Skin
No rashes or bruising

HEENT
PERRLA, EOMI, fundi sharp and well visualized

Neck
Thyroid not palpated

CV
Tachycardia; S_1, S_2 normal; no m/r/g

Lungs
Rapid, clear breath sounds

Abd
Non-tender; numerous BS

Gent/Rect
Deferred

Neuro
Mild tremor in hands; CN II–XII normal; DTRs 2+ bilaterally; sensory and motor function intact

Labs

Na 136 mEq/L	Hgb 14.8 g/dL	AST 20 IU/L
K 4.0 mEq/L	Hct 43.0%	ALT 25 IU/L
Cl 106 mEq/L	Plt $310 \times 10^3/mm^3$	Alk phos 40 IU/L
CO_2 24 mEq/L	WBC $6.3 \times 10^3/mm^3$	T. bili 0.9 mg/dL
BUN 12 mg/dL	Neutros 52%	T. chol 165 mg/dL
SCr 0.7 mg/dL	Lymphs 38%	T_3 resin uptake 42%
Glu 85 mg/dL	Monos 7%	T_4 total 9.6 μg/dL
	Eos 2%	TSH 0.7 μIU/mL
	Basos 1%	

ECG
NSR, mild tachycardia; no evidence of old MI

Pregnancy Test
Negative

Urine Drug Screen
Positive for benzodiazepines, otherwise neg

Assessment
Based on history, presentation, and normal labs and ECG, this patient meets diagnostic criteria for panic disorder. Because of her comorbid generalized anxiety disorder and depressive symptoms, she does not meet inclusion/exclusion criteria for our panic study.

DSM-IV Diagnosis

Axis I:	Panic disorder with agoraphobia
	Generalized anxiety disorder
	R/0 major depressive disorder, recurrent
Axis II:	Deferred
Axis III:	Irritable bowel syndrome, probably secondary to panic
	Meniere's syndrome, probably secondary to panic
Axis IV:	Daughter with ADHD
Axis V:	Global Assessment of Functioning (GAF): current 45

► Questions

Problem Identification

1. a. Create a list of the patient's drug-related problems.
   b. What information indicates the presence or severity of panic disorder in this patient?
   c. What medications would be expected to make this problem worse?

Desired Outcome

2. What are the goals of pharmacotherapy in this case?

Therapeutic Alternatives

3. a. What non-drug therapies might be useful for this patient?
   b. What feasible pharmacotherapeutic alternatives are available for treatment of panic disorder?

Optimal Plan

4. a. What drug, dosage form, dose, schedule, and duration of therapy are best for this patient?
   b. If initial treatment fails, what alternatives should be considered?

Outcome Evaluation

5. What clinical and laboratory parameters are necessary to evaluate the therapy for achievement of the desired therapeutic outcome and to detect or prevent adverse effects?

Patient Counseling

6. What information should be provided to the patient to enhance compliance, ensure successful therapy, and minimize adverse effects?

► Clinical Course

The patient was initially discouraged that she was not able to participate in the research study for the treatment of panic disorder. However, she was referred to a study program that allowed comorbid conditions to be present as long as the primary psychiatric problem was panic disorder. She was randomized in a double-blind trial comparing paroxetine versus imipramine versus phenelzine versus placebo in the treatment of panic and depression. She initially experienced some mild increase in generalized anxiety and had difficulty falling asleep (more than usual). The anxiety resolved, but the insomnia required zolpidem 5 mg po PRN for a week before her sleep normalized. A benzodiazepine, such as lorazepam, might be the drug of choice but was not allowed as it has potent antianxiety activity and could bias the study.

Over the next 12 weeks, she was tapered up to 6 tablets BID (paroxetine 60 mg, or imipramine 300 mg, or phenelzine 90 mg or placebo) with positive results. She had complete resolution of her panic attacks and a decrease in her HAM-D (17 item) score from 26 to 8. Side effects included mild sedation that was tolerable.

She continued in the study as a "responder" for the next 9 months. At this time, the medication was unblinded and the treating clinician was surprised to find her taking imipramine 300 mg/day. The clinician was almost certain she was receiving paroxetine because of so few side effects, but once again real life refused to follow the books.

Recently, she called EMS to her house when she "knew" she was having a heart attack. She soon realized and accepted it as a panic attack when the paramedics reminded her of her breathing exercises. She was also able to recall her clinician's words about cognitive therapy, repeating to herself over and over, "This is a panic attack. I've had these before. It will go away in 5 minutes and I will be fine."

She has continued to do well at a reduced dose of imipramine 150 mg at bedtime with no panic attacks, no anticipatory anxiety, reduced avoidance (she still refuses to shop in super-stores). She has no side effects except that she notices an occasional dry mouth when the clinician specifically asks her, "Do you have dry mouth?"

The clinical course of patients with panic disorder is quite variable. About a third do well, 50% continue to have mild and fluctuating symptoms of anxiety, and 20% do not do well.[4]

► Self-study Assignments

1. Research the medical literature on panic disorder and make a list of what "response" means and how it was defined.
2. Read two newsletters from the National Association of Anxiety Disorders' Web page, www.adaa.org.
3. Conduct an informal survey among your faculty, coworkers, and fellow students as to how long a benzodiazepine should be prescribed for panic disorder.
4. Discuss the following. Is a limited symptom attack with one symptom, such as "crushing chest pain" less of a problem than a six-symptom panic attack?

► Clinical Pearl

For some patients with panic disorder, the initial antidepressant dose may need to be extremely low, such as fluoxetine 1 mg. A 20-mg capsule of fluoxetine can be dissolved in 100 mL of water or juice and refrigerated for 14 days. A 5-mL dose will provide 1 mg.

References

1. Kessler RC, McGonagle KA, Zhao S, et al. Lifetime and 12-month prevalence of DSM-III-R psychiatric disorders in the United States. Results from the National Comorbidity Survey. Arch Gen Psychiatry 1994;51:8–19.
2. Lydiard RB. Anxiety and the irritable bowel syndrome: psychiatric, medical, or both? J Clin Psychiatry 1997;58(suppl 3):51–58.
3. Giesecke ME. Overcoming hypersensitivity to fluoxetine in a patient with panic disorder. Am J Psychiatry 1990;147:532–533.
4. Katschnig H, Amering M, Stolk JM, et al. Long-term follow-up after a drug trial for panic disorder. Br J Psychiatry 1995;167:487–494.

67   OBSESSIVE-COMPULSIVE DISORDER

► The Little Girl on the Swing   (Level II)

Lyle K. Laird, PharmD, BCPP

► After completing this case study, students should be able to:

- Identify the target symptoms of obsessive-compulsive disorder (OCD).
- Recommend appropriate pharmacotherapy for a patient suffering from OCD.
- Counsel a patient concerning the use of selective serotonin reuptake inhibitors.
- Discuss several nonpharmacotherapeutic approaches to the treatment of OCD.

☼ PATIENT PRESENTATION

Chief Complaint
"I worry about the police coming and arresting me because that little girl fell out of the swing I built and she might be hurt."

HPI
Drew Furchtbar is a 31 yo man who was referred for the first time to this Anxiety Disorders Clinic by his primary care doctor. For the past month, he has been in distress over multiple things in his life. Specifically, he is concerned about his own thoughts and behaviors. He stated, "I blow things out of proportion . . . but what if the little girl who fell out of the swing I built was hurt and now the police are going to arrest me? I call her house every day to ask her parents if she is OK, and they always say she is fine. And now they are upset with my calling." The girl fell when the rope broke and had the wind knocked out of her; there was no serious injury.

He goes on to state, "I know this is all strange, but I can't help myself and the thoughts continue no matter what I seem to do. I spend hours a day worrying about all of this! I get depressed and want to cry. I'm afraid of dying. I pace around my house and check the mail all the time." He has stated that he has considered suicide if anything had happened to the little girl.

He also reports other obsessions such as fearing that bumps in the road that he encounters while driving are actually bodies and worrying that he could contract HIV from a toilet seat by simply entering a public restroom. He has compulsive behaviors such as driving around the block for up to an hour searching for bodies he may have hit with his car and washing his hands for up to 10 minutes after entering a public restroom.

Mr. Furchtbar has several psychosocial stressors presently in his life including significant personal financial debt and the recent death of his mother. The patient is presently on medical leave from work as he is incapacitated by obsessive thoughts.

PMH

H/O kidney infections and peptic ulcer disease

FH

Positive for psychiatric illness; patient reports that all 3 siblings (2 sisters, 1 brother) have had "nervous breakdowns." His brother also suffers from alcoholism as did his father. A niece has a problem with worries and obsessions.

SH

Mr. Furchtbar is 1 of 4 children. He completed high school but did not attend college. He completed a program in electronics at a local technical school. For the past 10 years, he has been working for a local department store. He denies using street drugs or prescription medications but admits to drinking "several glasses" of wine when he is nervous. He relates that the wine seems to help at times in decreasing his overall level of anxiety. He smokes about 5 cigarettes a day and sometimes drinks up to 8 cups of coffee a day.

ROS

He reports a recent loss of appetite and difficulty sleeping (generally difficulty falling asleep and awakening in the middle of the night) unless he takes a hypnotic. No cough, exertional dyspnea, palpitations, chest pain, or edema. Denies epigastric pain, constipation, diarrhea, or abnormal stools. No nocturia or dysuria.

Meds

Clomipramine 250 mg po Q HS for the past 6 weeks
Flurazepam 30 mg po Q HS PRN sleep

All

Penicillin (H/O rash and hives)

PE

Gen

Alert, cooperative male in NAD, oriented to all spheres

VS

BP 130/85, P 100, RR 21, T 98.4°F, Ht 68″, Wt 60 kg

HEENT

PERRLA; EOMI; normal fundi; TMs clear; nares clear; pharynx WNL

Neck

Supple, thyroid normal size without nodules

Cor

Regular rate; normal S_1, S_2; no m/r/g

Resp

Breath sounds clear throughout

Abd

BS (+), soft and nontender, no palpable viscera or masses

Ext

(−) CCE; skin on both hands dry, cracked and appears to have been bleeding recently

Neuro

No localizing signs; negative Babinski and Romberg; DTRs active and equal bilaterally

Labs

Na 140 mEq/L	Hgb 15 g/dL	WBC $9.5 \times 10^3/mm^3$	AST 15 IU/L	T. chol 155 mg/dL
K 4.7 mEq/L	Hct 43.1%	Neutros 71%	ALT 18 IU/L	Ca 8.9 mg/dL
Cl 101 mEq/L	RBC $4.85 \times 10^6/mm^3$	Lymph 25%	Alk Phos 50 IU/L	Phos 4.5 mg/dL
CO_2 25 mEq/L	MCV 85.9 μm^3	Monos 3%	GGT 22 IU/L	Osm 287 mOsm/kg
BUN 18 mg/dL	MCH 33.4 pg	Eos 1%	T. bili 0.9 mg/dL	T_3 uptake 39%
SCr 0.8 mg/dL	MCHC 34.4 g/dL		T. Prot 7.8 g/dL	T_4 total 10.8 μg/dL
Glu 95 mg/dL	Plt $200 \times 10^3/mm^3$		Alb 4.0 g/dL	TSH 2.2 μIU/mL

UA

Color yellow, appearance slightly cloudy, Glu (−), bili (−), ketones (−), SG 1.025, blood (−), urobilinogen (−), nitrite (−), leukocyte esterase (−)

ECG

Sinus rhythm with borderline first degree A-V block; QTc = 436 mSec, ventricular rate 94

Assessment

Obsessive-compulsive disorder

▶ Questions

Problem Identification

1. *a. Create a list of the patient's drug-related problems.*
   b. What signs, symptoms, or laboratory parameters indicate the presence of OCD in this patient?

Desired Outcome

2. *What are the goals of the pharmacotherapy for OCD in this case?*

Therapeutic Alternatives

3. *a. What non-drug therapies might be useful for this patient?*
   b. What feasible pharmacotherapeutic alternatives are available for the treatment of OCD?

Optimal Plan

4. *What drug, dosage form, dose, schedule, and duration of therapy are best for this patient?*

Outcome Evaluation

5. *What clinical and laboratory parameters are necessary to evaluate the therapy for achievement of the desired therapeutic outcome and to detect or prevent adverse effects?*

Patient Counseling

6. *What information should be provided to the patient to enhance compliance, ensure successful therapy, and minimize adverse effects?*

▶ Clinical Course

The patient's medication regimen was changed from clomipramine to fluvoxamine. The clomipramine dosage was carefully tapered over a 1-month period. At the end of the taper, fluvoxamine 50 mg po Q HS was begun. (*Note:* an alternative strategy is to start the fluvoxamine a week or more before the end of the clomipramine taper.) Prior to starting the clomipramine taper, a Y–BOCS evaluation was obtained and a total score of 30 was recorded on the 10-item scale. The patient returned for follow-up medication and CBT assessments on a monthly basis. Since the patient was tapered off of the clomipramine just before starting the fluvoxamine, his clinical condition worsened slightly, with an increase in the level of anxiety and depression. The fluvoxamine was ultimately titrated over an 8-week period to a maximum dose of 300 mg/day. He also participated in a CBT regimen. Sleep was reported to improve somewhat over the first several weeks of fluvoxamine therapy. The patient reported early in the fluvoxamine trial that he felt "buzzed" after drinking only one cup of coffee, whereas previously he had been able to drink as much coffee as he wanted. He was advised to minimize his daily intake of coffee; he soon ceased complaining of the activating caffeine effects. Over a period of 10 weeks, the patient's Y–BOCS scores went from 30 to 16, and although he continued to periodically obsess about contamination and engaged in some hand-washing, he reported that the thoughts that the little girl had been hurt were gone. His appetite and sleep were essentially normalized and he no longer thought about suicide. He is being continued on the maximum dose of flu-

voxamine while continuing to see his therapist and going to the clinic's pharmacist for medication checks.

▶ Follow-up Questions

1. *Why is it important to taper the clomipramine?*
2. *Why is it important to minimize the use of the hypnotic?*
3. *Why was he apparently so intolerant of coffee when he was placed on fluvoxamine?*
4. *When is a decrease in the Y–BOCS score considered clinically significant?*

▶ Self-study Assignments

1. What is the importance of a positive family history of OCD when making a diagnosis of this anxiety disorder?
2. Investigate the cardiovascular effects of the antidepressants. For example, how are the TCAs different in this respect from the newer SSRIs?
3. Find a sample of the Y–BOCS rating scale on the Internet. What do the specific numbers obtained through its use indicate? For example, what does a total score of "30" mean? Is this indicative of a minimally, moderately, or severely impaired individual?
4. Investigate the costs of cognitive-behavioral therapy versus pharmacotherapy for OCD.
5. Perform a literature search on the treatment of schizophrenia plus OCD symptoms (i.e., sometimes called "schizo-obsessive" disorder). How is this presentation different from the "typical" version of OCD? How is schizo-obsessive disorder treated with medications?

▶ Clinical Pearl

Optimal therapy for OCD often includes non-pharmacologic modalities, such as cognitive-behavioral intervention; treatment regimens should be considered for a long-term basis.

References

1. American Psychiatric Association. Diagnostic and Statistical Manual of Mental Disorders (DSM-IV), 4th ed. Washington, DC, American Psychiatric Association, 1994.
2. Greist JH. An integrated approach to treatment of obsessive compulsive disorder. J Clin Psychiatry 1992;53 (suppl):38–41.
3. Laird LK, Lydiard RB, Morton WA, et al. Cardiovascular effects of imipramine, fluvoxamine, and placebo in depressed outpatients. J Clin Psychiatry 1993;54:224–228.
4. Laird LK. Issues in the monopharmacotherapy and polypharmacotherapy of obsessive-compulsive disorder. Psychopharmacol Bull 1996;32:569–578.
5. McDougle CJ. Update on pharmacologic management of OCD: Agents and augmentation. J Clin Psychiatry 1997;58 (suppl 12):11–17.
6. Goodman WK, Price LH, Rasmussen SA, et al. The Yale–Brown Obsessive Compulsive Scale. I. Development, use, and reliability. Arch Gen Psychiatry 1989;46:1006–1011.
7. Goodman WK, Price LH, Rasmussen SA, et al. The Yale–Brown Obsessive–Compulsive Scale. II. Validity. Arch Gen Psychiatry 1989;46:1012–1016.

68 INSOMNIA

▶ ## In Search of Safe and Restful Sleep   (Level II)

Penny S. Shelton, PharmD, BCPP, FASCP
Mollie Ashe Scott, PharmD, BCPS

▶ After completing this case study, students should be able to:

- Recognize and differentiate primary insomnia versus insomnia associated with a psychiatric diagnosis.
- Identify and understand the psychosocial, disease-related, and drug-induced causes of insomnia.
- Recognize when non-pharmacologic treatments for insomnia are preferred over drug therapy.
- Recommend appropriate pharmacologic treatment for insomnia.

☀ PATIENT PRESENTATION

Chief Complaint
"I don't sleep well at all."

HPI
Perry Francis is a 67 yo man who reports to an ambulatory care clinic for help with his insomnia. He is noticeably tired, nervous, and apprehensive. The patient is accompanied by his daughter. The patient states that he has not slept well in months. He has difficulty getting to sleep because of "all the things running through my head," and he also awakens very early (usually 3:00 AM) and cannot go back to sleep. He was recently widowed (about 3 months ago). He takes a daily mid-afternoon nap and dozes while watching television at night. He also states that he has been using Sominex for 1 month without relief.

The patient describes his health as poor. He states that he has had an overwhelming fear of dying for the past 1–2 months. He states that he has always been somewhat of a worrier but since the death of his wife, he has had significant problems with insomnia and his "nerves." Over the past month, he has had two episodes of a severe overwhelming sense of impending doom, shortness of breath, palpitations, and a choking sensation. Each episode occurred at night while home alone and lasted approximately 20 minutes. The daughter thinks he is depressed and bought him an "herbal remedy" for his depression approximately 2 months ago.

PMH
Osteoarthritis (right hip and right knee) × 6 years
Hypercholesterolemia diagnosed 4 years ago during hospitalization for MI
Hypothyroidism × 10 years
H/O generalized anxiety disorder (intermittent symptoms since age 25)
S/P MI 4 years ago

FH
Mother and father died in MVA when the patient was 24 years old. No siblings.

SH
Recently widowed (3 months ago). Good family support (1 daughter and 1 son). Patient was a truck driver who has been retired for 4 years. He now works part-time as a sales clerk at a hardware store 4 days/week. There is financial hardship, and the patient is seriously concerned about his finances. (+) cigarette smoker (20 pack-year history). H/O Seconal addiction when in his early 30s. Moderate EtOH user in his youth; none in the past 10 years until he recently began drinking 1 glass of wine in the evenings to help him rest.

ROS
Patient reports frequent episodes of sweating and tachypnea during times when he is "upset." He occasionally feels his heart "racing" but has had no chest pain since his MI. He reports periodic constipation that has been worse in the past month; no nausea, vomiting, or abdominal pain. He also reports symptoms of urinary frequency, nocturia 2 to 3 times/night, and trouble starting a urine stream, which have been worse in the past few weeks. He has right hip and knee pain and stiffness, particularly upon awakening and after sitting. His weight has been stable.

Meds
Pravachol 10 mg po Q HS
Synthroid 125 μg po QD × 4 years
EC ASA 325 mg po QD
Sominex 1–2 tablets each night × 1 month
St. John's wort 2 grams po daily × 2 months

PE

Gen
Elderly WDWN man who looks younger than his stated age. He appears anxious and is easily startled.

VS
BP 120/76, P 98, RR 12, T 98.7°F; Wt 81.6 kg; Ht 5′11″

Skin
Normal skin color and turgor, but moist from perspiration; no lesions noted

HEENT
Normocephalic, PERRLA, EOMI

Neck/LN
Supple with normal size thyroid, (−) JVD, (−) adenopathy

Lungs
CTA bilaterally

CV
Normal S_1, S_2; no m/r/g

Abd
NTND, no HSM

GU/Rect
Enlarged, non-tender prostate; heme (−) stool

Ext

No CCE; normal muscle bulk and tone; muscle strength 5/5 and equal in all extremities; femoral, popliteal, dorsalis pedis, and posterior tibial pulses 2+ and equal bilaterally

Neuro

Oriented to person, place, and time; CN II–XII intact

Labs

			Fasting Lipid Panel
Na 140 mEq/L	Hgb 14 g/dL	AST 54 IU/L	
K 4.1 mEq/L	Hct 43%	ALT 52 IU/L	T. chol 242 mg/dL
Cl 105 mEq/L	RBC $4.7 \times 10^6/mm^3$	LDH 112 IU/L	LDL 158 mg/dL
CO_2 28 mEq/L	Plt $262 \times 10^3/mm^3$	GGT 47 IU/L	HDL 47 mg/dL
BUN 11 mg/dL	WBC $6.2 \times 10^3/mm^3$	T. Bili 0.3 mg/dL	TG 185 mg/dL
SCr 0.7 mg/dL	TSH 0.25 μIU/mL	T. prot 7.1 g/dL	
Glu 81 mg/dL	Free T_4 4.1 ng/dL	Alb 4.0 g/dL	

ECG

Left bundle branch block

Assessment

1. Insomnia
2. Anxiety disorder (GAD vs. panic disorder)
3. Benign prostatic hyperplasia (symptomatic)
4. Osteoarthritis (right hip/knee)
5. Dyslipidemia
6. Social stressors

▶ Questions

Problem Identification

1. a. Create a drug-related problem list for the patient.
   b. What information (signs, symptoms, laboratory values) indicates the presence or severity of insomnia?
   c. Could any of the patient's problems have been caused by drug therapy?
   d. What additional information is needed to satisfactorily assess this patient?

Desired Outcome

2. What are the goals of pharmacotherapy in this case?

Therapeutic Alternatives

3. a. What non-pharmacologic therapies might be useful for this patient?
   b. What feasible pharmacotherapeutic alternatives are available for treatment of insomnia?

Optimal Plan

4. a. What drug, dosage form, dose, schedule, and duration of therapy are best for this patient?
   b. What alternatives would be appropriate if the initial therapy fails or cannot be used?

Outcome Evaluation

5. What clinical and laboratory parameters are necessary to evaluate the therapy for achievement of the desired therapeutic outcome and to detect or prevent adverse effects?

Patient Counseling

6. What information should be provided to the patient to enhance compliance, ensure successful therapy, and minimize adverse effects?

▶ Follow-up Question

1. What other medication adjustments should be made at this time?

▶ Self-study Assignments

1. Describe how aging affects normal sleep architecture.
2. Develop a pharmacotherapy plan for the treatment of his symptomatic benign prostatic hyperplasia.
3. If you were chair of the P & T committee for a health care system and were asked to choose only three agents for the treatment of insomnia for the new formulary, which agents would you include and why?

▶ Clinical Pearl

Insomnia is often a symptom of an underlying medical or psychiatric problem; correcting the cause and implementing good sleep hygiene practices may minimize the need for hypnotic agents.

References

1. Woelk H, Burkard G, Grunwald J. Benefits and risks of the hypericum extract LI 160: Drug monitoring study with 3250 patients. J Geriatr Psychiatry Neurol 1994;7(suppl 1):S34–S38.

2. Nowell PD, Buysse DJ, Reynolds CF III, et al. Clinical factors contributing to the differential diagnosis of primary insomnia and insomnia related to mental disorders. Am J Psychiatry 1997;154:1412–1416.

3. Lechin F, van der Dijs B, Benaim M. Benzodiazepines: Tolerability in elderly patients. Psychother Psychosom 1996;65:171–182.

4. Roger M, Attali P, Coquelin JP. Multicenter, double-blind, controlled comparison of zolpidem and triazolam in elderly patients with insomnia. Clin Ther 1993;15:127–136.

5. Scharf MB, Sachais BA. Sleep laboratory evaluation of the effects and efficacy of trazodone in depressed insomniac patients. J Clin Psychiatry 1990;51(suppl): 13–17.

6. Chase JE, Gidal BE. Melatonin: Therapeutic use in sleep disorders. Ann Pharmacother 1997;31:1218–1226.

SECTION 7

Endocrinologic Disorders

Robert L. Talbert, PharmD, FCCP, BCPS, Section Editor

---

69 TYPE 1 DIABETES MELLITUS

▶ **Carolyn Carter's Ketoacidosis   (Level II)**

Scott Jacober, DO, CDE
Linda A. Jaber, PharmD

▶ After completing this case study, students should be able to:

- Identify laboratory parameters necessary for the diagnosis and monitoring of diabetic ketoacidosis (DKA).

- Identify anticipated electrolyte abnormalities associated with DKA and their treatment.

- Recommend appropriate initial IV insulin doses and insulin infusion concentrations.

- Identify therapeutic decision points in DKA treatment and provide parameters for altering therapy at those decision points.

- Determine when patients may be converted from IV to subcutaneous insulin therapy and calculate the dose of insulin that should be administered.

- Provide patient counseling for sick day management of patients with diabetes mellitus.

☀ PATIENT PRESENTATION

Chief Complaint
"I have been throwing up since last night and feel weak and dizzy."

HPI
Carolyn Carter is a 33 yo mother of 1 son with a history of type 1 DM of 23 years' duration. Last night before supper, she took her usual dose of lispro insulin for a blood glucose measurement of 182 mg/dL. She began feeling nauseated several hours after supper, and she began vomiting at 11:00 p.m. Her blood glucose at that time was 368 mg/dL. She took her usual bedtime NPH insulin and supplemented this with additional lispro insulin to compensate for the hyperglycemia. She tried sipping water and diet soda but was unable to keep any fluids down. She vomited 6 more times that evening before falling asleep for several hours. She was weak on awakening the next morning, tried eating and drinking, but was unable to keep anything down again and vomited another 3 times. She contacted her physician by phone, who noted heavy breathing interrupting her speech and instructed her to seek transportation to the hospital ED. She did not test her urine for ketones but did take her prescribed insulin dose supplemented with additional lispro insulin for the hyperglycemia (glucose 424 mg/dL) at breakfast time, even though she was unable to eat. She denies fevers, chills, or diarrhea, but several children in her son's class have been ill recently with fever, vomiting, and diarrhea. She also denies cough, sore throat, and dysuria.

Carolyn was last treated with laser therapy for proliferative diabetic retinopathy 8 years ago and was told she had stable non-proliferative diabetic retinopathy at her last ophthalmologic examination 3 months ago. Her last screen for microalbuminuria 9 months ago was negative. She has no paresthesias of the feet or hands and has never had a foot ulcer. She denies any chest pain, history of hypertension, and intermittent claudication. Her last cholesterol measurement was 178 mg/dL with an HDL of 62 mg/dL. Her diabetic pregnancy 4 years ago resulted in a healthy newborn son. She has had a history of hypoglycemic coma but no episodes in the past 2 years. Her glucose control has been suboptimal with an HbA$_{1c}$ performed 3 months ago of 10.1%. She is prescribed a 1600-calorie ADA diet (3 meals and HS snack).

Meds

Insulin according to the schedule in Table 69–1.

Urinary ketones: if moderate, add 5 units lispro insulin; if large, add 10 units lispro insulin

PMH

Type 1 DM diagnosed 23 years ago; hospitalized 3 times for DKA in the past 10 years

PSH

C-section 4 years ago

FH

Father age 66 has HTN; mother deceased at 58 from breast CA; 1 brother age 36 with type 1 DM and HTN; 4 other healthy siblings; 1 healthy son age 4

SH

Divorced homemaker living alone with her 4-year-old. Does not smoke, drink, or abuse drugs.

ROS

HEENT—Awakened with blurry vision and dizziness on postural change but denies vertigo, head trauma, ear pain, tinnitus, dysphagia, odynophagia.

CV—No complaints of chest pain, orthopnea, peripheral edema, or heart murmur.

RESP—No complaints of cough, wheezing, dyspnea.

GI—Vomiting as noted above but no complaints of abdominal pain, constipation, diarrhea, or food intolerance.

GU—Had polyuria (large volumes every 2 hours) last night but has not urinated since awakening. No complaints of dysuria or hematuria.

OB-GYN—G_1P_1. Denies current pregnancy and has ongoing menses which began 3 days ago. Menses flows for 5 days and is regular every 30 days. Not sexually active and denies any vaginal discharge, pain, or itching.

Neuro—Has never had a seizure or weakness in an arm or leg. No complaints of headache, paresthesias, dysesthesias, or anesthesias.

Derm—No history of chronic rashes, sweating abnormalities, or recent skin lesions. Has had mild lipohypertrophy at old thigh injection sites but tries to avoid these areas.

Endo—Denies a history of goiter and has no heat or cold intolerance. Her weight has not fluctuated by more than 5 lb in the past 4 years.

TABLE 69–1. The Patient's Lispro and NPH Insulin Schedule (units)

Blood Glucose (mg/dL)	Lispro Insulin Doses			
	Breakfast	Lunch	Supper	Bedtime
< 80	4		7	
81–150	5		8	
151–200	6		9	1
201–250	7	2	10	2
251–300	8	3	11	3
301–350	9	4	12	4
351–400	10	5	13	5
> 400	11	6	14	6
NPH insulin	16	—	—	14

PE

Gen

Mildly overweight Caucasian woman with a female body habitus looking her stated age, with deep respirations, alcohol or ketones on her breath and not confused, but questionably appropriate.

VS

BP 124/86 supine & 110/84 sitting, P 128, RR 28, T 99.1°F; Ht 5′4″; Wt 155 lb

Skin

Lipohypertrophy is present on both lateral thighs.

HEENT

NCAT, PERRLA, EOM intact. Fundi reveal old laser scars bilaterally without vitreous hemorrhage and rare dot/blot hemorrhages and hard exudates bilaterally. Mucous membranes are dry, pharynx is erythematous without tonsillar exudates. Ears are unremarkable.

Neck

Thyroid is palpable but not enlarged. No masses are present.

LN

Cervical, axillary, and femoral lymph nodes are non-palpable.

CV

PMI is normal and non-displaced. S_1 and S_2 are normal without S_3, S_4, murmur, or rub. RRR. Carotid, femoral, and dorsalis pedis pulses are 3/4. There are no carotid, abdominal or femoral bruits.

Chest

Lungs are CTA & P. There is full excursion of the chest without any tenderness.

Abd

Soft, NT without organomegaly or masses. Bowel sounds are decreased.

Rect

Anus is normal. No masses or hemorrhoids are noted. Stool is Hemoccult negative.

Ext

There is no pretibial edema. Feet are without ulcers, callus, or other lesions.

Neuro

DTRs bilaterally are 3/4 for the biceps, brachioradialis, quadriceps, and Achilles. Plantars are downgoing bilaterally. Vibratory perception at the 1st MTP bilaterally is slightly depressed. Muscle strength is 5/5.

Labs

Na 127 mEq/L	Hgb 15.2 g/dL	WBC 6.0×10^3/mm³
K 6.1 mEq/L	Hct 45.5%	Neutros 71%
Cl 96 mEq/L	RBC 5.08×10^6/mm³	Bands 11%
CO_2 6.0 mEq/L	Plt 259×10^3/mm³	Lymphs 14%
Anion gap 25 mEq/L	MCV 89.5 μm³	Monos 4%
BUN 22 mg/dL	MCHC 33.3 g/dL	Serum pregnancy: negative
SCr 1.4 mg/dL		
Glu 645 mg/dL		
Acetone: 3+		

ABG
On room air: pH 7.05; pco$_2$ 7.6; po$_2$ 139; HCO$_3$ 2.0, O$_2$ sat 98%

UA
SG 1.018, pH 5.5, glu 3+, prot 2+, ketones 3+, blood 3+, RBCs 50–100/hpf

Chest X-ray
Normal

ECG
Sinus tachycardia

Assessment
1. Diabetic ketoacidosis precipitated by viral gastroenteritis
2. Type 1 DM complicated by proliferative diabetic retinopathy (s/p laser therapy) now stabilized to non-proliferative diabetic retinopathy and a history of hypoglycemic coma

---

▶ Questions

Problem Identification

1. *What problems beyond hyperglycemia are encountered in DKA that may require intervention?*

Desired Outcome

2. *What are the goals of therapy for this patient?*

Therapeutic Alternatives

3. *What therapies are available to correct the presenting metabolic derangements of DKA?*

Optimal Plan

4. *Outline your specific plan for providing the IV fluids and medications that should be administered to this patient.*

Outcome Evaluation

5. a. *What monitoring of therapy is necessary for the plan that you outlined for the patient?*
   b. *What changes in the therapeutic regimen should be considered when the blood glucose drops below 300 mg/dL or the potassium drops into the low normal range?*
   c. *When is the DKA considered to be resolved, and when can IV insulin therapy be converted to subcutaneous therapy?*
   d. *Outline a plan for converting the patient from IV to subcutaneous insulin after resolution of the DKA.*

Patient Counseling

6. *How should patients be counseled about self-management on a "sick day" (i.e., when they are anorectic, nauseated, or vomiting)?*

▶ Self-study Assignments

1. Describe the medical complications associated with DKA and DKA treatment.
2. DKA is usually associated with reduced serum bicarbonate concentrations. However, the routine use of sodium bicarbonate supplementation is quite controversial. Review the risks and benefits of bicarbonate therapy. In what situations should it be recommended?

3. Two metabolic disorders, DKA and hyperosmolar hyperglycemic nonketotic coma, are commonly encountered in patients with diabetes. Compare and contrast the two disorders as to the cardinal features, precipitating factors, pathophysiology, and treatment strategies.[4]

▶ Clinical Pearl

Although patients with type 2 diabetes are able to suppress ketogenesis under basal conditions, they may develop DKA in the presence of a precipitating factor such as severe infection (e.g., sepsis).

References

1. DeFronzo RA, Matsuda M, Barrett EJ. Diabetic ketoacidosis: A combined metabolic-nephrologic approach to therapy. Diabetes Rev 1994;2:209–238.
2. Foster DW, McGarry JD. The metabolic derangements and treatment of diabetic ketoacidosis. N Engl J Med 1983;309:159–169.
3. Morris LR, Murphy MB, Kitabchi AE. Bicarbonate therapy in severe diabetic ketoacidosis. Ann Intern Med 1986;105:836–840.
4. Ennis ED, Stahl EJB, Kreisberg RA. The hyperosmolar hyperglycemic syndrome. Diabetes Rev 1994;2:115–126.

70 TYPE 2 DIABETES MELLITUS

▶ Establishing Optimal Control   (Level II)

Milissa A. Rock, RPh, CDE
Jean-Venable (Kelly) R. Goode, PharmD, BCPS

▶ After completing this case study, students should be able to:

- Identify the goals of therapy for the treatment of type 2 diabetes mellitus (DM).
- Discuss the risk factors and comorbidities associated with type 2 DM.
- Compare options for drug therapy management of type 2 DM including mechanisms of action, combination therapies, comorbidities, and patient-friendly treatment plans.

- Develop an individualized drug therapy management plan including dosage regimens, therapeutic end points, and monitoring parameters.
- Provide patient counseling regarding medications, adherence to the treatment plan, monitoring the disease state, blood glucose control, and seeking advice from health care providers when necessary.

☀ PATIENT PRESENTATION

Chief Complaint
"I'm here for my regular check up. I don't have any problems today."

HPI
John McGuire is a 68 yo man who comes to the diabetes outpatient clinic for a follow-up visit. His blood glucose logbook indicates that he has been monitoring his blood glucose levels twice a day (before breakfast and dinner) with a range of 140 to 175 mg/dL. He reports adherence to an 1800-calorie meal plan and 40 minutes of walking on a treadmill every morning.

PMH
Type 2 DM × 5 years
HTN × 13 years
Hyperlipidemia × 1 year

FH
Maternal grandmother had DM; father had emphysema; no family history of CAD.

SH
Married, retired factory worker, active in church and a social club. No current tobacco use (stopped 40 years ago), consumes about 7–14 alcoholic drinks per week.

ROS
Denies nocturia, polyuria, polydipsia, nausea, constipation, diarrhea, signs or symptoms of hypoglycemia, paresthesias, and dyspnea. Reports occasional blurry vision and occasional lower leg pain.

Meds
Glynase 6 mg po QD × 1 year
Glucophage 1 gram po BID × 6 months
Zestril 20 mg po QD
EC ASA 81 mg po QD

All
NKDA

PE

Gen
WDWN mildly obese, elderly Caucasian man in NAD

VS
BP 182/82, P 80, RR 16, T 38.6°C; Wt 82.2 kg, Ht 66.5″

HEENT
PERRLA, EOMI, R & L fundus exam without retinopathy

CV
RRR, no m/r/g

Lungs
Clear to A & P

Abd
NT/ND

Genit/Rect
Deferred

MS/Ext
Carotids, femorals, popliteals, right dorsalis pedis pulses 2+ throughout, left dorsalis pedis 1+; feet show thick calluses on MTPs

Neuro
DTRs 2+ throughout, feet with normal sensation (5.07 monofilament) and vibration

Labs

Na 139 mEq/L	Ca 9.8 mg/dL	*Fasting Lipid Profile*
K 5.3 mEq/L	Phos 3.3 mg/dL	T. chol 238 mg/dL
Cl 102 mEq/L	AST 19 IU/L	LDL-C 168 mg/dL
CO$_2$ 22 mEq/L	ALT 13 IU/L	HDL-C 42 mg/dL
BUN 23 mg/dL	Alk phos 43 IU/L	Trig 170 mg/dL
SCr 1.2 mg/dL	T. bili 1.0 mg/dL	Free thyroxine index 3.4 U
Glu (random) 289 mg/dL		HbA$_{1c}$ 8.2%

UA
(−) protein, (−) microalbuminuria

Assessment
The patient reports adherence to diet, exercise, and drug therapy as prescribed. His glycemic control has improved somewhat (FBG and pre-dinner BG previously 170 to 200 mg/dL) with addition of Glucophage 6 months ago. His cholesterol levels have also improved (T. chol 268 mg/dL 10 months ago). Blood pressure has remained consistently high for the past 10 months. He has lost 1.6 kg in the last 3 months. His glycemic control, blood pressure, and lipid profile have not improved adequately in response to a combination of nutrition therapy utilizing the NCEP Step II diet (2 visits with a dietitian) and drug therapy implemented for the last 6 months.

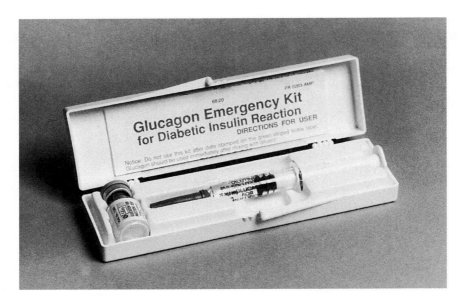

Figure 70–1. The Glucagon Emergency Kit for the treatment of hypoglycemia.

▶ Questions

Problem Identification

1. a. *What are this patient's drug-related problems?*
   b. *What findings indicate poorly controlled diabetes in this patient?*

Desired Outcome

2. a. *What are the goals of treatment for the management of type 2 diabetes in this patient?*
   b. *What individual patient characteristics should be considered in determining the goals of treatment?*

Therapeutic Alternatives

3. a. *What non-pharmacological interventions should be recommended for this patient?*
   b. *What pharmacologic interventions could be considered for this patient?*

Optimal Plan

4. a. *What pharmacotherapeutic regimen would you recommend for this patient?*
   b. *What alternative therapies might be appropriate if the initial plan fails?*

Outcome Evaluation

5. *What parameters should be monitored to evaluate the efficacy and possible adverse effects associated with the optimal regimen you selected?*

Patient Counseling

6. *What information should be given to the patient regarding diabetes mellitus and his treatment plan to increase adherence,* *minimize adverse effects, and improve outcomes? Include information on use of a glucagon emergency kit (see Figure 70–1).*

▶ Follow-up Questions

1. *What are the measurable objectives and long-term goals for treating hypertension and hyperlipidemia in this patient?*
2. *What non-pharmacological and pharmacological interventions would you consider to reach these goals?*

▶ Self-study Assignments

1. Discuss the phenomenon known as syndrome X and the role that insulin resistance is postulated to play in its sequelae.
2. Explore the advantages and disadvantages of using combination oral agents (based on different mechanisms and sites of action) in the management of type 2 diabetes and the rationale for delaying the initiation of insulin therapy.
3. Discuss combination therapy using various oral hypoglycemic agents with insulin.

▶ Clinical Pearl

The addition of a second oral agent is usually preferred over titrating to a maximum sulfonylurea dose to minimize adverse effects, improve therapeutic outcomes, decrease hyperinsulinemia, preserve pancreatic function, and postpone the need for exogenous insulin.

References

1. American Diabetes Association. Standards of medical care for patients with diabetes mellitus. Diabetes Care 1998;21(suppl 1):S24–S39.

2. Expert Panel on Detection, Evaluation, and Treatment of High Blood Cholesterol in Adults. Summary of the second report of the National Cholesterol Education Program (NCEP) Expert Panel on detection, evaluation, and treatment of high blood cholesterol in adults (Adult Treatment Panel II). JAMA 1993;269:3015–3023.

3. Joint National Committee on Prevention, Detection, Evaluation, and Treatment of High Blood Pressure. The sixth report of the Joint National Committee on Prevention, Detection, Evaluation, and Treatment of High Blood Pressure. Arch Intern Med 1997;157:2413–2446.

4. Melander A. Oral antidiabetic drugs: An overview. Diabet Med 1996;13(9 suppl 6):S143–S147.

5. Saltiel AR, Olefsky JM. Thiazolidinediones in the treatment of insulin resistance and type II diabetes. Diabetes 1996;45:1661–1669.

71   HYPERTHYROIDISM: GRAVES' DISEASE

▶ **Gland Central**   **(Level I)**

Kristine E. Santus, PharmD
Tara L. Posey, PharmD

▶ After completing this case study, students should be able to:

- Describe the signs, symptoms, and laboratory parameters associated with hyperthyroidism and relate them to the pathophysiology of the disease.
- Select and justify appropriate patient-specific initial and follow-up pharmacotherapy for patients with hyperthyroidism.
- Develop a plan for monitoring the pharmacotherapy for hyperthyroidism.
- Provide appropriate counseling information to patients receiving drug therapy for hyperthyroidism.

☀ PATIENT PRESENTATION

Chief Complaint
"My stomach hurts. I think I may have an ulcer."

HPI
Elaine Marywood is a 58 yo woman who presents with her daughter to the walk-in clinic with complaints of epigastric pain that radiates to the chest and occurs mostly at night. The pain is exacerbated by spicy foods and caffeine and is relieved by milk and antacids. She reports a 50-pound weight loss over the past year, 10 pounds of which occurred over the past month, despite a good appetite. She began experiencing palpitations a few months ago that come and go but are not associated with CP. However, she does note that her heart seems to "beat too fast" for the amount of activity she is doing. She has also had difficulty swallowing solid food for the past few months and has been unable to sleep for the past 3 days. She has noticed that her legs have been swollen for approximately 2 weeks and her neck "pulsates." Her daughter reports that the patient is "more nervous and hyper than usual."

PMH
Patient entered menopause 10 years ago.

FH
She has a daughter with hyperthyroidism and a half-sister with Graves' disease. Her father had arthritis and multiple MIs; her mother had breast cancer; her grandmother had leukemia.

SH
She lives with her husband and smokes $\frac{1}{2}$ ppd × 35 years (she may have smoked more in the past). She does not drink alcohol.

ROS
She notes that her hair has become more fine and thinner in distribution recently. She has no visual changes, CP, or dyspnea. She has occasional N/V/D.

Meds
None

All
PCN (rash)

PE

Gen
The patient is a thin, tan-appearing WF in NAD.

VS
BP 120/80, P 120–160 irreg, RR 18, T 37.1°C; Wt 118 lb., Ht 5'2"

Skin
Hyperpigmented on upper back and lower extremities, warm and moist. Hair is fine and sparse on crown of head.

HEENT
PERRL, EOMI, (+) lid lag, mild proptosis (no ophthalmoplegia), mild lid retraction

Neck/LN
Supple, (+) smooth, symmetrically enlarged thyroid, (+) thyroid bruit, (+) JVD to jaw, prominent pulsations in neck vessels

Lungs
CTA bilaterally, no wheezes or rales

CV
Irregularly irregular rhythm, tachycardic without murmurs; (+) carotid bruits bilaterally

Abd
Soft, NT/ND; (+) BS; no HSM or masses; mild navel erythema with some slight crusting with no exudate. Aortic pulsations palpable.

Rectal
Guaiac (−) stool

Ext

2+ pitting edema bilaterally in LE, 2+ DP pulses bilaterally, no calf tenderness. No cyanosis. Fingernails and toenails are flaking. Thumbnails have prominent ridges.

Neuro

A & O × 3; hyperreflexia at knees; no proximal muscle weakness or tremor.

Labs

Na 140 mEq/L	Hgb 8.8 g/dL	RDW 16.4%	AST 32 IU/L	Total T_4 24.3 μg/dL
K 3.8 mEq/L	Hct 27.4%	WBC $5.5 \times 10^3/mm^3$	ALT 29 IU/L	TSH < 0.018 μIU/mL
Cl 106 mEq/L	RBC $3.48 \times 10^6/mm^3$	Polys 45%	T. bili 0.8 mg/dL	T_3 resin uptake 49%
CO_2 25 mEq/L	Plt $156 \times 10^3/mm^3$	Lymphs 39%	Amylase 54 IU/L	Total T_3 720 ng/dL
BUN 9 mg/dL	MCV 78.8 μm³	Monos 13%	Ca 8.5 mg/dL	Free thyroxine index 41.3
SCr 0.4 mg/dL	MCH 25.3 pg	Eos 2%	Mg 1.5 mEq/L	
Glu N/A	MCHC 32.1 g/dL	Basos 1%	Phos 4.3 mg/dL	

ECG

Atrial fibrillation; sinus tachycardia (rate of 118)

Assessment

58 yo white female with goiter, probable hyperthyroidism, and new onset atrial fibrillation. Most likely cause is Graves' disease.

► Questions

Problem Identification

1. a. Create a list of the patient's drug-related problems.
   b. What signs, symptoms, and laboratory values indicate the presence or severity of hyperthyroidism?

Desired Outcome

2. What are the goals of pharmacotherapy in this case?

Therapeutic Alternatives

3. a. What non-drug therapies might be useful for this patient?
   b. What feasible pharmacotherapeutic alternatives are available for the treatment of hyperthyroidism in this patient?

Optimal Plan

4. What drug, dosage form, dose, schedule, and duration of therapy are best for this patient?

Outcome Evaluation

5. What clinical and laboratory parameters are necessary to evaluate the response to therapy and to detect or prevent adverse effects?

Patient Counseling

6. What information should be provided to the patient to enhance compliance, ensure successful therapy, and minimize adverse effects?

► Clinical Course

The patient is started on the treatment you recommended and returns for a 1-month follow-up visit. The following information is obtained.
VS: BP 120/80, P 98 irreg., RR 18, T 37.0°C.

Labs

Hgb 10.2 g/dL	WBC $4.6 \times 10^3/mm^3$	AST 26 IU/L	Total T_4 16.9 μg/dL
Hct 30.7%	Polys 61%	ALT 33 IU/L	TSH < 0.018 μIU/mL
MCV 83.0 μm³	Lymphs 26%	Alk phos 326 IU/L	*Thyroid antibodies*
MCH 27.5 pg	Monos 10%	T. bili 1.3 mg/dL	Thyroglobulin 176 IU/mL
MCHC 33.1 g/dL	Eos 2%	PT 14.4 sec	Tperox 158 IU/mL
RDW 16.7%	Basos 1%	INR 1.3	

► Follow-up Questions

1. What interventions, if any, would you suggest at this point?
2. If the patient subsequently becomes hypothyroid but clinical signs indicate that the patient still has Graves' disease, what plan should be implemented?

► Self-study Assignments

1. Develop a monitoring protocol for the pharmacotherapy of hyperthyroidism.
2. Design a systematic approach for a patient counseling technique for the drug therapy of hyperthyroidism.

► Clinical Pearl

Hyperthyroidism in pregnant women must be treated to avoid fetal complications or death. Because surgery and radioactive iodine are contraindicated in pregnancy, pregnant women should be treated with PTU, as it does not cross the placental barrier as efficiently as methimazole. The lowest dose possible should be used to avoid fetal hypothyroidism and goiter.

References

1. Vanderpump VMJ, Ahlquist JA, Franklyn JA, et al. Consensus statement for good practice and audit measures in the management of hypothyroidism and hyperthyroidism. BMJ 1996;313:539–544.

2. Kallner G, Vitols S, Ljunggren JG, et al. Comparison of standardized initial doses of two antithyroid drugs in the treatment of Grave's disease. J Intern Med 1996:239:525–529.

3. Hashizume K, Ichikawa K, Sakurai A, et al. Administration of thyroxine in treated Grave's disease: Effects on the level of antibodies to thyroid-stimulating hormone receptors and on the risk of recurrence in hyperthyroidism. N Engl J Med 1991;324:947–953.

4. Self TH, Straughn AB, Weisburst MR. Effect of hyperthyroidism on hypoprothombinemic response to warfarin. Am J Hosp Pharm 1976;33:387–399.

72 HYPOTHYROIDISM

► The Battle to Control the Thermostat
(Level II)

Tara L. Posey, PharmD

► After completing this case study, the student should be able to:

- Recognize the signs and symptoms of hypothyroidism.
- Identify the goals of therapy for hypothyroidism.
- Develop an appropriate treatment plan for thyroid replacement based on individual patient characteristics.
- Select an appropriate agent for thyroid replacement therapy.
- Thoroughly counsel a patient taking thyroid replacement therapy.

☀ PATIENT PRESENTATION

Chief Complaint
"I still feel very tired, even after my gynecologist said my iron levels are normal."

HPI
Maria Petrine is a 53 yo woman who presents to her PCP complaining of feeling tired for the last 6 months. Two months ago she had significant menstrual blood loss treated with a D & C and iron replacement for iron-deficiency anemia. She stated that she was told that once her anemia was treated she should feel better. Upon further questioning, she admits that at times she feels unable to cope with job-related stress like she used to and has difficulty participating in recreational activities outside of work because she is tired. She also reports that her skin seems more dry and itchy in the scalp, breast, abdomen, and buttock area. She also states that she has difficulty warming up and is always turning up the heat despite her husband's requests to turn it down.

PMH
Iron-deficiency anemia
HTN × 4 years
Perimenopausal

FH
Positive for CVD, CAD; father died of CVA at age 55, mother is alive with HTN and had an MI at 60; she has one brother with type 2 DM and a sister with HTN.

SH
Married, lives with her husband of 30 years; has 4 children who are now healthy adults. Works as a secretary in a middle school × 10 years. Drinks an occasional glass of wine; (–) tobacco or drug use.

ROS
Occasional headaches relieved with non-aspirin pain reliever; (–) tinnitus, vertigo, or infections; occasional body aches which she attributes to inactivity; (–) change in urinary frequency or stool habits; (–) skeletal muscle complaints; reports cold extremities; (–) history of seizures, MS changes, or LOC.

Meds
Atenolol 50 mg po QD
$FeSO_4$ 300 mg po BID
EC ASA 325 mg po QD

All
NKDA

PE

Gen
Well-appearing, middle-aged, slightly obese, Caucasian woman in NAD

VS
BP 130/82, P 70, RR 18, T 36.4°C; Wt 80 kg, Ht 5′2″

Skin
Dry appearing skin and scalp; (–) rashes or lesions

HEENT
NCAT; PERRLA, trace periorbital edema; (–) sinus tenderness; (–) signs of infection or sore throat

Neck/LN
(–) thyroid nodules or goiter; (–) lymphadenopathy

Lungs/Thorax
CTA

Breasts
(–) lumps/masses; yearly mammograms via gynecologist negative to date

CV
RRR, normal S_1, S_2; (–) S_3 or S_4

Abd
NT/ND

Neuro
A & O × 3; CN II–XII intact; DTRs 2+

Labs

Na 145 mEq/L	Hgb 16 g/dL	Serum Fe 50 μg/dL
K 4.0 mEq/L	Hct 42%	TIBC 250 μg/dL
Cl 101 mEq/L	RBC 5.2×10^6/mm^3	T. sat 35%
CO_2 26 mEq/L	WBC 6.0×10^3/mm^3	TSH 10.2 μIU/mL
BUN 10 mg/dL	MCV 88 μm^3	Free T_4 0.7 ng/dL
SCr 0.8 mg/dL	MCH 29 pg	T. chol 225 mg/dL
Glu 96 mg/dL	MCHC 33 g/dL	

Assessment

Middle-aged woman with signs, symptoms, and laboratory tests suggesting hypothyroidism.

► Questions

Problem Identification

1. a. Identify this patient's drug-related problems.
   b. What information (signs, symptoms, laboratory values) indicates the presence of hypothyroidism?
   c. Could any of the patient's problems have been caused by drug therapy?

Desired Outcome

2. What are the goals of pharmacotherapy in this patient?

Therapeutic Alternatives

3. a. What non-drug therapies might be useful for this patient?
   b. What feasible pharmacotherapeutic alternatives are available for treatment of hypothyroidism?

Optimal Plan

4. What drug, dosage form, dose, schedule, and duration of therapy are best for this patient?

Outcome Evaluation

5. What clinical and laboratory parameters are necessary to evaluate thyroid replacement therapy to achieve euthyroidism and prevent adverse effects?

Patient Counseling

6. What information should be provided to the patient to enhance compliance, ensure successful therapy, and minimize adverse effects?

► Follow-up Questions

1. How should this patient's elevated cholesterol be handled at this point?
2. Assume that the patient returns for a routine exam in 6 months and her cholesterol is still elevated. How should this be assessed?

► Self-study Assignments

1. What medications can interfere with thyroid hormone replacement?

2. What are the mechanisms of these interactions?
3. How should these interactions be managed?

► Clinical Pearl

Overzealous thyroid replacement can put patients at risk for serious side effects. It is important to start with low doses and titrate upward slowly. Thyroid requirements may change over time, so regular monitoring should be performed.

References

1. Dong BJ, Hauck WW, Gambertoglio JG, et al. Bioequivalence of generic and brand-name levothyroxine products in the treatment of hypothyroidism. JAMA 1997;277:1205–1213.
2. Singer PA, Cooper DS, Levy EG, et al. Treatment guidelines for patients with hyperthyroidism and hypothyroidism. Standards of Care Committee, American Thyroid Association. JAMA 1995;273:808–812.

73 CUSHING'S SYNDROME

► When One Gland Affects Another

Jerry D. Smith, PharmD
John G. Gums, PharmD

► After completing this case study, students should be able to:

- Recognize and differentiate the signs, symptoms, and laboratory changes associated with the various forms of Cushing's syndrome.

- Recognize the biochemical, anatomic, and emotional changes that can occur with Cushing's syndrome.

- Recommend appropriate treatment regimens for patients with Cushing's syndrome.

- Suggest appropriate adjunctive pharmacotherapy to other health care providers for patients with Cushing's disease.

- Provide patient counseling on proper dosing, administration, and adverse effects of treatment for Cushing's disease.

☀ PATIENT PRESENTATION

Chief Complaint
"I have been tired and weak lately."

HPI
Susan Taylor is a 31 yo woman who presents to her family physician complaining of fatigue and weakness. She also reports weight gain (50 lb over 2 years) and depression with insomnia.

PMH
Patient has been healthy with no other major medical illnesses. She had 2 healthy children by uncomplicated vaginal deliveries.

FH
Mother is alive at age 54 with type 2 DM; father is living at age 56 with HTN. She has 2 sisters, one is healthy, and the other has depression.

SH
Patient does not smoke, and drinks occasionally. She is a photographer. Children are ages 6 and 3.

ROS
(+) for fatigue, weakness, occasional back pain, and weight gain; also reports episodes of sadness, depressed mood, and insomnia; skin bruises easily; occasional headache, blurred vision, and heartburn; no CP, wheezing, or SOB. Normal menstruation with regular periods.

Meds
Triphasil-21 as directed
Unisom PRN sleep
Advil PRN headache
St. John's wort 300 mg po TID (self-initiated 3 weeks ago)

All
Sulfa → rash

PE

Gen
WDWN obese, Cushingoid-appearing Caucasian female in NAD

VS
BP 160/100, HR 85, RR 14, T 37.0°C; Wt 181 lb., Ht 5'3"

Skin
Thin skin with some bruising and scratches; purple striae visible on abdomen

HEENT
Rounded face; moderate facial hair; PERRLA; EOMI; funduscopic exam shows normal retinal background, optic cup-to-disk ratios 0.4; visual fields appear to be grossly intact; OP moist and pink

Neck/LN
Supple; (−) JVD, bruits, adenopathy, or thyromegaly

Chest
CTA bilaterally

Breasts
No lumps or masses

CV
RRR, no m/r/g

Abd
Obese, soft, NT, (−) masses or organomegaly

Genit/Rect
Guaiac (−); normal external genitalia; no masses

MS/Ext
Appears to have decreased strength bilaterally; DTR 1–2+ and symmetric throughout all 4 extremities; no CCE

Neuro
Oriented × 3; flat affect; CN II–XII intact

Labs

Na 138 mEq/L	Hgb 13.4 g/dL	AST 9 IU/L	TSH 2.33 μIU/mL
K 3.3 mEq/L	Hct 38.5%	ALT 7 IU/L	HbA$_{1c}$ 7.1%
Cl 105 mEq/L	RBC 4.0 × 10^6/mm^3	Alk Phos 180 IU/L	*Fasting Lipid Profile*
CO$_2$ 25 mEq/L	Plt 264 × 10^3/mm^3	T. bili 0.5 mg/dL	T. chol 261 mg/dL
BUN 12 mg/dL	WBC 5.8 × 10^3/mm^3	Alb 4.5 g/dL	HDL 62 mg/dL
SCr 0.9 mg/dL		UA 5.6 mg/dL	Trig 396 mg/dL
Glu 160 mg/dL			

Assessment
Patient appears to have Cushing's syndrome and should be evaluated by an endocrinologist.

▶ Clinical Course

The patient was seen by an endocrinologist for further evaluation. An MRI revealed an enlarged pituitary gland; the same finding was seen on a focused repeat MRI. There was no focal inhomogeneity that would suggest an isolated adenoma (i.e., the tumor cannot be localized). Baseline 24-hour urinary 17-OHCS was 19 mg, UFC was 156 μg, and 2-day low-dose DST revealed 17-OHCS of 17 mg and UFC of 135 μg. A 2-day high-dose DST showed 17-OHCS of 9 mg and UFC of 82 μg. Plasma ACTH levels on two consecutive days at 1:00 PM were 143 and 150 pg/mL.

The risks and benefits of all the treatments were explained to Ms. Taylor. She preferred to undergo radiation treatments rather than exploratory-type surgery. She indicated that she would like to have more children and would prefer to try other treatments prior to surgery.

▶ Questions

Problem Identification

1. a. Create a list of this patient's drug-related problems.
   b. What information (signs, symptoms, laboratory values) indicates the presence or severity of Cushing's syndrome?

Desired Outcome

2. What are the goals of pharmacotherapy in this case?

Therapeutic Alternatives

3. a. What non-drug therapies might be useful for this patient?
   b. What feasible pharmacotherapeutic alternatives are available for the treatment of Cushing's disease?

Optimal Plan

4. a. What drug, dosage form, dose, schedule, and duration of therapy are best for treating this patient's Cushing's disease?
   b. In addition to treatment for Cushing's disease, what other changes in this patient's drug therapy may be beneficial?

Outcome Evaluation

5. What clinical and laboratory parameters are necessary to evaluate the therapy for achievement of the desired therapeutic outcome and to detect or prevent adverse events?

Patient Counseling

6. What information should be provided to the patient to enhance compliance, ensure successful therapy, and minimize adverse events?

▶ Follow-up Question

1. How do the dexamethasone dosage and procedures for collecting urinary/plasma steroid levels differ in the 2-day versus the overnight dexamethasone suppression test for the diagnosis of Cushing's syndrome?

▶ Self-study Assignments

1. Many of the tests used in the differential diagnosis of Cushing's syndrome require drug therapy (e.g., DST, metyrapone testing). Create a table to assist health care providers in performing these tests correctly (include possible adverse events, timing, critical values, and evaluation of the results).
2. Compare the retail costs in your area for each of the pharmacotherapeutic alternatives for the treatment of Cushing's syndrome. Write a brief summary of your findings, and describe whether this information would cause you to change your recommendation for the initial drug therapy for this patient.
3. Describe methods that may be used to minimize drug-induced Cushing's syndrome.

▶ Clinical Pearl

Most patients with Cushing's disease are treated with transphenoidal surgery due to its high cure rate (80%). Pharmacotherapy is usually used as adjunctive therapy rather than primary therapy.

References

1. Tsigos C, Chrousos GP. Differential diagnosis and management of Cushing's syndrome. Annu Rev Med 1996;47:443–461.
2. Engelhardt D. Steroid biosynthesis inhibitors in Cushing's syndrome. Clin Investig 1994;72:481–488.

---

74 ADDISON'S DISEASE

▶ The Unintentional Tan   (Level II)

Cynthia P. Koh-Knox, PharmD
Bruce C. Carlstedt, PhD

▶ After completing this case study, students should be able to:

- Recognize the clinical presentation, symptoms, and laboratory changes associated with Addison's disease.
- Optimize pharmacologic and nonpharmacologic therapy for patients with Addison's disease.
- Counsel patients and family members on the proper administration of medication, side effects, and adverse effects of corticosteroids and mineralocorticoids, and the importance of adherence to therapy.
- Compare corticosteroids with respect to relative glucocorticoid and mineralocorticoid potencies.

☀ PATIENT PRESENTATION

Chief Complaint

"I've been nauseated and exhausted for the past few days . . . "

HPI

Carol Sanders is a 42 yo woman who presents to her sister's internist with nausea, anorexia, and progressive fatigue for the past several days. She and her family are summer vacationing and camping in Utah, but she has not felt well enough to hike and climb for the past six 6 days.

PMH

Hypothyroidism × 15 years

FH

Father had DM for 50 years; mother had HTN; has 3 sisters with hypothyroidism and 1 sister with hyperthyroidism.

SH

Married to a university professor; works as an occupational therapist; has 3 three teenage children; drinks wine with dinner occasionally and socially; non-smoker.

Meds

Levothyroxine 0.088 mg po QD (her own doctor at home has been progressively decreasing her dose)

All

NKDA

ROS

Several months of nausea, anorexia, profound fatigue, 6-pound weight loss. She has significant tanning of her skin, although she denies excessive exposure to the sun. Denies fever, night sweats, visual disturbances, or changes in menstrual cycle.

PE

Gen
Tired-looking, tanned woman in NAD

VS
BP 96/73, P 87 sitting; BP 80/60, P 110 standing; RR 22; T 96.4°F; Ht 66″, Wt 140 lb

Skin
Normal texture; pigmented skin creases on palms of hands; generalized tanned appearance even in nonexposed areas; darkened scar on left shin

HEENT
WNL except dry mucous membranes; TMs intact

Neck
Supple without thyromegaly or adenopathy

Lungs
Clear, normal breath sounds

Breasts
Very dark areolae, no masses

CV
RRR, no m/r/g

Abd
NT; no HSM

GU
Normal external female genitalia

MS/Ext
No CCE; normal ROM

Neuro
A & O × 3

Labs

Fasting, drawn at 9:10 AM:

Na 127 mEq/L	Hgb 15.1 g/dL	AST 50 IU/L	T. chol 152 mg/dL
K 5.0 mEq/L	Hct 46.2%	ALT 84 IU/L	Trig 100 mg/dL
Cl 98 mEq/L	RBC $5.33 \times 10^6/mm^3$	Alk Phos 115 IU/L	Fe 82 μg/dL
CO_2 30 mEq/L	Plt $281 \times 10^3/mm^3$	GGT 82 IU/L	TSH 0.015 μIU/mL
BUN 15 mg/dL	WBC $4.5 \times 10^3/mm^3$	LDH 164 IU/L	Free T_4 1.9 ng/dL
SCr 1.1 mg/dL	Neutros 43%	T. bili 1.5 mg/dL	Cortisol 1.4 mcg/dL
Glu 102 mg/dL	Lymphs 42%	D. bili 0.5 mg/dL	ETA-HCG QUAL neg
Ca 9.1 mg/dL	Monos 12%	T. prot 7.2 g/dL	ACTH 2096 pg/mL
Phos 4.1 mg/dL	Eos 2%	Alb 4.3 g/dL	
UA 3.2 mg/dL	Basos 1%		

UA

Clear, yellow, SG 1.015, pH 7.0

Other

No CT scan or ECG performed.

Assessment

1. Primary adrenal insufficiency, most likely due to an autoimmune disease.
2. History of hypothyroidism with recent progressive decreases in levothyroxine dosage.

► Questions

Problem Identification

1. a. Create a list of the patient's drug-related problems.
   b. What information (signs, symptoms, laboratory values) indicates the presence or severity of Addison's disease?

Desired Outcome

2. What are the goals of pharmacotherapy in this case?

Therapeutic Alternatives

3. a. What non-drug therapies might be useful for this patient?
   b. What feasible pharmacotherapeutic alternatives are available for the treatment of Addison's disease?
   c. What psychosocial considerations are applicable to this patient?

Optimal Plan

4. What drug, dosage form, dose, schedule, and duration of therapy are best for this patient?

Outcome Evaluation

5. What clinical and laboratory parameters are necessary to evaluate the therapy for achievement of the desired therapeutic outcome and to detect or prevent adverse effects?

Patient Counseling

6. *What information should be provided to the patient to enhance compliance, ensure successful therapy, and minimize adverse effects?*

▶ Self-study Assignments

1. What are the signs and symptoms of an acute adrenal crisis, and what is the treatment?
2. Differentiate the glucocorticoids with respect to duration of activity, glucocorticoid potency, and mineralocorticoid potency.
3. What are the biologic functions of cortisol and aldosterone?
4. Explain why the skin becomes pigmented in adrenal insufficiency.

▶ Clinical Pearl

A normal adrenal gland produces a larger amount of cortisol in the morning than in the evening; thus, corticosteroid replacement therapy in Addison's disease is dosed to mimic this diurnal rhythm.

References

1. Corrigan EK. Addison's disease. NIH publication no. 90-3054. Internet website: http://wellweb.com/INDEX/qaddison.htm
2. Margulies P. Addison's disease: The facts you need to know. Internet website: http://medhlp.netusa.net/www/nadf3.htm
3. Stoffer SS. Addison's disease: How to improve patients' quality of life. Postgrad Med 1993;93(4):265–266, 271–278.
4. McDermott MT, Georgittis WJ, Asp AA. Adrenal crisis in active duty service members. Mil Med 1996;161:624–626.
5. Cronin CC, Callaghan N, Kearney PJ, et al. Addison disease in patients treated with glucocorticoid therapy. Arch Intern Med 1997;157:456–458.

75 HYPERPROLACTINEMIA

▶ Preconceived Ideas (Level I)

Amy M. Heck, PharmD
Karim A. Calis, PharmD, MPH, BCPS, BCNSP, FASHP

▶ After completing this case study, students should be able to:

- Recognize the signs and symptoms of hyperprolactinemia.
- Recommend appropriate treatment options for hyperprolactinemia.
- Outline a plan to monitor the response to the pharmacologic treatment of hyperprolactinemia.

☀ PATIENT PRESENTATION

Chief Complaint
"I have not had my period for almost a year."

HPI
Laura Barnett is a 31 yo woman with a history of oligomenorrhea (menstrual cycle every 2 to 6 months) since menarche at age 14. She presents to her gynecologist after 11 months of amenorrhea and a small amount of milky discharge from her left breast, which she first noticed 1 to 2 months ago. The patient and her husband would like to start a family, but she is concerned that she may be unable to have children. The patient states that she and her husband have not used birth control for over 1 year, and she has had several negative home pregnancy tests.

PMH
GERD
Migraine headaches (1 to 2 episodes per month)

FH
Father died at age 58 from an AMI, mother (age 62) has type 2 DM and HTN. She also has 2 brothers (ages 33 and 35) who are alive and well.

SH
The patient is employed as a fifth-grade elementary school teacher. She does not smoke and drinks less than 1 drink of alcohol per month. She has been married for 18 months and lives with her husband.

ROS
Galactorrhea of the left breast and amenorrhea for 11 months as described above. No visual defects. No active GERD or migraine symptoms.

Meds
Omeprazole 20 mg po QD
Sumatriptan 6 mg SC PRN migraine
Acetaminophen 500 mg po PRN
Ginseng tea occasionally HS "to relieve stress"

All
PCN (hives)

PE

Gen
The patient is a WDWN Caucasian woman in NAD

VS
BP 118/68, P 70, RR 12, T 37.1°C; Ht 67″, Wt 65 kg

Skin
Normal, intact, warm and dry

HEENT
PERRLA, EOMI, normal funduscopic exam, normal visual fields

Neck/LN
Normal thyroid, no lymphadenopathy

CV
RRR, S_1 and S_2 normal, no m/r/g

Lungs/Chest
Clear to A & P

Breasts
Galactorrhea of left breast, no masses

Abd
Soft, non-tender, no organomegaly, (+) bowel sounds

GU
LMP 11 months ago, normal pelvic exam and Pap smear

MS/Ext
Normal range of motion, no edema, pulses 2+ throughout

Neuro
A & O × 3, bilateral reflexes intact, normal gait, CN II–XII intact

Labs

Na 139 mEq/L	AST 21 IU/L	TSH 2.2 μIU/mL
K 4.1 mEq/L	ALT 36 IU/L	T_3 110 ng/dL
Cl 102 mEq/L	Alk Phos 110 IU/L	Total T_4 7.6 μg/dL
CO_2 26 mEq/L	T. bili 0.4 mg/dL	Free T_4 1.2 ng/dL
BUN 12 mg/dL		Serum β-HCG negative
SCr 0.7 mg/dL		
Glu 86 mg/dL		

Serum prolactin on three separate days: 142, 123, and 131 μg/L

Other
MRI of the pituitary gland revealed a 6-mm pituitary adenoma.

Diagnosis
Hyperprolactinemia due to a microprolactinoma.

► Questions

Problem Identification

1. a. *Create a list of this patient's drug-related problems.*
   b. *What signs, symptoms, and laboratory values indicate the presence of hyperprolactinemia?*
   c. *Could this patient's hyperprolactinemia be drug-induced?*

Desired Outcome

2. *What are the goals of treatment for a woman with hyperprolactinemia?*

Therapeutic Alternatives

3. a. *What non-drug therapies can be considered for the treatment of hyperprolactinemia?*
   b. *What pharmacotherapeutic options are available for the treatment of hyperprolactinemia in this woman?*

Optimal Plan

4. *What medication regimen would you recommend for this patient?*

Outcome Evaluation

5. a. *What clinical and laboratory parameters are necessary to monitor the patient's response to therapy?*
   b. *If the initial therapy you recommend is effective, how soon can the patient hope to become pregnant?*

Patient Counseling

6. *What information should be provided to the patient to enhance compliance, ensure successful therapy, and minimize adverse effects?*

► Clinical Course

The patient was started on the regimen that you recommended, and she returned to the clinic 4 weeks later complaining of significant nausea and abdominal pain that was temporally associated with medication administration. Serum prolactin concentrations measured 10 minutes apart were 120 μg/L, 131 μg/L, and 115 μg/L. Galactorrhea and amenorrhea were unchanged.

► Follow-up Questions

1. *Identify the possible reasons for the patient's poor initial response to therapy.*
2. *Given the new patient information, what alternative therapies should be considered?*
3. *How long will this patient require drug treatment for the prolactinoma?*

► Clinical Pearl

Although dopamine agonists are the mainstay of therapy for hyperprolactinemia, about 8% to 12% of patients do not respond to these agents because of poor compliance, suboptimal dosing, or the presence of a treatment-resistant prolactinoma.

► Self-study Assignments

1. If this patient eventually becomes pregnant, should dopamine agonist therapy be continued?
2. Is this patient a candidate for hormone replacement therapy?
3. How would the management of hyperprolactinemia be different if the patient were diagnosed with a macroprolactinoma instead of a microprolactinoma?

References

1. Webster J. A comparative review of the tolerability profiles of dopamine agonists in the treatment of hyperprolactinaemia and inhibition of lactation. Drug Saf 1996;14:228–238.
2. Webster J, Piscitelli G, Polli A, et al. The efficacy and tolerability of long-term cabergoline therapy in hyperprolactinaemic disorders: An open, uncontrolled multicentre study. European Multicentre Cabergoline Study Group. Clin Endocrinol 1993;39:323–329.
3. Webster J, Piscitelli G, Polli A, et al. A comparison of cabergoline and bromocriptine in the treatment of hyperprolactinemic amenorrhea. Cabergoline Comparative Study Group. N Engl J Med 1994;331:904–909.
4. Yuen BH. Etiology and treatment of hyperprolactinemia. Semin Reprod Endocrinol 1992;10:228–235.
5. Cunnah D, Besser M. Management of prolactinomas. Clin Endocrinol 1991;34:231–235.
6. Molitch ME. Pathologic hyperprolactinemia. Endocrinol Metab Clin North Am 1992;21:877–901.
7. Sarapura V, Schlaff WD. Recent advances in the understanding of the pathophysiology and treatment of hyperprolactinemia. Curr Opin Obstet Gynecol 1993;5:360–367.

SECTION 8

Gynecologic Disorders

Barbara G. Wells, PharmD, FASHP, FCCP, BCPP, Section Editor

76 CONTRACEPTION

► I Need the Pill   (Level II)

Carla B. Frye, PharmD, BCPS

► After completing this case study, students should be able to:

- Discuss the advantages and disadvantages of the various forms of contraception.

- Compare and contrast the marketed oral contraceptive (OC) combinations and be able to select the best product for an individual patient.

- Develop strategies for managing the possible side effects of OCs and prepare appropriate alternative treatment plans.

- Provide specific patient counseling on the administration, expected side effects, and drug interactions with OCs.

☼ PATIENT PRESENTATION

Chief Complaint
"I need the pill."

HPI
Laurie Prentice is a 17 yo high school student who comes to the Family Practice Center for contraceptive counseling. She has been "going steady" with her 18 yo boyfriend, and they have been having unprotected sex for a few months with occasional condom use. The patient began menses at age 14, with irregular cycles of 25 to 38 days in length. Her last menses was 2 weeks ago.

PMH
Seizure disorder beginning at age 4 following a minor MVA in which she was not restrained and impacted the automobile's dashboard. She is currently controlled on seizure medications and has been seizure-free for 3 years.

FH
Mother has type 1 diabetes and migraines. Grandmother died from complications of breast cancer diagnosed at age 60. Paternal family history is positive for hyperlipidemia and cardiovascular disorders; father (age 38) has familial hypercholesterolemia, and grandfather died at age 52 of MI.

SH
Lives at home with mother, father, and two younger brothers. She is typically a "B" to "C" student. Sexually active for about 6 months. She denies smoking, alcohol, or drug abuse. At age 14 she became a lacto-ovo vegetarian. Participates in high school track team as a long-distance runner and also runs cross country.

ROS
Menstrual periods are the most irregular during cross-country season when she runs 30 to 50 miles per week. No complaints of headache. No symptoms of diabetes (no polyuria or urinary frequency) or cardiovascular disorders (BP has always been normal to low, no palpitations).

Meds
Tegretol XR 300 mg po BID

All
NKDA

PE

Gen
WDWN female, thin and pale in appearance, well-muscled legs

VS
BP 130/65, P 58, RR 13, T 37°C; Ht 5′4″, Wt 110 lb

HEENT
NC/AT; PERRLA; EOMI; TMs intact; oral mucosa clear

Breasts
Equal in size without nodularity or masses and are non-tender

CV
NSR without murmurs, rubs or gallops

Lungs
CTA, no wheezing

Abd
Soft, NT, no masses or organomegaly

GU
Normal vaginal exam w/o tenderness or masses

Ext
Normal ROM; muscle strength 5/5 throughout; pulses 2+

Neuro
A & O × 3; CN II–XII intact; DTRs 2+; Babinski (−)

Labs
Negative Pap smear and urine pregnancy test; carbamazepine level 7 μg/mL

Assessment
Sexually active teenager requesting birth control

► Questions

Problem Identification

1. a. Create a list of this person's potential drug-related problems.
   b. What medical problems are absolute contraindications to hormonal contraceptive use, and do any of those conditions apply to this patient?
   c. What medical problems are relative contraindications to hormonal contraceptive use, and do any of these apply to this patient?
   d. What other information should be obtained before finalizing a pharmacotherapeutic plan?

Desired Outcome

2. What are the goals of pharmacotherapy in this case?

Therapeutic Alternatives

3. a. What non-drug methods of contraception might be useful for this patient, considering the advantages and disadvantages of each?
   b. What pharmacotherapeutic alternatives are available for prevention of pregnancy in this patient, and what are the advantages or disadvantages of each (see Table 76–1 and Figure 76–1)?

Optimal Plan

4. What method, dose, schedule, and duration of therapy will be best for this patient?

Outcome Evaluation

5. What clinical and laboratory parameters are necessary to evaluate the therapy for efficacy and adverse effects?

Patient Counseling

6. What information should be provided to the patient to enhance compliance, ensure successful therapy, and minimize adverse effects?

TABLE 76–1. Comparative First-Year Contraceptive Failure Rates With Typical Use Versus Perfect Use[a]

Method	Percent of Women Experiencing an Accidental Pregnancy Within the First Year of Use		Percent of Women Continuing Use at One Year
	Typical Use	*Perfect Use*	
Chance	85	85	—
Spermicides	26	6	40
Cervical cap	20–40	9–26	42–56
Diaphragm	20	6	56
Female condom	21	5	56
Male condom	14	3	61
Combined OCs	3	0.1	72
Progestin-only OCs	3	0.5	72
IUD	0.1–2.0	0.1–1.5	81
Depo-Provera	0.3	0.3	70
Female sterilization	0.5	0.5	100

[a] Trussel J, Kowal D. The essentials of contraception: Efficacy, safety, and personal considerations. In: Hatcher RA, Trussell J, Stewart F, et al, eds. *Contraceptive Technology,* 17th ed. New York, Ardent Media, 1998:216.

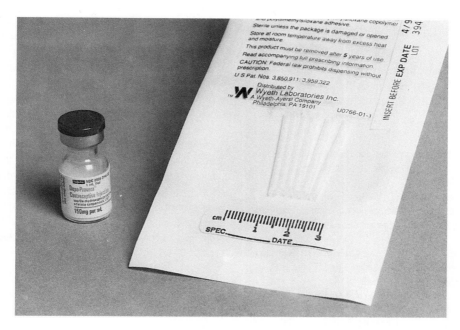

Figure 76–1. Two long-acting methods of contraception: medroxyprogesterone acetate suspension (Depo-Provera) for IM injection (left) and levonorgestrel capsule implants (Norplant System) for subdermal implantation (right).

▶ **Clinical Course**

Laurie returns to the clinic in 3 months complaining of never having a period since beginning the pill.

▶ **Follow-up Questions**

1. *What are the most likely causes of amenorrhea in this patient?*
2. *How could this problem be evaluated?*
3. *If her pregnancy and other diagnostic tests are negative, what are the pharmacotherapeutic alternatives for treating the amenorrhea?*
4. *If she had developed breakthrough bleeding when she initiated her OC, what could be some of the possible causes?*

5. *If breakthrough bleeding is not caused by a concomitant medical condition, how can it be managed?*

▶ **Self-study Assignments**

1. In a case such as the one described, review what might be done to adjust the patient's seizure medication to avoid drug interactions.
2. Compare the costs of each method of birth control and prepare a report that contains your conclusions as to which method provides the best efficacy at the most reasonable cost.
3. Visit a pharmacy and review the various home pregnancy tests; determine how you would counsel a patient to use each one, and evaluate them for ease of use (see Figure 76–2).

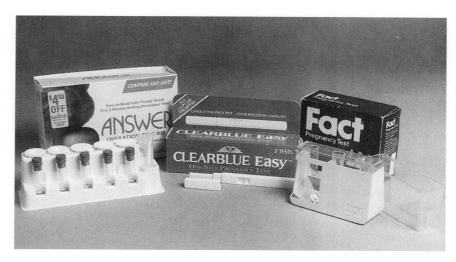

Figure 76–2. Several examples of home pregnancy test kits.

Caution patients taking oral contraceptives about the potential for drug interactions. Drugs that reduce absorption, induce metabolism, or alter gut bacteriologic flora can reduce oral contraceptive efficacy.

References

1. Hatcher RA, Guillebaud J. The pill: Combined oral contraceptives. In: Hatcher RA, Trussell J, Stewart F, et al, eds. Contraceptive Technology, 17th ed. New York, Ardent Media, 1998:405–465.
2. Lewis MA, Spitzer WO, Heinemann LA, et al. Third generation oral contraceptives and risk of myocardial infarction: An international case-control study. Transitional Research Group on Oral Contraceptives and the Health of Young Women. BMJ 1996;312:88–90.
3. American Diabetes Association. Report of the expert committee on the diagnosis and classification of diabetes mellitus. Diabetes Care 1998;21(suppl 1):S5–S19. Also see www.diabetes.org/diabetescare/supplement198.
4. National Cholesterol Education Program: Second report of the National Cholesterol Education Program (NCEP) Expert Panel on detection, evaluation, and treatment of high blood cholesterol in adults (Adult Treatment Panel II). Circulation 1994;89:1329–1445.

77   PREMENSTRUAL DYSPHORIC DISORDER

▶ **Dual Identity**   (Level II)

Donna M. Jermain, PharmD, BCPP

▶ After completing this case study, students should be able to:

- Recognize and differentiate the symptoms of premenstrual dysphoric disorder (PMDD) from other psychiatric disorders.
- Develop a pharmacotherapeutic plan for treatment of PMDD.
- Recommend alternative treatment options for patients with PMDD.
- Counsel patients on the expected benefits and possible adverse effects of the drugs used to treat PMDD.

☼ PATIENT PRESENTATION

Chief Complaint
"I feel like two different people."

HPI

Sharon Beck is a 38 yo woman who was referred to the PMS clinic by her obstetrician–gynecologist. She states that she is frightened because for some months she has felt suicidal just prior to her menses. Upon further questioning, she states that 7 to 10 days prior to menses she is unable to concentrate at work, and she cries at anything including commercials, especially the Hallmark ones. She feels depressed, and she is extremely irrita-ble with her co-workers, husband, and children. She describes feeling tired, uncoordinated, anxious, and out of control. She also has irresistible chocolate cravings and experiences weight gain, bloating, backaches, cramps, breast tenderness, and headaches. Other concerns include confusion and mood swings.

She relates the story of how severe her cravings are. During the most recent ice storm she was experiencing these symptoms and risked her life by driving on ice to get chocolate. During this time, she was convinced that her family and friends would be better off if she were dead. However, she states that "the moment I see blood I feel like a new woman." Her mood improves, and her symptoms resolve. "I am normally a happy person," she says. She also states that she really believes she is "normal" when she starts her menses. She describes her PMS symptoms as getting worse with age and much worse after the birth of her second child. She brought to clinic the daily calendars she has completed to document her symptoms (see Table 77–1).

PMH
Tubal ligation after her second child 4 years ago.

FH
Her father has CAD and her mother has DM.

TABLE 77–1. A Portion of the Daily Calendar Used by the Patient to Document Her PMDD Symptoms.[a]

Symptom	Before Treatment	After Treatment
Fatigue, lack of energy	4	1
Poor coordination	3	1
Feeling out of control, overwhelmed	3	1
Crying	4	1
Headache	3	0
Anxiety	3	0
Aches	4	0
Irritability, persistent anger	3	1
Mood swings	3	1
Bloating, weight gain	4	0
Food cravings, increased appetite	4	0
Nervous tension	3	1
Cramps	3	0
Depression, feeling sad or blue	3	1
Breast tenderness	2	0
Insomnia or hypersomnia	3	1
Confusion, difficulty concentrating	3	1
How much distress or concern have your symptoms caused you today?	3	1

[a] Data shown are the last day before the onset of menses. Scale: 0, not present; 1, mild; 2, moderate; 3, severe; 4, very severe.

SH

She has been married for 12 years. She has 2 children, a daughter 9 years old and a son 4 years old. She denies tobacco use but admits to drinking alcohol socially. She works as a secretary.

ROS

She states she has had a headache for the past 2 days and that she feels somewhat nauseated.

Meds

Ibuprofen 800 mg PRN for headaches.

All

She has cedar fever (an allergy to mountain juniper).

PE

Gen

She is a healthy appearing, mildly overweight female in NAD

VS

BP 114/60, P 83, RR 18, T 99.0°F; Ht 5′6″; Wt 77.3 kg

Skin

Warm and dry

HEENT

PERRLA, throat pink, no nasal discharge

Neck/LN

Supple; no palpable nodes, thyroid not enlarged

Lungs

CTA

Breasts

Mild fibrocystic changes

CV

RRR; S_1, S_2 normal; no S_3 or S_4 heard; no murmurs or rubs

Abd

Mildly obese, NT/ND

Genit/Rect

She declined examination, as she just had a pelvic exam one week ago

MS/Ext

Normal ROM, pedal pulses strong

Neuro

WNL; CN II–XII intact, DTRs 2+ throughout

Labs

Hgb 13.2 g/dL	WBC $5.2 \times 10^3/mm^3$	*Fasting Lipid Profile*
Hct 38.1%	Neutros 73%	T. Chol 240 mg/dL
RBC $4.4 \times 10^6/mm^3$	Lymphs 18%	LDL 175 mg/dL
MCV 97.7 μm^3	Monos 9%	HDL 41 mg/dL
MCH 33.0 pg	Eos 0%	Trig 121 mg/dL
MCHC 33.7 g/dL	Basos 0%	
RDW 12.8%		TSH 1.7 μIU/mL
Plt $155 \times 10^3/mm^3$		

Assessment

1. PMDD
2. Mild obesity
3. History of headaches
4. Elevated fasting lipid panel

▶ Questions

Problem Identification

1. a. What are the patient's drug-related problems?
   b. What pattern of symptoms does this patient have that are consistent with PMDD requiring treatment?
   c. Which symptoms does this patient have that are amenable to drug therapy?

Desired Outcome

2. What are the goals of treatment for PMDD in this case?

Therapeutic Alternatives

3. What non-pharmacologic and pharmacotherapeutic choices are available for persons with PMDD?

Optimal Plan

4. Outline a pharmacotherapeutic plan to treat this patient's PMDD.

Outcome Evaluation

5. What clinical parameters are necessary to evaluate the therapy for achievement of the desired therapeutic outcome and to detect or prevent adverse effects?

Patient Counseling

6. What information should be provided to the patient to enhance compliance, ensure successful therapy, and minimize adverse effects?

▶ Clinical Course

The patient was asked to return to clinic 1 month after being started on the treatment you recommended. During the initial 2 to 3 days of treatment, she had some nausea but considered it to be mild. She noted that her irritability, depressive feelings, feelings of losing control, and food cravings were markedly decreased. She is hopeful that she may be able to stick to a diet now that her chocolate cravings are not as severe. She states that her husband and children noted the improvement because she responded to them as she would have during her "non-PMS" days. She even notes that her cramps and breast tenderness did not seem as severe. Her daily calendars also reflect the improvement (see Table 77–1).

▶ **Follow-up Questions**

1. *What is your assessment of the patient's response to the intervention?*
2. *How long would you recommend that she continue therapy?*

▶ **Clinical Pearl**

The diagnosis and recommendation for luteal phase dosing of PMDD should be based on prospective daily calendars to assure that there is no co-morbidity such as a depressive disorder.

▶ **Self-study Assignments**

1. Review the textbook chapter "Hyperlipidemia" and outline your recommendations for lowering her total and LDL cholesterol levels.
2. Based upon the individual's PMS symptoms, develop a monitoring tool that would allow the patient and you to record and track the changes in her individual symptoms. This monitoring tool should also include space for her to document adverse effects.

References

1. Halbreich U, Smoller JW. Intermittent luteal phase sertraline treatment of dysphoric premenstrual syndrome. J Clin Psychiatry 1997;58:399–402.
2. Freeman EW, Rickels K, Sondheimer SJ, et al. A double-blind trial of oral progesterone, alprazolam, and placebo in treatment of severe premenstrual syndrome. JAMA 1995;274:51–57.
3. Freeman EW, Rickels K, Sondheimer SJ, et al. Nefazodone in the treatment of premenstrual syndrome: A preliminary study. J Clin Psychopharmacol 1994;14:180–186.
4. Halbreich U, Rojansky N, Palter S. Elimination of ovulation and menstrual cyclicity (with danazol) improves dysphoric premenstrual syndromes. Fertil Steril 1991;56:1066–1069.
5. Mezrow G, Shoupe D, Spicer D, et al. Depot leuprolide acetate with estrogen and progestin add-back for long-term treatment of premenstrual syndrome. Fertil Steril 1994;62:932–937.

78 HORMONE REPLACEMENT THERAPY

▶ **Reaching the Climacteric**   (Level II)

Alka Z. Somani, PharmD

▶ After completing this case study, students should be able to:

• Identify the hallmark signs and symptoms of menopause and differentiate them from other possible causes.

• Recommend appropriate first-line and alternative therapy to prevent the symptoms of menopause.

• Develop a comprehensive monitoring plan for patients who are started on hormone replacement therapy.

• Counsel patients effectively on the treatment options, benefits, and risks of hormone replacement therapy.

☀ PATIENT PRESENTATION

Chief Complaint
"It was too hard to remember to take the Provera, and I had problems with spotting, so I stopped taking the medicines. Now I have hot flashes again."

HPI
Esther R. Thorpe is a 50 yo woman who started to experience hot flashes and associated nausea a few months ago. Her PCP prescribed Premarin and cyclic Provera. He also advised Esther to exercise and take a calcium supplement, but she chose to increase the calcium in her diet instead. She had a pelvic exam, mammogram, and endometrial biopsy within the last month. The endometrial biopsy was performed because of a previous suspicious Pap smear.

PMH
HTN × 10 years
Hypercholesterolemia × 5 years, controlled by diet

FH
Father died of presumed heart disease in his 50s; mother died of an unknown cancer in her 60s. Patient is the oldest of 4 sisters; the others are ages 46, 43, and 41 and are A & W.

SH
Husband died in his 50s after a second heart attack. Patient has 3 adult children who are all in good health. She graduated from high school and works as a bank teller. She enjoys walking on her treadmill and watching her grandchild. She denies the use of illicit drugs, does not smoke, and drinks alcohol occasionally. She tries to follow a low-salt and low-cholesterol diet but admits that it is difficult. She has increased her intake of calcium containing food (milk, yogurt and cheese) to 3–4 servings per day.

Meds
Procardia XL 30 mg po QD
Acetaminophen 325 mg 1–2 po QD PRN for joint pain after exercise
Premarin 0.625 mg po QD days 7–30 of every month
Provera 5 mg po QD days 1–7 of every month

All
NKDA. "Dust" causes patient to sneeze.

ROS
Non-contributory except for complaints noted above. LMP 3 months ago.

PE

Gen
The patient is an alert and oriented woman who looks her stated age and is in NAD

VS
BP 130/85, P 85, RR 16, T 37.0°C; Wt 150 lb, Ht 5'8"

Skin
Warm, dry

HEENT
PERRLA; EOMI; funduscopic exam reveals no AV nicking, hemorrhages, or exudates; oropharynx clear; TMs intact

Neck/LN
Supple, no JVD or thyromegaly

Breasts
No lumps

CV
RRR, normal S_1 and S_2; no m/r/g

Resp
CTA

Abd
NT/ND, (+) BS; no HSM

GU/Rect
Pelvic exam with pain and mucosal atrophy; stool guaiac (−)

MS
Full ROM, pulses 2+ throughout; muscle strength 5/5 bilaterally

Neuro
CN II–XII intact; normal sensory and motor levels; DTRs 2+; Babinski (−)

Labs

			Fasting Lipid Profile
Na 131 mEq/L	Hgb 13 g/dL	Ca 10.1 mg/dL	
K 3.9 mEq/L	Hct 39%	AST 42 IU/L	T. chol 198 mg/dL
Cl 95 mEq/L	WBC $8.0 \times 10^3/mm^3$	ALT 33 IU/L	LDL 125 mg/dL
CO_2 24 mEq/L	Plt $216 \times 10^3/mm^3$	GGT 36 IU/L	HDL 37 mg/dL
BUN 20 mg/dL		TSH 2.6 µIU/mL	Trig 180 mg/dL
SCr 1.3 mg/dL		FSH 38 mIU/mL	
Glu 105 mg/dL			

Other
Pap smear, mammogram, and endometrial biopsy: Normal

Pregnancy Test
Negative

Assessment
50 yo postmenopausal woman who requires HRT but is unable to tolerate breakthrough bleeding secondary to the regimen prescribed.

▶ Questions

Problem Identification

1. a. Create a list of the patient's drug-related problems.
   b. What information (signs, symptoms, laboratory values) indicates the presence or severity of this patient's problems as she begins menopause?

Desired Outcome

2. What are the benefits and risks of hormone replacement therapy for this patient?

Therapeutic Alternatives

3. a. What non-drug therapies might be useful for this patient?
   b. What feasible pharmacotherapeutic alternatives are available for treatment of menopause (see Figure 78–1)?

Optimal Plan

4. What drug, dosage form, dose, schedule, and duration are best for this patient?

Outcome Evaluation

5. What clinical and laboratory parameters are necessary to evaluate the therapy for achievement of the desired therapeutic outcome and to detect or prevent adverse effects?

Patient Counseling

6. What information should be provided to the patient to enhance compliance, ensure successful therapy and minimize adverse effects?

▶ Clinical Course

The patient received the regimen you recommended every day with no further complaints. However, her triglyceride levels continued to elevate over the next 6 months from 180 to 395 mg/dL. Her physician is concerned that the medication is going to eventually increase Esther's triglycerides to a dangerous level (> 500 mg/dL) and asks for your advice.

▶ Follow-up Question

1. What changes in the patient's therapy, if any, should be considered at this point?

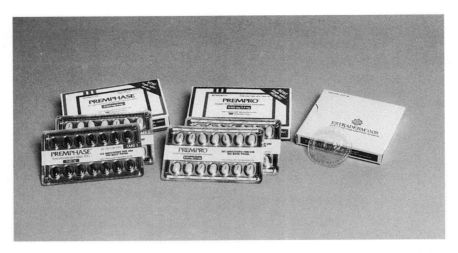

Figure 78–1. Premphase, Prempro, and Estraderm products for hormone replacement therapy.

▶ Clinical Pearl

It is important to give progesterone along with estrogen in postmenopausal women with an intact uterus to decrease the risk of endometrial cancer.

▶ Self-study Assignments

1. Identify the therapeutic alternatives to prevent postmenopausal osteoporosis in women who cannot receive estrogen therapy.
2. Perform a literature search on combined estrogen-progesterone therapy and its effects on cholesterol and cardiac risk.

References

1. Belchetz PE. Hormonal treatment of postmenopausal women. N Engl J Med 1994;330:1062–1071.
2. Writing group for the PEPI Trial. Effects of estrogen or estrogen/progestin regimens on heart disease risk factors in postmenopausal women. The Postmenopausal Estrogen/Progestin Interventions (PEPI) Trial. JAMA 1995;273:199–208.
3. Weiss NS, Ure CL, Ballard JH, et al. Decreased risk of fractures of the hip and lower forearm with postmenopausal use of estrogen. N Engl J Med 1980;303:1195–1198.
4. Birge SJ. Is there a role for estrogen replacement therapy in the prevention and treatment of dementia? J Am Geriatr Soc 1996;44:865–870.
5. Paganini-Hill A, Henderson VW. Estrogen replacement therapy and risk of Alzheimer's disease. Arch Intern Med 1996;156:2213–2217.
6. Calle EE, Miracle-McMahill HL, Thun MJ, et al. Estrogen replacement therapy and risk of fatal colon cancer in a prospective cohort of postmenopausal women. J Natl Cancer Inst 1995;87:517–523.
7. Vingerling JR, Dielemans I, Witteman JC, et al. Macular degeneration and early menopause: A case-control study. BMJ 1995;310:1570–1571.
8. Lobo RA. Benefits and risks of estrogen replacement therapy. Am J Obstet Gynecol 1995;173:982–989.
9. Lufkin EG, Ory SJ. Relative value of transdermal and oral estrogen therapy in various clinical situations. Mayo Clin Proc 1994;69:131–135.

SECTION 9

Immunologic Disorders

Gary C. Yee, PharmD, FCCP, Section Editor

---

79 SYSTEMIC LUPUS ERYTHEMATOSUS

▶ **More Than Just Skin Deep** (Level II)

Thomas W. Redford, PharmD
Ralph E. Small, PharmD, FCCP, FASHP, FAPhA

▶ After completing this case study, students should be able to:

- Describe the clinical and laboratory features of lupus nephritis.
- Recommend appropriate therapy for lupus nephritis.
- Define the monitoring parameters for disease activity, drug efficacy, and drug toxicity.

☀ PATIENT PRESENTATION

Chief Complaint
"I've had a red rash on my arms for the past 3 days."

HPI
Linda Fields is a 46 yo woman admitted from Rheumatology Clinic with increased serum creatinine. She was diagnosed with SLE 2 years ago after she presented with arthralgias and rash. At the beginning of this year, she was found to have proteinuria with RBCs and RBC casts in her urine. Her BUN and creatinine were 20 and 0.9 mg/dL, respectively. Renal biopsy revealed segmental proliferative glomerulonephritis and membranous glomerulonephritis compatible with lupus nephritis. She was treated with prednisone without significant improvement in her proteinuria. At this visit, she complains of a 3-day history of erythematous rash on her arms. She denies taking OTC drugs or NSAIDs.

PMH
HTN × 7 years
Acute sinusitis 1 year ago
Ovarian cyst removal 20 years ago

FH
Father died of MI; mother alive in her 70s.

SH
Employed as a teacher; married 20 years; no tobacco use; occasional EtOH use.

Meds
Enalapril 10 mg po BID
Prednisone 10 mg po QD

All
PCN (rash)

ROS
No fever, chills, or sweats; no arthralgias or myalgias.

PE

Gen
Slightly obese woman in NAD

VS
BP140/80, P 70, RR 20, T 38.2°C; Wt 64 kg

203

Skin
Erythematous rash on upper extremities

HEENT
PERRLA; EOMI; disks flat, no hemorrhages or exudates; oropharynx without lesions

Neck/LN
Supple without adenopathy

CV
RRR, grade IV systolic murmur

Abdomen
Soft, non-tender

Ext
Peripheral pulses intact; joint examination reveals no active synovitis or arthritis; no CCE

Neuro
A & O × 3; sensory and motor levels normal; CN II–XII intact; DTRs 2+; Babinski negative

Labs

Na 140 mEq/L	Hgb 10.5 g/dL	C4 14 mg /dL
K 4.9 mEq/L	Hct 32%	C3 66 mg/dL
Cl 107 mEq/L	WBC $6.3 \times 10^3/mm^3$	Anti-ds DNA antibody 584 mg/dL
CO_2 24 mEq/L	Plt $280 \times 10^3/mm^3$	
BUN 52 mg/dL	ESR 53 mm/hr	
SCr 2.0 mg/dL		
Uric acid 8.3 mg/dL		

UA
Many RBCs, RBC casts, 3+ proteinuria

Renal biopsy
Much more proliferative changes than on previous biopsy and increased interstitial fibrosis

Assessment
Acute worsening of lupus nephritis; exacerbation of SLE.

► Questions

Problem Identification

1. a. *Create a list of the patient's drug-related problems.*
   b. *What information indicates worsening lupus nephritis?*

Desired Outcome

2. *What are the goals of pharmacotherapy for lupus nephritis in this patient?*

Therapeutic Alternatives

3. a. *What nonpharmacologic therapies might be useful in this patient?*
   b. *What pharmacotherapeutic alternatives are used to manage patients with lupus nephritis?*

Optimal Plan

4. *Outline a specific pharmacotherapeutic plan for treating lupus nephritis in this patient.*

Outcome Evaluation

5. *How should this patient be monitored for efficacy and adverse effects?*

Patient Counseling

6. *What information should be provided to the patient regarding her drug therapy?*

► Clinical Course

The patient experienced a remission in her renal disease following the drug therapy you recommended, but her proteinuria failed to improve, suggesting that her mesangial renal histology was irreversible. She also tapered her prednisone but experienced a lupus flare with complications from vasculitis and reemergence of her lupus nephritis. Her prednisone dosage was increased and treatment of her lupus nephritis was reinstituted.

► Follow-up Question

1. *What other medications can be used to control this patient's non-renal disease manifestation (i.e., erythematous rash)?*

► Self-study Assignments

1. Recent animal experiments have suggested a number of strategies for treating lupus nephritis. Perform a literature search on experimental treatments for lupus nephritis.
2. Glucocorticoid-induced osteoporosis is a serious complication associated with long-term prednisone therapy. Perform a literature search and suggest strategies for ameliorating the long-term effects of prednisone.

► Clinical Pearl

Since UV light exacerbates SLE, drugs that induce photosensitivity should be avoided.

References

1. Austin HA III, Klippel JH, Balow JE, et al. Therapy of lupus nephritis. Controlled trial of prednisone and cytotoxic drugs. N Engl J Med 1986;314:614–619.

2. Liebling MR, McLaughlin K, Boonsue S, et al. Monthly pulses of methylprednisolone in SLE nephritis. J Rheumatol 1982;9:543–548.

3. Sztejnbok M, Stewart A, Diamond H, et al. Azathioprine in the treatment of systemic lupus erythematosus. A controlled study. Arthritis Rheum 1971;14:639–645.

4. Lewis EJ, Hunsicker LG, Lan SP, et al. A controlled trial of plasmapheresis therapy in severe lupus nephritis. The Lupus Nephritis Collaborative Study Group. N Engl J Med 1992;326:1373–1379.

SECTION 10

Bone and Joint Disorders

L. Michael Posey, RPh, Section Editor

80 OSTEOPOROSIS

▶ **These Brittle Bones**   (Level II)

   Carla B. Frye, PharmD, BCPS

▶ After completing this case study, students should be able to:

- Identify the risk factors for developing osteoporosis.

- Recommend appropriate non-pharmacologic measures for preventing or treating osteoporosis.

- Recommend the correct amount and form of calcium supplementation required to prevent or treat osteoporosis.

- Design a treatment regimen for hormonal and non-hormonal drug therapy in postmenopausal women.

- Provide appropriate patient education about osteoporosis and its therapy.

☀ PATIENT PRESENTATION

Chief Complaint
"That calcium supplement you recommended makes me nauseated."

HPI
Norma Johns is a 72 yo woman with a history of HTN, hyperlipidemia, COPD, hypothyroidism, and osteoporosis. She presents to the ambulatory medicine clinic for a follow-up visit for her HTN and osteoporosis. She has been experiencing episodes of nausea without vomiting since she began taking Oscal after her last clinic visit.

PMH
HTN first diagnosed at age 50. She has been treated with a variety of medications over the years, including thiazide and loop diuretics, β-blockers, and calcium channel blockers. She is currently in good control with BPs averaging 135/82.
S/P MI 13 years ago
Hyperlipidemia × 13 years; patient modified diet and took cholestyramine for several years
Hypothyroidism × 27 years, treated with levothyroxine
Osteoporosis diagnosed by DEXA scan 2 years ago
COPD diagnosed several years ago after MI; stable on Atrovent MDI
Appendectomy at age 15
Breast cancer with mastectomy of left breast and radiation therapy at age 40
Menopause at age 48
Right carotid endarterectomy 2 years ago

FH
Patient is of German and French descent. Paternal history (+) for CAD; father died at age 60 of "heart trouble." Maternal history (+) for stroke and vascular disorders; mother became menopausal before age 45.

SH
Widowed; G_2P_3; 2 ppd smoker, quit after MI; non-drinker.

ROS
Mild headaches and chronic back pain, treated with acetaminophen; vaginal dryness; hot flushes and night sweats occasionally; has noticed that her height has decreased by 2″ since she was 35; cold intolerant; denies shortness of breath or chest pain.

Meds

Procardia XL 120 mg po QD × 2 years
Atrovent inhaler 2 puffs TID × 4 years
Synthroid 75 μg po QD × 20 years
Atenolol 25 mg po QD × 10 years
Lipitor 10 mg po QD × 3 months
Oscal 500 po TID × 3 months

All

NKDA

PE

Gen

WDWN Caucasian woman in NAD

VS

BP 150/85, P 64, RR 17, T 37°C; Ht 5′3″, Wt 145 lb.

Skin

Fair complexion, color good, no lesions

HEENT

Normocephalic; smooth, red tongue; mucous membranes moist; PER-RLA; EOMI; eyes and throat clear; funduscopic exam reveals mild arteriolar narrowing, with AV ratio 1:3; no hemorrhages, exudates, or papilledema

Neck/LN

Supple, without obvious nodes; no JVD

Chest

Decreased breath sounds bilaterally; air movement decreased; no rales or rhonchi

Breasts

Mastectomy scar left breast; right breast normal

CV

RRR; no murmurs; normal S_1 and S_2, no S_3 or S_4

Abd

Soft, NT/ND, (+) BS

Genit/Rect

Deferred

MS/Ext

Prominent saphenous vein visible in left leg, with multiple varicosities bilaterally; tendon xanthoma noted in left Achilles; good pulses bilaterally

Neuro

CN II–XII intact; DTRs 2+; sensory and motor levels intact; toes downgoing

Labs

Na 145 mEq/L	TSH 3.492 μIU/mL	
K 4.1 mEq/L	*Fasting lipid profile*	*Lipids 3 months ago*
Cl 107 mEq/L	T. chol 224 mg/dL	T. chol 253 mg/dL
CO_2 24 mEq/L	Trig 260 mg/dL	Trig 320 mg/dL
BUN 24 mg/dL	HDL 43 mg/dL	HDL 30 mg/dL
SCr 1.1 mg/dL	LDL 165 mg/dL	LDL 180 mg/dL
Glu 98 mg/dL		

Other

DEXA of lumbar spine (4 mo ago): L2-4 = 0.780 g/cm^2 (−3.5 SD); right femoral neck = 0.615 g/cm^2 (−3.04 SD)

Assessment

1. Nausea due to Oscal
2. HTN and hypothyroidism well controlled
3. Familial combined hyperlipidemia responding to therapy
4. Osteoporosis requires further intervention

▶ Questions

Problem Identification

1. a. Create a list of the patient's drug-related problems.
   b. What information (signs, symptoms, laboratory values, risk factors) indicates the presence or severity of the patient's osteoporosis? Also identify her risk factors for developing osteoporosis.
   c. What additional information would be useful in determining the extent of the patient's osteoporosis and the need for aggressive therapy?

Desired Outcome

2. What are the goals of pharmacotherapy for osteoporosis in this case?

Therapeutic Alternatives

3. a. What non-drug therapies might be useful for this patient's osteoporosis?
   b. What feasible pharmacotherapeutic alternatives are available for treatment of the osteoporosis?

Optimal Plan

4. a. What drug, dosage form, dose, schedule, and duration of therapy are best for treating this patient's osteoporosis?
   b. What alternatives would be appropriate if the initial therapy fails or cannot be used?

Outcome Evaluation

5. What clinical and laboratory parameters are necessary to evaluate the therapy for achievement of the desired therapeutic outcome and to detect or prevent adverse effects?

Patient Counseling

6. *What information should be provided to the patient to enhance compliance, ensure successful therapy, and minimize adverse effects?*

► Clinical Pearl

In elderly patients, use calcium gluconate, citrate, or lactate instead of calcium carbonate, as these salt forms do not require an acidic gastric pH for dissolution.

► Self-study Assignments

1. Investigate the new drugs and drug classes under development for the treatment of osteoporosis.
2. Complete a pharmacoeconomic analysis of the various drugs used to treat osteoporosis. Which therapy is the most cost-effective?
3. Develop an exercise plan to prevent osteoporosis.

References

1. Cauley JA, Cummings SR, Seeley DG, et al. Effects of thiazide diuretic therapy on bone mass, fractures and falls. The Study of Osteoporosis Fractures Research Group. Ann Intern Med 1993;118:666–673.
2. Summary of the second report of the National Cholesterol Education Program (NCEP) expert panel on detection, evaluation, and treatment of high blood cholesterol in adults (adult treatment panel II). JAMA 1993;269:3015–3023.
3. Assessment of fracture risk and its application to screening for postmenopausal osteoporosis. Report of a WHO Study Group. World Health Org Tech Rep Ser 1994;843:1–18.
4. Ebeling PR, Atley LM, Guthrie JR, et al. Bone turnover markers and bone density across the menopausal transition. J Clin Endocrinol Metab 1996;81:3366–3371.

81 RHEUMATOID ARTHRITIS

► **Joint Project**   (Level II)

Ralph E. Small, PharmD, FCCP, FASHP, FAPhA
Thomas W. Redford, PharmD
Amy L. Whitaker, PharmD

► After completing this case study, students should be able to:

• Identify the signs and symptoms of rheumatoid arthritis (RA).

• Recommend appropriate drug therapy for the management of RA.

• Recognize alternative therapies for the treatment of pain and inflammation in patients with RA.

• Recommend appropriate non-pharmacological options for managing patients with RA.

• Counsel patients about the drug therapy used to treat RA.

☀ PATIENT PRESENTATION

Chief Complaint
"I have pain in all of my joints, a swollen left knee, and stiffness every morning."

HPI
Janet Hobbs is a 58 yo woman who presents to her rheumatologist with generalized arthralgias, a swollen left knee, and morning stiffness. These symptoms have been occurring with increasing severity for the past week. She presented with the same symptoms when she came to clinic 2 months ago.

PMH
RA × 6 years
S/P hysterectomy 4 years ago
HTN × 10 years

FH
Father died from complications after a traumatic fall at age 65. Mother died of hip fracture and pneumonia at age 78. No siblings.

SH
Housewife; married for 32 years; has 2 grown children with no known medical problems. Denies alcohol or tobacco use. Volunteers in the community extensively but has been doing less in the past 2 months.

ROS
Swelling in left knee; no rash, nausea, vomiting, or diarrhea; decreased ROM in hands; denies HA, chest pain, SOB, bleeding episodes, or syncopal attacks; fatigue experienced daily during afternoon hours; denies loss of appetite or weight loss; reports minor visual changes corrected with stronger prescription glasses.

Meds
HCTZ 25 mg po Q AM
Norvasc 10 mg po QD
Relafen 750 mg, 2 tabs Q HS
Prednisone 5 mg, $1/2$ tab po Q AM
Patient receives medications at a local community pharmacy. Medication profile indicates that she refills her medications on time the first of each month.

All
Penicillin (rash 25 years ago)

PE

Gen

Pleasant middle-aged Caucasian woman in moderate distress due to pain and swelling in knee

VS

BP 138/80, P 82, RR 14, T 98.8°F; Ht 66″, Wt 144 lb.

Skin

No rashes; normal turgor; no breakdown or ulcers

HEENT
Atraumatic; moon facies; PERRLA; EOMI; A-V nicking visible bilaterally; pale conjunctiva bilaterally; TMs intact; xerostomia

Neck/LN
Supple, no JVD or thyromegaly; no bruits; palpable lymph nodes

Chest
CTA

CV
RRR; normal S_1, S_2; no m/r/g

Abd
Soft, NT/ND; (+) BS

Breasts
Normal; no lumps

GU/Rect
Deferred

MS/Ext
Hands—mild RA changes; swelling 3,4,5 PIP joints bilaterally; pain 3,4 MCP joints on left; Boutonniere deformity 3,4 bilaterally; ulnar deviation bilaterally; decreased grip strength, L > R (patient is left-handed)
Wrists—good ROM
Elbows—good ROM; slight permanent contracture on right; fixed nodule at pressure point
Shoulders—decreased ROM (especially abduction) bilaterally
Hips—decreased ROM on right; atrophy of quadriceps, L > R

Knees—pain bilaterally; decreased ROM on left; effusion/edema on left
Feet—no edema; full plantar flexion and dorsiflexion; 3+ pedal pulses

Neuro
CN II–XII grossly intact; muscle strength 5/5 UE, 4/5 LE, DTRs 2/4 biceps & triceps, 1/4 patella

Labs
Na 135 mEq/L	Hgb 10.0 g/dL	CK < 20 IU/L
K 4.1 mEq/L	Hct 31%	ANA negative
Cl 101 mEq/L	WBC $13.5 \times 10^3/mm^3$	Wes ESR 47 mm/hour
CO_2 22 mEq/L	Plt $356 \times 10^3/mm^3$	RF positive, 1:1280
BUN 12 mg/dL	Ca 9.1 mg/dL	TSH 0.74 µIU/mL
SCr 0.8 mg/dL	Urate 5.1 mg/dL	
Glu 103 mg/dL	T. chol 219 mg/dL	

UA
Normal

Chest X-ray
No fluid, masses, or infection; no cardiomegaly

Synovial Fluid
From knee; white cells $23.0 \times 10^3/mm^3$, turbid in appearance

Assessment
58 yo woman in moderate distress with acute flare of RA (functional class II). RA not adequately controlled with current therapy. Patient is adherent with current medication regimen. HTN is controlled on present therapy.

▶ Questions

Problem Identification
1. a. List the patient's drug-related problems.
   b. What information (signs, symptoms, laboratory values) indicates the presence and severity of rheumatoid arthritis?
   c. What additional information is needed to assess the patient?

Desired Outcome
2. What are the goals of pharmacotherapy in this case?

Therapeutic Alternatives
3. a. What non-pharmacological modalities may be beneficial to this patient?
   b. What pharmacologic alternatives are available for the treatment of RA?
   c. What economic and psychosocial considerations are applicable to this patient?

Optimal Plan
4. What drug, dosage form, dose, schedule, and duration of therapy are best for this patient?

Outcome Evaluation
5. What clinical and laboratory parameters are necessary to evaluate the patient's drug therapy?

Patient Counseling
6. What information should be provided to the patient to enhance adherence, ensure successful therapy, and minimize adverse effects?

▶ Self-study Assignments

1. Perform a literature search and assess the current information about COX-2 selective inhibitors.
2. Write a list of the clinically significant drug interactions for NSAIDs and DMARDs, including methotrexate (see Figure 81–1).
3. Describe the rationale for the use of biologic agents as therapies for RA, and provide a summary of the results of clinical trials.

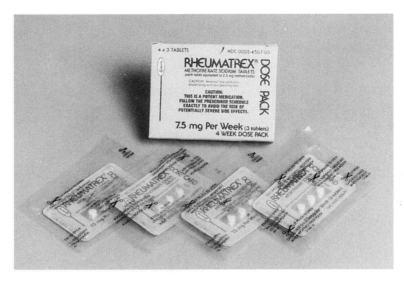

Figure 81–1. The Rheumatrex Dose Pack (7.5 mg/wk) for treatment of rheumatoid arthritis.

▶ Clinical Pearl

Treat with high-dose corticosteroids to obtain short-term benefit and relieve the flare of rheumatoid arthritis. Concurrently, or shortly thereafter, begin an NSAID and a DMARD to obtain long-term benefit and prevent disease flares and progression.

References

1. American College of Rheumatology Ad Hoc Committee on Clinical Guidelines. Guidelines for the management of rheumatoid arthritis. Arthritis Rheum 1996;39:713–722.
2. Cash JM, Klippel JH. Second-line drug therapy for rheumatoid arthritis. N Engl J Med 1994;330:1368–1375.
3. Brick JE, DiBartolomeo AG. Rethinking the therapeutic pyramid for rheumatoid arthritis. When are NSAIDs alone not enough? Postgrad Med 1992;91:75.
4. American College of Rheumatology Ad Hoc Committee on Clinical Guidelines. Guidelines for monitoring drug therapy in rheumatoid arthritis. Arthritis Rheum 1996;39:723–731.

82 OSTEOARTHRITIS

▶ Murder by Joints   (Level II)

Michael A. Oszko, PharmD, BCPS

▶ After completing this case study, students should be able to:

- Recognize the most common signs and symptoms of osteoarthritis.
- Design an appropriate pharmacotherapeutic regimen for treating osteoarthritis, taking into account a patient's other medical problems and drug therapy.

- Incorporate potential adjunctive therapies (both pharmacologic and non-pharmacologic) into the regimen of a patient with osteoarthritis.
- Assess and evaluate the efficacy of an analgesic regimen for a patient with osteoarthritis, and formulate an alternative plan if the regimen is inadequate or causes unacceptable toxicity.

☀ PATIENT PRESENTATION

Chief Complaint
"My joints are killing me."

HPI
Marjorie Harris is a 49 yo woman who presents to the Family Medicine Clinic for the first time complaining of increasing pain in her lower back, hips, and right knee. She has a long history of osteoarthritis and had most recently been seen by a local rheumatologist, who tried a variety of NSAIDs without apparent success. She began insisting that the rheumatologist provide her with increasing quantities of opioid analgesics, and he subsequently asked her to find another doctor. She is now seeking medical care from the Family Medicine Clinic.

Last fall, she broke her right ankle and a bone in her foot. Her foot was in a cast for 4 weeks, and she was on crutches for 2 months. During this time, she noted that her arthritic symptoms were becoming increasingly more bothersome. In addition, she states that although her arthritis usually improves with warmer weather, it didn't improve at all this past summer. She is a rather poor historian.

PMH
Osteoarthritis × 18 years
Morbid obesity × 21 years

Type 2 DM, insulin-requiring × 9 years
Hypercholesterolemia × 5 years
HTN × 5 years
Frequent UTIs
Depression with anxiety for many years

PSH

Appendectomy 27 years ago
T & A 33 years ago
TAH-BSO 14 years ago
Right lateral maleolus and first metatarsal fracture repair 9 months ago

FH

Mother alive with DM; father died at age 69 secondary to pancreatic cancer; no siblings.

SH

Unemployed; disabled, on Medicaid; no other insurance; no alcohol, tobacco, or illicit drug use.

ROS

Positive for pain in left shoulder; low back pain with "shooting pains" radiating to the buttocks and groin area; "deep, boring" pain originating in the right pretibial area and extending distally to the right ankle and toes. Negative for headache, neck stiffness, joint swelling, or erythema; no SOB or palpitations; denies urinary frequency or burning, constipation, diarrhea, or tarry stools. Fingerstick blood glucose concentrations are usually in the low 300s; no polyuria or blurred vision.

Meds

Lotensin 10 mg po Q AM
Novolin 70/30, 25 units SC Q AM and 15 units SC Q PM
Premarin 0.625 mg po Q AM
Elavil 200 mg po Q HS
Vicodin po PRN pain
Ambien 10 mg po Q HS PRN sleep
Xanax 0.5 mg po TID PRN anxiety
Claritin 10 mg po PRN

All

Demerol—"makes me goofy"
"Mycins"—unknown reaction
Various pain meds (unspecified)—nausea

PE

Gen

Well developed, obese, Caucasian woman in NAD

VS

BP 164/94, P 64, RR 16, T 37.1°C; Ht 5′3″, Wt 201 lb. No orthostatic changes

Skin

Warm, dry; no petechiae or rashes; feet without lesions, erythema, or edema

HEENT

NC/AT; PERRLA; funduscopic exam reveals sharp disks; no A-V nicking, hemorrhages or exudates; no scleral icterus; TMs intact; mucous membranes moist; poor dentition with gingival erythema; no lateral deviation of tongue; no pharyngeal edema or erythema

Neck

Supple; no thyromegaly or lymphadenopathy; no carotid bruits

Lungs

CTA

Breasts

Difficult to examine due to size; symmetrical; no apparent masses

CV

Distant heart sounds; PMI at 5th ICS/MCL; RRR; no m/r/g; no JVD or HJR

Abdomen

Obese, soft, non-tender; no guarding; (+) BS; no HSM

GU/Rect

Normal female genitalia; some mild vaginal atrophy; normal sphincter tone; guaiac (−) stool in rectal vault

MS/Ext

Back pain radiating to right buttock with straight leg raising at 60°; right hip pain with flexion > 90° and with internal and external rotation > 45°; both hips tender to palpation; right knee (+) crepitus; right ankle with full ROM, no swelling or edema

Neuro

CN II–XII intact; DTRs equal bilaterally except for slightly diminished Achilles reflexes bilaterally; no focal deficits; gait impaired secondary to hip pain. Slightly decreased sensation to pinprick and vibration on the distal half of right foot. Babinskis downgoing.

Psych

Oriented × 4; flat affect; appears at times to alternate between apathy and anger/frustration

Labs

Na 135 mEq/L	Hgb 13.7 g/dL	RDW 14.4%	Ca 11.2 mg/dL
K 4.8 mEq/L	Hct 39.7%	AST 38 IU/L	Phos 4.5 mg/dL
Cl 98 mEq/L	WBC $4.5 \times 10^3/mm^3$	Alk Phos 106 IU/L	Uric acid 7.2 mg/dL
CO_2 26 mEq/L	Plt $286 \times 10^3/mm^3$	T. prot 7.4 g/dL	ESR 46 mm/hour
BUN 9 mg/dL	MCV 85.3 μm^3	Alb 4.4 g/dL	
SCr 0.9 mg/dL	MCH 29.4 pg	T. chol 354 mg/dL	
Glu 248 mg/dL	MCHC 34.5 g/dL		

UA

SG 1.011; pH 6.5; WBC (−), RBC (−), leukocyte esterase (−), nitrite (−)

Urine Culture

$< 10^5$ Enterococcus, $< 10^4$ Corynebacterium (contaminant)

X-rays

Lumbar spine: advanced degenerative changes at L3-4 and at L4-5.
Right hip: moderate degenerative changes with some spurring of the femoral head and slight decrease in joint space.

Right knee: moderate degenerative changes. No effusion.
Right foot: completely healed lateral maleolus and first metatarsal bone.

Assessment

1. Pain secondary to moderate–severe osteoarthritis of the lumbar spine, hips, and right knee

2. Morbid obesity (175% of IBW, BMI = 35.7 kg/m^2)
3. HTN
4. DM
5. Hypercholesterolemia
6. Hx depression with anxiety
7. R/O possible narcotic abuse

▶ Questions

Problem Identification

1. a. *Create a list of the patient's drug-related problems.*
   b. *What information (signs, symptoms, laboratory values) indicates the presence or severity of the primary problem (osteoarthritis)?*
   c. *What additional information is needed to satisfactorily assess this patient?*

Desired Outcome

2. *What are the goals of pharmacotherapy for each of this patient's drug-related problems?*

Therapeutic Alternatives

3. a. *What non-drug therapies might be useful for this patient?*
   b. *What feasible pharmacotherapeutic alternatives are available for treatment of this patient's osteoarthritis?*

Optimal Plan

4. a. *What drug, dosage form, schedule, and duration of therapy are best for treating this patient's osteoarthritis?*
   b. *What alternatives would be appropriate if the initial therapy fails or cannot be used?*

Outcome Evaluation

5. *What clinical and laboratory parameters are necessary to evaluate the therapy for achievement of the desired therapeutic outcome and to detect or prevent adverse effects?*

Patient Counseling

6. *What information should be provided to the patient to enhance compliance, ensure successful therapy, and minimize adverse effects?*

Additional Case Questions

1. *What risk factors for coronary artery disease does this patient have? Should she be placed on aspirin as a cardioprotectant in light of the fact that she is taking either acetaminophen or an NSAID?*
2. *What effect might NSAID therapy have on this patient's antihypertensive therapy?*
3. *Is this patient a candidate for pharmacotherapy to treat her morbid obesity?*

▶ Self-study Assignments

1. Medicaid regulations concerning medications vary from state to state. Keep in mind that many NSAIDs are expensive and, based on this patient's insurance status (see social history), your choice of NSAID may be restricted by the state Medicaid formulary. What restrictions on NSAIDs are in place in your state? If a prescriber prescribes an NSAID that is not on the formulary, what options are available to the patient? Is therapeutic substitution an option? Can you obtain prior approval? Or will the patient have to pay "out of pocket"?

2. Using the Internet, identify one website that provides useful information to patients about osteoarthritis. Identify one site that you think provides misleading or potentially dangerous information to patients.

▶ Clinical Pearl

Osteoarthritis, unlike rheumatoid arthritis, is typically not an inflammatory condition; NSAIDs are used primarily for their analgesic effects rather than their anti-inflammatory effects.

References

1. Kraus VB. Pathogenesis and treatment of osteoarthritis. Med Clin North Am 1997;81:85–112.
2. Anderson JJ, Felson DT. Factors associated with osteoarthritis of the knee in the first national Health and Nutrition Examination Survey (HANES I). Am J Epidemiol 1988;128:179–189.
3. Felson DT, Zhang Y, Anthony JM, et al. Weight loss reduces the risk for symptomatic knee osteoarthritis in women. The Framingham Study. Ann Intern Med 1992;116:535–539.
4. McAlindon TE, Jacques P, Zhang Y, et al. Do antioxidant micronutrients protect against the development and progression of knee osteoarthritis? Arthritis Rheum 1996;39:648–656.
5. Bradley JD, Brandt KD, Katz BP, et al. Comparison of an antiinflammatory dose of ibuprofen, an analgesic dose of ibuprofen, and acetaminophen in the treatment of patients with osteoarthritis of the knee. N Engl J Med 1991;325:87–91.
6. Rich-Edwards JW, Manson JE, Hennekens CH, et al. The primary prevention of coronary heart disease in women. N Engl J Med 1995;332:1758–1766.
7. Pope JE, Anderson JJ, Felson DT. A meta-analysis of the effects of nonsteroidal anti-inflammatory drugs on blood pressure. Arch Intern Med 1993;153:477–484.

83 GOUT AND HYPERURICEMIA

▶ **The Professor's Lament**   (Level II)

Page H. Pigg, PharmD
Ralph E. Small, PharmD, FCCP, FASHP, FAPhA

▶ After completing this case study, students should be able to:

- Identify the risk factors for hyperuricemia.

- Recommend appropriate treatment for an acute attack of gouty arthritis.

- Recognize the importance of determining the presence of an over-producer versus underexcretor of uric acid.

- Recommend appropriate therapy for the treatment of chronic gouty arthritis.

☀ PATIENT PRESENTATION

Chief Complaint
"My toe hurts so bad, I can't put my shoe on!"

HPI
Garrett Simms is a 44 yo man seen by his physician for severe pain in his left great toe. The pain was noted after a night of "partying" at a work-related convention 2 days ago. The pain has been persistent and increasing since the initial morning and has awakened him from sleep 2 nights in a row. Currently, the patient can bear no weight on the affected foot without intolerable pain.

PMH
Occasional joint stiffness in the lower limbs
HTN × 9 years
Seasonal allergic rhinitis × several years

FH
His father (age 72) and mother (age 73) are both alive and healthy. His father has had HTN for 20+ years.

SH
Married with adult children. Works as a college professor. Non-smoker who is an occasional alcohol user (2–3 drinks per week).

ROS
No headache, dizziness, rhinorrhea, sneezing, itching, or generalized swelling or tenderness in the joints.

Med
Hydrochlorothiazide 25 mg po QD
Aspirin 325 mg po QD
Loratadine 10 mg po QD during allergy season
Acetaminophen 650 mg po QID since onset of pain

All
NKDA

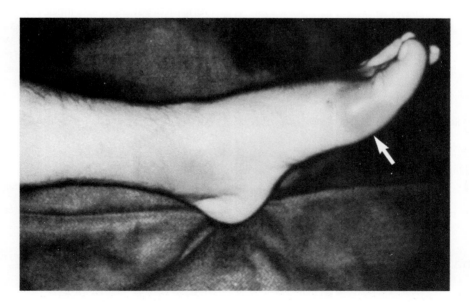

Figure 83–1. Swollen, erythematous, and painful left great toe due to an acute attack of gout. *(Reprinted from the Clinical Slide Collection on the Rheumatic Diseases, copyright 1991. Used by permission of the American College of Rheumatology.)*

PE

General
Healthy Caucasian man in acute distress

VS
BP 138/86, HR 89, RR 24, T 100.3°F; Wt 215 lb, Ht 5'11"

Neck/Nodes
Normal with no swelling, thyromegaly, or JVD

HEENT
PERRLA; no A-V nicking, hemorrhages or exudates

Lungs
CTA

CV
RRR, no m/r/g

ABD
Non-tender; obese; no HSM

MS/Ext
Left first MTP swollen, hot, tender, red (see Figure 83–1)

NEURO
A & O × 3; CN II–XII intact; DTRs 2+, Babinski (−)

Labs

Na 142 mEq/L	Hgb 15.3 g/dL	Uric acid 11.5 mg/dL
K 4.1 mEq/L	Hct 46.4%	West. ESR 18 mm/hr
Cl 101 mEq/L	WBC 12 × 10³/mm³	
CO$_2$ 24 mEq/L	60% PMNs	
BUN 12 mg/dL	3% Bands	
SCr 1.1 mg/dL	35% Lymphs	
Glu 101 mg/dL	2% Eos	

UA
Negative

X-ray
Left great toe—some soft tissue swelling; normal joint space

Other
Left great toe synovial fluid aspirate—PMNs and monosodium urate crystals (see Figure 83–2)

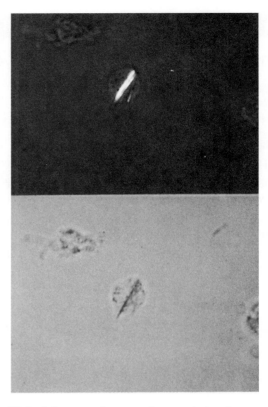

Figure 83–2. Monosodium urate crystals phagocytosed by a polymorphonuclear leukocyte in the joint fluid during an acute attack of gout. In the top section, compensated polarized light demonstrates two longer crystals (approximately 13 microns) and one shorter crystal (approximately 9 microns). The bottom section shows the same field under ordinary light. Here only one of the longer crystals is identifiable. This demonstrates the superiority of compensated polarized light over ordinary light microscopy when evaluating joint fluid for crystals. (*Reprinted from the Clinical Slide Collection on the Rheumatic Diseases. Copyright 1991. Used by permission of the American College of Rheumatology.*)

Assessment
1. Primary presentation of acute gout
2. HTN controlled on medical therapy
3. Allergic rhinitis controlled on medical therapy

▶ Questions

Problem Identification

1. a. Create a list of the patient's drug-related problems.
   b. What information (signs, symptoms, laboratory values) indicates the presence or severity of an acute gouty attack?
   c. Could any of the patient's problems have been caused by drug therapy?

Desired Outcome

2. What are the goals of pharmacotherapy in this case?

Therapeutic Alternatives

3. a. *What non-drug therapies might be useful for this patient?*
   b. *What feasible pharmacotherapeutic alternatives are available for treatment of the acute attack of gouty arthritis?*

Optimal Plan

4. *What drug, dosage form, dose, schedule, and duration of therapy are best for this patient?*

Outcome Evaluation

5. *What clinical and laboratory parameters are necessary to evaluate the therapy for achievement of the desired therapeutic outcome and to detect or prevent adverse effects?*

Patient Counseling

6. *What information should be provided to the patient to enhance compliance, ensure successful therapy, and minimize adverse effects?*

▶ Clinical Course

Mr. Simms responded completely to the initial therapy that you recommended, with total resolution of his joint pain in 5 days. Within 6 months after his initial presentation, he experienced 2 more episodes of acute gouty arthritis. Although his BP is adequately controlled on alternative therapy (an ACE inhibitor), he has not followed dietary guidelines, resulting in continued elevation of serum uric acid (>10.5 mg/dL) and inability to lose weight. He has also not tolerated colchicine prophylactic therapy that was initiated after resolution of his acute gout attacks due to persistent diarrhea. Short-term courses of an NSAID (naproxen) are effective in controlling his second and third acute attacks. A 24-hour urine collection was obtained after 3 days on a purine-free diet. The results revealed a urine uric acid value of 750 mg.

▶ Follow-up Questions

1. *Provide an interpretation of the urine uric acid value.*
2. *What recommendations do you have for further management of this patient?*

▶ Clinical Pearl

Oral colchicine can cause serious diarrhea resulting in dehydration and electrolyte disturbances; although IV colchicine avoids these GI effects, it may result in local extravasation injury.

▶ Self-study Assignments

1. Which uric acid lowering therapy would be most useful in the patient with chronic hyperuricemia and diminished renal function? Outline the rationale for your response, and prepare dosage regimens of the drug for patients with varying degrees of renal impairment.
2. Make a list of the NSAIDs that have FDA-approved labeling for the treatment of acute gouty attacks. Compare the dosage regimens used and contact a local pharmacy to determine which agents provide the most economical therapy.

References

1. Agudelo CA, Wise CM. Gout and hyperuricemia. Curr Opin Rheumatol 1991;3:684–691.
2. Star VL, Hochberg MC. Prevention and management of gout. Drugs 1993;45:212–222.
3. Edwards NL. Drugs to lower uric acid levels. How to avoid misuse in gouty arthritis. Postgrad Med 1991;89:111–113, 116.

Eyes, Ears, Nose, and Throat Disorders

L. Michael Posey, RPh, Section Editor

84 GLAUCOMA

▶ **Another Silent Disease** (Level II)

Tien T. Kiat-Winarko, PharmD, BSc

▶ After completing this case study, students should be able to:

- Recognize the importance of regular eye examinations and the difference between glaucoma and ocular hypertension.
- List the risk factors for developing open-angle glaucoma.
- Recommend conventional glaucoma therapy as well as new options in glaucoma management when indicated.
- Implement the basic ophthalmologic monitoring parameters used in glaucoma therapy.
- Counsel patients on their medication regimen and proper ophthalmic administration technique.

☼ PATIENT PRESENTATION

Chief Complaint
"My left eye is foggy, and I get blurred vision and headaches."

HPI
Lee Angeles is a pleasant 34 yo man with a history of advanced open-angle glaucoma who presents to his ophthalmologist with complaints of fogging and distortion of vision in the left eye lasting 6 to 12 hours. This occasion-

ally progresses to tunnel vision, with chronic sensitivity to fluorescent lights, and throbbing band-like squeezing headaches lasting for hours. He also complains of periodic distortion in the left eye for the past 3 months, sometimes associated with central area visual blurring.

He was in his usual state of health until he had a skydiving accident 9 years ago and fractured his thoracic spine at the level of T9-10. During that hospitalization, he complained of blurred vision. Ophthalmology consult was sought and he was ultimately diagnosed with advanced open-angle glaucoma. He was managed by a general ophthalmologist for several years, who prescribed Timoptic 0.5% ou BID, Propine 0.1% ou BID, and Ocusert Pilo-40 od and Ocusert Pilo-20 os Q week. He was subsequently referred to a glaucoma specialist due to worsening of his condition. He had undergone laser trabeculoplasty ou prior to his referral. The glaucoma specialist examined the patient, and a complete work-up was done on the initial visit.

Bilateral laser trabeculoplasty was performed 8 years ago with an initial decrease in IOP; however, IOP subsequently increased several months later. Filtering surgery was performed in Boston ou 7 years ago. Multiple prior brain MRIs revealed no abnormal findings. Other ocular history includes high myopia since childhood, history of dry eyes, and history of contact lens wear.

PMH
Childhood asthma that resolved at puberty

Depression due to chronic open-angle glaucoma and worsening of vision after completion of his PhD program

S/P ultrasonic renal lithotripsy secondary to nephrolithiasis associated with acetazolamide use

S/P tonsillectomy as a child

FH
Father, mother, and sister have glaucoma. Father has hypertension.

SH

PhD in molecular biology from Harvard. Single. No history of smoking. Drank 4 cans of beer per day × 3 years during post-graduate study. Currently drinks 2 to 3 cans of beer/week.

Meds

Betoptic 0.5% ou BID
Iopidine 0.5% os TID
Trusopt 2% os TID
FML 0.1% ou TID
Bion Tears ou BID
Nifedipine 10 mg po TID
Trental 400 mg po TID
Paxil 20 mg po QD
Also performs eye massage ou QID
Past medications include pilocarpine 4%, Timoptic 0.5%, Propine, Diamox sequels 500 mg, and Pred-Forte 1%

All

NKDA

ROS

Non-contributory. No heart, lung, or circulatory problems; no stroke or anemia.

PE

VS

BP 120/82, P 70, R 18

Eyes

Visual acuity—OD—hand motion at 3 inches with correction spectacles; OS—20/30
Slit lamp exam—Lid margins were without inflammation ou; conjunctiva without injection; normal tear break-up, did not stain with fluorescein; cornea clear and smooth; anterior chamber deep and quiet; lenses—clear ou; iris round without neovascularization or abnormality; no mass/nodules; filtering bleb is visible at 11 o'clock meridian.
Intraocular pressure—OD—14 mm Hg; OS—20 mm Hg
Vitreous examination—clear ou
Disks—OD—the disc appeared whitish, fully cupped and showed marked pallor; cup-to-disk (C/D) ratio = 1.0; OS—CD ratio = 0.99 with only a narrow rim present (normal C/D ratio = < 0.33)
Color vision—OD—unable to see; OS—WNL
Visual fields—OD—unable to see the Amsler grid; can only see hand motion at 3 inches away; OS—several paracentral scotomata with the Amsler grid; 20/30. Diurnal curve of IOP revealed pressures between 10 mm Hg and 21 mm Hg.

CV

RRR without m/r/g; carotid pulses are brisk and equal bilaterally without bruits

Neuro

Smell and corneal sensation are intact bilaterally. Facial symmetry, tone, and sensation are intact bilaterally. Cranial nerves VIII through XII were intact. Gait was intact. Finger-to-nose and rapid alternating movement tests were normal. Reflexes were symmetric and normal. Sensation was intact and symmetric to pinprick, proprioception, and light touch. Motor strength of all extremities was 5/5.

Labs

Na 138 mEq/L	Bun 10 mg/dL
K 3.3 mEq/L	SCr 0.9 mg/dL
Cl 99 mEq/L	FBG 126 mg/dL
CO_2 25 mEq/L	

Assessment

High myopia with advanced chronic juvenile open-angle glaucoma
No evidence of macular edema
No cataracts
S/P filtering procedure ou
Depression associated with chronic open-angle glaucoma

Plan

Increase eye massage to 8 times/day
Follow-up in 6 weeks
Repeat filtering surgery/trabeculectomy with mitomycin C to further lower IOP
Switch nifedipine to nimodipine for better CNS/ophthalmic absorption to increase blood flow
Counsel with neuro-ophthalmologist, retina ophthalmologist, and neurologist

► Questions

Problem Identification

1. a. Provide a list of this patient's drug-related problems.
   b. What risk factors for primary open-angle glaucoma (POAG) are present in this patient?
   c. What information (signs, symptoms) indicates the presence or severity of this patient's glaucoma?

Desired Outcome

2. What are the goals of pharmacotherapy in this case?

Therapeutic Alternatives

3. a. What non-drug therapies might be useful for this patient?
   b. What feasible pharmacotherapeutic alternatives are available for treatment of the patient's glaucoma?

Optimal Plan

4. a. Devise an optimal pharmacotherapeutic regimen for the treatment of this patient's glaucoma.
   b. What alternatives would be appropriate if the initial therapy fails or cannot be used?

Outcome Evaluation

5. *What clinical and laboratory parameters are necessary to evaluate the therapy for achievement of the desired therapeutic outcome and to detect or prevent adverse effects?*

Patient Counseling

6. *What information should the patient receive about the disease of glaucoma, proper medication administration technique, and possible side effects of treatment?*

▶ Self-study Assignments

1. Perform a literature search on the reason why antimetabolites such as mitomycin C and 5-FU are used in glaucoma surgery. What is the mechanism of action of these antimetabolites in trabeculectomy pressure-lowering surgery?
2. Perform a literature search and explain the rationale for using nimodipine and pentoxifylline in advanced open-angle glaucoma. How do these agents work to increase blood flow to the eye and retard the progression of nerve damage?
3. Under what circumstances should the product Ocusert-pilo be used? Compare the advantages and disadvantages of using this long-acting ocular insert.

References

1. Kane H, Gaasterland DE, Monsour M. Response of filtered eyes to digital ocular pressure. Ophthalmology 1997;104:202–206.
2. Liu JH. Circadian rhythm of intraocular pressure. J Glaucoma 1998;7:141–147.
3. Sacca SC, Rolando M, Marletta A, et al. Fluctuations of intraocular pressure during the day in open-angle glaucoma, normal-tension glaucoma and normal subjects. Ophthalmologica 1998;212:115–119.
4. Ichihara S, Tsuda Y, Hosomi N, et al. Nimodipine improves brain energy metabolism and blood rheology during ischemia and reperfusion in the gerbil brain. J Neurol Sci 1996;114:84–90.
5. Herbette LG, Mason PE, Sweeney KR, et al. Favorable amphiphilicity of nimodipine facilitates its interaction with brain membranes. Neuropharmacology 1994; 33:241–249.

85 ALLERGIC RHINITIS

▶ Reining in Rhinitis   (Level I)

W. Greg Leader, PharmD

▶ After completing this case study, students should be able to:

- Educate patients in appropriate measures to limit or avoid exposure to specific antigens.
- Compare and contrast available agents used to treat allergic rhinitis with respect to efficacy and safety.
- Develop a safe and effective therapeutic regimen for the management of allergic rhinitis.
- Select appropriate therapy for patients who have failed first-line therapy.

- Counsel patients with allergic rhinitis on appropriate medication use.

☀ PATIENT PRESENTATION

Chief Complaint
"My eyes and ears are itchy all the time; I'm sneezing a lot, and I have a draining sensation in the back of my throat that is causing me to gag; I also have a sore throat."

HPI
Celeste Boudreaux is a 32 yo woman who presents to the ambulatory care clinic stating that she has had a long history of seasonal allergy, and that she has had post-nasal drainage starting several days before the throat irritation began and continuing over the last 6 days. The patient denies fever, chills, or sinus pain. She states that she only has an occasional cough that is non-productive.

PMH
Perennial rhinitis
Eczema

FH
Father age 52, with a history of HTN and s/p MI; mother with DM and increased cholesterol; one sister with HTN.

SH
Married for 14 years with 2 children (ages 8 and 4). Lives in a turn-of-the-century farmhouse where she divides her time between caring for her children and her 6 horses and providing part-time horse riding lessons. Quit smoking 10 years ago; denies EtOH use.

Meds
Hismanal 10 mg po QD × 3 years
Ortho-Novum 1/35-28, 1 po QD
Hydrocortisone cream 1% PRN eczema

All
NKDA

ROS
No wheezing, shortness of breath, chest pain, abdominal discomfort, bowel or bladder symptoms, dysuria, or focal weakness. No complaints concerning her eczema.

PE

Gen
The patient appears tired but is in NAD and appears to be her stated age

VS
BP 120/68, P 80, RR 16, T 37.3°C; Ht 5'2", Wt 145 lb.

HEENT

NC/AT; PERRLA; EOMI. Conjunctivae are pink. TMs are intact. There is no epistaxis or nasal discharge. Mucous membranes are moist. There are no oropharyngeal lesions. There is mild erythema over the left anterior tonsillar pillar. Otherwise, no exudate or posterior pharynx swelling or masses noted.

Neck

Supple; no lymphadenopathy or thyromegaly

Chest

CTA bilaterally

Breasts

Normal

Heart

RRR without m/r/g

Abdomen

Soft, non-tender, (+) BS, obese; small areas of flaking skin noted

Extremities

No CCE, pulses 2+ throughout

Neuro

A & O × 3; 2+ reflexes throughout; 5/5 strength; CN I–XII intact

Assessment

This 32-year-old woman likely has posterior pharynx irritation due to post-nasal drainage.

Plan

1. Rhinitis: Discharge to home with Rx for Entex in an attempt to dry up the nasal drainage. The patient has been receiving Hismanal for several years without adequate relief of symptoms. We will consider adding cromolyn sodium vs. intranasal corticosteroid. The patient was instructed to return if the pain becomes worse, or if she has any worsening of swelling or difficulty in breathing, swallowing, eating, or drinking.
2. Eczema: Continue use of PRN hydrocortisone.
3. Health maintenance: Administer flu vaccine today.

► Questions

Problem Identification

1. a. *Create a list of the patient's drug-related problems.*
   b. *What information (signs, symptoms, laboratory values) indicates the presence or severity of allergic rhinitis?*
   c. *Could any of the patient's problems have been caused by drug therapy?*
   d. *What additional information from the patient history is needed to satisfactorily assess this patient?*

Desired Outcome

2. *What are the goals of pharmacotherapy in this case?*

Therapeutic Alternatives

3. a. *What non-drug therapies might be useful for this patient?*
   b. *What feasible pharmacotherapeutic alternatives are available for treatment of allergic rhinitis?*

Optimal Plan

4. a. *What drug, dosage form, dose, schedule, and duration of therapy are best for this patient?*
   b. *What alternatives would be available if the initial therapy fails?*

Outcome Evaluation

5. *What clinical and laboratory parameters are necessary to evaluate the therapy for achievement of the desired therapeutic outcome and to detect or prevent adverse effects?*

Patient Counseling

6. *What information should be provided to the patient to enhance compliance, ensure successful therapy, and minimize adverse effects?*

► Self-study Assignments

1. Outline a plan to initiate therapy with a first-generation antihistamine that will minimize the sedative effects experienced by the patient.
2. Search the literature on immunotherapy and prepare a table that summarizes the results of controlled clinical trials.
3. Make a recommendation as to a single first-generation antihistamine, second-generation antihistamine, and intranasal steroid to include on a hospital or health maintenance organization formulary. Support your recommendations with efficacy, safety, and economic data.

► Clinical Pearl

First-generation antihistamines are still the agents of choice for the treatment of seasonal allergic rhinitis because of comparable efficacy with the non-sedating agents and their lower cost.

References

1. Long WF, Taylor RJ, Wagner CJ, et al. Skin test suppression by antihistamines and the development of subsensitivity. J Allergy Clin Immunol 1985;76:113–117.

2. Simons FE, Watson WT, Simons KJ. Lack of subsensitivity to terfenadine during long-term terfenadine treatment. J Allergy Clin Immunol 1988;82:1068–1075.

3. Girard JP, Sommacal-Schopf D, Bigliardi P, et al. Double-blind comparison of astemizole, terfenadine and placebo in hay fever with special regard to onset of action. J Int Med Res 1985;13:102–108.

4. Gastpar H, Aurich R, Petzold U, et al. Intranasal treatment of perennial allergic rhinitis. Comparison of azelastine nasal spray and budesonide nasal aerosol. Arzneimittelforschung 1993;43:475–479.

5. International Rhinitis Management Working Group. International Consensus Report on the diagnosis and management of rhinitis. Allergy 1994;49(19 suppl):1–34.

SECTION 12

Dermatologic Disorders

L. Michael Posey, RPh, Section Editor

---

86 ACNE VULGARIS

▶ **The Graduate** (Level II)

Rebecca M. Law, PharmD
Wayne P. Gulliver, MD, FRCPC

▶ After completing this case study, students should be able to:

- Understand risk factors and aggravating factors in the pathogenesis of acne vulgaris.

- Understand the treatment strategies in acne, including appropriate situations for using non-prescription and prescription medications; and the use of topical and systemic therapies.

- Counsel patients with acne on systemic therapies.

- Monitor the safety and efficacy of selected systemic therapies.

☀ PATIENT PRESENTATION

Chief Complaint
"I can't stand this acne!"

HPI
Elaine Morgan is an 18 yo young woman with a history of facial acne since age 15. One month ago she completed a 3-month course of minocycline in combination with Differin (adapalene). Her acne has flared up again and she has again presented to her family physician for treatment.

PMH
Has irregular menses due to polycystic ovarian disease diagnosed 3 years ago, which has not required medical treatment. However, it has resulted in an acne condition that was initially quite mild; and she responded well to nonprescription topical products. In the past 2 years, the number of facial lesions has increased despite OTC, and later prescription, drug treatments. Initially, Benzamycin Gel was beneficial, but this had to be discontinued due to excessive drying. Differin was used next and it controlled her condition for about 6 months, then the acne worsened and oral antibiotics were added. Most recently, she has received two 3-month courses of minocycline over the past year. She has also noted some scarring and cysts in the past few months.

FH
Parents alive and well; 2 older brothers (ages 21 and 25). Father had acne with residual scarring.

SH
The patient is under some stress since she is graduating in a few weeks. She wants to do well in school so she will qualify for the best colleges. Both of her brothers graduated with honors. She is sexually active, and her boyfriend uses condoms.

Meds
None currently

All
NKDA

ROS
In addition to the complaints noted above, the patient has dysmenorrhea and mild hirsutism.

PE

Gen
Alert, moderately anxious teenager in NAD

VS
BP 110/70, RR 15, T 37°C, Ht 5′2″, Wt 45 kg

Skin
Comedones on forehead, nose, and chin. Papules and pustules on the nose and malar area. A few cysts on the chin. Scars on malar area. Increased facial hair.

HEENT
PERRLA, EOMI, fundi benign, TMs intact

Chest
CTA bilaterally

Cor
RRR without m/r/g, S_1 and S_2 normal

Abd
(+) BS, soft, non-tender, no masses

MS/Ext
No joint aches or pains; peripheral pulses present

Neuro
CN II–XII intact

Labs

Na 140 mEq/L	Hgb 13.0 g/dL	AST 21 IU/L	LDL-C 90 mg/dL
K 3.7 mEq/L	Hct 38%	ALT 39 IU/L	Trig 90 mg/dL
Cl 100 mEq/L	Plt 300 × 10³/mm³	LDH 105 IU/L	DHEAS 6 μmol/L
CO_2 25 mEq/L	WBC 7.0 × 10³/mm³	Alk phos 89 IU/L	Testosterone 2.0 ng/mL
BUN 12 mg/dL		T. bili 1.0 mg/dL	Prolactin 15 ng/mL
SCr 1.0 mg/dL		Alb 3.9 g/dL	FSH 150 mIU/mL
Glu 100 mg/dL		T. chol 170 mg/dL	LH 30 mIU/mL

▶ Questions

Problem Identification

1. a. Create a drug-related problem list for this patient.
   b. What signs and symptoms consistent with acne does this patient demonstrate?
   c. How does polycystic ovarian disease contribute to this patient's acne and other physical findings?

Desired Outcome

2. What are the treatment goals for this patient?

Therapeutic Alternatives

3. What feasible therapeutic alternatives are available for management of this patient's acne?

Optimal Plan

4. What treatment regimen is best suited for this patient?

Outcome Evaluation

5. How would you monitor the therapy you recommended for efficacy and adverse effects?

Patient Counseling

6. How would you counsel the patient about this treatment regimen to enhance compliance and ensure successful therapy?

▶ Self-study Assignments

1. Review the dysmorphic syndrome associated with acne.
2. Review the non-pharmacologic management of acne, including stress reduction and dietary changes.

▶ Clinical Pearl

In acne, scarring + cysts + 2 courses of oral antibiotics means "consider isotretinoin."

References

1. Leyden JJ. Therapy for acne vulgaris. N Engl J Med 1997;336:1156–1162.
2. Brogden RN, Goa KE. Adapalene: A review of its pharmacological properties and clinical potential in the management of mild to moderate acne. Drugs 1997;53:511–519.
3. al-Khawajah MM. Isotretinoin for acne vulgaris. Int J Dermatol 1996;35:212–215.
4. James M. Isotretinoin for severe acne. Lancet 1996;347:1749–1750.
5. Cheung AP, Chang RJ. Polycystic ovary syndrome. Clin Obstet Gynecol 1990;33:655–667.
6. Berson DS, Shalita AR. The treatment of acne: The role of combination therapies. J Am Acad Dermatol 1995;32(5 Pt 3):S31–S41.

87 PSORIASIS

▶ The Harried School Teacher   (Level II)

Rebecca M. Law, PharmD

▶ After completing this case study, students should be able to:

- Understand the pathophysiology of plaque psoriasis, including clinical presentation and skin changes.

- Understand the sequence of using topical, photochemical, and systemic treatment modalities for psoriasis.

- Compare the efficacy and adverse effects of various systemic therapies for psoriasis including methotrexate, acitretin, cyclosporine, azathioprine, hydroxyurea, and sulfasalazine.

- Select appropriate therapeutic regimens for patients with plaque psoriasis.
- Counsel patients with psoriasis about proper use of pharmacotherapeutic treatments, potential adverse effects, and necessary precautions.

☀ PATIENT PRESENTATION

Chief Complaint

"Nothing is helping my psoriasis."

HPI

Geraldine Kirk is a 55 yo woman with a 30+ year history of psoriasis who presented to the outpatient dermatology clinic 2 days ago with another flare-up of her psoriasis. She was admitted to the inpatient dermatology service for a severe flare-up of plaque psoriasis involving her arms, legs, elbows, knees, palms, abdomen, back, and scalp (see Figure 87–1).

She was diagnosed with plaque psoriasis at age 23. She initially responded to topical therapy with crude coal tar, later to topical cortico-

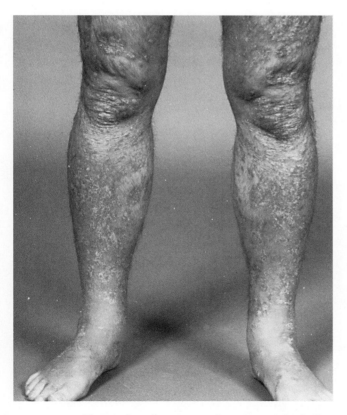

Figure 87–1. Example of severe plaque psoriasis involving the lower extremities in a male patient (not the patient discussed in this case). *(Photo courtesy of Wayne P. Gulliver, MD.)*

steroids with anthralin paste to thicker areas. She subsequently required photochemotherapy using psoralens with UVA phototherapy (PUVA) to control her condition. PUVA eventually became ineffective and 5 years ago she was started on oral methotrexate 5 mg once/week. Dosage escalations have kept her condition under fairly good control. Until recently, flare-ups have consisted of lesions to limited skin areas (mostly abdomen and legs) and were successfully treated with SCAT (short contact anthralin therapy). Recently, flare-ups have been more frequent and lesions have become more widespread. She has already been admitted twice for SCAT treatments in the past 4 months, most recently 6 weeks ago. Her current methotrexate dose is 25 mg once/week. This was increased from 20 mg once/week 6 months ago. Her cumulative lifetime dose of methotrexate is 2.2 g.

PMH

Menopause occurred at age 50; currently on HRT.

One episode of major depressive illness triggered by the death of her first husband, which occurred 21 years ago (age 34). She was treated by her family physician who prescribed amitriptyline. She has had no recurrences. She has no other chronic medical conditions and no other acute or recent illnesses.

FH

Parents alive and well. 2 sisters. No history of psoriasis, immune disorders, or malignancy.

SH

Patient is an elementary school teacher; non-smoker; social use of alcohol (glass of wine with dinner). She is married and has 3 children ages 11–17 with her second husband. There have been increasing tensions and anxiety at work recently due to restructuring of her school board.

Meds

Methotrexate 25 mg po Q Sunday
Conjugated estrogens 0.625 mg po QD
Medroxyprogesterone acetate 5 mg po QD

All

NKDA

ROS

Skin does not feel very itchy despite extensive scaling; she reports using a non-medicated moisturizer TID. No joint aches or pains. No complaints of shortness of breath. No spotting or breakthrough bleeding. No nausea, vomiting, or bloating from HRT. Occasional nausea associated with the weekly methotrexate dose. Has been feeling jumpy and stressed due to tensions at work but does not feel depressed.

PE

Gen

Alert, mildly anxious 55 yo Caucasian woman in NAD

VS

BP 145/88, P 85, T 37°C; Ht 5'5", Wt 65 kg

Skin

Confluent plaque psoriasis with extensive lesions on abdomen, arms, legs, back, and scalp. Thick crusted lesions on elbows, knees, palms, and soles. Lesions are red to violet in color, with sharply demarcated borders except where confluent, and are loosely covered with silvery-white scales. There are no pustules or vesicles.

HEENT
PERRLA, EOMI, fundi benign, TMs intact; extensive scaly lesions on scalp as noted

Neck/LN
No lymphadenopathy; thyroid non-palpable

Chest
CTA bilaterally

CV
RRR without m/r/g; S_1 and S_2 normal

Abd
(+) BS, soft, non-tender, no masses; extensive scaly lesions on skin as noted above

GU
WNL

Rect
Deferred

MS/Ext
No joint swelling, increased warmth, or tenderness; skin lesions as noted above; no nail involvement; peripheral pulses 2+ throughout

Neuro
A & O × 3; CN II–XII intact; DTRs 2+; toes downgoing

Labs

Na 143 mEq/L	Hgb 12 g/dL	AST 22 IU/L
K 3.9 mEq/L	Hct 34.0%	ALT 38 IU/L
Cl 101 mEq/L	Plt 250 × 10³/mm³	LDH 107 IU/L
CO_2 25 mEq/L	WBC 7.5 × 10³/mm³	Alk phos 98 IU/L
BUN 14 mg/dL		T. bili 1.0 mg/dL
SCr 1.0 mg/dL		Alb 3.7 g/dL
Glu 98 mg/dL		Uric acid 4 mg/dL
		T. chol 180 mg/dL

Other
Liver biopsy from previous admission (6 weeks ago): No evidence of fibrosis, hepatitis, or cirrhosis.

► Questions

Problem Identification

1. a. Create a list of this patient's drug-related problems.
    b. What signs and symptoms consistent with psoriasis does this patient demonstrate?
    c. What risk factors for a flare-up of psoriasis are present in this patient?
    d. Could the signs and symptoms be caused by any drug therapy she is receiving?

Desired Outcome

2. What are the goals of pharmacotherapy for psoriasis in this patient?

Therapeutic Alternatives

3. a. What non-pharmacologic alternatives are available for managing the patient's psoriasis?
    b. What feasible pharmacotherapeutic alternatives are available for controlling the patient's disease at this point?

Optimal Plan

4. What drug regimen is best suited for treating this flare of the patient's psoriasis?

Outcome Evaluation

5. How should you monitor the therapy you recommended for efficacy and adverse effects?

Patient Counseling

6. What information should be provided to the patient to enhance compliance and ensure successful therapy?

► Self-study Assignments

1. Perform a literature search to identify potential future topical therapies for psoriasis, such as NSAIDs, protein kinase C inhibitors, a methotrexate gel, and an implantable 5-fluorouracil formulation.
2. Perform a literature search to identify potential future systemic therapies for psoriasis, including glucosamine and immunomodulators such as monoclonal antibodies and cytokines.

► Clinical Pearl

The 3 "R"s of systemic therapy for psoriasis are Rotate Regimens Regularly.

References

1. Finzi AF. Individualized short-course cyclosporin therapy in psoriasis. Br J Dermatol 1996;135(suppl 48):31–34.
2. Berth-Jones J, Voorhees JJ. Consensus conference on cyclosporin A microemulsion for psoriasis, June 1996. Br J Dermatol 1996;135:775–777.
3. Jegasothy BV, Ackerman CD, Todo S, et al. Tacrolimus (FK506): a new therapeutic agent for severe recalcitrant psoriasis. Arch Dermatol 1992;128:781–785.

SECTION 13

Hematologic Disorders

Gary C. Yee, PharmD, FCCP, Section Editor

88 IRON DEFICIENCY ANEMIA

▶ **Bertha's Belly Pain** (Level I)

William E. Wade, PharmD, FASHP, FCCP
William J. Spruill, PharmD

▶ After completing this case study, the student should be able to:

- Recognize that the consumption of selected OTC products may lead to the development of iron deficiency anemia.

- Recognize common signs, symptoms, and laboratory manifestations associated with iron deficiency anemia.

- Select appropriate iron therapy for the treatment of iron deficiency anemia.

- Counsel patients on potential adverse effects associated with iron therapy.

☀ PATIENT PRESENTATION

Chief Complaint
"I have belly pain and feel tired all the time."

HPI
Bertha Swingdale is a 40 yo woman who presents to your pharmacy with the above complaint. With further questioning, she relates the onset of her GI complaints at the time she initiated self-medication with Aleve for "arthritis in her right knee." The stomach pain has progressively gotten worse over the past 2 months. She describes this pain as a burning sensation that usually begins 30 minutes to 1 hour after meals and may or may not be relieved by antacid administration. Upon reviewing her medication profile, you note that she has a prescription for PRN ranitidine. Further questioning reveals a history of PUD approximately 4 years ago. When asked what over-the-counter medications she is currently consuming and how long she has been taking them, she responds that she started taking Aleve 1 tablet twice daily 7 months ago for "arthritis" in her right knee. Due to a progression of her arthritis pain and a loss of adequate relief, she increased the dose of Aleve to 2 tablets twice a day 2 months ago. You suggest that she discontinue the Aleve, begin acetaminophen for her "arthritis," and see her family physician as soon as possible. You also recommend that she should not consume OTC medications in the future without first consulting her pharmacist or physician and that she not take doses in excess of the manufacturer's recommended dose.

▶ Clinical Course

Three days later, she is evaluated by her family physician, which provides the following additional information.

PMH
Osteoarthritis diagnosed after a recent fall; patient self-medicates with naproxen; history of heavy menses and PUD

FH
Father died from MI 8 years ago; mother had a history of PUD. She has 2 sisters, both living with no known medical problems. Two daughters without medical problems.

SH
Occasionally consumes alcohol; denies tobacco or illicit drug use.

ROS

Burning pain in stomach after meals; denies heartburn, melena, vomiting BRB; good appetite, has 1 daily BM; no weight changes over past 5 years; (+) fatigue; tires easily; (−) paralysis, fainting, numbness, paresthesia, or tremor; headache once every 3 to 4 months; has myopic vision; (−) tinnitus or vertigo; has hay fever in spring; (−) cough, sputum production, or wheezing; denies chest pain, edema, dyspnea, or orthopnea; denies nocturia, hematuria, dysuria, or Hx of stones; P_2G_2; onset of menses at age 11; heavy flow for past 8 years; last Pap smear 6 months ago; unilateral joint pain in right knee of recent onset; frequent early morning stiffness in RLE.

Meds

Aleve 2 tablets po BID
Mylanta PRN

All

"Mycins" (upset stomach)

PE

Gen

WDWN African-American woman in NAD who appears her stated age

VS

BP 120/78, P 82, RR 10, T 98.6°F; Ht: 5′6″, Wt 130 lb

Skin

Without lesions, bruising, or discoloration; decreased turgor

HEENT

NC/AT; EOM intact; (−) nystagmus; PERRLA; slightly pale conjunctiva; normal funduscopic exam without retinopathy; TMs intact; deviated nasal septum; no sinus tenderness; several dental caries; native teeth present; oropharynx clear

Neck/LN

Supple without masses; normal thyroid; (−) JVD

Lungs/Thorax

Trachea midline; clear to A & P; breath sounds equal bilaterally

Breasts

Symmetrical bilaterally; without masses or discharge; normal axilla

CV

RRR; PMI at 5th ICS, MCL; (−) bruits, murmurs, S_3 or S_4

Abd

Soft, but tender to palpation; no masses; normal peristalsis; without bruits

Genit/Rect

Normal external female genitalia, uterus, and adnexa; rectal exam (+) stool guaiac

MS/Ext

Spooning of finger nails; (−) CCE; changes consistent with DJD and limited ROM of lower right knee

Neuro

DTR 2+; normal gait

Labs

Na 140 mEq/L	Hgb 9.2 g/dL	WBC 6.5×10^3/mm³	AST 12 IU/L	Ca 9.2 mg/dL
K 4.5 mEq/L	Hct 27.6%	81% Segs	ALT 15 IU/L	Iron 36 μg/dL
Cl 102 mEq/L	RBC 3.4×10^6/mm³	2% Bands	T. bili 0.2 mg/dL	TIBC 705 μg/dL
CO_2 20 mEq/L	MCV 72 μm³	15% Lymphs	LDH 115 IU/L	Transferrin sat 19.6%
BUN 15 mg/dL	MCH 20 pg	1% Monos	T. prot 7.2 g/dL	Ferritin 9.8 ng/mL
SCr 0.7 mg/dL	MCHC 28 g/dL	1% Eos	Alb 4.5 g/dL	Vit. B_{12} 680 pg/mL
Glucose 105 mg/dL	RDW 16.1%		Chol 189 mg/dL	Folic acid 8.2 ng/mL

Other

Peripheral blood smear: hypochromic, microcytic red blood cells (see Figure 88–1).

UA

pH 4.8, SG 1.030, protein (−), glucose (−), ketones (−), RBC 1/lpf, WBC 3/lpf; casts (−)

Assessment

1. Iron deficiency anemia possibly secondary to NSAID-induced gastropathy and heavy menses.
2. DJD of right knee.

Plan

Refer to gastroenterologist.

▶ Clinical Course

Two days later, the patient is seen by a gastroenterologist and undergoes EGD with biopsy. The findings include extensive gastritis with multiple bleeding lesions; negative for *Helicobacter pylori*.

Final assessment: Iron deficiency anemia secondary to NSAID-induced gastritis.

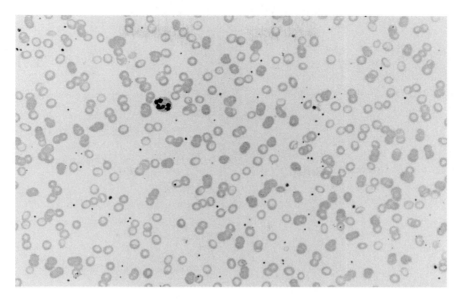

Figure 88–1. Blood smear with hypochromic microcytic red blood cells. *(Wright-Giemsa × 330; photo courtesy of Lydia C. Contis, MD.)*

► Questions

Problem Identification

1. a. *What potential drug-related problems does this patient have?*
   b. *What signs, symptoms, and laboratory findings are consistent with the finding of iron deficiency anemia secondary to blood loss?*
   c. *Could any of the patient's symptoms or laboratory abnormalities be drug-related?*

Desired Outcome

2. *What are the goals of pharmacotherapy for this patient's anemia?*

Therapeutic Alternatives

3. a. *What non-drug therapy may be effective in managing this anemia?*
   b. *What alternative drug therapy could be used to treat this patient's anemia?*

Optimal Plan

4. *Outline an optimal pharmacotherapy plan for this patient.*

Outcome Evaluation

5. *What clinical and laboratory parameters are necessary to evaluate the therapy for achievement of the desired therapeutic outcome and to detect and prevent adverse effects?*

Patient Counseling

6. *What information should be provided to the patient to enhance compliance, ensure successful therapy, and minimize adverse effects?*

► Clinical Course

In addition to the anemia therapy you recommended, Ms. Swingdale is given a prescription for ranitidine 150 mg po BID. Upon her return to the clinic 1 month later for evaluation, she complains of no adverse effects with her medications. At that time, she is instructed to return in 3 months. Laboratory values continue to improve and her next follow-up visit is in 6 months. Laboratory values at 1, 3, and 6 months into therapy are as shown in Table 88–1.

At the 6-month follow-up visit, it was decided to discontinue the anemia treatment.

TABLE 88–1. Laboratory Test Values

Test (units)	1 Month	3 Months	6 Months
RBC count ($\times 10^6/mm^3$)	3.6	4.0	4.3
Hgb (g/dL)	9.9	11.9	14.1
Hct (%)	29.9	35.9	42
MCV (μm^3)	78	86	90
MCH (pg)	24	29	31
MCHC (g/dL)	30	33	34
RDW (%)	15.8	14.9	12.8
Serum iron (μ/dL)	47	79	98
TIBC (μg/dL)	385	380	392
Transferrin sat (%)	24.2	31	42
Ferritin (ng/mL)	69	120	163
Stool guaiac	Negative	Negative	Negative

► Self-study Assignments

1. Make a list of all potential medications that should be avoided within close proximity of iron administration.
2. Perform a literature search to determine the status of the efficacy of ascorbic acid for increasing iron absorption from iron tablets.
3. What monitoring steps should be incorporated into your pharmaceutical care plan to:
   a. Check for recurrence of signs/symptoms of iron deficiency due to her history of heavy menses?
   b. Encourage the patient to avoid future NSAID therapy?
   c. Monitor for recurrence of signs and symptoms of gastropathy?
   d. Monitor for efficacy of new treatment (such as acetaminophen) for her osteoarthritis?

► Clinical Pearl

Therapeutic doses of iron must be given for 3 to 6 months to ensure repletion of all iron stores; the serum ferritin is the best parameter to monitor iron stores after correction of the hemoglobin and hematocrit.

References

1. Middleton E, et al. Studies on the absorption of orally administered iron from sustained release preparations. N Engl J Med 1966;274:136.
2. Bairiel I. Absorption of sustained release iron and the effects of ascorbic acid in normal subjects and after partial gastrectomy. BMJ 1974;4:505–508.
3. Swain RA, Kaplan B, Montgomery E. Iron-deficiency anemia—when is parenteral therapy warranted? Postgrad Med 1996;100:181–185.

89 VITAMIN B₁₂ Deficiency

► Treatment for Life   (Level I)

Barbara J. Mason, PharmD
Beata Saletnik, PharmD

► After completing this case study, students should be able to:

- Recognize the signs, symptoms, and laboratory abnormalities associated with B₁₂ deficiency anemia.
- Select an appropriate dosage regimen for treatment of B₁₂ deficiency anemia.
- Describe monitoring parameters for the initial and subsequent evaluations of patients with B₁₂ deficiency anemia.
- Counsel patients treated with vitamin B₁₂ therapy.

☀ PATIENT PRESENTATION

Chief Complaint
"I've been feeling terrible for a year."

HPI
Larry Wise is a 74 yo man who presents to the Veterans Affairs Medical Center (VAMC) for a routine check-up. Upon questioning he states that he has been feeling weak and terrible for a year now but has not had any weight loss.

PMH
Multiple DVT with resulting chronic venous insufficiency
Type 2 DM
HTN
Prostate cancer, s/p prostatectomy
S/P CVA
Hyperlipidemia
DJD

FH
Positive for DM; father died of stroke.

SH
Retired minister, married; no alcohol or tobacco use; lives near the VAMC and returns for frequent follow-up visits.

ROS
(−) SOB, headache, chest pain, joint pain, polyuria, or polydipsia.

Meds
Docusate sodium 100 mg po BID
Famotidine 20 mg po HS
Glipizide 20 mg po BID
Pravastatin 20 mg po HS
Quinapril 15 mg po QD
Pseudoephedrine 60 mg po QD
Warfarin sodium 5 mg po QD

All
Codeine (rash)

PE

Gen
This is an elderly pleasant Caucasian man in NAD

VS
BP 141/95, P 84; Wt 163 lb, BMI 24.1, Ht 5′9″

SKIN
Color and turgor normal, (−) vitiligo

HEENT
Left eye almost blind, retinal detachment, PERRLA, EOMI, fundi showed no cotton wool exudates; (−) photophobia, (−) glossitis

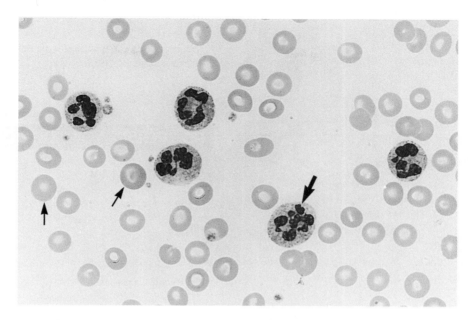

Figure 89–1. Blood smear of enlarged hypersegmented neutrophils, one with eight nuclear lobes (large arrow); and macrocytes (small arrows). *(Wright-Giemsa × 1650; photo courtesy of Lydia C. Contis, MD.)*

Neck

Supple, no lymphadenopathy or thyromegaly

Lungs

Bilateral BS, no wheezes or crackles

CV

RRR; III/VI systolic murmur heard best at the right sternal border; no rubs

Abd

Soft, non-tender, no masses, (+) bowel sounds

Ext

No lower leg edema, no warmth or pain, (−) paresthesias

Rectal

Good sphincter tone, guaiac (−) stool

Neuro

A & O × 3, CN right visual field intact, hearing intact, slight left facial weakness, sensory—decreased pinprick on right LE and UE, propriocep-

tion intact bilaterally, coordination intact, decreased vibratory sensation LE, (−) ataxia

Labs

Na 140 mEq/L	Hgb 11.3 g/dL	Retic (corr) 0.4%	AST 19 IU/L
K 4.2 mEq/L	Hct 33.5%	Iron 85 μg/dL	ALT 13 IU/L
Cl 106 mEq/L	RBC 3.95×10^6/mm^3	Ferritin 48 ng/mL	Alk Phos 77 IU/L
CO_2 24 mEq/L	Plt 221×10^3/mm^3	Transferrin 250 mg/dL	T. Chol 201 mg/dL
BUN 13 mg/dL	WBC 5.8×10^3/mm^3	Direct Coombs' (−)	LDL-chol 116 mg/dL
SCr 1.2 mg/dL	MCV 84.8 μm^3	EPO 26 Units/L	RBC folate 247 ng/mL
Glu 238 mg/dL	MCH 28.6 pg	B_{12} 177 pg/mL	TSH 2.93 μIU/mL
	MCHC 33.8 g/dL	INR 3.5	HbA$_{1c}$ 8.4%

Other

Peripheral blood smear shows anisocytosis, poikilocytosis, giant platelets, hypersegmented neutrophils, and macrocytic red blood cells with megaloblastic changes (see Figure 89–1).

Assessment

Cobalamin deficiency; mild hypoproliferative anemia secondary to pelvic XRT and/or prostate metastatic to marrow

---

▶ Questions

Problem Identification

1. a. *Create a drug-related problem list for this patient.*
   b. *What information indicates the presence or severity of the B_{12} deficiency?*
   c. *Could the B_{12} deficiency have been caused by drug therapy?*
   d. *What additional information is needed to assess this patient's B_{12} deficiency?*

Desired Outcome

2. *What are the goals of pharmacotherapy in this case?*

Therapeutic Alternatives

3. a. *What non-drug therapies might be useful for this patient?*
   b. *What feasible pharmacotherapeutic alternatives are available for treatment of the B_{12} deficiency?*

Optimal Plan

4. *What drug, dosage form, dose, schedule, and duration of therapy are best for this patient?*

Outcome Evaluation

5. *What clinical and laboratory parameters are necessary to evaluate the therapy for achievement of the desired therapeutic outcome and to detect or prevent adverse effects?*

Patient Counseling

6. *What information should be provided to the patient to enhance compliance, ensure successful therapy, and minimize adverse effects?*

► Follow-up Question

1. *If this patient had been taking the H_2-receptor antagonist (famotidine) for a documented history of gastritis, how might that have related to vitamin B_{12} deficiency?*

► Self-study Assignments

1. Defend the argument that all patients at risk for vitamin B_{12} deficiency should be put on monthly vitamin B_{12} injections rather than periodically monitoring laboratory tests to identify B_{12} deficiency. Have a debate with a classmate who defends the opposite point of view.
2. Describe the potential relationship between vitamin B_{12} deficiency and premature cerebrovascular disease, peripheral and coronary vascular disease, and ventricular dysfunction.
3. What is the rationale for screening for iron deficiency in patients with pernicious anemia?

► Clinical Pearl

Patients with inconclusive evidence of B_{12} deficiency (e.g., low serum vitamin B_{12} levels, nonspecific symptoms, and normal hemoglobin) may merit treatment for a few months; a positive symptomatic response suggests that vitamin B_{12} deficiency was the underlying cause.

References

1. Carmel R. Pernicious anemia: The expected findings of very low serum cobalamin levels, anemia, and macrocytosis are often lacking. Arch Intern Med 1988; 148:1712–1714.
2. Metz J, Bell A, Flicker L, Bottligliera T, et al. The significance of subnormal serum vitamin B_{12} concentration in older people: A case control study. J Am Geriatr Soc 1996;44:1355–1361.
3. Reisner E Jr, Weiner L, Schittone M, et al. Oral treatment of pernicious anemia with Vitamin B_{12} without intrinsic factor. N Engl J Med 1955;253:502–506.
4. Thompson R, Ashby D, Armstrong E. Long-term trial of oral vitamin B_{12} in pernicious anemia. Lancet 1962;2:577–579.

90 FOLIC ACID DEFICIENCY

► The Piano Man   (Level I)

Beata Saletnik, PharmD
Barbara J. Mason, PharmD

► After completing this case study, students should be able to:

- Identify the potential concurrent risks that may facilitate the development of folic acid deficiency (e.g., medications, concurrent disease states, dietary habits).
- Recommend appropriate treatment guidelines for folic acid deficiency anemia.
- Counsel patients with folic acid deficiency to appropriately use pharmacologic and non-pharmacologic therapies to correct their deficiency.
- Understand the relevant parameters that need to be assessed to evaluate the outcomes of therapy.

☼ PATIENT PRESENTATION

Chief Complaint
"I have been more irritable and restless lately."

HPI
Kenneth Johnson is a 90 yo man with a long history of bipolar disorder who presents to his retirement group meeting at the mental health clinic with the above complaint. He states that he has been waking up frequently at night, dreaming about the past. He also reports the presence of visual hallucinations and racing thoughts.

PMH
Bipolar disorder; on lithium in the past with lithium toxicity about 1 year ago
BPH; s/p TURP 11 years ago
Osteoarthritis
Mild memory loss
Questionable compliance with medications in the past

SH
Retired; lives with girlfriend; enjoys singing and playing the piano at senior centers; no alcohol or tobacco.

Meds

Acetaminophen 325 mg, 2 po Q 6 H PRN
Ascorbic acid 250 mg po BID
Docusate sodium 100 mg po BID
Prazosin 1 mg po BID
Divalproex 500 mg po BID with food

All

NKDA

ROS

(+) Right knee pain; (−) glossitis, paresthesias, or muscle weakness.

PE

Gen

Elderly Caucasian man, appears younger than stated age of 90, cooperative, oriented × 3, slight rambling speech, easily redirectable

VS

BP 165/82, P 59, RR 18, T 96.3°F

Skin

Seborrheic keratoses over back area

HEENT

NC/AT; actinic keratoses on face, PERRLA, EOMI, probable immature cataract left eye, decreased hearing bilaterally, decreased movement through left nostril, dentures present, (−) glossitis

Neck

Normal motion of the neck; trachea in midline; thyroid normal size; no bruit, masses, or other abnormalities

Thorax

Lungs normal to inspection and CTA

CV

RRR without murmur

Abd

NT/ND, bowel tones (+)

Ext

Enlarged ankles bilaterally, distal portion right index finger disfigured, right knee enlarged with decreased ROM; (−) paresthesias, (−) ataxia

Neuro

CN II–XII grossly intact; muscle strength in LE equal bilaterally; decreased in LUE compared to RUE; DTRs absent in LE bilaterally; vibratory sense normal

Labs

Na 142 mEq/L	Hgb 12.8 g/dL	MCV 97.4 μm^3	AST 16 IU/L
K 4.0 mEq/L	Hct 38.4%	MCH 32.6 pg	ALT 7 IU/L
Cl 112 mEq/L	RBC $3.94 \times 10^6/mm^3$	MCHC 33.5 g/dL	Alk Phos 87 IU/L
CO_2 27 mEq/L	Plt $216 \times 10^3/mm^3$	Vitamin B_{12} 221 pg/mL	T. bili 0.4 mg/dL
BUN 24 mg/dL	WBC $4.99 \times 10^3/mm^3$	RBC Folate 33 ng/mL	Alb 3.3 g/dL
SCr 1.1 mg/dL	Serum Iron 67 μg/L		
Glu 93 mg/dL	RDW 12.8%		

▶ Questions

Problem Identification

1. a. What drug-related problems exist in this patient?
   b. What signs, symptoms, and laboratory values indicate this patient has anemia secondary to folate deficiency?
   c. Could the patient's folate deficiency have been caused by drug therapy?
   d. What additional information is needed to satisfactorily assess this patient?
   e. Why is it important to differentiate folate deficiency from vitamin B_{12} deficiency, and how is this accomplished?

Desired Outcome

2. What are the goals of pharmacotherapy for this patient's anemia?

Therapeutic Alternatives

3. a. What non-drug therapies may be used to correct this patient's folic acid deficiency?
   b. What pharmacotherapeutic alternatives are available for the treatment of this patient's anemia?
   c. What economic or psychosocial issues are applicable to this patient and may contribute to the development of folic acid deficiency?

Optimal Plan

4. What is the most appropriate drug, dosage form, dose, schedule, and duration of therapy for the resolution of this patient's anemia?

Outcome Evaluation

5. What parameters should be used to evaluate the efficacy and adverse effects of folic acid replacement therapy in this patient?

Patient Counseling

6. What information would you provide to this patient about his folic acid replacement therapy?

▶ Self-study Assignments

1. Discuss the controversy associated with the fortification of food with folic acid.
2. What is the dual interaction between phenytoin and folic acid, and how should this interaction be managed?
3. What is the role of folic acid and homocysteine in the development of cardiovascular disease?

► Clinical Pearl

Folate deficiency is often a manifestation of acute, chronic alcoholism due to poor dietary intake and the impairment of enterohepatic recycling of folate secondary to toxic effects of alcohol on hepatic parenchymal cells.

References

1. Lewis DP, Van Dyke DC, Willhite LA, et al. Phenytoin–folic acid interaction. Ann Pharmacother 1995;29:726–735.
2. Tucker KL, Mahnken B, Wilson PW, et al. Folic acid fortification of the food supply: Potential benefits and risks for the elderly population. JAMA 1996;276:1879–1885.
3. Campbell NR. How safe are folic acid supplements? Arch Intern Med 1996;156:1638–1644.
4. Swain RA, St. Clair L. The role of folic acid in deficiency states and prevention of disease. J Fam Pract 1997;44:138–144.

91 SICKLE CELL ANEMIA

► One Crisis After Another   (Level I)

R. Donald Harvey III, PharmD, BCPS
Celeste C. Lindley, PharmD, MS, FASHP, FCCP, BCPS

► After completing this case study, students should be able to:

- Recognize the clinical characteristics associated with an acute sickle cell crisis.
- Recommend optimal analgesic therapy based on patient-specific information.
- Identify optimal end points of pharmacotherapy in sickle cell anemia patients.
- Discuss the role of erythropoietin in sickle cell anemia.
- Recommend treatment that may reduce the frequency of sickle cell crises.

☀ PATIENT PRESENTATION

Chief Complaint
"My arms, legs, and back have been hurting for two days."

HPI
Jennifer Davis is a 23-year-old African-American woman with sickle cell anemia who presents with a 2-day history of pain localized to her arms, legs, and back. Her pain has been unrelieved by 2 oxycodone/acetaminophen tablets taken every 6 hours. Currently she rates her pain intensity at 9 out of 10. She is 12 weeks' pregnant with her first child.

PMH
Sickle cell anemia diagnosed at age 9 months. She has approximately 5 to 10 crises per year requiring hospitalization.
Chronic renal insufficiency secondary to rhabdomyolysis from toxic shock syndrome 1 year prior to admission.
Lack of endogenous erythropoietin production.
Osteomyelitis of the right great toe 2 months prior to admission.
Coagulase negative staphylococcal bacteremia 5 months prior to admission.
Endocarditis 2 years prior to admission.
Left foot drop and deformity secondary to neurologic damage sustained during admission for toxic shock syndrome.

FH
Mother and father alive and well, both with sickle cell trait. Two sisters also with sickle cell trait.

SH
Currently unemployed, separated from her husband, lives at home with her mother and father.

ROS
Denies cough, fever, shortness of breath, or chest pain.

Meds
Folic acid 1 mg po QD
Ferrous sulfate 325 mg po TID
Erythropoietin 4000 U SC M,W, F (begun 6 weeks prior to admission)
Percocet 1–2 tablets Q 6 H PRN

All
Penicillin (hives)
Morphine (reported as hallucinations)

PE

Gen
She is a thin, well-developed African-American woman in moderate distress

VS
BP 123/48, P 90, RR 17, T 37.3°C; 54 kg, O_2 sat 100% on 2 liters O_2

HEENT
PERRL, EOMI, oral mucosa soft and moist; normal sclerae and funduscopic exam

Skin
Normal turgor, no rashes or cellulitis noted

Neck
Supple, no lymphadenopathy or thyromegaly

CV
RRR, II/VI SEM, no rubs or gallops

Lungs
CTA bilaterally

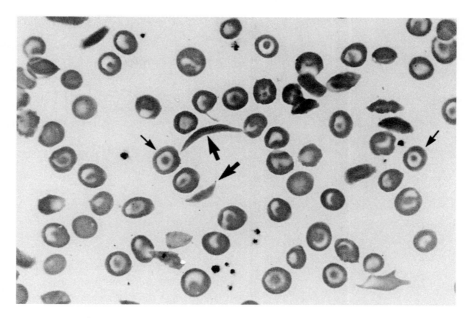

Figure 91–1. Peripheral blood with sickle cells (large arrows) and target cells (small arrows). *(Wright-Giemsa × 1650; photo courtesy of Lydia C. Contis, MD.)*

Abd

Hypoactive bowel sounds; soft, NT/ND; no hepatomegaly, splenomegaly, or masses

Ext

Pulses 2+ bilaterally, no edema or ulcers, right great toe slightly enlarged

Neuro

A & O × 3; normal strength, reflexes intact

Labs

Na 137 mEq/L	Hgb 4.1 g/dL	AST 21 IU/L	Ca 8.6 mg/dL
K 4.4 mEq/L	Hct 11.5%	ALT 11 IU/L	Mg 1.8 mEq/L
Cl 108 mEq/L	Plt 223 × 10³/mm³	Alk Phos 77 IU/L	Phos 3.5 mg/dL
CO₂ 18 mEq/L	WBC 9.6 × 10³/mm³	LDH 957 IU/L	(+) anti-E red cell antibody
BUN 18 mg/dL	MCV 88 μm³	T. bili 0.9 mg/dL	
SCr 2 mg/dL	Retic 4.1%	Alb 3.5 g/dL	
Glu 81 mg/dL			

Other

EPO <5 mIU/mL (normal > 25) (obtained 2 months prior to admission)
Peripheral blood smear: sickle forms present, Howell–Jolly bodies present (see Figure 91–1).

Chest X-ray

Clear

ECG

Normal sinus rhythm

Echocardiogram

Normal LV function; mild TR, MR

Assessment

A 23-year-old, 12 weeks' pregnant African-American woman in sickle cell crisis.

► Questions

Problem Identification

1. a. *Create a list of the patient's drug-related problems.*
   b. *What signs, symptoms, and laboratory values are consistent with an acute sickle cell crisis in this patient?*
   c. *What additional information is needed to satisfactorily assess this patient?*

Desired Outcome

2. *What are the goals of pharmacotherapy in this case?*

Therapeutic Alternatives

3. a. *What non-drug therapies might be useful for this patient?*
   b. *What feasible pharmacotherapeutic alternatives are available for treatment of the patient's pain and chronic anemia?*

Optimal Plan

4. *Outline a detailed therapeutic plan to treat all facets of this patient's acute sickle cell crisis. For all drug therapies, include the dosage form, dose, schedule, and duration of therapy.*

Outcome Evaluation

5. *a. What clinical and laboratory parameters are necessary to evaluate therapy for achievement of the desired therapeutic outcome and to detect or prevent adverse effects?*

▶ Clinical Course

The plans you recommended have been initiated and on the second day of hospitalization the patient's pain is markedly improved. It is discovered that the patient's hemoglobin and hematocrit were 4.6 g/dL and 13.3% 2 months prior to admission. An erythropoietin concentration will be obtained upon return to the clinic 1 week after discharge.

b. Considering this information, what changes (if any) in the pharmacotherapeutic plan are warranted?

Patient Counseling

6. *What information should be provided to the patient to enhance compliance, ensure successful therapy, and minimize adverse effects?*

▶ Follow-up Question

1. *What therapies may be effective in reducing the frequency of crises in this patient who presently has up to 10 episodes per year?*

▶ Self-study Assignments

1. Determine the likelihood of the patient's offspring having sickle cell trait and/or disease if the father has:
   a. Normal hemoglobin
   b. Sickle cell trait
   c. Sickle cell disease
2. Describe the complications associated with frequent crises in each organ system.
3. Discuss the role of prophylactic antibiotics in the management of sickle cell anemia.

▶ Clinical Pearl

Allogeneic bone marrow transplantation has proven curative in pediatric sickle cell anemia patients. Approximately 20% of patients have a matched sibling donor, and matches may also be found through the National Marrow Donor Program.

References

1. King KE, Ness PM. Treating anemia. Hematol Oncol Clin North Am 1996;10:1305–1320.
2. El-Shafei AM, Dhaliwal JK, Sandhu AK, et al. Indications for blood transfusion in pregnancy with sickle cell disease. Aust NZ J Obstet Gynecol 1995;35:405–408.
3. Howard RJ. Management of sickling conditions in pregnancy. Br J Hosp Med 1996;56:7–10.
4. Tang R, Shimomura SK, Rotblatt M. Meperidine-induced seizures in sickle cell patients. Hosp Formul 1980;15:764–772.
5. Bourantas K, Makrydimas G, Georgiou J, et al. Preliminary results with administration of recombinant human erythropoietin in sickle cell/β-thalassemia patients during pregnancy. Eur J Haematol 1996;56:326–328.

PART THREE

Diseases of Infectious Origin

Joseph T. DiPiro, PharmD, FCCP, Section Editor

92 USING LABORATORY TESTS IN INFECTIOUS DISEASES

▶ **No More Vanco for Me** (Level I)

Steven J. Martin, PharmD, BCPS

▶ After completing this case study, students should be able to:

- Discuss the use of minimum inhibitory concentrations (MICs) and minimum bactericidal concentrations (MBCs) in antimicrobial agent selection and dosing for specific bacterial pathogens.

- Identify infections for which bactericidal concentrations of antimicrobial agents are required.

- Outline the interpretation of checkerboard synergy testing.

- Describe the appropriate serum sampling times for SBT testing, including mono- and combination-antimicrobial regimens.

☀ PATIENT PRESENTATION

Chief Complaint
"My back pain is getting worse and I have a bit of a fever."

HPI
Wilma Freeman is a 59 yo woman who has been admitted to the neurosurgery service at the University Medical Center with complaints of worsening back pain and a low-grade fever. Five months PTA, she developed severe back pain and was found to have an epidural abscess over the lumbar area. *Staphylococcus aureus* (methicillin-resistant) was cultured sequentially from her blood, and she was treated with 6 weeks of IV vancomycin therapy. During the third week of vancomycin, she developed a raised, red, blotchy rash over most of her body that ultimately led to desquamation of the outer dermal layer on her anterior torso, shoulders, face, neck, and all 4 extremities. A dermal biopsy showed toxic epidermal necrolysis, thought to be secondary to vancomycin. She was given corticosteroids both topically and systemically, and she continued the vancomycin therapy to completion.

PMH
Asthma
HTN
CAD
S/P cholecystitis
S/P pneumonia × 2 in the past
Surgical history includes a cholecystectomy, hysterectomy, and hemorrhoidectomy

FH
Her mother is deceased secondary to breast cancer (age 53); father is deceased secondary to MI (age 67). She has one daughter, age 27.

SH
Married housewife, living at home with husband; no alcohol, tobacco, or illicit drug use.

ROS
(+) lower back pain and difficulty walking; (−) chest pain, SOB, wheezing, abdominal pain, or tenderness; (−) difficulty with urination or bowel movements; (−) skin eruptions, rashes, or other skin damage.

Meds

Propranolol 20 mg po BID

Premarin 0.9 mg po Q AM

Diphenhydramine 50 mg po TID

Nitroglycerin SR 6.5 mg po Q 8 H

Nitroglycerin 0.4 mg SL PRN

Temazepam 30 mg po Q HS

Naproxen sodium 550 mg po BID

Acetaminophen 650 mg with codeine 30 mg 1–2 tablets po QID PRN

All

Vancomycin (rash and desquamation)

Penicillin (rash and hives)

Cephalexin (rash, hives, and difficulty breathing)

Sulfa-containing products (rash)

PE

Gen

The patient is an obese woman in considerable pain and mild distress. She experienced several chills during the examination.

VS

BP 134/78, P 102, RR 22, T 100.4°F, Wt 113.3 kg, Ht 5′6″

Skin

Warm and slightly diaphoretic

HEENT

NC/AT; PERRLA; conjunctiva pink; sclerae clear; EOMI; disk margins sharp, no arteriolar narrowing, A-V nicking, hemorrhages, or exudates; ear canals clear and drums negative; good auditory acuity; nares normal; teeth intact, tongue midline and negative, tonsils intact and normal, pharynx negative

Neck/LN

Trachea midline, thyroid palpable, no nodes

Chest

CTA bilaterally, no added sounds

CV

RRR, normal S_1 and S_2, no heaves, thrills, or bruits

Abd

Obese but symmetrical; soft, non-distended; no masses or tenderness; liver, spleen, and kidneys not felt; no CVA tenderness

Back

A 3.5×5.5 cm area over the superior lumbar spine was tender to touch; no abscess

Genit/Rect

Not performed

MS/Ext

Full ROM in all 4 extremities, no muscle weakness perceived

Neuro

Mental status intact; CN II–XII intact; motor 5/5 in both upper extremities, 4/5 over both legs secondary to pain; no sensory deficits; reflexes normal; plantars downgoing; cerebellar—no dysmetria; no neck rigidity

Labs

Na 138 mEq/L	Hgb 12.7 g/dL	WBC $11.4 \times 10^3/mm^3$	RDW 15%
K 4.1 mEq/L	Hct 38.4%	68% Neutros	ESR 26 mm/hr
Cl 100 mEq/L	RBC $4.7 \times 10^6/mm^3$	9% Bands	PT 11.6 sec
CO_2 26 mEq/L	MCV 81.8 μm^3	16% Lymphs	aPTT 28.1 sec
BUN 11 mg/dL	MCH 27.1 pg	7% Monos	
SCr 0.9 mg/dL	MCHC 33.1 g/dL		
Glu 116 mg/dL	Plt $255 \times 10^3/mm^3$		

Assessment

R/O recurrence of spinal abscess

R/O vertebral osteomyelitis

Plan

Collect 2 sets of blood cultures (anaerobic and aerobic) from 2 separate sites

Obtain an MRI of the spine to determine the presence of infection in the bone

---

▶ Questions

Problem Identification

1. a. *Create a list of this patient's drug-related problems.*
   b. *What subjective and objective data indicate the presence of infection?*

Desired Outcome

2. *What are the desired treatment goals for this patient's current medical problems?*

▶ Clinical Course

The patient is emotional in refusing vancomycin therapy. She is reluctant to try any antimicrobial therapy until a definitive diagnosis is made. On the day after admission, the microbiology laboratory identifies *S. aureus* from both sets of blood cultures (aerobic and anaerobic bottles). Preliminary susceptibility testing reveals the following information (Table 92–1).

Therapeutic Alternatives

3. a. *The microbiology laboratory provided both a minimum inhibitory concentration (MIC) and an interpretation of that MIC for each antimicrobial agent tested. How are the MIC and the interpretation correlated?*

TABLE 92–1. Preliminary Susceptibility Testing Results

Antibiotic	Interpretation	MIC (μg/mL)
Cephalothin	R	> 32
Clindamycin	R	> 4
Erythromycin	R	> 8
Gentamicin	S	4
Ampicillin	R	≥ 32
Penicillin	R	≥ 4
Oxacillin	R	≥ 4
Rifampin	S	1
Tetracycline	I	8
Ciprofloxacin	R	≥ 4
Trimethoprim-sulfamethoxazole	S	≤ 2/38
Vancomycin	S	4
Quinupristin/dalfopristin[a]	S	2

[a] Investigational at the time of this writing.

b. *Should the laboratory be asked to provide minimum bactericidal concentration (MBC) data for these antibiotics? If so, how would those data be of value in selecting antimicrobial therapy?*

c. *What additional testing should be performed in the microbiology laboratory to provide information that might be helpful in choosing antimicrobial therapy for this patient? How should this information be interpreted?*

Optimal Plan

4. *The patient was started on quinupristin/dalfopristin 850 mg IV Q 8 H after meeting criteria for compassionate use from the drug's manufacturer. In addition, she was started on rifampin 300 mg po Q 12 H.*

Outcome Evaluation

5. a. *Determination of serum concentrations for either of these antibiotics is not readily available. What other laboratory testing could be used to determine more precisely the efficacy of this regimen in vivo? How is it interpreted? What is the pharmacist's role in performing this test?*

b. *Outline a follow-up plan for monitoring the efficacy of this therapeutic regimen.*

▶ Self-study Assignments

1. What combination of antimicrobial agents is likely to demonstrate additive effects or synergy *in vitro* against gram-positive bacteria? Gram-negative bacteria?

2. When should the microbiology laboratory be asked *not* to report results of susceptibility testing? What role does the pharmacist play in this situation?

▶ Clinical Pearl

The pharmacist often plays the role of data manager, coordinating the efforts of the microbiology laboratory, the infectious disease or other medical subspecialties, the nursing staff, the patient, and the pharmacy department to ensure maximum benefit from drug therapy.

References

1. National Committee for Clinical Laboratory Standards. Performance Standards for Antimicrobial Disk Susceptibility Tests, 6th ed. Approved Standard. NCCLS, 940 West Valley Road, Suite 1400, Wayne, PA 19087-1898, 1997.
2. Dworkin R, Modin G, Kunz S, et al. Comparative efficacies of ciprofloxacin, pefloxacin, and vancomycin in combination with rifampin in a rat model of methicillin-resistant *Staphylococcus aureus* chronic osteomyelitis. Antimicrob Agents Chemother 1990;34:1014–1016.
3. National Committee for Clinical Laboratory Standards. Methodology for the Serum Bactericidal Test: Tentative Guideline. NCCLS document M21-T (ISBN 1-56238-143-1) NCLS, 771 East Lancaster Avenue, Villanova, PA 19085, 1992.

93 BACTERIAL MENINGITIS

▶ Trouble on Day One   (Level II)

Sherry Luedtke, PharmD

▶ After completing this case study, students should be able to:

- Identify risk factors and common presenting signs and symptoms of bacterial meningitis in infants.
- Differentiate common bacterial pathogens associated with bacterial meningitis in newborns versus older children and adults.
- Recommend appropriate empiric antimicrobial therapy for bacterial meningitis in infants.
- Identify appropriate parameters for monitoring antimicrobial therapy for treatment of bacterial meningitis in infants.

☀ PATIENT PRESENTATION

Chief Complaint
Unobtainable.

HPI
Jason is a 37-week gestation, 3504 g infant male with respiratory distress. He was delivered via spontaneous vaginal delivery to a 25 yo G_1P_1 Caucasian woman. The delivery was uncomplicated with initial Apgar scores of 9/9. The infant was transferred to normal nursery with some mild grunting and retracting that required supplemental oxygen for the first 2 hours of life. He was later taken to the mother to feed. Six hours later, he developed

tachypnea, grunting, retracting, and became hypotensive. Two boluses of 10 mL/kg NS were administered with little improvement in perfusion. He was placed on dopamine, blood cultures were drawn, antibiotics were initiated, and he was transferred to a nearby neonatal intensive care unit.

Maternal History

Uncomplicated prenatal course and delivery. Premature rupture of the membranes for 41 hours prior to delivery. Rubella immune, HbsAg (−), GBS (−), RPR (−). Maternal meds: prenatal vitamins, iron supplement. Mother denies alcohol use, tobacco, and use of illicit drugs.

Meds

Ampicillin 350 mg IV Q 12 H (200 mg/kg/day)
Cefotaxime 174 mg IV Q 12 H (50 mg/kg/dose)
Dopamine 5 μg/kg/min

PE

Gen

Appears to be large, a well-developed male newborn, with dusky undertones and tachypnea on oxygen hood

VS

BP 85/37, HR 148, RR 77, T 98.2°F; Wt 3504 g; length 53 cm; HC 34.7 cm

Skin

Grayish-pink color

HEENT

No nasal flaring, sutures overriding (Note: open/bulging sutures or "pulsatile" sutures may be seen in some cases, which is indicative of elevated cerebrospinal fluid pressure.)

Neck/LN

Clavicles intact

Chest

Lungs clear bilaterally; chest wall rise is symmetrical; there is grunting and mild intercostal retractions

CV

RRR, grade I/VI systolic murmur LLSB

Abd

Soft, distended, (+) BS, liver 1 cm below RCM, 3 vessel cord (Note: 2-vessel umbilical cords in neonates are associated with an increased incidence of other congenital anomalies, such as cleft palate and heart defects.)

GU/Rect

Normal uncircumcised external genitalia, testes descended; rectal midline, patent anus

Ext

20 digits, brachial pulses palpable, capillary refill > 4 sec

Neuro

Mildly hypotonic, responds to stimuli

Labs

		WBC Differential	CBG	
Na 138 mEq/L	Hgb 18.7 g/dL	8% Neutros	pH 7.26	Ca 8.3 mg/dL
K 3.9 mEq/L	Hct 54.7%	13% Bands	po_2 57.3 mm Hg	T. bili 2.2 mg/dL
Cl 109 mEq/L	Plt 297 × 10³/mm³	76% Lymphs	pco_2 29.6 mm Hg	
CO_2 21 mEq/L	WBC 3.2 × 10³/mm³	1% Eos	HCO_3 25.2 mEq/L	
SCr 1.3 mg/dL		2% Basos	BE −2.9 mEq/L	
Glu 103 mg/dL				

Other

Urine and CSF serology: *H. influenzae* type B (−), *S. pneumoniae* (−), Group B Streptococcus (+), *N. meningitis* (−), *N. meningitis* B/*E. coli* (−) CSF chemistry/cell count: color/appearance hazy, glucose 40 mg/dL, protein 281 mg/dL, WBC 306/mm³ (5% Lymphs, 62% Monos, 33% Neutros), RBC 16/mm³

Cultures

Blood, urine, CSF pending

Chest X-ray

Minimal interstitial prominence suggesting retained lung fluid

Assessment

1. Group B streptococcus meningitis
2. Hypoperfusion
3. Metabolic acidosis
4. Neutropenia

▶ Questions

Problem Identification

1. a. *What drug-related problems does this infant have?*
   b. *What risk factors does this patient have for bacterial meningitis?*
   c. *What clinical findings indicate the presence of meningitis and its severity?*
   d. *Is there any drug-related therapy that may have prevented the infection?*

Desired Outcome

2. *What are the goals of drug therapy in this situation?*

Therapeutic Alternatives

3. a. *What non-drug therapies might be useful in this patient?*
   b. *Describe the antimicrobial alternatives available for the management of meningitis in this patient.*

▶ **Clinical Course**

Blood cultures returned positive for group B streptococcus. CSF cultures (drawn after antibiotics were initiated) were negative and urine cultures were positive for group B streptococcus. Sensitivity studies revealed an MIC < 0.12 µg/mL to ampicillin.

Optimal Plan

4. *Given this new information, what therapy would you recommend for the management of this infant?*

Outcome Evaluation

5. *Describe the monitoring parameters necessary to evaluate the efficacy and safety of the therapy.*

▶ **Clinical Course**

The infant was treated with the regimen you recommended, and his perfusion, muscle tone, respiratory distress, and metabolic acidosis improved within the first 24 hours of treatment. Supplemental oxygen was removed at that time. Forty-eight hours after initiation of antibiotic therapy, a repeat CBC showed completed resolution of the infant's leukopenia. A repeat lumbar puncture performed on day 5 of therapy was clear. The patient was discharged on day 7 of therapy to receive an additional 7 days as an outpatient. Audiometry testing performed after completion of antibiotic therapy was normal. The child had no evidence of neurologic impairment due to the infection at follow-up evaluations.

▶ **Self-study Assignments**

1. Review the recommendations for early-onset group B streptococcal prophylaxis in infants.
2. Discuss the role of the erythrocyte sedimentation rate and C-reactive protein measurements in the evaluation of sepsis and meningitis in infants.
3. Describe the management of SIADH in infants with meningitis.

▶ **Clinical Pearl**

Infants may become colonized and/or infected with group B streptococcus despite negative maternal group B streptococcal cultures.

References

1. Feigin RD, McCracken GH Jr, Klein JO. Diagnosis and management of meningitis. Pediatr Infect Dis J 1992;11:785–814.
2. American Academy of Pediatrics Committee on Infectious Diseases and Committee on Fetus and Newborn. Revised guidelines for prevention of early-onset group B streptococcal (GBS) infection. Pediatrics 1997;99:489–496.
3. Gerdes JS, Polin RA. Sepsis screen in neonates with evaluation of plasma fibronectin. Pediatr Infect Dis J 1987;6:443–446.
4. Taketomo CK, Hodding JH, Kraus DM. Pediatric Dosage Handbook, 3rd ed. Hudsen, OH, Lexi-Comp, 1996.

94 COMMUNITY-ACQUIRED PNEUMONIA

▶ **Vern's Visit to the Hospital**   (Level I)

Patrick P. Gleason, PharmD, BCPS

▶ After completing this case study, students should be able to:

- Recognize the common signs and symptoms of community-acquired pneumonia.
- Establish the goals of pharmacotherapy and monitoring parameters for a patient with community-acquired pneumonia.
- Know which pathogens are commonly associated with community-acquired pneumonia.
- Be able to recommend an effective and economical antimicrobial regimen including specific antimicrobial agent(s), route of administration, and dose(s).
- Identify the patient parameters associated with clinical stability in order to convert from IV to oral antimicrobial therapy.

☀ PATIENT PRESENTATION

Chief Complaint
"My cough is getting worse, and now it hurts."

HPI
Vern Johnson is a 28 yo man who presents with a 2-day history of left-sided pleuritic chest pain, dyspnea, orthopnea, intermittent fever and chills, and a cough productive of yellow sputum, which became brown yesterday. The pleuritic chest pain radiates to the proximal LUE during coughing. He experienced no nausea but did have one episode of emesis yesterday. He also states that he had one episode of rhinorrhea this morning and had a sore throat, which has now resolved.

PMH
Asthma since childhood, which is under good control despite the fact that he ran out of his albuterol inhaler and has not been using it for some time.

FH
Positive for HTN and negative for CAD, asthma, DM, and cancer

SH
Patient denies tobacco or drug use. Denies having received a blood transfusion. Reports occasional alcohol use.

ROS

In addition to the findings reported in the HPI, he is currently experiencing a mild headache and reports intermittent headaches, occasional dysuria, and a decreased appetite. He reports normal BMs without blood and noted no blood in his emesis. He reports no dysphagia, weakness, or any known infectious contacts.

Meds

Albuterol inhaler PRN (not used for an undetermined period of time)

All

NKDA; patient reports seasonal allergies

PE

Gen

This is a well-developed, thin, African-American man lying in bed; tachypneic but does not appear to be uncomfortable

VS

BP 100/60, P 120, RR 24, T 37.3°C

Skin

Warm, dry

HEENT

NC/AT; EOMI; PERRLA; hearing is intact to finger rub on the right and grossly intact on the left. Nose is without discharge. Oropharynx is benign with no obvious mucosal lesions, although the tongue does deviate slightly to the right.

Neck/LN

Neck is supple and without adenopathy or thyromegaly

Lungs/Thorax

The right side is CTA. The LUL is CTA with significantly decreased breath sounds. There are E-to-A changes in the LLL and across the middle of the right lung field.

CV

Tachycardic and regular; no murmurs appreciated

Abd

Normoactive BS; soft; NT except at the upper border of the LUQ near the site of the patient's pleuritic chest pain

Genit/Rect

Deferred

MS/Ext

Strength is 4–5/5 throughout and symmetrical. Pulses are 1+ bilaterally

Neuro

A & O × 3; CNs II–XII intact; DTRs 2+; Babinski (−)

Labs

Na 142 mEq/mL	Hgb 14.2 g/dL	Ca 8.2 mEq/L
K 3.7 mEq/mL	Hct 42%	Mg 1.3 mEq/L
Cl 99 mEq/ml	WBC $14.7 \times 10^3/mm^3$	Phos 2.7 mg/dL
CO_2 20 mEq/L	72% Neutros	CPK 256 IU/L
BUN 7 mg/dL	12% Bands	
SCr 0.9 mg/dL	14% Lymphs	
Glu 126 mg/dL	2% Monos	

UA

Hazy urine; SG 1.018, pH 5.0, protein > 300 mg/dL, trace ketones, moderate blood, 2 WBC/hpf, 4 RBC/hpf, no bacteria

Chest X-ray

Consolidation of the inferior segments of the LLL as well as the superior segment of the LLL. Remainder of the lungs are clear. Heart size is WNL.

Sputum Gram Stain

Many WBC, few epithelial cells, moderate gram-positive cocci in chains and pairs.

Sputum and Blood Cultures

Pending

Assessment

1. LLL pneumonia, probably pneumococcal.
2. Urine (+) for protein and ketones with elevated CPK of uncertain etiology.

▶ Questions

Problem Identification

1. a. Create a list of the patient's drug-related problems.
    b. What information (signs, symptoms, laboratory and other diagnostic tests) indicate the presence of community-acquired pneumonia?
    c. What signs and symptoms indicate the severity of community-acquired pneumonia in this patient?
    d. What additional information is needed to satisfactorily assess this patient?

Desired Outcome

2. What are the goals of pharmacotherapy in this case?

Therapeutic Alternatives

3. What feasible pharmacotherapeutic alternatives are available for treatment of community-acquired pneumonia?

Optimal Plan

4. a. What drug, dosage form, dose, schedule, and duration of therapy are best for this patient?

► Clinical Course

The patient was admitted and treated with the single-drug antimicrobial regimen you recommended. He continued to have fevers to 40°C for 48 hours after treatment was initiated. A thoracentesis was performed because of new small bilateral layering pleural effusions; the results disclosed a peripneumonic effusion. Attempts to place a drainage catheter were unsuccessful.

   b. *What changes in the antimicrobial therapy would you recommend, since the initial treatment is apparently failing?*

Outcome Evaluation

   5. a. *What clinical and laboratory parameters are necessary to evaluate the therapy for achievement of the desired therapeutic outcome and to detect or prevent adverse events?*
   b. *At what point is it suitable to change from IV to oral therapy?*

► Clinical Course

The patient improved after the changes in therapy you recommended were implemented. On the sixth hospital day, he was discharged on azithromycin 500 mg po × 2 capsules once, then 500 mg po once daily for 4 days to be completed as an outpatient.

Patient Counseling

   6. *What information should be provided to the patient about azithromycin to enhance compliance, ensure successful therapy, and minimize adverse events?*

► Clinical Pearl

Initiation of antimicrobial therapy within 8 hours of presentation to the hospital or emergency department is associated with decreased mortality from pneumonia.

► Self-study Assignments

   1. Perform a literature search or use the Internet to identify the most recent treatment guidelines from the American Thoracic Society for treating community-acquired pneumonia.
   2. Determine appropriate pharmacotherapy recommendations for empiric outpatient treatment of community-acquired pneumonia.
   3. Determine the role of newer macrolide and fluoroquinolone antimicrobials for the treatment of this disease.

References

1. Fine MJ, Auble TE, Yealy DM, et al. A prediction rule to identify low-risk patients with community-acquired pneumonia. N Engl J Med 1997;336:243–250.
2. Bartlett JG, Breiman RF, Mandell LA, et al. Community-acquired pneumonia in adults: Guidelines for management. The Infectious Diseases Society of America. Clin Infect Dis 1998;26:811–838.
3. Metlay JP, Fine MJ, Schulz R, et al. Measuring symptomatic and functional recovery in patients with community-acquired pneumonia. J Gen Intern Med 1997;12:423–430.
4. Ramirez JA, Srinath L, Ahkee S, et al. Early switch from intravenous to oral cephalosporins in the treatment of hospitalized patients with community-acquired pneumonia. Arch Intern Med 1995;155:1273–1276.
5. Meehan TP, Fine MJ, Krumholz HM, et al. Quality of care, process, and outcomes in elderly patients with pneumonia. JAMA 1997;278:2080–2084.

95 OTITIS MEDIA

► Ears and Tears   (Level II)

Carla Wallace, PharmD, BCPS

► After completing this case study, students should be able to:

- Identify the signs and symptoms of acute otitis media (AOM).
- Identify risk factors that are associated with an increased incidence of AOM.
- Identify the most likely pathogens associated with AOM.
- Identify antibiotics used to treat AOM, their spectrum of activity, and adverse effects.
- Recommend appropriate antibiotic therapy for AOM based on patient presentation and history.
- Recognize when prophylactic antibiotic therapy for AOM is required.
- Counsel parents about recommended drug therapy using appropriate non-technical terminology.

PATIENT PRESENTATION

Chief Complaint
"My son has a fever."

HPI
Joseph Wilder is a 15-month-old Caucasian male who is brought to his pediatrician in early January with a 2-day history of fever and decreased appetite. Mom states that his temperature the last 2 nights has been up to 101°F. Joseph is also coughing at night.

PMH
Former 37 week, 3.2 kg healthy infant at birth.
Routine immunizations are up-to-date. He also received the influenza vaccine in October at 12 months with a second vaccine in November.
Diagnosed with asthma at 13 months old.
First episode of acute otitis media (AOM) at age 4 months. Otitis media × 7 over past year; most recent episode 14 days ago treated with Augmentin × 10 days. The current episode is the first episode of the new year. In addition to penicillin derivatives, Joseph has received cephalosporins and macrolides in the past. The only adverse effect has been significant diarrhea with Augmentin.

FH

Parents both in good health. No siblings.

SH

Joseph lives at home with his parents, who are both employed. He attends day care. Parents are non-smokers. There is a pet dog in the home.

Meds

Albuterol solution 0.25 mL with 2 mL cromolyn nebulized BID
Beclomethasone MDI with spacer 2 puffs BID
Tylenol PRN for the last 2 days

All

NKDA

PE

Gen

WDWN male, now crying

VS

BP 100/60, HR 152, RR 50, T 36.2°C; Wt 13.2 kg, Ht 84 cm

HEENT

Both right and left TMs erythematous, bulging and non-mobile; throat is erythematous; nares patent

Neck

Supple

Chest

Bilateral wheezes

CV

RRR

Abd

Soft, non-tender

GU

Tanner stage I

Ext

No c/c/e; moves all extremities well; warm, pink, no rashes

Neuro

Responsive to stimulation, 2+ DTRs; no clonus, CNs intact

Assessment

Bilateral AOM with asthma exacerbation

▶ Questions

Problem Identification

1. a. *Create a drug-related problem list for this patient.*
   b. *What subjective and objective data support the diagnosis of AOM?*
   c. *What information indicates the type and severity of otitis media?*
   d. *What risk factors for OM are present in this child?*

Desired Outcome

2. *What are the goals of pharmacotherapy for OM in this child?*

Therapeutic Alternatives

3. a. *What bacterial organisms typically cause OM?*
   b. *What pharmacotherapeutic alternatives are available for treatment of AOM in this patient?*
   c. *Other than antibiotics, what other drug or non-drug therapies may be beneficial to this patient?*

Optimal Plan

4. *Which of the above alternatives would you recommend to treat this child's AOM? Include the dose, duration of therapy, and rationale.*

Outcome Evaluation

5. *How should the therapy you recommended be monitored for efficacy and adverse effects?*

Patient Counseling

6. *How would you provide important information about this therapy to the child's mother?*

▶ Follow-up Questions

1. *Will this child benefit from further antibiotic treatment after this course of therapy for AOM? Include the rationale for your response and suggest appropriate drug regimens.*
2. *How should Joseph's acute exacerbation of asthma be addressed? Provide specific recommendations for therapy.*

▶ Clinical Pearl

Target treatment for AOM on the causative organisms, but individualize the therapy for each specific infant or child. If the patient will not take the medication because it tastes bad, or if parents can only manage 1 dose a day, use this information to select the best antibiotic.

▶ Self-study Assignments

1. Describe a scenario in which it would be appropriate to use ceftriaxone to treat AOM.
2. Which vaccines have been studied in the prevention of recurring OM? Provide an assessment of their efficacy.

References

1. Barnett ED, Teele DW, Klein JO, et al. Comparison of ceftriaxone and trimethoprim-sulfamethoxazole for acute otitis media. Pediatrics 1997;99:23–28.
2. Chamberlain JM, Boenning DA, Waisman Y, et al. Single-dose ceftriaxone versus 10 days of cefaclor for otitis media. Clin Pediatr (Phila) 1994;33:642–646.
3. Varsano I, Volovitz B, Horev Z, et al. Intramuscular ceftriaxone compared with oral amoxicillin-clavulanate for treatment of acute otitis media in children. Eur J Pediatr 1997;156:858–863.
4. Adler M, McDonald PJ, Trostmann U, et al. Cefdinir versus amoxicillin/clavulanic acid in the treatment of suppurative acute otitis media in children. Eur J Clin Microbiol Infect Dis 1997;16:214–219.
5. Rosenfeld RM. An evidence-based approach to treating otitis media. Pediatr Clin North Am 1996;43:1165–1181.

96 STREPTOCOCCAL PHARYNGITIS

▶ **It's Not Just a Sore Throat** (Level I)

Denise L. Howrie, PharmD
Elaine McGhee, MD

▶ After completing this case study, students should be able to:

- Identify patient-specific information including signs and symptoms, medical history, and findings on physical examination that support the diagnosis of Group A β-hemolytic streptococcal (GABHS) pharyngitis.
- Describe appropriate diagnostic tools for evaluating infectious pharyngitis.
- Compare commonly-prescribed antibacterial agents with regard to spectrum, efficacy, and appropriateness of selection for GABHS pharyngitis.
- List common causes of anti-infective treatment failure in GABHS pharyngitis and recommend appropriate management strategies.

☀ PATIENT PRESENTATION

Chief Complaint
"My throat hurts."

HPI
Katie Smith is a 5 yo girl who has been ill for 2 days with sore throat and fever of 100.8°F (axillary). Her appetite has been decreased for solid foods, but fluid intake has been adequate; she has also complained that her head hurts and she feels hot. There have been no vomiting or cold symptoms. No one else in the family is ill at the present time.

PMH
Katie was the 8-lb, 7-oz product of a full-term pregnancy who was breastfed and supplemented with formula
Hospitalizations: age 2 months for dacrocystitis
Development: normal for age
3 episodes of otitis media (last episode 10 months ago)
1 episode of pneumonia at age 9 months
Immunizations: up to date

FH
Non-contributory

ROS
Negative except for complaints noted in the HPI

Meds
None

All
NKDA

PE

VS
BP 92/50, HR 124, RR 20, T 100.3°F (oral); Wt 49.5 lb

Gen
Child is alert and oriented but irritable and uncooperative

Skin
No rashes

HEENT
Tonsils 3+, bright red, without exudate; soft palate erythematous; tongue with strawberry appearance; TMs translucent

Neck/LN
Several small mobile anterior lymph nodes

Chest
CTA

CV
RRR, S_1 and S_2 normal, no murmurs

Abd
Soft, normal bowel sounds, no HSM

MS
Muscle strength and tone 5/5

CNS
CN II–XII intact, DTRs 2+

Labs
Rapid streptococcal antigen test positive

Assessment
A 5-year-old female with her first episode of GABHS pharyngitis

---

▶ Questions

Problem Identification

1. a. Create a list of the patient's drug-related problem(s).
   b. What information indicates the presence or severity of pharyngitis?
   c. How can the diagnosis of streptococcal pharyngitis best be made in a timely manner?

Desired Outcome

2. State the goals of treatment of GABHS pharyngitis in this case.

Therapeutic Alternatives

3. a. What non-drug therapies may be helpful in this child?
   b. What therapeutic alternatives are available for treatment of pharyngitis?

Optimal Plan

4. a. What drug, dosage form, dose, schedule, and duration of therapy are best for this patient?
   b. What alternatives would be appropriate if the initial therapy cannot be used?
   c. If the child's symptoms recur after completion of the prescribed regimen, what options are then available?

Outcome Evaluation

5. What clinical and laboratory parameters are necessary to evaluate the therapy for achievement of the desired outcome and to detect or prevent adverse effects?

Patient Counseling

6. What information should be provided to the patient's parents to enhance compliance, ensure success of therapy, and minimize adverse effects?

▶ Clinical Pearl

Because patients generally improve within a few days of treatment, non-adherence with the total duration of therapy is a major issue in GABHS pharyngitis.

▶ Self-study Assignments

1. Survey 10 patients in a community pharmacy setting to estimate compliance with antibacterial agents, including reason for use, du-

ration of treatment prescribed, number of days and/or doses taken as prescribed, and factors that influenced the individual's decision to adhere or not adhere with instructions. Should you modify your counseling strategies? If so, how?

2. Using various measurement devices, simulate dosage preparation and measurements for common pediatric oral antibacterial liquids. How do the various devices compare for accuracy, ease of use, and reliability?

References

1. Gerber MA. Strep pharyngitis: Update on management. Contemporary Pediatr 1997;14:156–165.
2. Schwartz B, Marcy SM, Phillips WR, et al. Pharyngitis—principles of judicious use of antimicrobial agents. Pediatrics 1998;101S:171–174.
3. Dajani AS. Current therapy of Group A streptococcal pharyngitis. Pediatr Ann 1998;27:277–280.
4. Pichichero ME, Cohen R. Shortened course of antibiotic therapy for acute otitis media, sinusitis and tonsillopharyngitis. Pediatr Infect Dis J 1997;16:680–695.

97 RHINOSINUSITIS

▶ Head Case   (Level II)

Aaron D. Killian, PharmD, BCPS

▶ After completing this case study, students should be able to:

- Describe the differences in clinical features between acute, recurrent, chronic, infectious, and inflammatory rhinosinusitis.
- Recommend specific drug therapy for the treatment of rhinosinusitis based upon patient symptoms, objective data, anticipated etiology/microbial resistance patterns, and clinical response.
- Given a case scenario, identify specific factors that predispose a patient to rhinosinusitis.
- List specific monitoring parameters for each of the antibiotics and adjunctive therapeutic agents recommended for the treatment and chronic maintenance of rhinosinusitis.
- Provide pertinent patient information (including non-antibiotic therapy) for the outpatient management of rhinosinusitis.

☼ PATIENT PRESENTATION

Chief Complaint
"When I bent down to tie my shoes yesterday, it felt as though my head was going to explode."

HPI

Alvin Kuchinsky is a 25 yo man who c/o generalized malaise with intermittent, migratory arthralgias for the past 6 months. He recalls having low-grade fevers about once a month, each episode lasting for a couple of days. He describes frequent awakenings at night, difficulty in concentrating during the day, and the sensation that his head is "swimming." He experiences a constant pressure of moderate severity, most often in the left temporal region, but sometimes bilaterally with forehead involvement as though his head was in a "vice grip." He reports intermittent left supra/retro-orbital tenderness as though someone were "pushing or poking" at his eye. Infrequently, the tenderness is associated with discomfort in the gums around his upper molars. Patient also c/o occasional cramping and diarrhea.

PMH

Rheumatic fever 17 years ago
? Viral meningitis 6 months ago; left sphenoid opacification found incidentally on CT
Giant papillary conjunctivitis (GPC) induced by contact lenses 6 months ago

PSH

Bilateral upper and lower wisdom teeth extraction 4 years ago
Benign familial dysplastic nevi excision ($\times$ 7) 1 year ago

FH

Father with pernicious anemia $\times$ 12 years; mother has had RA $\times$ 27 years; one sister who has Graves' disease who underwent subtotal thyroidectomy 1 year ago.

SH

Denies alcohol, smoking, and IVDU. Lives alone and moved from Buffalo to Chicago about $1\frac{1}{2}$ years ago. HIV status unknown.

Meds

MVI 1 tablet po QD
Clemastine fumarate 1 mg po BID PRN itchy eyes and sneezing $\times$ 1 month
Levocabastine 0.05% 1 gtt ou QID PRN
Naproxen 500 mg po BID PRN

All

NKDA

PE

Gen
White male with darkened circles beneath eyes bilaterally ("shiners")

VS
BP 122/78, HR 73, RR 18, T 100.3°F; Wt 66 kg, Ht 5'7"

HEENT
PERRLA; funduscopy normal. Tortuous, injected conjunctivae with mild peripheral hyperemia; anicteric sclerae. Intranasal exam reveals slight, non-significant right septal deviation. Mild nasal crusting and mucosal hypertrophy (R > L) without evidence of polyp formation. Thick, mucus-filled post-nasal discharge; no oral lesions; tympanic membranes intact.

Neck
Supple, mild stiffness, no JVD or lymphadenopathy

Chest
CTA; equal air entry bilaterally; no crackles or wheezing

CV
S_1, S_2 normal; no S_3 or S_4; regular rate and rhythm

Abd
Soft, non-tender, no HSM

Ext
No C/C/E

Neuro
Oriented to person, place, and time. Mild hyperaesthesia of left maxillary and ophthalmic dermatomes. Deep sensation and visual fields intact. CN II–XII intact.

Labs

Na 134 mEq/L	Hgb 14.2 g/dL	WBC $12.9 \times 10^3/mm^3$
K 3.9 mEq/L	Hct 42%	65% Neutros
Cl 99 mEq/L	Plt $349 \times 10^3/mm^3$	4% Bands
CO_2 27 mEq/L		19% Lymphs
BUN 6 mg/dL		3% Monos
SCr 0.7 mg/dL		8% Eos
Glu 115 mg/dL		1% Basos

Sinus CT Scan
Pending

► Questions

Problem Identification

1. a. *Identify all of the drug-related problems of this patient.*

   b. *What clinical and laboratory features are consistent with a diagnosis of infectious rhinosinusitis rather than nasal allergy (inflammatory rhinosinusitis) in this patient? (Note: Rhinosinusitis is used instead of the term sinusitis since the nose and sinuses are both generally involved in the inflammatory process.)*

   c. *Are this patient's signs and symptoms consistent with acute, recurrent acute, or chronic rhinosinusitis?*

   d. *What factors predispose this patient to the development of rhinosinusitis?*

Desired Outcome

2. What are the goals of pharmacotherapy in this patient?

Therapeutic Alternatives

3. a. What are the most likely causative pathogens in this patient?
b. What antibiotics are available for the acute empiric therapy of rhinosinusitis?

Optimal Plan

4. a. Based on the patient's presentation, what would you recommend as initial antibiotic and anti-inflammatory therapy? Include drug(s), dosage form(s), schedule(s), and duration(s) of therapy.
b. What adjunctive measures can be employed to optimize this patient's medical therapy?

Outcome Evaluation

5. How should these new medications be monitored for efficacy and adverse effects?

Patient Counseling

6. How would you counsel the patient about his new therapeutic regimen?

▶ Clinical Course

The patient is given prescriptions for the regimens you recommended. One month later, he returns complaining of increased nasal congestion. He describes an awful "metallic" taste during therapy but feels that his infection has improved from 3/10 to 5/10 (where 1 = significant illness, 10 = no illness). He continues to exhibit ocular allergy and left-sided ocular discomfort with temporal pressure consistent with maxillary sinus involvement. The previous CT scan revealed mucosal thickening, bilateral ethmoid involvement (L > R), a left maxillary air fluid level, and mild frontal disease. The patient agrees to proceed with aggressive medical therapy and will consider functional endoscopic sinus surgery if there is no further improvement. Amoxicillin/clavulanic acid 500 mg po TID is added for an additional 3 weeks. Five days later, the patient complains of mild nausea, chills, significant abdominal cramping, and 6 episodes of clear, watery diarrhea over the past 48 hours.

▶ Follow-up Question

1. If the current regimen cannot be continued, what would you recommend and why?

▶ Self-study Assignments

1. Perform a literature search on the adverse effects associated with long-term use of intranasal corticosteroids.
2. Compare the microbial resistance patterns of *S. pneumoniae* in your geographic locale with those reported in the epidemiologic data by Doern and co-workers.[6]
3. Create an algorithm for the outpatient management of acute and chronic rhinosinusitis.

▶ Clinical Pearl

Patients with suspected sinus disease should be thoroughly evaluated for nasal/sinus allergy, because improperly controlled allergic rhinosinusitis (seasonal or perennial) may prevent the resolution of sinus infection and lead to chronic rhinosinusitis.

References

1. Spector SL. The allergy-sinusitis link: Treatment of sinusitis with an allergic component. Hosp Med 1997;33(suppl):28–34.
2. Leopold DA. Management of rhinosinusitis. Hosp Med 1997;33(suppl):40–44.
3. Gwaltney JM Jr. Sinusitis: Pathogenesis and antimicrobial resistance. Hosp Med 1997;33(suppl):35–44.
4. Ramadan HH. What is the bacteriology of chronic sinusitis in adults? Am J Otolaryngol 1995;16:303–306.
5. Nord CE. The role of anaerobic bacteria in recurrent episodes of sinusitis and tonsillitis. Clin Infect Dis 1995;20:1512–1524.
6. Doern GV, Brueggemann A, Holley HP Jr, et al. Antimicrobial resistance of Streptococcus pneumoniae recovered from outpatients in the United States during the winter months of 1994 to 1995: Results of a 30-center national surveillance study. Antimicrob Agents Chemother 1996;40:1208–1213.
7. Sydnor TA Jr. Antibiotic therapy in bacterial sinusitis: New options. Hosp Med 1997;33(suppl):45–49.

98 PRESSURE SORES

▶ When Life Gets You Down (Level III)

Richard S. Rhodes, PharmD
Catherine A. Heyneman, PharmD, MS

▶ After completing this case study, students should be able to:

- Comprehend the etiology and pathophysiology of pressure sores (decubitus ulcers).
- Understand pressure ulcer risk assessment and classification.
- Identify conditions or risk factors that predispose individuals to pressure ulceration.
- Recommend different options for treating decubitus ulcers.
- Define goals, strategies, and interventions for prevention of decubitus ulcers.

PATIENT PRESENTATION

Chief Complaint
"I have raw places on my back and rear that really hurt."

HPI
William Anderson, an 82 yo man just admitted to the Hill Side Nursing Home, complains of constant pain on his lower back and buttock. The pain started approximately 4 weeks ago and has gotten progressively worse. His

wife noticed that he had several sores that started as areas of redness and have evolved to open wounds displaying small amounts of drainage.

PMH

COPD × 11 years
Urinary overflow incontinence × 10 years
Depression × 2 years
DJD; hip fracture 7 years ago
Trace heme (+) stool → (−) × 3 in the last year

FH

Father and brother were mine workers and died at ages 68 and 62 from complications of silicosis. Mother died of "old age" at age 88.

SH

Retired at age 65 after 45 years as a mine worker, completed high school. 60+ year h/o cigarette use which continues; heavy EtOH abuse × 50+ years. Married for 52 years; wife is 72 yo and in relatively good health but is unable to provide adequate care for her husband at home; one son. Patient has spent all of his time in bed for the past 9 months due to chronic illnesses (depression, DJD, COPD). His wife is physically unable to assist with his ambulation.

Meds

Nortriptyline 50 mg po QD
Ipratropium bromide MDI 2 puffs QID
Baclofen 10 mg po QD
Lorazepam 0.5 mg po TID
Acetaminophen 325 mg po Q 4–6 H PRN

All

NKDA

ROS

In addition to complaints noted above, he also has pain in his joints that hurt too much to get out of bed. Because the pain occurs with any physical activity and because of his difficulty breathing on exertion he wants to "just stay in bed." He reports trouble sleeping and also feels sad and depressed most of the time. He states he doesn't belong here and he feels he was admitted to the nursing home because no one wanted him.

PE

Gen

Ill-appearing, frail, elderly man; pale, weak, slightly over weight, rigid in appearance, slightly confused; responds to questions slowly, in apparent discomfort

VS

BP 152/76, P 85, RR 30, T 98.6°F; Wt 210 lb, Ht 5′10″

Skin

Overall fair to poor skin turgor, diffuse macular rash on the ischial and sacral area. The sacral area revealed 2 areas of denuded skin above and on either side of the anal opening, measuring 1 × 2 cm (right buttock) and 3 × 3 cm (left buttock) surrounded by 2 cm of erythema around the outer edges, with creamy, yellowish, sloughing of necrotic tissue with slight drainage and no signs of infection. These shallow craters involving the epidermis are characteristic of stage II decubitus ulcers. Immediately over and covering the coccyx is a stage I decubitus ulcer displaying a small 1 × 1 cm erythematous area of tender, intact skin.

HEENT

PERRLA, EOMI; TMs intact, oropharynx clear, funduscopic exam normal; tongue and mucous membranes slightly dry, nares and throat clear

Lungs/Thorax

Breath sounds decreased bilaterally, chest is resonant on percussion, diffuse breath sounds on auscultation, wheezes present bilaterally on inspiration and expiration, slight rhonchi without rales

CV

Normal heart sounds, RRR, no m/r/g

Abd

Soft, NT/ND, normal BS, no masses

Genit/Rect

Normal male genitalia, slightly enlarged prostate, normal sphincter tone, guaiac (−)

MS/Ext

No CCE, normal appearing musculature for patient's age, stiffness in hands and knees consistent with DJD, peripheral pulses palpable (PPP) bilaterally. Hand stiffness bilaterally, slight swelling of MCPs and PIPs of right hand. Knee stiffness, but no visible swelling or inflammation of either knee; ↓ ROM. Wrists, elbows, shoulders, and ankles have normal ROM, without swelling.

Neuro

Oriented to person and place, slightly confused, memory intact, diminished DTRs (L > R), no motor or sensory deficits, CNs intact

Labs

Sodium 139 mEq/L	Hgb 13.2 g/dL	AST 52 IU/L	T. chol 218 mg/dL
Potassium 5.2 mEq/L	Hct 43.0%	ALT 44 IU/L	Trig 60 mg/dL
Chloride 101 mEq/L	Plt 276 × 10³/mm³	Alk Phos 68 IU/L	Uric acid 4.0 mg/dL
CO_2 24 mEq/L	WBC 11.0 × 10³/mm³	GGT 22 IU/L	Iron 88 µg/dL
BUN 11 mg/dL	63% Neutros	LDH 208 IU/L	T_4 5.9 µg/dL
SCr 1.3 mg/dL	25% Lymphs	T. bili 1.1 mg/dL	TSH 1.8 µIU/mL
Glu 122 mg/dL	10% Monos	T. prot 6.0 g/dL	
Ca 8.5 mg/dL	2% Eos	Alb 3.1 g/dL	
Phos 2.7 mg/dL	1% Basos	Glob 2.5 g/dL	

UA

Color yellow, appearance clear; glucose (−), ketones (−), bilirubin (−), SG 1.02, blood (−), pH 5.5, urobilinogen 0.2 mg/dL, nitrite (−), leukocyte esterases (−)

ABG

pH 7.37, po$_2$ 71 mm Hg, pco$_2$ 44 mm Hg, HCO$_3$ 26 mEq/L, BE −1 mEq/L, O$_2$ sat 92%, to$_2$ 16.0 vol %, tHgb 14.3 g/dL, CO-Hgb 6%

▶ Questions

Problem Identification

1. a. *Create a list of the patient's drug-related problems.*
   b. *Which of the patient's medical problems contributes to the development of pressure sores?*
   c. *List other risk factors (whether or not they are present in this patient) that predispose individuals to the development of pressure sores.*

Desired Outcome

2. *What are the goals of treatment for this patient's pressure sores?*

Therapeutic Alternatives

3. a. *What therapeutic interventions are available for treatment of the patient's pressure sores?*
   b. *What economic issues should be considered when making plans to prevent or treat pressure sores?*

Optimal Plan

4. a. *What drug dosage form, dose, schedule, and duration of therapy are best for this patient?*
   b. *What alternatives would be appropriate if the initial therapy fails or cannot be used?*

Outcome Evaluation

5. *What clinical and laboratory parameters are necessary to evaluate the therapy for achievement of the desired therapeutic outcome and to detect or prevent adverse effects?*

Patient Counseling

6. *What information should be provided to the patient to enhance compliance, ensure successful therapy, and minimize adverse effects?*

▶ Clinical Course

After the treatment you recommended was initiated, the sacral ulcer above and on the left side of the anal opening was completely healed on the 12th day of therapy. The ulcer on the right was healed after 22 days of treatment. The stage I pressure sore on the coccyx evolved to a stage II decubitus ulcer and was healed after 4 weeks using the same treatment as the others. Sertraline was started at 50 mg po Q HS, baclofen was increased to 10 mg po TID, albuterol MDI 2 puffs QID PRN was added, and acetaminophen 1 gram po QID was given on a regular schedule. These changes decreased sedation, increased mobility, improved breathing, and controlled the incontinence. Osteoarthritis, difficulty sleeping, and anxiety all improved with better control of the patient's disease states.

▶ Self-study Assignments

1. Describe the phases of wound healing and the etiology and pathophysiology of pressure sores.

2. Perform a search of the most recent literature and develop institutional policies and procedures for the prevention and treatment of pressure sores.
3. Concerning the prevention and treatment of pressure sores, describe in your own words how you would educate a patient and/or family on the following: risk factors, signs and symptoms of infection, pressure relief, body positioning, incontinence care, nutrition support, skin care, and dressing changes.
4. Describe the classification and staging of decubitus ulcers.

▶ Clinical Pearl

The Agency for Health Care Policy and Research (AHCPR) publishes guidelines for clinicians and consumers on the prevention and treatment of pressure sores (http://www.ahcpr.gov).

References

1. Maklebust J, Sieggreen MY. Pressure ulcer treatment. In: Pressure Ulcers: Guidelines for Prevention and Nursing Management, 2nd ed. Springhouse, PA, Springhouse Corporation, 1996:77–94.
2. Yarkony GM. Pressure ulcers: A review. Arch Phys Med Rehabil 1994;75:908–917.
3. Evans JM, Andrews KL, Chutka DS, et al. Pressure ulcers: Prevention and management. Mayo Clin Proc 1995;70:789–799.
4. Maklebust J, Sieggreen MY. Pressure ulcer treatment. In: Pressure Ulcers: Guidelines for Prevention and Nursing Management, 2nd ed. Springhouse, PA, Springhouse Corporation, 1996:104–121.
5. Leigh IH, Bennett G. Pressure ulcers: Prevalence, etiology, and treatment modalities: a review. Am J Surg 1994;167(1A):25S–30S.
6. Kertesz D, Chow AW. Infected pressure and diabetic ulcers. Clin Geriatr Med 1992;8:835–852.

99 DIABETIC FOOT INFECTION

▶ Watch Your Step   (Level II)

Renee-Claude Mercier, PharmD

▶ After completing this case study, students should be able to:

- Recognize the signs and symptoms of diabetic foot infections and identify the risk factors and the most likely pathogens associated with these infections.
- Recommend appropriate antimicrobial regimens for diabetic foot infections, including patients with drug allergies or renal insufficiency.
- Recommend appropriate home IV therapy and proper counseling to patients.
- Outline monitoring parameters for achievement of the desired pharmacotherapeutic outcome and prevention of adverse effects.

- Counsel diabetic patients about adequate blood glucose control as part of an overall plan for good foot health.

☀ PATIENT PRESENTATION

Chief Complaint
"I stepped on a piece of metal and now my foot is swollen."

HPI
Fredine Littlehorse is a 39 yo woman who presents to the ED complaining of a sore and swollen foot. A few days ago she stepped on a piece of metal and later noticed redness and soreness in the area which increased over the next several days.

PMH
Type 2 DM × 12 years
Depression
Obesity
Hypothyroidism

FH
Father has HTN and mother is deceased secondary to breast cancer.

SH
The patient is a housewife and is now living in a women's shelter because her husband physically abuses her. She has been more depressed lately because her son was sentenced to jail for 10 years. She denies alcohol, tobacco, or illicit drug use. She admits to non-adherence with her medications and glucometer due to poor and unstable living conditions.

Meds
Novolin 70/30 60 units Q AM and Q PM
Klonopin 1 mg po BID
Micronase 10 mg po BID
Imipramine 200 mg po QHS
Synthroid 0.05 mg po QD

All
NKDA

ROS
Negative

PE

Gen
The patient is an obese Native American woman with a dull affect but in NAD

VS
BP 138/81, P 92, RR 20, T 37.4°C; Ht 61″, Wt 111 kg

Skin
Warm, coarse, and very dry

HEENT
PERRLA; EOMI; funduscopic exam is normal with absence of hemorrhages or exudates. TMs are clouded bilaterally but with no erythema or bulging. Oropharynx shows poor dentition but is otherwise unremarkable.

Neck/LN
Neck is supple; normal thyroid; no JVD; no palpable lymph nodes

Chest
CTA

Heart
RRR, normal S_1 and S_2 with a grade I/VI systolic murmur at the sternal border

Abd
Distended, (+) BS, no guarding, no hepatosplenomegaly or masses felt

Ext
2+ edema of right foot with markedly diminished sensation of the right foot. Area of redness and induration 4 × 5 cm from portal of entry. Dorsalis pedis pulse present. Pulses 3+ throughout. Normal range of motion. Poor nail care with some fungus and overgrown toenails.

Neuro
A & O × 3. CN II–XII intact. Motor system intact (overall muscle strength 4–5/5). Sensory system exam showed a decreased sensation to light touch of the lower extremities (both feet); intact upper body sensation.

Labs

Na 136 mEq/L	Hgb 12.6 g/dL
K 3.6 mEq/L	Hct 37.8%
Cl 98 mEq/L	Plt 390 × 10³/mm³
CO_2 24 mEq/L	WBC 20.45 × 10³/mm³
BUN 4 mg/dL	71% PMNs
SCr 0.5 mg/dL	8% Bands
Glu 181 mg/dL	15% Lymphs
HbA_{1c} 11.8 %	6% Monos

X-ray
Right foot: There is a metallic foreign body approximately 2 cm in length in the soft tissue inferior to the third metatarsal. No evidence of adjacent periosteal reactions or erosions to suggest radiographic evidence of osteomyelitis. No definite subcutaneous air is evident. Presence of vascular calcifications.

▶ Clinical Course

On the day of admission, the patient went to surgery for an I & D and removal of the foreign body. Blood and tissue specimens were sent for culture and sensitivity testing.

► Questions

Problem Identification

1. a. Create a list of the patient's drug-related problems.
   b. What signs, symptoms, or laboratory values indicate the presence of an infection?
   c. What risk factors for infection does the patient have?
   d. What organisms are most likely involved in this infection?

Desired Outcome

2. What are the therapeutic goals for this patient?

Therapeutic Alternatives

3. a. What non-drug therapies might be useful for this patient?
   b. What feasible pharmacotherapeutic alternatives are available for the empiric treatment of the foot infection?
   c. What economic and social considerations are applicable to this patient?

Optimal Plan

4. Outline a drug regimen that would provide optimal initial empiric therapy for the infection.

Outcome Evaluation

5. a. What clinical and laboratory parameters are necessary to evaluate your therapy for achievement of the desired therapeutic outcomes and monitoring for adverse effects?

► Clinical Course

Ms. Littlehorse received the empiric therapy you recommended until the tissue cultures were reported positive for methicillin-sensitive *Staphylococcus aureus*. The blood cultures were all found to have no growth. The patient remained hospitalized for an additional 2 weeks and received a more directed antimicrobial regimen and multiple surgical debridements of the wound. The cellulitis slowly improved over this time and multiple x-rays did not suggest osteomyelitis. She was then discharged to complete her antimicrobial regimen on an outpatient basis. Even though her social conditions were not at first favorable, a secure and comfortable place to live was found for her. Over the next 2 weeks, she received wound care at home and showed significant but slow progress in healing of the wound.

   b. What therapeutic alternatives are available for treating this patient once results of cultures are known to contain MSSA?
   c. Design an optimal drug treatment plan for treating her MSSA infection while she remains hospitalized.
   d. Design an optimal pharmacotherapeutic plan for completion of her treatment once she has been discharged from the hospital.

Patient Counseling

6. What information should be provided to the patient to enhance compliance, ensure successful therapy, and minimize adverse effects with IV nafcillin?

► Self-study Assignments

1. Review in more detail different therapeutic options available for home IV therapy, including the antimicrobial agents suitable for use, types of IV lines available, and contraindications to home IV therapy.
2. Outline the patient counseling you would provide for successful home IV therapy.
3. Describe how you would educate this diabetic patient about proper foot care to prevent further skin or tissue breakdown.

► Clinical Pearl

Treatment of diabetic foot infections with antimicrobial agents alone is often inadequate; local wound care (incision, drainage, debridement and amputation), good glycemic control, and immobilization of the limb are often required.

References

1. Lipsky BA, Pecoraro RE, Wheat LJ. The diabetic foot: Soft tissue and bone infection. Infect Dis Clin North Am 1990:4:409–432.
2. Lipsky BA, Pecoraro RE, Larson SA, et al. Outpatient management of uncomplicated lower-extremity infections in diabetic patients. Arch Intern Med 1990;150:790–797.
3. Lipsky BA, Baker PD, Landon GC, et al. Antibiotic therapy for diabetic foot infections: Comparison of two parenteral-to-oral regimens. Clin Infect Dis 1997;24:643–648.

100   INFECTIVE ENDOCARDITIS

► If the Heart Could Tell   (Level II)

Renata Smith, PharmD
Keith A. Rodvold, PharmD, FCCP, BCPS

► After completing this case study, students should be able to:

- Identify the symptoms of infective endocarditis.
- Select appropriate antimicrobial therapy based on a particular organism and drug allergies.
- Develop a penicillin desensitization protocol.
- Discuss common adverse reactions of the chosen drug therapy and monitoring parameters.
- Identify candidates for home IV therapy of infective endocarditis.
- Counsel patients who are being discharged home on oral therapy.

PATIENT PRESENTATION

Chief Complaint
"I really feel bad. I'm sick to my stomach, and I've had 2 seizures today."

HPI
Eddie Garry is a 39 yo man who reports vomiting, diarrhea, anorexia, and 30-pound weight loss within 1 month prior to admission. He also had 2 seizures at home on the day of admission and 2 more in the ED.

PMH
SLE × 5 years
Endocarditis 2 months ago
Thrombocytopenia for > 2 months
Seizures due to heroin withdrawal

FH
Mother and sister both had blood clots in the leg; sister had a PE. A sister and uncle also have SLE. Grandmother had HTN and DM.

SH
IVDA (heroin) × 25 years with last use 3 days PTA; EtOH 6-pack/day × 15 years; 20 pack-year tobacco history.

Meds
Prednisone 20 mg po Q AM

All
Penicillin

ROS
Noncontributory except for complaints noted above.

PE

Gen
Patient is a cachectic African-American man in mild distress.

VS
BP 81/54, P 118, RR 24, T 102.0°F; Ht 5'11.5", Wt 54 kg

Skin/Nails
No evidence of petechiae, Janeway lesions, Osler nodes, or splinter hemorrhages; (+) nail clubbing

HEENT
Anicteric sclerae, PERRLA, pink conjunctivae, dry oral mucosa, no Roth spots

Neck
No lymphadenopathy, JVD, or thyromegaly

CV
RRR, normal S_1 S_2, (+) S_3, II-III/VI SEM at left lower sternal border

Lungs
Crackles in RLL; no wheezing

Abd
Soft with mild diffuse tenderness; (+) hepatomegaly, (−) splenomegaly

GU/Rect
Normal; guaiac (−) stool

Ext
Reflexes bilaterally 3/5 UE, 2/5 LE, Babinski decreased; no edema

Neuro
Non-focal; A & O × 3, (+) asterixis

Labs

Na 133 mEq/dL	Hgb 11.1 g/dL	WBC 25.4 × 10³/mm³	RDW 17.3%
K 3.6 mEq/dL	Hct 32.6%	88% Neutros	ESR 23 mm/hr
Cl 91 mEq/dL	RBC 4.35 × 10⁶/mm³	3% Bands	
CO_2 21 mEq/L	Plt 60 × 10³/mm³	7% Lymphs	
BUN 45 mg/dL	MCV 81.1 μm³/cell	2% Monos	
SCr 2.0 mg/dL	MCH 26.3 pg		
Glu 145 mg/dL	MCHC 34 g/dL		

Urine Toxicology Screen
(+) opiates, (+) barbiturates, and (+) cocaine

ECG
Non specific T-wave changes; increased QT interval

Two-dimensional Echocardiogram
3-cm vegetation on the tricuspid valve with severe tricuspid regurgitation. Moderate left ventricular hypertrophy.

Blood Cultures
(+) × 4 for *Staphylococcus aureus*.

Questions

Problem Identification

1. a. Identify all of the drug-related problems of this patient.
   b. What signs, symptoms, and other information indicates the presence of endocarditis in this patient?
   c. What risk factors does this patient have for developing endocarditis?
   d. Based on this patient's risk factors and location of the vegetation, does this patient have right-sided or left-sided endocarditis?
   e. What additional information (laboratory tests or patient information) is needed to satisfactorily assess this patient?

Desired Outcome

2. *What are the goals of pharmacotherapy for infective endocarditis?*

▶ Clinical Course

The patient was started on empiric vancomycin with doses adjusted for his decreased renal function until susceptibilities for the *S. aureus* isolate became available. Susceptibility testing subsequently showed the organism to be sensitive to oxacillin, vancomycin, gentamicin, trimethoprim-sulfamethoxazole, ofloxacin, and cefazolin. The organism was resistant to penicillin. When questioned about his penicillin allergy, the patient reported that he gets a bad rash, "swells up," and gets short of breath.

Therapeutic Alternatives

3. a. *Identify the therapeutic alternatives for the treatment of* S. aureus *endocarditis based on the organism's susceptibilities. Include the drug name, dose, dosage form, schedule, and duration of therapy in your answer.*

   b. *What non-drug therapies might be used to treat this patient's endocarditis?*

Optimal Plan

4. a. *What is the most appropriate treatment plan for this patient (give drug name, dose, dosage form, schedule, and duration of therapy).*

▶ Clinical Course

After 8 days of IV vancomycin therapy, the patient's blood cultures are still positive. The organism continues to have the same susceptibilities.

   b. *What is an appropriate, non-surgical, therapeutic alternative for this patient?*

   c. *Explain how you would desensitize this patient to penicillin, and provide your new treatment recommendations assuming that desensitization is successful.*

Outcome Evaluation

5. a. *What clinical and laboratory parameters should be monitored to evaluate the efficacy of therapy and to prevent adverse reactions?*

▶ Clinical Course

The patient has been treated for 8 days with vancomycin followed by 2 weeks of the therapy chosen in question 4.c. Blood cultures became negative 4 days after the new regimen was instituted. He is afebrile (T$_{max}$ 97.3°F), his white count is normalizing (WBC 10.4×10^3/mm^3 with no bands), he is feeling much better, and he wishes to leave the hospital now.

   b. *Based on your assessment of this patient's response and his past history, what alternatives are available for completing his course of therapy?*

Patient Counseling

6. *If this patient is discharged home to complete his regimen on oral antibiotics, what information should be provided to him to enhance adherence and ensure successful therapy?*

▶ Self-study Assignments

1. Outline the most recent treatment guidelines for streptococcal and enterococcal endocarditis.
2. What would be the most appropriate antibiotic prophylaxis for this patient if he returns to the hospital to have his tricuspid valve replaced (include the drug name, dosage form, dose, and duration of therapy)?

▶ Clinical Pearl

A minimum of two sets of blood cultures should be obtained from two different sites prior to initiation of antibiotics in patients with infective endocarditis. Once a patient receives antibiotics, blood cultures may become non-diagnostic.

References

1. Cunha B, Gill V, Lazar JM. Acute infective endocarditis: Diagnostic and therapeutic approach. Infect Dis Clin North Am 1996;10;811–834.
2. Wilson WR, Karchmer AW, Dajani AS, et al. Antibiotic treatment of adults with infective endocarditis due to streptococci, enterococci, staphylococci, and HACEK microorganisms. JAMA 1995;274:1706–1713.
3. DiNuble MJ. Short-course antibiotic therapy for right-sided endocarditis caused by *Staphylococcus aureus* in injection drug users. Ann Intern Med 1994;121: 873–876.
4. Chambers HF. Short-course combination and oral therapies of *Staphylococcus aureus* endocarditis. Infect Dis Clin North Am 1993;7:69–80.
5. Pryka RD, Rodvold KA, Erdman SM. An updated comparison of drug dosing methods. Part IV: Vancomycin. Clin Pharmacokinet 1991;20:463–476.
6. Rehm SJ. Outpatient intravenous antibiotic therapy for endocarditis. Infect Dis Clin North Am 1998;12:879–901.
7. Heldman AW, Hartert TV, Ray SC, et al. Oral antibiotic treatment of right-sided staphylococcal endocarditis in injection drug users: Prospective randomized comparison with parenteral therapy. Am J Med 1996;101:68–76.
8. Lawlor MT, Sullivan MC, Levitz RE, et al. Treatment of prosthetic valve endocarditis due to methicillin-resistant *Staphylococcus aureus* with minocycline. J Infect Dis 1990;161:812–814.

101 PULMONARY TUBERCULOSIS

▶ Someone to Watch Over Me   (Level I)

Susan Shaffer, PharmD
Dennis M. Williams, PharmD, FASHP, FCCP, BCPS

▶ After completing this case study, students should be able to:

- Recognize the signs and symptoms of active tuberculosis (TB).
- Recommend initial empiric drug therapy for a patient with active TB.
- Describe appropriate monitoring parameters to assess the effectiveness and toxicity of anti-TB drug therapies.

- Recognize common adverse events of drugs used to treat TB.
- Identify treatment options for patients with drug-resistant organisms.

☀ PATIENT PRESENTATION

Chief Complaint
"I have this constant cough that's getting worse, and I have no energy."

HPI
Jerry Fritz is a 50 yo man who presents to the Medicine Clinic complaining of a 2-month history of a persistent cough that has become productive over the past 3 weeks. He also complains of malaise, fever, night sweats, and a 20-pound weight loss over the past 2 months.

PMH
Seizure disorder since age 10
HTN × 5 years

FH
His mother and father died in an MVA 20 years ago; one brother died at age 52 of heart disease; one sister, age 47, is still living with no known medical problems.

SH
Single, no children. He has been residing at homeless shelters for 2 months. He lost his job as a security guard 2 years ago and could not afford to continue paying rent for his apartment. He has spent time in and out of various shelters as well as nights on the street. He denies smoking or IV drug use. He had a 20-year history of alcohol abuse but has been sober for 10 years.

Meds
Phenytoin 300 mg po Q HS
Hydrochlorothiazide 25 mg po QD
Patient reports that he tries to be compliant with his therapies and takes them regularly except when he is unable to get his refills; over the past 2 months, he went 3 or 4 days without medication.

All
NKDA

ROS
Unremarkable except for complaints of recurrent headaches and intermittent abdominal pain. No seizures for 8 months.

PE

Gen
Thin, emaciated African-American man who appears older than stated age. Appears fatigued, but otherwise in NAD.

VS
BP 138/88, P 84, RR 16, Temp 38.3°C; Wt 51 kg

Skin
Cool to touch; multiple bruises on extremities; moles on trunk

HEENT
PERRLA; EOMI; funduscopic exam with grade 2, mild arterial narrowing, no hemorrhages or exudates; TMs occluded bilaterally with wax. Pharynx shiny, no exudates.

Neck
Supple; no lymphadenopathy, bruits, or JVD; no thyromegaly

Chest
Diffuse rhonchi in upper lobes, decreased breath sounds on left, with pleural rub

CV
RRR; no m/r/g

Abd
(+) BS; non-tender; no masses; liver edge palpable

Genit/Rect
No masses or discharge; rectal tone decreased, prostate slightly enlarged, Heme (+) stool

MS/Ext
No CCE; muscle strength 3–4/5 throughout; peripheral pulses present

Neuro
Sluggish, but A & O × 3; no focal abnormalities; CN II–XII intact; DTRs 2+; Babinski downgoing bilaterally

Labs

Na 138 mEq/L	Hgb 13 g/dL	WBC 4.5×10^3/mm³	AST 72 IU/L
K 3.8 mEq/L	Hct 39%	62% PMNs	ALT 56 IU/L
Cl 96 mEq/L	RBC 4.1×10^6/mm³	34% Lymphs	Alk Phos 120 IU/L
CO₂ 23 mEq/L	MCV 98 μm³	4% Monos	GGT 60 IU/L
BUN 30 mg/dL	MCH 32 pg		T. bili 1.0 mg/dL
SCr 1.3 mg/dL	Retic 0.4%		PT 14 sec
Glu 126 mg/dL			

Other
Consent for HIV testing obtained.

Chest X-ray
Profound bilateral upper lobe infiltrates, bases spared; 1-cm circular lesion in left lower lobe (? old granuloma); small left pneumothorax with effusion.

CT Chest
Small posterior peritracheal and hilar nodes; left pleural thickening and small pneumothorax. Cavity (3 × 4 cm) in left posterior segment, no air fluid level.

▶ Clinical Course

The patient was admitted and placed on respiratory isolation. An intermediate-strength PPD tuberculin skin test (Mantoux method) was placed. Candida and mumps were used as controls. Sputum samples were sent for

AFB, fungi, and bacteria. After 48 hours, the PPD skin test was read as a 12-mm area of induration. Subsequently, 3 sputum Gram stain specimens were reported to contain 3+ AFB.

Assessment

Active pulmonary tuberculosis.

▶ Questions

Problem Identification

1. a. Create a list of the patient's drug-related problems.
   b. What signs, symptoms, and other findings are consistent with active TB infection?
   c. What factors place this patient at increased risk for acquiring TB?

Desired Outcome

2. What are the goals of therapy for this patient with active TB?

Therapeutic Alternatives

3. a. What non-drug therapies might be useful in this patient?
   b. What drug therapies are available for the treatment of active TB?
   c. What economic and social considerations are applicable to this patient?

Optimal Plan

4. a. What drug, dosage form, dose, schedule, and duration of therapy are best for this patient?
   b. What alternatives to daily administration of medicines exist?

Outcome Evaluation

5. What clinical and laboratory parameters are necessary to evaluate the therapy for achievement of the desired therapeutic outcome and to detect or prevent adverse effects?

Patient Counseling

6. What information should be provided to the patient to enhance compliance, ensure successful therapy, and minimize adverse effects?

▶ Clinical Course

This patient is treated with the regimen you recommended under respiratory isolation in the hospital. The results of his HIV test were negative. After 14 days, his presenting symptoms have improved, and 3 consecutive sputum specimens have been negative for AFB. Because he had 3 negative smears, he was removed from respiratory isolation and subsequently discharged to home. After 6 weeks, the results of his initial cultures are available. *Mycobacterium tuberculosis* is present, and the sensitivity report indicates INH-resistant organisms. The organism is sensitive to all other agents.

▶ Follow-up Questions

1. How should the presence of INH resistance influence the drug therapy?
2. After 3 months of therapy, an increase in the patient's AST and ALT are noted (AST 160 IU/L; ALT 190 IU/L). Other liver enzymes and total bilirubin are normal. The patient reports no new complaints. What changes would you make to the current therapy and monitoring plan?
3. What potential drug interactions should be evaluated? How should they be managed?
4. How should close contacts of the patient be treated (considering that he has INH-resistant organisms)?

▶ Self-study Assignments

1. How would therapy be different if the patient was HIV positive? A child or adolescent? A pregnant woman?
2. Discuss how the treatment would have been different if the patient had multidrug resistant organisms.
3. How would the treatment of extrapulmonary TB differ from the treatment of pulmonary TB?
4. What are the BCG vaccines? In what situations would BCG be recommended?

▶ Clinical Pearl

All patients receiving treatment for active TB should be considered for directly observed therapy (DOT). With adequate drug therapy for TB, nearly all patients with drug-susceptible organisms will become bacteriologically negative, recover, and remain well.

References

1. Bass JB Jr, Farer LS, Hopewell PC, et al. Treatment of tuberculosis and tuberculosis infection in adults and children. American Thoracic Society and the Centers for Disease Control and Prevention. Am J Respir Crit Care Med 1994;149: 1359–1374.
2. American Thoracic Society. Control of tuberculosis in the United States. Am Rev Respir Dis 1992;146:1623–1633.

Note: A document entitled "Core Curriculum on Tuberculosis: What the Clinician Should Know," (3rd ed, 1994) is available from the Centers for Disease Control and Prevention on the Internet at http://www.cdc.gov/nchstp/tb/pubs/core-curr.htm

102 *CLOSTRIDIUM DIFFICILE*–ASSOCIATED DIARRHEA

▶ **When One Antibiotic Requires Another**   (Level I)

Margaret B. Zak, PharmD

▶ After completing this case study, students should be able to:

- Recognize the interaction between host factors, local defense, and the use of antibiotic agents as they apply to the development of *Clostridium difficile* diarrhea.
- Identify the signs and symptoms of *C. difficile* diarrhea.
- Recommend specific drug therapy for the treatment of primary therapy and relapse of *C. difficile* diarrhea.
- Establish appropriate monitoring parameters for evaluating response and managing side effects of therapy for *C. difficile* diarrhea.
- Effectively counsel patients on therapy for *C. difficile* diarrhea who are being discharged.

☼ PATIENT PRESENTATION

Chief Complaint
None.

HPI
Thomas Smithers is brought to the ED by ambulance after his sister found him to be "acting confused" and lethargic. The patient is a 70 yo man with a history of numerous medical problems including type 2 DM and recent right great toe amputation 15 days prior for which he was receiving 14 days of oral Augmentin therapy. He was taking his normal dose of glipizide XL but has not been eating well for a few days prior and has not eaten at all today because of an upset stomach.

PMH
Type 2 DM
CRI secondary to diabetic nephropathy (baseline SCr 1.9 mg/dL)
HTN
CAD
CHF
PVD
BPH

FH
Not obtainable (patient unable to recollect).

SH
Single, lives with sister; occasional alcohol (1 beer per week); no tobacco or illicit drug use.

ROS
Occasional fevers; no chills, weight loss or headaches. He reports changes in vision secondary to cataracts; denies runny nose, cough or sore throat. He denies chest pain, shortness of breath, or palpitations. No urinary urgency or hesitancy. He reports cramping and abdominal tenderness that is relieved by bowel movements. Greenish, watery diarrhea (5 to 10 stools daily) without hematochezia or melena started about 5 days ago. His sister denies any history of past neurologic problems.

Meds
Bumex 2 mg po QD
Isosorbide mononitrate 60 mg po QD
Slow-Mag 64 mg po QD
Hismanal 10 mg po QD
Glipizide XL 5 mg po QD
Augmentin 500 mg po BID × 14 days (course completed 1 day PTA)

All
NKDA

PE

Gen
The patient is confused and lethargic but easily aroused

VS
BP 140/70, P 89, RR 24, T (oral) 36.9°C; Ht 5′11″, Wt 113 kg

Skin
Dry with some hyper-pigmentation noted on the lower extremities

HEENT
NC/AT; PERRLA; disks flat, no hemorrhages or exudates. EOMI. Pharynx is dry but clear and without erythema.

Neck/LN
Supple with no JVD, bruits, or lymphadenopathy; normal thyroid

Chest
Occasional bibasilar crackles

CV
RRR. Normal S_1, S_2 with grade II/VI SEM. PMI displaced laterally.

Abd
Mildly distended with diffuse tenderness; (+) guarding; hyperactive BS × 4 quadrants

Genit/Rect
Enlarged prostate; rectal exam not performed

MS/Ext
Poor LE pulses bilaterally; cold to touch. Trace pre-tibial edema with hyper-pigmentation on anterior tibia. Bilateral venous stasis ulcers on both LE, red and warm to touch. Right great toe amputation. Strength 5/5 and equal throughout.

Neuro
Alert and oriented to person. Poor immediate and recent memory with intact comprehension and repetition. Cranial nerves II–XII intact. Deep

tendon reflexes 2+ and equal throughout. Decreased sensation to light touch, pinprick with stocking distribution.

Labs

Na 140 mEq/L	WBC 10.7×10^3/mm^3
K 3.3 mEq/L	51% Neutros
Cl 97 mEq/L	30% Bands
CO$_2$ 31 mEq/L	13% Lymphs
BUN 43 mg/dL	6% Monos
SCr 2.2 mg/dL	Mg 1.7 mEq/L
Glu 35 mg/dL	

Chest X-ray

Difficult to read because of poor quality; cannot rule out pulmonary edema.

EKG

NSR; no acute ST wave changes, and no change from previous EKG.

UA

(+) protein; no bacteria or WBCs

Urine Culture

Pending

Blood Cultures

2 sets pending

Stool Cultures

Pending

Fecal Leukocytes

Pending

C. difficile Culture

Pending

Assessment

1. Altered mentation secondary to hypoglycemia
2. Diarrhea; etiology to be determined
3. Wound infection (recent history of toe amputation and LE ulcers)
4. Probable dehydration

▶ Clinical Course

The patient is admitted, and dextrose 50% is given IV until the glucose level is continuously maintained between goal levels of 115 to 140 mg/dL. Aggressive IV fluid management with 10% dextrose and normal saline is given until hypoglycemia and dehydration resolve. Hypokalemia is corrected, and magnesium supplementation is continued. The following microbiology data are subsequently reported:

- Urine culture: no growth
- Blood cultures × 2: no growth
- Stool cultures: (−) for *Salmonella, Shigella, Campylobacter,* and *E. coli.*0157:H7.
- Fecal leukocytes: positive
- *C. difficile* stool culture: positive (final report on day 3 after admission)

▶ Questions

Problem Identification

1. a. Create a complete list of the patient's drug-related problems at the time of admission.
   b. What signs, symptoms, and laboratory values are consistent with C. difficile *diarrhea in this patient?*
   c. Which antibiotics have been shown to cause C. difficile *diarrhea?*

Desired Outcome

2. What are the goals of pharmacotherapy in this case?

Therapeutic Alternatives

3. a. What non-drug therapies may be useful for the treatment of C. difficile *in this patient?*
   b. What feasible pharmacotherapeutic alternatives are available for treatment of C. difficile *diarrhea?*

Optimal Plan

4. a. What drug, dosage form, dose, schedule, and duration of therapy are best suited for this patient?

   b. The patient was placed on the regimen you recommended. However, after 7 days his diarrhea is still present (5 to 7 watery stools per day) and a repeat C. difficile *stool culture is reported as positive. What possible explanations do you have for his treatment failure?*
   c. What changes, if any, should be made in the pharmacotherapeutic plan for the patient at this time?

Outcome Evaluation

5. What clinical and laboratory parameters are necessary to evaluate the therapy for achievement of the desired therapeutic outcome and to detect or prevent adverse effects?

Patient Counseling

6. What information should be provided to the patient to enhance compliance, ensure successful therapy, and minimize adverse effects?

▶ Self-study Assignments

1. Several treatment options exist for the treatment of recurrent *C. difficile*–associated diarrhea. Review the literature and write down three potential regimens that you would recommend (include

drugs, routes, dosages, and duration), and determine the cost to the patient of each regimen based on pharmacy prices in your area.

2. Some patients are asymptomatic carriers of *C. difficile*. Perform a literature search and determine what evidence exists to support the treatment of these patients.

3. Review the endoscopic findings associated with *C. difficile* colitis. What percentage of patients with *C. difficile* diarrhea have positive endoscopic findings?

▶ Clinical Pearl

Oral vancomycin is usually not absorbed; however, there have been several case reports of significant vancomycin absorption in patients with long-standing colitis and renal failure.

References

1. Teasley DG, Gerding DN, Olson MM, et al. Prospective randomised trial of metronidazole versus vancomycin for *Clostridium difficile*-associated diarrhea and colitis. Lancet 1983;2:1043–1046.

2. Centers for Disease Control and Prevention. Preventing the spread of vancomycin resistance—a report from the hospital infection control practices advisory committee. Fed Reg 1994;59(94):25758–25763.

3. Kelly CP, Pothoulakis C, LaMont JT. *Clostridium difficile* colitis. N Engl J Med 1994:330:257–262.

4. Fekety R. Guidelines for the diagnosis and management of *Clostridium-difficile*-associated diarrhea and colitis. Am J Gastroenterol 1997;92:739–750.

5. Fekety R, Silva J, Kauffman C, et al. Treatment of antibiotic-associated *Clostridium difficile* colitis with oral vancomycin: Comparison of two dosage regimens. Am J Med 1989;86:15–19.

103 INTRA-ABDOMINAL INFECTION

▶ **Like Mother, Like Son**   (Level II)

Renee-Claude Mercier, PharmD

▶ After completing this case study, students should be able to:

- Recognize the signs and symptoms of bacterial peritonitis.
- Identify the bacteria commonly found in the different parts of the GI tract.
- Recommend appropriate empiric therapy for primary bacterial peritonitis.
- Establish a long-term plan for the patient regarding alcohol abuse and hepatitis C, including monitoring parameters and counseling.

☀ PATIENT PRESENTATION

Chief Complaint
"My belly hurts so bad I can barely move."

HPI
John Chavez is a 67 yo Hispanic man who was brought to the ED by his wife. She stated that he has been suffering from nausea, vomiting, severe abdominal pain, and has been acting "goofy" for the last 2–3 days. His intake of food and fluids has been minimal over the past several days. He is a well-known patient of the ED who often presents with alcohol intoxication and severe hepatic encephalopathy.

PMH
Cirrhosis with ascites for the last 3 years
Hepatic encephalopathy
GERD
HTN
Cholecystectomy 10 years ago
Hepatitis C (+) since June 1997

FH
Mother was alcoholic; died 10 years ago in car accident. Father's history unknown.

SH
Retired construction worker; EtOH abuse with 10–12 cans of beer per day × 20 years; denies use of tobacco or illicit drugs; poor compliance with medications and dietary restrictions.

Meds
Lactulose 30 mL po QID PRN
Procardia XL 60 mg po QD
Maalox 30 mL po QID PRN
Axid 150 mg po BID

All
NKDA

ROS
Patient reports heartburn in addition to complaints noted above.

PE

Gen
Elderly man who appears older than his stated age and is in severe pain

VS
BP 154/82, P 102, RR 32, T 39.4°C; current weight 92 kg, IBW 68 kg

Skin
Jaundiced, warm, coarse, and very dry. Facial spider angiomata present.

HEENT
Yellow sclera; PERRLA; EOMI; funduscopic exam is normal. Tympanic membranes are clouded bilaterally but with no erythema or bulging. Oropharynx showed poor dentition but was otherwise unremarkable.

Neck
Supple; normal size thyroid; no JVD or palpable lymph nodes

Chest
Lungs are CTA; shallow and frequent breathing

Heart

Tachycardia, normal S_1 and S_2 with no S_3 or S_4

Abd

Distended; pain upon pressure or movements; pain is sharp and diffuse throughout abdomen; (+) guarding. Unable to palpate liver or spleen. Decreased bowel sounds.

Ext

Unremarkable

Genit/Rect

Prostate normal size; guaiac (−) stool

Neuro

A & O × 2 (time and person); lethargic and apathetic, slumped posture, slowed movements. CN II–XII intact. Motor system intact; overall muscle strength equal to 4–5/5), poor coordination and gait. Sensory system intact. Reflexes 3+.

Labs

Na 142 mEq/L	Hgb 14.1 g/dL	AST 290 IU/L
K 3.9 mEq/L	Hct 42.6%	ALT 320 IU/L
Cl 96 mEq/L	Plt $250 × 10^3$/mm³	Alk Phos 350 IU/L
CO_2 20 mEq/L	WBC $18.25 × 10^3$/mm³	T. bili 3.2 mg/dL
BUN 44 mg/dL	73% Neutros	D. bili 1.4 mg/dL
SCr 1.2 mg/dL	9% Bands	
Glu 101 mg/dL	13% Lymphs	
	5% Monos	

Abdominal X-ray

No evidence of free air.

Chest X-ray

No infiltrates; heart normal size and shape.

Blood Cultures

Pending × 2

Paracentesis

Ascitic fluid: leukocytes 720/mm³, protein 2.5 g/dL. Gram-stain: numerous PMNs, no organisms.

Assessment

Primary bacterial peritonitis

▶ Clinical Course

Due to the recent low intake of food and fluids and the high BUN-to-creatinine ratio, the patient was thought to be dehydrated and was given 1 L/hr of 0.9% NaCl in the ED. His breathing became progressively worse, and he had to be intubated and transferred to the intensive care unit.

▶ Questions

Problem Identification

1. a. Create a list of the patient's drug-related problems.
   b. What signs, symptoms, and laboratory values indicate the presence of primary bacterial peritonitis?
   c. What risk factors for infection are present in this patient?
   d. What organisms are the most likely cause of this infection?

Desired Outcome

2. What are the therapeutic goals for this patient?

Therapeutic Alternatives

3. a. What non-drug therapies might be useful for this patient?
   b. What feasible pharmacotherapeutic alternatives are available for the treatment of the primary bacterial peritonitis?

Optimal Plan

4. a. Given this patient's condition, which drug regimens would provide optimal therapy for the infection?
   b. In addition to antimicrobial therapy, what other drug-related interventions are required for this patient?

Outcome Evaluation

5. What clinical and laboratory parameters are necessary to evaluate the therapy for achievement of the desired therapeutic outcome and to detect or prevent adverse effects?

Patient Counseling

6. What information should be provided to the patient to enhance compliance, ensure successful therapy, and minimize adverse effects?

▶ Clinical Course

After 48 hours of IV antibiotics, Mr. Chavez was extubated. The blood cultures were reported positive for *E. coli* sensitive to ampicillin, ampicillin/sulbactam, TMP-SMX, gentamicin, cefazolin, and ceftizoxime. The ascitic fluid culture did not grow any organisms. The antibiotic regimen was simplified to ampicillin 2 g IV Q 6 H for a total of 10 days. After 3 days of antimicrobial treatment, repeat blood cultures were negative. He rapidly improved, and upon discharge his mental status had returned to baseline.

▶ Self-study Assignments

1. What are the main differences (clinical manifestations, pathogens involved, diagnosis methods, and treatment) between primary and secondary bacterial peritonitis?

2. What are risk factors, clinical signs and symptoms, modes of transmission, diagnostic methods, prognosis, and therapeutic options associated with Hepatitis C?

► Clinical Pearl

Bacteremia is present in up to 75% of patients with primary peritonitis due to aerobic bacteria but is rarely found in those with peritonitis due to anaerobes.

References

1. Conn HO, Fessel JM. Spontaneous bacterial peritonitis in cirrhosis: Variations on a theme. Medicine (Baltimore) 1971;50:161–197.
2. Felisart J, Rimola A, Arroyo V, et al. Cefotaxime is more effective than is ampicillin-tobramycin in cirrhotics with severe infections. Hepatology 1985;5:457–462.
3. Bohnen JM, Solomkin JS, Dellinger EP, et al. Guidelines for clinical care: Anti-infective agents for intra-abdominal infection. A Surgical Infection Society policy statement. Arch Surg 1992;127:83–89.

104 PELVIC INFLAMMATORY DISEASE AND OTHER SEXUALLY TRANSMITTED DISEASES

► Frankie and Jenny Were Lovers   (Level II)

Denise L. Howrie, PharmD
Pamela J. Murray, MD, MPH

► After completing this case study, students should be able to:

- Identify relevant information from patient history, physical examination, and laboratory data suggestive of the diagnosis of a sexually transmitted disease (STD).
- List major complications of STDs and appropriate strategies for prevention and/or treatment.
- Discuss other health issues that may be present in patients referred for treatment of STDs.
- Provide appropriate treatment plans for patients with STDs, including drug(s), doses, and monitoring.
- Develop patient counseling strategies regarding drug treatment and possible adverse effects.

► Patient Presentation #1

Chief Complaint
"My lady and I don't feel good."

HPI
Frankie Mason is a 28 yo man who presents to a health clinic with complaints of 5 days of painful urination and increasing amounts of discolored urethral discharge. Today he noted 4 painful blisters on the penis. He is single, sexually active with 2 to 3 frequent partners, and admits to unprotected sex "at least once" in the past 2 weeks. He denies IV drug use, is heterosexual, and has no active medical problems. He denies oral or rectal intercourse.

PMH
History of genital herpes 2 years ago, otherwise negative.

FH
Non-contributory.

SH
Denies cigarette use; has 2–4 beers "on weekends," may be unreliable in keeping follow-up appointments because he states, "I don't like doctors."

ROS
Occasional headaches; denies stomach pain, constipation, vision problems, or allergies.

Meds
None

All
NKDA

PE

Gen
Patient is a well-developed male in NAD, very talkative

VS
BP 104/80, HR 72, RR 12, T 37.6°C; Wt 78 kg

Skin
No rashes or other lesions seen

HEENT
No erythema of pharynx or oral ulcers

Neck/LN
No lymphadenopathy, neck supple

Chest
Normal breath sounds, good air entry

CV
RRR, no murmurs

Abd
No tenderness or rebound, no HSM

Genit/Rect
Tanner Stage V, testes descended, non-tender, without erythema. Thick gray-white urethral discharge; 4 small erupting vesicles on penile tip and glans; negative rectal exam; no scrotal tenderness or swelling

MS/Ext
No inguinal or other lymphadenopathy, no lesions or rashes, muscle strength and tone normal

Neuro
CN II–XII intact, DTRs 2+ bilaterally and symmetrical

Urethral Smear
15 WBC/hpf, Gram stain (+) for intracellular gram-negative diplococci (see Figure 104–1); rare flagellated organisms by saline prep microscopy

Assessment
1. Urethritis due to gonococcal and trichomonas infections
2. Recurrent genital herpes

▶ Patient Presentation #2

Chief Complaint
"I feel sick to my stomach."

HPI
Jenny Klein is a 22 yo female sexual partner of Frankie who reports a 1-day history of increasingly severe dysuria, lower abdominal pain, fever, nausea, emesis × 2, and vaginal discharge. She is sexually active with "only Frankie," has no previous history of urinary or genital infection, and denies IV drug use. She is unaware of Frankie's multiple sexual partners. Her last menses ended 10 days ago and last intercourse was 7 days ago without use of a condom. She noted the vaginal discharge yesterday, which she describes as thick and yellow. She denies oral or rectal intercourse.

PMH
Negative

FH
HTN in maternal grandmother; history of depression

SH
Denies nicotine or recreational drug use; occasional 1–2 glasses of wine; does not use hormonal contraception, reports occasional use of condoms; no routine medical care

ROS
Occasional painful menses self-treated with acetaminophen

Meds
None

All
NKDA

PE

Gen
Well-developed woman in moderate-to-severe abdominal discomfort

VS
BP 110/76, HR 120, RR 16, T 102.5°F; Wt 52 kg

Skin
No rashes seen

HEENT
No erythema of pharynx or oral ulcers

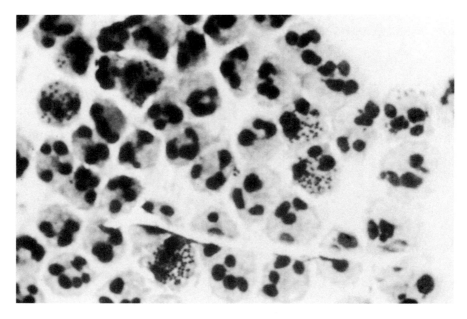

Figure 104–1. Gram-negative intracellular diplococci (*Neisseria gonorrhoeae*).

Neck/LN
No lymphadenopathy, neck supple

Chest
Normal breath sounds, good air entry; breasts Tanner Stage V

CV
RRR, no murmurs

Abd
Guarding of right and mid-lower quadrants with palpation

Genit/Rectal
Pubic hair Tanner Stage V. Vulva with no ulcers visible; large amount of thick, moderate erythema with mild excoriations. Vagina with yellow-white discharge and mild erythema. Cervix shows extensive yellow-white discharge from the os and erythema; no masses on bimanual exam; cervical motion tenderness; adnexal tenderness and fullness

MS/Ext
No adenopathy, lesions or rashes; no arthritis or tenosynovitis

Neuro
CN II–XII Intact, DTRs 2+ and symmetrical bilaterally

Labs

Na 138 mEq/L	Hgb 12.2 g/dL	WBC $12.75 \times 10^3/mm^3$
K 4.2 mEq/L	Hct 37%	66% Neutros
Cl 102 mEq/L	Plt $250 \times 10^3/mm^3$	12% Bands
BUN 22 mg/dL		10% Lymphs
SCr 0.9 mg/dL		12% Monos
Glu 106 mg/dL		

Other
Examination of vaginal discharge: pH 6.0, no yeast or hyphae seen; KOH prep negative, whiff test negative; flagellated organisms and increased WBC seen by saline prepared microscopy; negative for clue cells.

UA
Rare WBC/hpf, protein 100 mg/dL, Gram stain (−)

Assessment
1. PID
2. Infection of the genital tract: cervicitis, vaginitis, and urethritis

▶ Questions

Problem Identification

1. a. For each patient, create a list of drug-related problems.
   b. What information indicates the presence or severity of each STD in each patient?
   c. Should any additional tests be performed in these patients?
   d. What complications of infection can be reduced or avoided with appropriate therapy?

Desired Outcome

2. State the goals of treatment for each patient.

Therapeutic Alternatives

3. What therapeutic options are available for treatment of each patient?

Optimal Plan

4. a. What treatment regimen (drug, dosage form, dose, schedule, and duration) is appropriate for these patients?
   b. What alternatives would be appropriate if the initial therapy cannot be used?

Outcome Evaluation

5. a. What clinical and laboratory parameters are necessary to evaluate the therapy for achievement of the desired outcome and to detect or prevent adverse effects?

▶ Clinical Course

Two days later, the following test results are received. Frankie: *Chlamydia* PCR positive, urethral discharge culture positive for *Neisseria gonorrhoeae*. Jenny: *Chlamydia* PCR positive, vaginal discharge culture positive for *Neisseria gonorrhoeae*.

   b. What changes, if any, in antibacterial therapy are required?

Patient Counseling

6. What information should be provided to Frankie to enhance compliance, ensure success of therapy, and minimize adverse effects?

▶ Clinical Pearl

Effective antibacterial therapy of pelvic inflammatory disease may reduce the frequency of serious long-term complications including sterility and chronic pain syndrome in women.

▶ Self-study Assignments

1. Using the Internet, review information from the Centers for Disease Control and two other reputable sites that can be accessed by patients for information about STDs. Compare the quality of the information provided. Who would be the likely audiences for each site?
2. Calculate patient costs of two regimens each for treatment of herpes

genitalis, chlamydial urethritis, and gonococcal urethritis. How do cost and convenience compare for the various regimens?

3. Provide a comprehensive plan for patient counseling about the use of male condoms.

References

1. Lappa S, Moscicki A. The pediatrician and the sexually active adolescent: A primer for sexually transmitted diseases. Pediatr Clin North Am 1997;44: 1405–1445.
2. Carson DS, Wild SW. Pelvic inflammatory disease. US Pharmacist 1997;22: 187–196.
3. Centers for Disease Control and Prevention. 1998 Guidelines for Treatment of Sexually Transmitted Diseases. MMWR 1998;47(No. RR-1):1–116. http://www.cdc.gov/diseases/diseases.html

105 LOWER URINARY TRACT INFECTION

▶ Yearning and Burning   (Level I)

Christine A. Lesch, PharmD
Keith A. Rodvold, PharmD, FCCP, BCPS

▶ After completing this case study, students should be able to:

- Recognize the usual symptoms of an uncomplicated urinary tract infection (UTI) in females.
- Select specific drug therapy for the treatment of an uncomplicated UTI after consideration of patient symptoms, objective findings, and expected clinical response.

- Describe monitoring parameters to ensure efficacy and prevent toxicity during treatment.
- Counsel patients about how to take the regimen, noting relationship with meals, proper storage, and potential side effects.

PATIENT PRESENTATION

Chief Complaint
"Over the past 24 hours I've been alternating between urinating frequently to needing to urinate and not being able to."

HPI
Jacqueline Michaels is a 21 yo woman who presents to the University Family Practice Clinic with a 24-hour history of dysuria, frequency, and urgency. She also complains of constipation. She denies being sexually active.

PMH
UTI 6 months ago
Bulimia; states that she has been trying to eat better and is not vomiting anymore

FH
Non-contributory

SH
Non-smoker, lives with her mother

ROS
Denies flank pain or fever

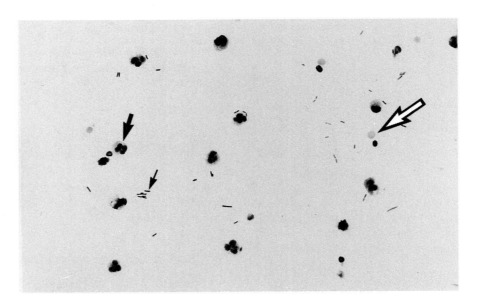

Figure 105–1. Urine sediment with neutrophils (solid arrow), bacteria (small arrow), and occasional red blood cells (open arrow). *(Wright-Giemsa × 1650; photo courtesy of Lydia C. Contis, MD.)*

Meds
None

All
Bactrim → rash

PE

Gen
Cooperative woman in no distress

VS
BP 110/60, P 68, R 18, T 96.2°F; Wt 57 kg, Ht 67″

Skin
Mild facial acne

HEENT
PERRLA, EOMI, fundi benign, TMs intact

Back
No CVA tenderness

Chest
CTA

CV
RRR

Abd
Soft, (+) bowel sounds, no organomegaly or tenderness

Pelvic
No vaginal discharge or lesions; LMP 2 weeks ago

Ext
Pulses 2+ throughout; full ROM

Neuro
A & O × 3; CN II–XII intact; reflexes 2+, sensory and motor levels intact

Labs
Not obtained

UA
WBC 10–15 cells/hpf, RBC 1–5 cells/hpf, bacteria 2–5/hpf, nitrite negative

Assessment
Acute cystitis

▶ Questions

Problem Identification

1. a. What clinical and laboratory features are consistent with the diagnosis of an acute uncomplicated lower UTI (cystitis) in this patient?
   b. How does one differentiate cystitis from urethritis (caused by Chlamydia trachomatis, Neisseria gonorrhoeae, or herpes simplex virus) or vaginitis (due to Candida or Trichomonas species)?
   c. Should a urine culture be obtained in this patient experiencing her second episode of cystitis?
   d. What are the most likely pathogens and frequency of occurrence causing this patient's infection?
   e. What factors can increase the risk of developing a UTI?
   f. Create a list of this patient's drug-related problems.
   g. Since this is her second episode of an uncomplicated UTI, should she receive prophylactic antibiotics to prevent further episodes?

Desired Outcome

2. What are the goals of pharmacotherapy in this case?

Therapeutic Alternatives

3. a. What are the desirable characteristics of an anti-infective agent selected for the treatment of this uncomplicated UTI?
   b. What feasible pharmacotherapeutic alternatives are available for empiric first-line and second-line treatment of an uncomplicated UTI?

c. Which non-pharmacologic therapies may be useful in treating uncomplicated UTIs? Conflicting evidence exists that certain behaviors may decrease the risk of UTI.

Optimal Plan

4. What drug, dosage form, dose, schedule, and duration of therapy are best for this patient?

Outcome Evaluation

5. What clinical and laboratory parameters are necessary to evaluate the therapy for achievement of the desired therapeutic outcome and to detect or prevent adverse effects?

Patient Counseling

6. What information should be provided to the patient to enhance compliance, ensure successful therapy, and minimize adverse effects?

▶ Self-study Assignments

1. List potential therapeutic methods to prevent cystitis in patients who experience more than 2 episodes a year (recurrent cystitis).
2. Perform a literature search to obtain information on the use of cranberry juice for the reduction of bacteriuria and pyuria. What is your assessment of its effectiveness, and in what situations should it be recommended?
3. Provide your assessment and recommendation on the role of phenazopyridine in treatment of UTIs.

Fluoroquinolones should be reserved for patients intolerant, allergic, or resistant to first-line agents to avoid the emergence of resistant organisms.

References

1. Hooton TM, Stamm WE. Diagnosis and treatment of uncomplicated urinary tract infections. Infect Dis Clin North Am 1997;11:551–581.
2. Stapleton A, Stamm WE. Prevention of urinary tract infection. Infect Dis Clin North Am 1997;11:719–733.
3. Wong ES, McKevitt M, Running K, et al. Management of recurrent urinary tract infections with patient-administered single-dose therapy. Ann Intern Med 1985;102:302–307.
4. Norrby SR. Short-term treatment of uncomplicated lower urinary tract infections in women. Rev Infect Dis 1990;12:458–467.
5. Hooton TM, Winter C, Tiu F, et al. Randomized comparative trial and cost analysis of 3-day antimicrobial regimens for treatment of acute cystitis in women. JAMA 1995;273:41–45.

106   ACUTE PYELONEPHRITIS

► **The Stone Glazer**   (Level III)

Margaret E. McGuinness, PharmD

► After completing this case study, students should be able to:

- Differentiate the signs, symptoms, and laboratory findings associated with pyelonephritis from those seen in lower urinary tract infections.
- Recognize patient risk factors that predispose to development of pyelonephritis.
- Recommend appropriate empiric antimicrobial and symptomatic pharmacotherapy for a patient with suspected pyelonephritis.
- Make appropriate adjustments in pharmacotherapy based on patient response and culture results.
- Design a monitoring plan for a patient with pyelonephritis that allows objective assessment of the response to therapy.

☀ PATIENT PRESENTATION

Chief Complaint
"I feel tired and sick, and my back aches. It hurts to pass urine."

HPI

Simon Wyeth is a 75 yo man with a history of small cell cancer of the prostate, last treated with combination chemotherapy 2 weeks ago. He presents with a 2-day history of feeling exhausted, with at least 4 episodes of vomiting, nausea, constant back pain, and chills. He has no constipation, diarrhea, or chest pain. He was feeling well prior to the onset of the vomiting. Since then, he has become progressively weaker, and in the last 12 hours has hardly been able to get out of his chair. He has eaten nothing in 24 hours.

FH

Mother died at age 82 with cancer; father died at age 74 with "heart disease"; brother died at age 67 of bladder cancer; has 6 other siblings who are alive and well.

SH

120 pack-year smoking history, non-smoker × 20 years; no alcohol or IVDA. Monogamous relationship with his wife of 50 years. Interests include stone glazing, reading, and classical music.

PMH

Small cell cancer of prostate diagnosed 6 months ago. Patient presented at that time with flank pain, difficulty urinating, intermittent hematuria, and a prostate mass on physical exam. No metastases identified in liver (CT scan of chest and abdomen), bone (bone scan), or brain (CT scan). Has received 4 cycles of carboplatin and etoposide without incident.

CAD (s/p MI 15 years ago)

Bradycardia; pacemaker placed 3 years ago

Hiatal hernia with occasional reflux symptoms; drug and diet therapy control symptoms

Osteoarthritis of both knees

Type 2 DM × 5 years, diet controlled

Benign essential tremor

ROS

Patient has occasional headaches after chemotherapy for which he takes Tylenol #3. He has significant osteoarthritis in both knees that limits his mobility and prevents him sleeping through the night. He has nocturia that has improved since receiving chemotherapy. He has no shortness of breath except when walking more than 1 mile.

Meds

Nitroglycerin 0.4 mg PRN SL chest pain

Metamucil 1 tablespoon po QD constipation

Salsalate 750 mg po TID

Tylenol #3 1–2 tablets po Q 6 H PRN pain

Plendil ER 5 mg po BID for CAD management

Pepcid 20 mg po BID

Aspirin EC 325 mg po BID

Quinine sulfate 325 mg po PRN cramps

All

Penicillin → developed a rash in the late 1950s. Repeat courses have also been associated with rashes, most recently after the first course of chemotherapy when treated with amoxicillin for LRTI.

PE

Gen

Alert and oriented elderly male who appears ill, wrapped in blankets and cold to touch

He is able to walk without assistance but is slow due to pain in back and weakness.

VS
BP 121/68, P 73, RR 22, T 38.4°C; O_2 sat 98% on 1L, 93% room air; Ht 5'10", Wt 83.5 kg

HEENT
NCAT, EOMI; funduscopic exam with no evidence of exudates or cotton wool spots; pharynx clear and dry

Skin
No tenting; dry

Neck
Flat JVP; small left supraclavicular lymph node palpable

Chest
CTA, mild expiratory wheezes

CV
RRR, normal S_1 and S_2, no S_3

Abd
Mildly obese, active bowel sounds, tender on deep inspiration in all 4 quadrants. Mild rebound tenderness. No guarding or hepatomegaly.

Back
(+) CVAT. No paraspinal or spinal tenderness; complains of pain on bending forward.

Genit/Rect
Normal male genitalia; normal sphincter tone; pain on palpation of prostate, which is nodular with mass evident on left side.

Ext
No CCE; dry flaky skin on lower legs bilaterally. Pulses 2+ bilaterally.

Neuro
A & O × 3, CN II–XII intact; confused at times during interview; sensory and perception intact; (–) Romberg; normal gait; DTRs 4/5; muscle strength 4/5 all groups.

Labs and UA on Admission
See Table 106–1 and Figure 106–1.

Chest X-ray
No infiltrates seen

Abdominal Ultrasound
Bilateral hydronephrosis; no gross change from 6 months ago

CT Abdomen
Patchy contrast retention in both kidneys suggestive of inflammation; no focal abscess; 3.5-cm infrarenal aortic aneurysm; no adenopathy; prostate unchanged from 3 months ago.

Assessment
1. Pyelonephritis.
2. R/O sepsis.
3. Volume depletion.
4. Type 2 DM, poorly controlled.
5. Small cell cancer of the prostate; appears stable at present. Will delay chemotherapy (due in 1 week) given current infection.

TABLE 106–1. Laboratory Tests and Urinalyses on Days 1 Through 3 of Hospitalization.

Parameter (units)	Day 1 (12:30 PM)	Day 2 (5:00 AM)	Day 3 (5:00 AM)
Serum Chemistry			
Na (mEq/L)	134	136	138
K (mEq/L)	3.1	3.2	3.6
Cl (mEq/L)	99	101	105
CO_2 (mEq/L)	27	28	28
BUN (mg/dL)	35	30	28
SCr (mg/dL)	1.8	1.6	1.4
Glu (mg/dL)	220	174	129
Hematology			
Hgb (g/dL)	10.3	9.5	8.8
Hct (%)	34.8	29.2	25.9
Plt (× 10^3/mm³)	119	76	46
WBC (× 10^3/mm³)	20.2	18.5	15.6
PMN/B/L/M[a] (%)	82/10/8/0	85/9/3/3	80/5/13/2
Urinalysis			
pH	5.0	5.0	5.0
WBC/hpf	518	72	70
RBC/hpf	413	644	341
Appearance	Turbid, red	Clear, red	Clear
Protein (mg/dL)	> 300	100	100
Blood	Large	Large	Moderate
Glucose (mg/dL)	100	Negative	Negative
Ketones	Trace	Negative	Negative
Leukoesterase	Positive	Positive	Negative
Nitrite	Positive	Positive	Positive
Bacteria	Many	Few	Nil

[a] PMN, polymorphonuclear leukocytes; B, bands; L, lymphocytes; M, monocytes.

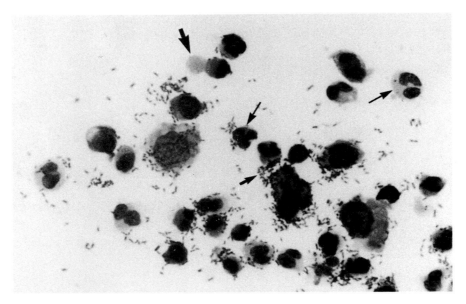

Figure 106–1. Urine sediment with red blood cells (large arrow) and numerous neutrophils (line arrows) and bacteria (small arrow). *(Wright × 1650; photo courtesy of Lydia C. Contis, MD.)*

► Questions

Problem Identification

1. a. *Create a list of the patient's drug-related problems.*
   b. *What information (signs, symptoms, laboratory tests) indicates the presence and severity of pyelonephritis in this patient?*
   c. *List any potential contributing factors, including drug therapy, that may have predisposed this patient to developing pyelonephritis.*
   d. *What additional information is needed to fully assess the patient?*

Desired Outcome

2. *What are the goals of pharmacotherapy in this patient?*

Therapeutic Alternatives

3. a. *What non-drug therapies might be useful for this patient?*
   b. *What organisms are commonly associated with pyelonephritis?*
   c. *What feasible pharmacotherapeutic alternatives are available for the empiric treatment of pyelonephritis?*

Optimal Plan

4. *Outline an antimicrobial regimen that will provide appropriate empiric therapy for pyelonephritis in this patient.*

Outcome Evaluation

5. a. *What clinical and laboratory parameters are necessary to evaluate the antibiotic therapy for achievement of the desired therapeutic outcomes and to detect or prevent adverse effects?*

► Clinical Course

The patient was started on the empiric antimicrobial regimen you recommended. He remained febrile for the next 2 days and required acetaminophen Q 6 H for back and abdominal pain. The antibiotic dose was adjusted for his renal function (calculated CL_{cr} on admission: 36 mL/min). On day 3 of hospitalization, he was much improved and had begun to eat a normal diet. Laboratory tests for days 2 and 3 are included in Table 106–1. He had 2 or 3 episodes of loose stools that were cultured but did not show any evidence of infection. Culture results on day 3 (late in the day) are shown in Table 106–2.

TABLE 106–2. Culture Results of Blood and Urine on Day 3

Organism, *Escherichia coli*	Blood	Urine
Sensitive to		
	Ampicillin	Ampicillin
	Ampicillin/sulbactam	Ampicillin/sulbactam
	Cefazolin	Cefazolin
	Cefpodoxime	Cefpodoxime
	Ceftriaxone	Ceftriaxone
	Ceftazidime	Ceftazidime
	Piperacillin	Piperacillin
	Ciprofloxacin	Ciprofloxacin
	Gentamicin	Gentamicin
	TMP-SMX	TMP-SMX

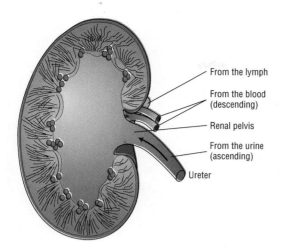

Figure 106–2. Routes of infection for pyelonephritis.

From the lymph
From the blood (descending)
Renal pelvis
From the urine (ascending)
Ureter

b. *What recommendations, if any, do you have for changes in the initial drug regimen?*

Patient Counseling

6. *What information should be provided to the patient upon discharge to enhance adherence, ensure successful therapy, and minimize adverse effects?*

▶ Clinical Pearl

Pyelonephritis can be managed with many different drugs; choose drugs that are bactericidal and cleared in active form by the kidney. Drugs suitable for once-daily therapy help to reduce treatment costs.

▶ Self-study Assignments

1. Develop a protocol for switching patients from IV to oral therapy when treating pyelonephritis.
2. Perform a literature search to find clinical trials comparing drug therapy in pyelonephritis and compare inclusion criteria, drug regimens, outcomes, and costs of therapy.
3. Develop a clinical pathway that could be used for the management of suspected pyelonephritis.

References

1. Bailey RR, Begg EJ, Smith AH, et al. Prospective, randomized controlled study comparing two dosing regimens of gentamicin/oral ciprofloxacin switch therapy for acute pyelonephritis. Clin Nephrol 1996;46:183–186.
2. Sandberg T, Alesig K, Eilard T, et al. Aminoglycosides do not improve the efficacy of cephalosporins for treatment of acute pyelonephritis in women. Scand J Infect Dis 1997;29:175–179.
3. Jinnah F, Islam MS, Rumi MA, et al. Drug sensitivity pattern of *E. coli* causing urinary tract infection in diabetic and non-diabetic patients. J Int Med Res 1996;24:296–301.

107 SYPHILIS

▶ **Hitting Below the Belt** (Level I)

Alex K. McDonald, PharmD
Dennis M. Williams, PharmD, FASHP, FCCP, BCPS

▶ After completing this case study, students should be able to:

- Identify activities or behaviors that put an individual at risk for contracting a sexually transmitted disease (STD).
- Describe the tests used to diagnose syphilis and evaluate treatment.
- Recommend appropriate therapies for the treatment of syphilis.
- Counsel patients receiving treatment for an STD.
- Discuss the association between syphilis and HIV infection.

☀ PATIENT PRESENTATION

Chief Complaint
"I'm here for a follow-up visit because I am pregnant."

HPI
Irene Sanchez is a 28 yo woman who presents for prenatal care. Her last normal menstrual period was 14 weeks ago. She is a single mother of 2 children.

PMH
Unremarkable. This is her third pregnancy (G_3P_2). She has delivered 2 other healthy babies who are now 9 and 6 years old.

FH
Both parents live in Mexico. Father is in good health. Mother has HTN and DM.

SH
Single woman who has been living with her brother and his family in a trailer for 2 years; works at a textile mill. She reports being sexually active since age 14 with numerous sexual partners but currently is not sexually active. The apparent father has left the area. Denies use of tobacco or alcohol.

ROS
Complaints of nasal congestion, heartburn, and episodes of N/V on most mornings for past 3 weeks. Patient denies previous skin lesions, rashes, or alopecia.

Meds
None

All
NKDA

PE

Gen
WDWN pregnant Hispanic woman who appears anxious but in NAD

VS
BP 130/70, P 90, RR 18, T 37°C; Wt 62.7 kg (baseline 60 kg)

Skin
Warm, dry, non-jaundiced; without bruising or lesions; hair quantity, distribution, and texture unremarkable

HEENT
NC/AT; TMs pearly gray revealing good cone of light bilaterally; PERRLA; EOMI; optic disk margins appropriately sharp; nasal mucous membranes moist; no oropharyngeal lesions

Neck
Supple; no lymphadenopathy, bruits, JVD, or thyromegaly

Chest
CTA bilaterally

Breast
No masses or dimples; no axillary lymphadenopathy

CV
RRR; no m/r/g

Abd
(+) BS; nontender; no masses or organomegaly; 15-week fundal height with (+) fetal heart sounds (rate 140 bpm).

Neuro
A & O × 3; no focal abnormalities; CN II–XII intact.

Labs

Na 141 mEq/L	Hgb 14.3 g/dL
K 4.6 mEq/L	Hct 36.0%
Cl 101 mEq/L	WBC 5.5×10^3/mm^3
CO_2 28 mEq/L	Plt 225×10^3/mm^3
BUN 13 mg/dL	
SCr 0.9 mg/dL	
Glu 87 mg/dL	

Assessment
28 yo Hispanic woman who is 14 weeks pregnant. As per current CDC guidelines, will screen serologically for syphilis during the early stages of this pregnancy.

▶ Clinical Course

A positive RPR titer of 1:16 is reported the afternoon of the physical examination. This result is confirmed 2 days later with a positive FTA-ABS test. HBsAg (–), *Chlamydia* (–), GC culture (–), Pap smear (–). There are no signs/symptoms of syphilis.

▶ Questions

Problem Identification

1. What information (signs, symptoms, laboratory values) indicates the presence or stage of syphilis?

Desired Outcome

2. What are the goals of pharmacotherapy in this case?

Therapeutic Alternatives

3. a. What non-drug recommendations should be given to this patient?
   b. What pharmacotherapeutic alternatives are available for this patient?

Optimal Plan

4. a. What is the recommended treatment (drug, dose, and duration) for this patient?
   b. What alternatives would you recommend if this patient were allergic to your first suggestion?

Outcome Evaluation

5. What clinical and laboratory parameters are necessary to evaluate the therapy for achievement of the desired therapeutic outcome and to detect or prevent adverse effects?

Patient Counseling

6. a. What information should be provided to the patient to enhance compliance, ensure successful therapy, and minimize adverse effects?
   b. What information should be provided to the patient to prevent a future sexually transmitted disease?

▶ Clinical Course

The patient subsequently delivered a uterine pregnancy at 41 weeks. At delivery, her RPR titer was 1:4 and an MHA-TP was reactive. The infant's RPR was nonreactive.

▶ Follow-up Questions

1. What are potential explanations for this finding?
2. What further assessment and treatment should be considered for the patient?
3. What assessment and treatment should be considered for the infant?

► ## Self-study Assignments

1. What other therapies are currently being investigated as treatment for syphilis?
2. What tests or procedures are indicated to diagnose neurosyphilis?
3. How would the presence of neurosyphilis alter the recommended treatment regimen?

► ## Clinical Pearl

There is no acceptable alternative to penicillin for the treatment of syphilis in pregnant women allergic to penicillin.

Reference

1. Centers for Disease Control and Prevention. Syphilis. 1998 guidelines for treatment of sexually transmitted diseases. MMWR 1998;47(RR-01):28–49. www.cdc.gov

108 GENITAL HERPES AND CHLAMYDIAL INFECTIONS

► ### Double Trouble   (Level II)

Suellyn J. Sorensen, PharmD, BCPS

► After completing this case study, students should be able to:

- Identify subjective and objective data consistent with genital herpes and *Chlamydia*.
- Recommend appropriate therapies for the treatment of genital herpes and *Chlamydia*.
- Provide effective and comprehensive counseling for patients with genital herpes and *Chlamydia*.
- Identify drug interactions of clinical significance and provide recommendations for managing them.

☀ PATIENT PRESENTATION

Chief Complaint
"I have painful blisters in my genital area and I have terrible headaches and muscle aches."

HPI
Lisa Flint is a 20 yo nulligravida woman who presents to the county health STD clinic for evaluation of genital lesions that have been present for 3 days. She has also noticed a white non-odorous vaginal discharge that has lasted 14 days. She admits to anal and vaginal intercourse with 2 regular partners in the last 60 days. It has been 5 days since her last sexual encounter.

PMH
Recurrent UTIs; most recent 3 months ago
Vaginal candidiasis; most recent 6 months ago
Gonorrhea 5 years ago
Trichomonas vaginalis 2 years ago

FH
Mother type 2 DM; father died at age 50 of an acute MI.

SH
Lives with her boyfriend and works at a Mexican restaurant. She admits to occasional use of alcohol and marijuana.

Meds
Loestrin-21 1 tablet po QD
Multivitamin with iron 1 tablet po QD
Ibuprofen 200 mg po PRN
Ciprofloxacin 250 mg po QD

All
Penicillin (hives and tongue swelling)

ROS
(−) cough, (−) night sweats, (−) weight loss, (+) diarrhea; (−) dysuria or urinary frequency, (+) anorectal pain; LMP 6 weeks ago

PE

Gen
Thin young woman in NAD

VS
BP 136/71, P 78, RR 17, T 37.2°C; Wt. 51 kg, Ht 65″

Skin
Dry, no lesions, normal color and temperature

HEENT
PERRLA, EOMI without nystagmus

Neck
Supple; no adenopathy, JVD, or thyromegaly

Chest
Air entry equal, no crepitations or wheezing

CV
RRR, normal S_1 and S_2, no S_3 or S_4, no murmurs or rubs

Abd
Soft, mild tenderness to palpation in RLQ, (+) bowel sounds, no HSM

Genit/Rect

Tender inguinal adenopathy. External exam clear for nits and lice, several extensive shallow small painful vesicular lesions over vulva and labia, swollen and red. Vagina red, rugated, moderate amounts of creamy white discharge. Cervix pink, covered with above discharge, non-tender, ~3 cm. Corpus non-tender, no palpable masses. Adnexa with no palpable masses or tenderness. Rectum with no external lesions; (+) diffuse inflammation and friability internally, no masses.

Ext

Peripheral pulses 2+ bilaterally, DTRs 2+, no joint swelling or tenderness

Neuro

Alert and oriented, CN II–XII intact

Labs

Na 135 mEq/L	Hgb 12.9 g/dL	WBC $6.3 \times 10^3/mm^3$	RPR non-reactive
K 4.0 mEq/L	Hct 37.3%	64% PMNs	Preg test: hCG pending
Cl 102 mEq/L	Plt $255 \times 10^3/mm^3$	2% Bands	HIV serology: ELISA pending
CO_2 27 mEq/L		1% Eos	
BUN 11 mg/dL		24% Lymphs	
SCr 0.9 mg/dL		9% Monos	
Glu 72 mg/dL			

Other

Vaginal discharge—whiff test (−); pH < 4.5; wet mount *Trichomonas* (−), clue cells (−), monilia (+)

▶ Clinical Course

The following results were reported 5 days later.
- Viral culture of genital vesicular fluid: HSV2 isolated
- Vulval swab DFA monoclonal stain: HSV2 isolated
- Rectal and cervical bacterial cultures: *Neisseria gonorrhoeae* (−)
- Rectal and cervical cultures: *Chlamydia trachomatis* (+)

▶ Questions

Problem Identification

1. a. Create a list of the patient's drug-related problems.
   b. What subjective and objective clinical data are consistent with a primary genital herpes infection?
   c. Could any of the patient's problems have been caused by drug therapy?

Desired Outcome

2. What are the goals of pharmacotherapy in this case?

Therapeutic Alternatives

3. a. What non-drug therapies might be useful for this patient?
   b. What feasible pharmacotherapeutic alternatives are available for treatment of genital herpes and Chlamydia?

Optimal Plan

4. What drug, dosage form, dose, schedule, and duration of therapy are best for treating this patient's genital herpes and chlamydial infections?

Outcome Evaluation

5. What clinical and laboratory parameters are necessary to evaluate the therapy for achievement of the desired therapeutic outcome and to detect or prevent adverse effects?

Patient Counseling

6. What information should be provided to the patient to enhance compliance, ensure successful therapy, and minimize adverse effects?

▶ Follow-up Questions

1. Six months later Lisa calls the STD clinic complaining of genital lesions that look and feel the same as the lesions she had 6 months earlier when seen and treated in the clinic. Should this episode of recurrent genital herpes be treated? If so, what therapies would be appropriate?
2. Is daily suppressive therapy indicated because she had a recurrent episode?
3. When is Chlamydia treatment indicated for sex partners?
4. What additional pharmacotherapeutic interventions should be made to address the problems that were identified in question 1.a.?

▶ Self-study Assignments

1. Determine if there is a role for vaccines in the future management of herpes simplex disease.
2. Recommend alternative agents for the treatment of acyclovir-resistant herpes.
3. Explain the relationship between herpes simplex and HIV infections.
4. Describe herpes simplex complications that may require hospitalization, and recommend an appropriate treatment regimen.

▶ Clinical Pearl

Many cases of genital herpes are transmitted by persons who have asymptomatic viral shedding and are unaware that they have the infection.

References

1. Centers for Disease Control and Prevention. Genital herpes simplex (HSV) infection; Chlamydial infection. 1998 guidelines for treatment of sexually transmitted diseases. MMWR 1998;47(RR-01):20–26, 53–59. Also see http://www.cdc.gov/
2. Anon. Drugs for non-HIV viral infections. Med Lett 1997;39:69–76.
3. Valtrex Caplets Package Insert. Research Triangle Park, NC, Glaxo Wellcome, 1997.

109 OSTEOMYELITIS

▶ **My Brother's Kicker**   (Level I)

Edward P. Armstrong, PharmD, BCPS, FASHP
Victor A. Elsberry, PharmD, BCNSP
Leslie L. Barton, MD

▶ After completing this case study, students should be able to:

- List the most common presenting signs and symptoms of acute osteomyelitis.
- Suggest alternative treatment approaches for acute osteomyelitis in pediatric patients.
- Outline a treatment plan for empiric therapy of acute osteomyelitis.
- List monitoring parameters for antibacterial treatment of osteomyelitis, including efficacy and toxicity of therapy.

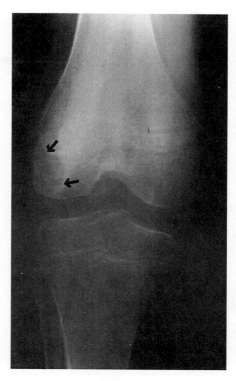

Figure 109–1. Lytic lesion of the distal right femur indicating osteomyelitis.

☀ PATIENT PRESENTATION

Chief Complaint
"My knee still hurts."

HPI
John Grant is an 8 yo boy referred to the Infectious Disease Clinic because of persistent right knee pain 1 month after being kicked in the right knee by his brother. The day after the incident, he was seen in urgent care because of right knee pain and was sent home with symptomatic therapy. He returned to urgent care 1 week later (3 weeks ago) because of persistent tenderness in that knee.

He was again sent home only to be seen 1 week later (2 weeks ago), at which time physical examination suggested and x-rays confirmed the diagnosis of osteomyelitis of the distal right femur (see Figure 109–1). He had a WBC count of $8.0 \times 10^3/mm^3$, ESR of 21 mm/hr, and tenderness over the right lateral femoral condyle. He underwent aspiration of the lesion, which revealed no pus. He was started on home IV therapy with cefazolin 500 mg IV Q 6 H. He had continued to play soccer during the first 2 weeks after his injury.

He was seen 1 week ago because of increasing knee pain after 1 week of antibiotic therapy. He denied any systemic symptoms and was afebrile. His ESR had risen to 48 mm/hr; x-rays showed an increased size of the femoral lytic lesion. Aspiration of the knee joint revealed purulent fluid. The bone culture and the knee aspirate revealed no growth. Arthroscopic surgery of the knee was performed and cefazolin was continued.

Three days ago at an office visit with the orthopedic surgeon, his mother reported mild improvement of the pain. She related that his pain had diminished during the preceding 3 days; he could now sleep through the night. He was still unable to bear weight on his right leg and was only able to ambulate with crutches. His ESR was 56 mm/hr.

PMH
No prior history of serious diseases or infections. Immunizations are up-to-date.

FH
No family history of early childhood deaths secondary to severe infection.

SH
Mother and father live in the household and are well, as are 3 siblings. There are 3 dogs in the home.

ROS
No positive findings with regard to head, eyes, ears, nose, throat, cardiorespiratory systems, skin lesions, or recent illness. No recent travel. No other significant trauma.

Meds
Cefazolin 500 mg IV every 6 hours

All
NKA

PE

Gen
His general appearance is that of a thin, apprehensive male in no distress unless his right knee is flexed, extended, or palpated

VS
BP 93/50, P 104, RR 22, T 36.0°C; Wt 26.6 kg, Ht 52″

Skin
No lesions

HEENT
Eyes without corneal lesions, normal fundi; throat and pharynx without exudate; nose without discharge or congestion

Neck/LN
No lymphadenopathy or thyromegaly

Lungs/Thorax
Chest was clear to percussion and auscultation

CV
Normal S_1 and S_2, no murmurs present

Abd
Soft without hepatosplenomegaly

Genit/Rect
Genitalia are normal; circumcised male

MS/Ext
Swollen, slightly tender right knee held in flexion with marked decreased ROM. He has developed some tightness around the joint and is unable to bear weight on standing and preferred use of a posterior splint.

Neuro
Reflexes 2+; plantar reflexes downgoing; no cerebellar or sensoral abnormalities; normal strength and tone except where unmeasurable at the right knee.

Assessment
Continued distal femoral osteomyelitis and adjacent septic arthritis of the right knee, secondary to delayed and partial treatment of the staphylococcal infection. The persistently elevated ESR and slow resolution of knee symptoms are of concern.

► Questions

Problem Identification

1. a. Create a list of the patient's drug-related problems.
   b. What information (signs, symptoms, laboratory values) indicates the presence or severity of acute osteomyelitis?

Desired Outcome

2. What are the goals of pharmacotherapy in this case?

Therapeutic Alternatives

3. a. What non-drug therapies might be useful for this patient?
   b. What feasible pharmacotherapeutic alternatives are available for the empiric treatment of acute osteomyelitis?

Optimal Plan

4. What drug, dosage form, dose, schedule, and duration of therapy are best for this patient?

► Clinical Course

An x-ray taken after low-dose antibiotic treatment showed a persistent lesion (see Figure 109–2). The I.D. consultant continued the cefazolin but changed the regimen to 100 mg/kg/24 hours in 3 divided doses. She recommended clinical re-evaluation with repeat WBC and ESR in 1 week. If his ESR is the same, or (preferably) lower, cefazolin is to be discontinued and oral cephalexin 100 mg/kg/day in 4 divided doses initiated. Re-evaluation of the patient after 1 week of oral therapy was planned.

Ten days later, the patient was again seen in the Pediatric Infectious Disease Clinic where clinical evaluation revealed no additional findings. The patient continued to be afebrile and his ESR was 12 mm/hr. He was still on crutches, but he had recently removed the right posterior leg splint. His mother had been helping him perform some passive range-of-motion exercises. His right leg was still maintained in a flexed position at the knee. He had full range of motion at the right hip but decreased flexion and extension at the right knee. The gastrocnemius circumference was slightly diminished on the right side, but strength on both plantar flexion and dorsiflexion of the right foot was normal. He had been tolerating the oral antibiotic regimen without apparent abdominal discomfort, diarrhea, or rash. Oral cephalexin was to be continued for at least 3 additional weeks at the same dose of 100 mg/kg/day.

Outcome Evaluation

5. What clinical and laboratory parameters are necessary to evaluate the therapy for achievement of the desired therapeutic outcome and to detect or prevent adverse effects?

Patient Counseling

6. What information should be provided to the patient's caregiver to enhance compliance, ensure successful therapy, and minimize adverse effects?

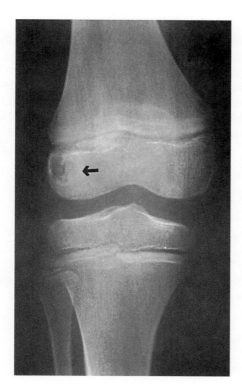

Figure 109–2. Persistent lesion of the distal right femur after low-dose antibiotic treatment.

▶ Clinical Pearl

The ultimate prognosis of acute osteomyelitis is based on the speed of diagnosis, prompt initiation of appropriate antimicrobial therapy, and surgical drainage, if needed.

▶ Self-study Assignments

1. Plan alternative IV and oral treatment regimens in the event that the patient could not tolerate the antibiotic initially used.
2. Compare optimal oral treatment strategies for osteomyelitis in adults with those in children.

References

1. Burnett MW, Bass JW, Cook BA. Etiology of osteomyelitis complicating sickle cell disease. Pediatrics 1998;101:296–297.
2. Nelson JD. Skeletal infections in children. Adv Pediatr Infect Dis 1991;6:59–78.
3. Dagan R. Management of acute hematogenous osteomyelitis and septic arthritis in the pediatric patient. Pediatr Infect Dis J 1993;12:88–92.
4. Lew DP, Waldvogel FA. Osteomyelitis. N Engl J Med 1997;336:999–1007.

110   GRAM-NEGATIVE SEPSIS

▶ **Bottomed Out**   (Level II)

Mary M. Hess, PharmD

▶ After completing this case study, students should be able to:

- Recognize the signs and symptoms that are present in patients with sepsis.
- Recommend appropriate treatments for sepsis-induced hypotension.
- Design an empiric antimicrobial regimen for the initial treatment of presumed sepsis, based on the potential sources of infection and the most common organisms involved in those sources.
- React appropriately to changes in the sepsis patient's medical condition and adjust pharmacotherapeutic regimens properly.
- Interpret culture and sensitivity data correctly and recommend rational changes in antimicrobial therapy based on this information.

☀ PATIENT PRESENTATION

Chief Complaint
Not available.

HPI
Thomas Jackson is a 77 yo man who is brought to the ED by a family member who states that the patient has been experiencing progressive weakness and DOE. The family decided to bring him to the ED when he was unable to respond to them appropriately.

PMH
CHF, s/p pacemaker insertion 3 weeks PTA
Alcoholic cirrhosis

SH
(+) Tobacco (amount unknown); (+++) alcohol (amount unknown)

FH
Noncontributory

All
NKDA

ROS
Noncontributory

PE

VS
BP 76/Palp, P 74 (reg), RR 20, T 35.6°C; Ht 6'1", Wt 81 kg

HEENT

PERRLA; EOMI; optic disks flat; TMs intact; oropharynx clear

Neck

11 cm JVD, (--) bruits

CV

RRR, (+) S_3, pacemaker present

Resp

Minimal basilar crackles; mechanically ventilated with FiO_2 50%, assist control mode, tidal volume 700 mL, PEEP 5 mm Hg, RR 20 breaths/minute

Abd

Soft, NT/ND; (−) BS; protuberant abdomen with ascites

Genit/Rect

Normal male genitalia: heme (−) stool

Ext

1–2+ pitting edema; 1+ pulses; normal ROM throughout

Neuro

A & O × 3 (lethargic but oriented); CN II–XII intact; ? asterixis; Babinski (−)

Labs

Na 135 mEq/L	Hgb 11 g/dL	Ca 8.4 mg/dL
K 6.5 mEq/L	Hct 31.6%	Mg 1.7 mEq/L
Cl 102 mEq/L	Plt 57 × 10³/mm³	Phos 4.1 mg/dL
CO_2 23 mEq/L	WBC 11.3 × 10³/mm³	Alb 2.5 g/dL
BUN 46 mg/dL	73% Polys	PT 27.1 sec
SCr 2.3 mg/dL	15% Bands	aPTT 63.1 sec
Glu 169 mg/dL	6% Lymphs	INR 5.1
	6% Monos	

ECG

Wide complex paced rhythm.

ABG

pH 7.24, $Paco_2$ 35 mm Hg, Pao_2 47 mm Hg, HCO_3 27 mEq/L

Assessment

Unresponsiveness, respiratory decompensation, hypotension, and hyperkalemia in a patient with known cirrhosis; R/O sepsis.

Plan

Stabilize the patient emergently and transfer to ICU.

► Clinical Course

In the ED, the patient was given normal saline 2 L for hypotension. Treatment of hyperkalemia included administration of calcium chloride 1 ampule (1 g calcium), $NaHCO_3$ 1 syringe (50 mEq), $D_{50}W$ 1 syringe, regular insulin 10 units, and furosemide 40 mg IV. Cultures were obtained from urine, blood × 2, and sputum. He was electively intubated for airway protection. He was then transferred to the medical ICU for further treatment.

► Questions

Problem Identification

1. a. Devise a drug-related problem list for this patient.
   b. What clinical signs does this patient exhibit that are consistent with infection? What elements must be present to confirm the presence of sepsis?

Desired Outcome

2. What are the short-term and long-term goals of therapy when managing a patient with sepsis?

Therapeutic Alternatives

3. a. What are the treatment alternatives for sepsis-induced hypotension?
   b. What colloids are commercially available?
   c. Outline a reasonable alternative antibiotic regimen for empiric treatment of this patient (include dosing and duration of therapy). In formulating your answer, consider the potential sources of infection and the most common infecting organisms for those sources.

► Clinical Course, Day #1

After the patient was admitted to the medical ICU, medications initiated by the ICU team included:

Vitamin K_1 20 mg IV QD × 5 days
Kayexalate 30 g po × 2 doses
Ofloxacin 400 mg IV Q 12 H
Ticarcillin/clavulanate 3.1 g IV Q 6 H
Gentamicin 350 mg IV × 1
Famotidine 20 mg IV Q 12 H
Thiamine 100 mg IV QD
Folic acid 1 mg IV QD

The 2 L of NS given in the ED for hypotension resulted in minimal improvement in blood pressure. Therefore, dopamine 800 mg/250 mL was initiated at a rate of 5 µg/kg/min. The patient's repeat serum potassium after treatment in the ED was 4.7 mEq/L. One hour after starting the dopamine drip, his VS are: BP 87/42, P 74 (paced), RR 20.

Optimal Plan

4. a. *Based on this information, what do you recommend as the next therapeutic intervention?*
    b. *One hour after your recommendation was implemented, his BP was 85/45 and pulse was 74. What is the next therapeutic option to achieve your BP goal?*

▶ Clinical Course, Day #2

The patient remained stable on the dopamine and vasopressor regimens you selected. His maximum temperature for 24 hours has been 39.7°C. The past 24-hour fluid intake was 3175 mL and urine output was 500 mL. His current laboratory values are as follows.

Na 146 mEq/L	Hgb 11 g/dL
K 4.2 mEq/L	Hct 31.4%
Cl 111 mEq/L	Plt $36 \times 10^3/mm^3$
CO_2 26 mEq/L	WBC $9.4 \times 10^3/mm^3$
BUN 37 mg/dL	70% Polys
SCr 1.3 mg/dL	16% Bands
Glu 97 mg/dL	6% Lymphs
	8% Monos

ABG

pH 7.4, $Paco_2$ 34 mm Hg, Pao_2 68 mm Hg, HCO_3 26 mEq/L

Microbiology Report

Sputum: many gram-negative rods
Urine: no growth
Blood cultures, 2 bottles: no growth × 48 hours

c. *What adjustments in therapy do you recommend for the patient at this point?*

▶ Clinical Course, Day #3

The patient's BP has remained stable throughout the weaning of the α-agonist. He still remains on maximum dopamine rates. Laboratory data are the same as yesterday with the exception that his WBC is $12.2 \times 10^3/mm^3$ with 84% polys, 5% bands, 5% lymphs, and 6% monos. The gram-negative rod in the sputum has been identified as *Klebsiella*. The sensitivities are pending. The maximum temperature for the past 24 hours has been 37.5°C. The fluid intake is 2780 mL; urine output is 1100 mL.

d. *What is your plan at this point?*

▶ Clinical Course, Day #3 (continued)

Later in the day, sensitivity results return:

Culture type: sputum
Date of culture: 3 days prior
Report: heavy *Klebsiella pneumoniae*

Sensitivities

Ticarcillin/clavulanic acid	R
Aztreonam	S
Ampicillin/sulbactam	R
Ofloxacin	R
Piperacillin	S
Gentamicin	S
Tobramycin	S
Ceftazidime	S
Cefepime	S
Trovafloxacin	S

e. *What adjustments, if any, do you want to make now that all of the information is available?*

▶ Clinical Course, Day #4

The patient has been successfully weaned from all vasopressors. His laboratory parameters are returning to normal, and he is undergoing weaning trials from the ventilator.

f. *What are your final recommendations regarding the antimicrobial therapy?*

Outcome Evaluation

5. *What parameters should be monitored to evaluate the efficacy and toxicity of your interventions?*

▶ Clinical Course, Day #7

The patient was extubated from the ventilator and transferred to a general medicine unit. His therapy was converted to an oral agent and he is ready to be discharged tomorrow.

Patient Counseling

6. *What information should be provided to the patient about his antimicrobial regimen upon discharge?*

▶ Self-study Assignments

1. Review hemodynamic monitoring parameters and their correlation with various shock states.
2. Describe what is meant by concentration-dependent versus concentration-independent microbial killing.
3. Review mechanisms of antimicrobial resistance by organism and drug class. Create a list of antimicrobial agents to which organisms are more likely to develop resistance.

▶ Clinical Pearl

Preservation of perfusion to the organ systems is crucial to prevent the development of multiorgan system failure. Antimicrobial therapy should be initiated during the process of stabilizing the patient.

References

1. Bone RC, Balk RA, Cerra FB, et al. Definitions for sepsis and organ failure and guidelines for the use of innovative therapies in sepsis. The ACCP/SCCM Consensus Conference Committee. Chest 1992;101:1644–1655.
2. Boucher BA, Coffey BC, Kuhl DA, et al. Algorithm for assessing renal dysfunction risk in critically ill trauma patients receiving aminoglycosides. Am J Surg 1990; 160:473–480.
3. Yim JM, Vermeulen LC Jr, Erstad BL, et al. Albumin and nonprotein colloid solution use in U.S. academic health centers. Arch Intern Med 1995;155:2450–2455.
4. Vermeulen LC Jr, Ratko TA, Erstad BL, et al. A paradigm for consensus. The University Hospital Consortium guidelines for the use of albumin, nonprotein colloid, and crystalloid solutions. Arch Intern Med 1995;155:373–379.
5. Nicolau DP, Freeman CD, Belliveau PP, et al. Experience with a once-daily aminoglycoside program administered to 2,184 adult patients. Antimicrob Agents Chemother 1995;39:650–655.

111 SYSTEMIC FUNGAL INFECTION

▶ **Solving a Budding Problem**   (Level III)

Aaron D. Killian, PharmD, BCPS

▶ After completing this case study, students should be able to:

- Describe the pathogenesis and potential sequelae of hematogenous fungal infections in hospitalized patients.
- Given a case scenario, identify risk factors that predispose a patient to systemic fungal infection.
- Differentiate fungal colonization from invasion/dissemination.
- Recommend empiric antifungal therapy based upon patient history/clinical condition, site of infection, and antifungal resistance patterns.
- List specific monitoring parameters for antifungal use in critically ill patients.

☀ PATIENT PRESENTATION

Chief Complaint
"My chest feels so tight, and I just can't seem to breathe anymore."

HPI
Wanda Stevenson is a 57 yo woman admitted with a COPD exacerbation. Ten days into her hospital stay, she experienced increased wheezing, severe tachypnea, and accessory muscle use. She also began to produce thick, yellowish sputum, and treatment was initiated for a *Serratia marcescens* nosocomial pneumonia. After failing both BIPAP and CPAP, she was sedated with lorazepam, paralyzed with pancuronium, and intubated. A nasogastric tube was placed for enteral feedings, and 2 days later the patient produced 600 mL of dark, reddish-black aspirate that was guaiac positive. On day 18, the patient developed diminished bowel sounds with a distended abdomen and mild RUQ tenderness. She also exhibited intermittent episodes of delirium and a "hypoventilation" syndrome of unknown origin. Gastric residual was 75 mL at last check. A right internal jugular (IJ) line and urinary catheter were placed 10 and 14 days ago, respectively.

PMH
COPD
Depression
Hypercholesterolemia
HTN
Hypothyroidism

PSH
Non-contributory

FH
Mother alive with hypothyroidism × 25 years; father alive with hypertension × 30 years.

SH
Denies alcohol and IVDU; 45 pack-year smoker. Lives alone.

Meds
Heparin 5000 units SC Q 12 H
KCl 20 mEq NG QD
Metoclopramide 10 mg IV Q 6 H
Furosemide 20 mg IV Q 6 H
Methylprednisolone 60 mg IV Q 6 H
Terazosin 5 mg NG BID
Levothyroxine 0.05 mg IV QD
Theophylline 200 mg NG TID
Simvastatin 20 mg NG QD
Lorazepam continuous IV infusion 2 mg/hr
Morphine 2 mg IV Q 2 H
Piperacillin 3 g IV Q 4 H
Gentamicin 400 mg IV Q 24 H
Enteral feeding (Pulmocare) at 30 mL/hr

All
Iodinated compounds → maculopapular rash
Meperidine → hypotension with rash
Metronidazole → peripheral neuropathies
Terfenadine → occasional palpitations
Erythromycin → unknown reaction

PE

Gen
Morbidly obese Caucasian woman with vitiligo of extremities. APACHE II = 12.

VS
BP 115/75, HR 122, RR 26–30 (pre-intubation), T 101.7°F; Wt 128 kg, Ht 73″

Skin

Slight monilial overgrowth on skin folds lateral to vaginal area

HEENT

PERRLA; funduscopy reveals clear disk margins without exudates. Patient orotracheally intubated; ocular lubricant applied bilaterally

Neck

Supple without stiffness or lymphadenopathy; mild JVD

Chest

No consolidation; diminished breath sounds with wheezes bilaterally

CV

S_1, S_2 normal with regular rate and rhythm; no S_3, S_4, or murmurs

Abd

Absent bowel sounds; (+) RUQ tenderness; mild abdominal wall tenderness (without rebound)

Ext

1+ pitting edema of extremities; no clubbing or cyanosis. Significant atonia of left arm; grip strength 1/5 in both upper extremities

Neuro

Oriented to person, place, and time. Plantar reflexes downgoing. DTRs depressed bilaterally. Patient moves to noxious stimuli

Labs

Na 139 mEq/L	Hgb 14.5 g/dL	WBC $21.1 \times 10^3/mm^3$	Mg 2.5 mEq/L
K 3.5 mEq/L	Hct 42.5%	89% Neutros	Ca 8.8 mEq/L
Cl 98 mEq/L	Plt $239 \times 10^3/mm^3$	5% Lymphs	Phos 5.2 mg/dL
CO_2 32 mEq/L		3% Monos	Alb 2.5 g/dL
BUN 93 mg/dL		0% Eos	LDH 1229 IU/L
SCr 1.3 mg/dL		3% Basos	CK 209 IU/L
Glu 267 mg/dL			

UA

Yellow, hazy, SG 1.022, pH 5.5; no protein, bilirubin, albumin, glucose, or ketones; nitrite and leukocyte esterase negative; few bacteria; 10–25 RBC/hpf; 0–2 WBC/hpf, 0–1 squamous epithelial cells/hpf

Tracheal Aspirate

0–1 WBCs, no bacteria seen, moderate yeast

ABG

pH 7.39, Pco_2 52 mm Hg, Po_2 87 mm Hg, HCO_3 31 mEq/L, Sao_2 88% (60% Fio_2, tidal volume 700 mL, pressure support 15 cm H_2O, PEEP 5 cm H_2O, assist control 14 breaths/min)

Abdominal Flat Plate

Colonic dilatation; right colonic/ileal air-fluid level; no pneumoperitoneum.

CT Head

Right maxillary sinusitis.

► Questions

Problem Identification

1. *a. Identify the patient's initial drug-related problems and provide recommendations for managing each of them.*

► Clinical Course

The patient continues to have low-grade fevers, and her WBC increases to $42.0 \times 10^3/mm^3$ with 80% PMNs, 10% bands, 5% lymphs, 3% monos, 1% eos, and 1% basos. An abdominal CT is performed that reveals no abscesses. She is evaluated by the gastroenterology and surgical services, both of which agree to an exploratory laparotomy. Subsequently, she is found to have a perforated cecum, and a right hemicolectomy is performed. Enteral feedings are temporarily discontinued and TPN is initiated. Five days after the operation, the patient's SCr increases to 1.9 mg/dL, her WBC increases from 23 to $32 \times 10^3/mm^3$, and she develops moderate hypotension. Microscopic analysis of the patient's urine reveals 60 to 80 WBCs, light bacteria, and the presence of $> 10^5$ CFU/mL *Candida* on 2 successive cultures. One set of blood cultures taken on the day of surgery is now positive (1 of 2 tubes) for *Staphylococcus epidermidis*.

b. What risk factors for disseminated fungal infection are present in this patient?

c. Does this patient meet the criteria for colonization or invasive/disseminated fungal infection?

Desired Outcome

2. *What are the goals of pharmacotherapy in this patient?*

Therapeutic Alternatives

3. *a. What non-drug measures would you recommend for treatment of this fungal infection?*

► Clinical Course

The patient's right IJ catheter is removed, the catheter tip is sent for culture, and a new central line is placed in the left IJ. Four days later, 1 set of blood cultures (right IJ) is positive (1 of 2 tubes) for *S. epidermidis* and the most recent cultures (left IJ) are positive for yeast with "germ tubes" (see Figure 111–1). The patient is started on fluconazole 400 mg IV QD.

b. What are the most likely causative pathogens in this patient?

► Clinical Course

The patient continues to be hypotensive, and the previous catheter-tip culture reveals 6 CFU of *S. epidermidis*. The latest blood and urine cultures are both positive for *Candida albicans*.

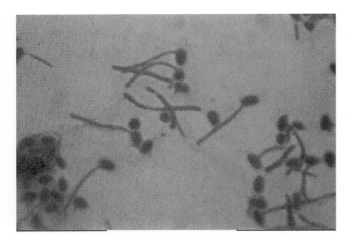

Figure 111–1. Germ tubes of *Candida albicans*. (Reproduced with permission from Beneke ES, Rippon JW, Rogers AL. Human mycoses: A scope publication. *Upjohn, 1986.*)

c. *What pharmacotherapeutic agents are available for the acute therapy of this infection?*

d. *What is the significance of the catheter tip cultures and the continued positive blood and urine cultures?*

Optimal Plan

4. *What drug therapy (including dose and route of administration) would you recommend for this patient?*

Outcome Evaluation

5. *How should the antifungal regimen be monitored for efficacy and adverse effects?*

► Clinical Course

The patient responds well to the antifungal therapy with resolution of the hypotension, fevers, leukocytosis, and candidemia/candiduria. However, after 7 days of therapy, her serum creatinine increases to 2.3 mg/dL.

► Follow-up Questions

1. *Would liposomal amphotericin B be an appropriate alternative to consider at this time?*

2. *How much longer should therapy be continued?*

► Self-study Assignments

1. Conduct a literature search on candiduria as an early marker of disseminated fungal infection.

2. Compare the types of fungal pathogens that would be expected in patients with candidemia due to hematologic malignancy versus patients with solid tumors or non-oncologic illnesses.

3. Evaluate the role of amphotericin B in fat emulsion in the treatment of systemic fungal infections.

4. Develop an algorithm for the management of patients with candidemia using the consensus guidelines on the management and prevention of severe candidal infections.[7]

► Clinical Pearl

A reduction in the incidence of amphotericin B nephrotoxicity may be achieved by administering saline boluses before and after the infusion. Patients receiving extended-spectrum penicillins such as ticarcillin (5.2 mEq sodium/g), mezlocillin (1.85 mEq sodium/g), and piperacillin (1.98 mEq sodium/g) may not require as much additional saline to minimize nephrotoxicity.

References

1. Burchard KW, Minor LB, Slotman GJ, et al. Fungal sepsis in surgical patients. Arch Surg 1983;118:217–221.
2. Dean DA, Burchard KW. Fungal infection in surgical patients. Am J Surg 1996;171:374–382.
3. Slotman GJ, Shapiro E, Moffa SM. Fungal sepsis: Multisite colonization versus fungemia. Am Surg 1994;60:107–113.
4. Fisher JF, Newman CL, Sobel JD. Yeast in the urine: Solutions for a budding problem. Clin Infect Dis 1995;20:183–189.
5. Maki DG. Infections caused by intravascular devices used for infusion therapy: Pathogenesis, prevention, and management. In: Infections Associated With Indwelling Devices, 2nd ed. American Society for Microbiology, 1994:155–211.
6. Uzun O, Anaissie EJ. Problems and controversies in the management of hematogenous candidiasis. Clin Infect Dis 1996;22(suppl 2):S95–S101.
7. Edwards JE Jr, Bodey GP, Bowden RA, et al. International conference for the development of a consensus on the management and prevention of severe candidal infections. Clin Infect Dis 1997;25:43–59.

112　DERMATOPHYTOSIS

► Skin and Nails　　　　　　　　　　(Level II)

Winnie M. Yu, PharmD, BCPS

► After completing this case study, students should be able to:

- Identify the risk factors for tinea pedis and onychomycosis.
- Know the pathogens associated with tinea pedis and onychomycosis.
- Discuss the risks and benefits of the therapeutic alternatives available for the treatment of tinea pedis and onychomycosis.
- Develop a patient-specific therapeutic plan for the management of tinea pedis and onychomycosis.

☀ PATIENT PRESENTATION

Chief Complaint
"My feet are killing me. White flakes are growing on my feet again. Why are my toenails brittle and yellow?"

HPI
Harold White is a 46 yo man who presents to the dermatology clinic for evaluation of his feet. He is a tenured professor who travels frequently for conferences and meetings. Two months ago when he was out of town attending a conference, he experienced mild itching and redness on his feet. He went to the gift shop in his hotel and bought some hydrocortisone cream, which gave him some relief. However, 1 week after the conference, white flakes appeared on both of his feet, and he realized that it was a recurrence of his athlete's foot. Today, he complains that the itching still bothers him and is not relieved by tolnaftate and hydrocortisone creams. He also complains that his toenails have turned yellow and brittle. He states that he never skips his daily jogging, even though it has been raining for the past 2 weeks. He wants a cure as soon as possible because he has to travel again next week for another presentation.

PMH
Athlete's foot 6 months ago
Osteoarthritis of both knees × 2 years
Hypercholesterolemia × 3 years
HTN × 5 years
Recurrent PUD diagnosed 4 months ago
S/P cholecystectomy 4 years ago

FH
Father died at age 48 of CAD; mother is alive with HTN.

SH
Professor in political science; has jogged at least 1 mile/day for 30 years; drinks 1 glass of wine with dinner; likes traveling and gourmet dining.

ROS
Denies fever, chills, fatigue, numbness and tingling in extremities, or recent trauma to his feet. Complains of brittle and yellow toenails and dry, scaling, and itchy feet.

Meds
Aspirin 81 mg po QD × 1 year
Pravastatin 20 mg po QD × 1 year
Atenolol 50 mg po QD
Omeprazole 20 mg po QD
Hydrocortisone 0.5% cream applied TID PRN to itchy feet
Tolnaftate cream applied BID PRN to itchy feet
Ibuprofen 200 mg po Q 4 H PRN knee pain
Multiple vitamins 1 tablet po QD
Echinacea 1 capsule po QD

All
Citrus foods and juices (upset stomach)

PE

GEN
Pleasant, talkative, anxious man who is wearing a suit and a pair of old, foul-smelling tennis shoes

VS
BP 145/89, P 95, RR 18, T 37.8°C, Ht 66″, Wt 78 kg

Skin
Moist and soft

HEENT
PEERLA, EOMI, oropharynx clear, moist mucous membranes, normal fundi

Neck/LN
Neck supple, normal lymph nodes and thyroid gland, no JVD

Lungs/Chest
Normal breath sounds, chest CTA

CV
RRR, normal S_1 and S_2, no murmur

Abd
Soft and non-tender, no guarding or HSM

GU/Rect
Normal male genitalia, rectal exam not performed

MS/Ext
Mild erythematous skin; fine silvery white flakes on the plantar surfaces of both feet; dry scales and hyperkeratotic skin covering the soles of both feet. Yellow-brown discoloration and thickening of the first, second, and third toenails of both feet; brittle toenails. Patellar crepitus of both knees; no synovial thickening or inflammation; normal range of motion; 2+ pulses throughout.

Neuro
Intact, A & O × 3, normal DTRs, CNs intact, normal plantar flexion

Labs (one month ago)

			Fasting Lipid Panel
Na 145 mEq/L	Hgb 13.8 g/dL	AST 20 IU/L	
K 3.8 mEq/L	Hct 41.4%	ALT 30 IU/L	T. chol 250 mg/dL
Cl 110 mEq/L	Plt 160 × 10³/mm³	Alk phos 78 IU/L	LDL 175 mg/dL
CO_2 25 mEq/L	WBC 9.8 × 10³/mm³	GGT 89 IU/L	HDL 54 mg/dL
BUN 22 mg/dL		T. bili 1.2 mg/dL	
SCr 1.1 mg/dL			
Glu 98 mg/dL			

Other
Microscopy of toenail debris—KOH preparation viewed with dark-field illumination reveals branching and filamentous hyphae consistent with dermatophyte infection.
Fungal culture of toenail debris—pending.

Assessment
46 yo man with tinea pedis and onychomycosis.

► Questions

Problem Identification

1. a. *Create a list of the patient's drug-related problems.*
   b. *What are the subjective and objective signs and symptoms of tinea pedis and onychomycosis in this patient?*
   c. *What are the common pathogens associated with tinea pedis and onychomycosis?*
   d. *What are the risk factors for tinea pedis and onychomycosis in this patient?*

Desired Outcome

2. *What are the goals of treatment for tinea pedis and onychomycosis in this patient?*

Therapeutic Alternatives

3. a. *What non-drug therapies might be useful for this patient?*
   b. *What feasible pharmacotherapeutic alternatives are available for treatment of the tinea pedis and onychomycosis?*

Optimal Plan

4. *What drug, dosage form, dose, schedule, and duration of therapy are best for this patient?*

Outcome Evaluation

5. *What clinical and laboratory parameters are necessary to evaluate the therapy for achievement of the desired therapeutic outcome and to detect or prevent adverse effects?*

Patient Counseling

6. *What information should be provided to the patient to enhance compliance, ensure successful therapy, and minimize adverse effects?*

► Clinical Course

The patient's symptoms of athlete's foot slowly resolved over 4 weeks, and appearance of his toenails improved after 3 months of therapy.

► Follow-up Questions

1. *What are the cardiovascular risk factors in this patient?*
2. *How does his risk factor status affect your management of his hypercholesterolemia?*

► Self-study Assignments

1. What is the role of oral azole therapy in the treatment of tinea pedis?
2. Discuss the advantages and disadvantages of using itraconazole over fluconazole for the management of onychomycosis.
3. What are the potential benefits of using a topical cream instead of a topical gel for the management of tinea pedis?

► Clinical Pearl

Tinea pedis is a risk factor for onychomycosis. Management of onychomycosis requires long-term treatment and is associated with high rates of relapse.

References

1. Elewski BE, Hay RJ. Update on the management of onychomycosis: Highlights of the Third Annual International Summit on Cutaneous Antifungal Therapy. Clin Infect Dis 1996;23:305–313.
2. Odom R. Pathophysiology of dermatophyte infections. J Am Acad Dermatol 1993;28(5 Pt 1):S2–S7.
3. Gupta AK, Scher RK, De Doncker P. Current management of onychomycosis. Dermatol Clin 1997;15:121–135.
4. Como JA, Dismukes WE. Oral azole drugs as systemic antifungal therapy. N Engl J Med 1994;330:263–272.
5. Abdel-Rahman SM, Nahata MC. Oral terbinafine: A new antifungal agent. Ann Pharmacother 1997;31:445–456.

113 BACTERIAL VAGINOSIS

► Competition Among Bacteria   (Level I)

Charles D. Ponte, PharmD, BCPS, CDE, FAPhA, FASHP, FCCP

► After completing this case study, students should be able to:

- Identify predisposing factors associated with bacterial vaginosis.
- List the common clinical and diagnostic findings associated with bacterial vaginosis.
- Develop a therapeutic plan for the management of bacterial vaginosis.
- Describe the role of the pharmacist in the overall management of infectious vaginitis.

☼ PATIENT PRESENTATION

Chief Complaint
"I'm here for a follow-up visit."

HPI
Brenda Singer is a 20 yo woman who comes to the University Health Service for follow-up visit for cervicitis. She was diagnosed 1 week ago and started on doxycycline 100 mg po BID × 7 days. At that time, a test for *Chlamydia* was non-reactive. She states that she has completed her course of doxycycline without any problems. Her sexual partners have been informed and are scheduled for treatment. She has abstained from sexual activity during this time and denies that she is pregnant. Her last period was approximately 4 weeks ago. She continues to take birth control pills.

PMH
Non-contributory

FH
Non-contributory

SH
Is a student in the College of Business and Economics. Has multiple sex partners; partners rarely use condoms. Smokes 1/2 pack of cigarettes per day since age 16. Alcohol use is mostly beer, mixed drinks on occasion.

ROS
Non-contributory except that she has noticed a small amount of thin white mucus on her underclothing.

Meds
Ortho-Cyclen 1 tablet po QD (no problems)
Doxycycline 100 mg po BID × 7 days (completed with no problems)
Multivitamins 1 po QD

All
Dogs → itchy eyes and sneezing; house dust → watery eyes, sneezing; sulfas → measles-like pruritic rash

PE
Limited due to follow-up of specific gynecologic complaint.

Gen
Patient is a healthy appearing 20 yo woman in NAD.

VS
BP 100/70, P 80, RR 16, T 37°C; Ht 5'6", Wt 113 lb

Genit/Rect
External genitalia WNL; vagina with a small amount of thin white mucus; positive whiff test; pH 5.0. Cervix—not completely visualized; appears clear with a small amount of mucoid discharge from the os. Uterus small, non-tender, anteverted, no cervical motion tenderness. Adnexa without tenderness or masses.

Labs
Microscopic examination of vaginal secretions: 20–25 WBC/hpf; 10–15 clue cells/hpf; 0 Lactobacilli/hpf; 15–20 squamous epithelial cells/hpf

Assessment
Resolving cervicitis
Bacterial vaginosis

► Questions

Problem Identification

1. a. *Create a list of the patient's drug-related problems.*
   b. *What clinical or laboratory information indicates the presence of bacterial vaginosis (see Table 113–1)?*
   c. *What is the pathophysiologic basis for the development of bacterial vaginosis?*
   d. *Could the patient's problem have been caused by drug therapy?*

Desired Outcome

2. *What are the goals of pharmacotherapy in this case?*

Therapeutic Alternatives

3. a. *What feasible pharmacotherapeutic alternatives are available for the treatment of bacterial vaginosis?*
   b. *What economic, psychosocial, and ethical considerations are applicable to this patient?*

TABLE 113–1. Characteristics of Different Types of Vaginitis

Characteristic	*Candida*	Bacterial	*Trichomonas*	Chemical
Pruritus	++	+/–	+/–	++
Erythema	+	+/–	+/–	+
Abnormal discharge	+	+	+/–	–
Viscosity	Thick	Thin	Thick/thin	–
Color	White	Gray	White, yellow, green-gray	–
Odor	None	Foul, "fishy"	Malodorous	–
Description	Curd-like	Homogeneous	Frothy	–
pH	3.8–5.0	>4.5	5.0–7.5	–
Diagnostic tests	KOH prep. shows long, thread-like fibers of mycelia microscopically	+ "whiff test," "clue cells"	Pear-shaped protozoa, cervical "strawberry" spots	–

Optimal Plan

4. a. *What drug, dosage form, dose, schedule, and duration of therapy are best for this patient?*
   b. *What alternatives would be appropriate if the initial therapy fails or cannot be used?*

Outcome Evaluation

5. *What clinical and laboratory parameters are necessary to evaluate the therapy for achievement of the desired therapeutic outcome and to detect or prevent adverse effects?*

Patient Counseling

6. *What information should be provided to the patient to enhance compliance, ensure successful therapy, and minimize adverse effects?*

▶ Clinical Course

After completion of the treatment you recommended, the patient returns to the clinic for follow-up. She voices no complaints except that she has been experiencing some vaginal itching and painful intercourse. Physical examination reveals whitish cottage-cheese-like material adherent to the vaginal mucosa. The vulva also appears erythematous. Microscopic analysis of vaginal secretions revealed hyphae and budding yeast. No white cells are noted. Vaginal pH is normal. The patient is diagnosed with vaginal candidiasis.

▶ Follow-up Questions

1. *What is the most likely cause of this patient's vaginal candidiasis?*
2. *What other issues should be addressed with the patient during this follow-up visit?*
3. *What is the role of the pharmacist in the management of patients with infectious vaginitis?*

▶ Self-study Assignments

1. Discuss the management of a patient who fails a specific course of treatment for bacterial vaginosis.
2. Discuss the pros and cons of screening asymptomatic pregnant women for the presence of bacterial vaginosis.
3. Describe the best therapeutic approach for a woman diagnosed with bacterial vaginosis who is breast-feeding her infant.
4. Discuss the role of sexual transmission in the pathogenesis of bacterial vaginosis.

▶ Clinical Pearl

Avoid condom or diaphragm use with clindamycin 2% vaginal cream. The vehicle is petroleum-based (mineral oil) and will weaken the integrity of latex products, increasing the risk of pregnancy.

References

1. Joesoef MR, Schmid GP. Bacterial vaginosis: Review of treatment options and potential clinical indications for therapy. Clin Infect Dis 1995;20(suppl 1): S72–S79.
2. Sobel JD. Vaginitis. N Engl J Med 1997;337:1896–1903.
3. Ries AJ. Treatment of vaginal infections: Candidiasis, bacterial vaginosis, and trichomoniasis. J Am Pharm Assoc 1997;NS37:563–569.
4. Centers for Disease Control and Prevention. Diseases characterized by vaginal discharge. 1998 guidelines for treatment of sexually transmitted diseases. MMWR 1998;47(RR-01):70–79. www.cdc.gov

114 ANTIMICROBIAL PROPHYLAXIS FOR SURGERY

▶ To Be Able to Walk Down the Aisle
(Level II)

Susan J. Skledar, RPh, MPH
Paige Robbins Gross, RPh

▶ After completing this case study, students should be able to:

- Understand the risk factors that may predispose a patient to surgical wound infection.
- Know the major causative organisms for surgical wound infection for most surgical procedures.
- Recommend appropriate antimicrobial regimens for prophylaxis of surgical wound infection.
- Outline monitoring parameters for post-operative surgical wound infection.
- Understand the importance of optimal timing of pre-surgical antimicrobial doses in relation to incidence of post-operative surgical wound infection.

☀ PATIENT PRESENTATION

Chief Complaint
"My left knee is getting more painful, and it is starting to affect my daily activities. Before I could get by with taking my pain pills, but now the pills don't work anymore and I feel like I am getting more and more crippled."

HPI
Holly Robertson is a 68 yo woman who presents for pre-operative assessment and preparation for a left total knee replacement for degenerative osteoarthritis. Previously, her osteoarthritis was controlled with a narcotic/non-narcotic combination agent and NSAIDs as needed. Her pain is increasingly intolerable, and her mobility has decreased.

PMH
Osteoarthritis × 10 years

Asthma × 10 years, which she attributes to her exposure to chemicals while being a hairdresser. Her asthmatic episodes have never required hospitalization but did require brief corticosteroid treatment about 1 year ago. Asthma is currently well controlled on her present regimen.

Postmenopausal state

Seasonal allergies

Hysterectomy 1976

Cystocele 1993

Arthroscopy of left knee in June 1997, complicated 1 week later by an invasive staphylococcal infection for which she received 6 weeks of IV vancomycin therapy.

FH

She has one child who is alive and well. Her mother died in her 80s from stroke and diabetes. Her father died at age 60 from an acute MI.

SH

She does not smoke or drink. She is widowed and is presently engaged.

ROS

She denies any pain or discomfort in her right knee. No headaches, visual blurring, or history of thyroid problems, GI or GU difficulties, HTN, DM, heart disease, PUD, DVT, or PE. Patient receives regular mammograms, which have been WNL.

Meds

Premarin 0.625 mg po QD

Serevent inhaler 2 puffs QID

Aerobid inhaler 2 puffs QID

Claritin 10 mg po QD

Ambien 10 mg po Q HS

Voltaren 75 mg po QD

Vicodin 1–2 tablets po Q 4–6 H PRN

All

Penicillin and cephalexin → severe hives; sulfa → confusion

PE

Gen

WDWN woman in NAD; appears younger than her stated age

VS

BP 110/70; P 80, regular; RR 16; T 98°F

HEENT

NC/AT; EOMI; PERRLA; ENT all WNL

Neck

Supple; no enlargement or nodal involvement; no bruits; thyroid normal

Thorax

CTA & P

Breasts

Exam deferred

CV

RRR; S_1 and S_2 normal without m/r/g

Abd

Soft, NT/ND; (+) BS; no bruits or organomegaly

Ext

The left knee incision from prior arthroscopy is well healed and is slightly warm; no edema or pus. Sensation not impaired.

Neuro

A & O × 3; CN II–XII intact. Strength is equal throughout.

Labs

Na 140 mEq/L	Hgb 11.8 g/dL	WBC 8.0×10^3/mm^3
K 4.0 mEq/L	Hct 34.7%	77% Polys
Cl 100 mEq/L	Plt 250×10^3/mm^3	15% Lymphs
CO_2 23 mEq/L		5% Monos
BUN 18 mg/dL		3% Eos
SCr 0.8 mg/dL		
Glu 95 mg/dL		

ECG

NSR; no abnormalities noted

Assessment

A recent aspiration and biopsy of her left knee shows no evidence of recurrent staphylococcal infection. Due to increasing pain and decreasing mobility, the patient is a candidate for a left total knee replacement. Her asthma is well controlled on her current regimen, which will be maintained. She is also at low risk for cardiovascular complications. Therefore, the patient is a suitable candidate to undergo this procedure.

▶ Questions

Problem Identification

1. a. Prepare a complete drug-related problem list for the patient.
   b. What are the risk factors for surgical wound infection (SWI) in patients undergoing surgical procedures?
   c. What organisms are the most likely causes of infection in orthopedic surgery patients?
   d. What recent event in this patient's PMH should be a caution for close monitoring of this patient for postoperative SWI?

Desired Outcome

2. What are the therapeutic goals for this patient?

Therapeutic Alternatives

3. a. What non-pharmacologic interventions should be considered in this patient pre- and post-surgery?

b. *What pharmacotherapeutic alternatives are available to minimize post-operative wound infection in this type of surgery?*

c. *What pharmacotherapeutic alternatives are available to manage postoperative pain for this patient?*

Optimal Plan

4. *What antimicrobial drugs, dosage form, schedule, and duration of therapy are best for this patient?*

Outcome Evaluation

5. *What clinical and laboratory parameters are necessary to evaluate therapy for achievement of desired outcomes and to detect and prevent adverse drug reactions?*

▶ Clinical Course

The patient tolerated surgery well, and drains were inserted prior to closure without complication. She did not show signs of infection post-operatively. She received the antimicrobial regimen you recommended for 2 days after surgery, and her postoperative pain was adequately controlled with the IV and then oral treatment you suggested. She was discharged on post-operative day 4 with a normal temperature and normal WBC and differential. Her discharge pain prescription was for Vicodin 1 to 2 tablets Q 4 to 6 H, and she was told to follow-up in 1 week with her orthopedic surgeon. Because she has no cardiovascular risks, diabetes, or history of DVT/PE, she was not discharged on an anticoagulant.

Patient Counseling

6. *What information should be provided to the patient to enhance compliance, ensure successful therapy, and minimize adverse events?*

▶ Self-study Assignments

1. Describe the sequence of pain management for this patient from PCA to oral pain medications.
2. Review recommendations for surgical prophylaxis for other types of surgical procedures.
3. Review the typical length of stay and expected course of recovery for a patient undergoing a total joint replacement, focusing on the difference between joint replacements and hip fractures.

▶ Clinical Pearl

Patients who receive antimicrobials within 3 hours *after* incision have a surgical wound infection rate almost 3 times that of patients who receive the first dose within 2 hours *before* incision.

References

1. Classen DC, Evans RS, Pestotnik SL, et al. The timing of prophylactic administration of antibiotics and the risk of surgical-wound infection. N Engl J Med 1992;326:281–286.
2. Lizan-Garcia M, Garcia-Caballero J, Asensio-Vegas A. Risk factors for surgical-wound infection in general surgery: A prospective study. Infect Control Hosp Epidemiol 1997;18:310–315.
3. Page CP, Bohnen JM, Fletcher JR, et al. Antimicrobial prophylaxis for surgical wounds. Guidelines for clinical care. Arch Surg 1993;128:79–88.
4. Antimicrobial prophylaxis in surgery. Med Lett 1997;39:97–102.
5. Silver A, Eichorn A, Kral J, et al. Timeliness and use of antibiotic prophylaxis in selected inpatient surgical procedures. The Antibiotic Prophylaxis Study Group. Am J Surg 1996;171:548–552.
6. Deacon JM, Pagliaro AJ, Zelicof SB, et al. Prophylactic use of antibiotics for procedures after total joint replacement. J Bone Joint Surg 1996;78:1755–1770.

115 PEDIATRIC IMMUNIZATION

▶ Ensuring a Healthy Start   (Level II)

Daniel T. Casto, PharmD, FCCP

▶ After completing this case study, students should be able to:

- Develop a plan for administering any needed vaccines, when given a patient's age, immunization history, and medical history.
- Recognize the differences in Hib-conjugate vaccines currently in use in the United States.
- Explain when the use of DTaP is preferred over DTwP, and why IPV is preferred over OPV.
- Describe appropriate use of hepatitis B and varicella vaccines.
- Counsel a child's parents on the risks associated with pediatric vaccines and ways to minimize adverse effects.
- Recognize inappropriate reasons for deferring immunization.

☀ PATIENT PRESENTATION

Chief Complaint
"My daughter was in the hospital because of seizures, and they told me to come here today to have her checked."

HPI
Jennifer Thomas is a 6.5-month-old girl who is being seen in the General Pediatrics Clinic for the first time, in follow-up to a recent hospitalization for an episode of convulsions. Three weeks ago, the child experienced a 10-minute tonic-clonic seizure after waking up from a nap. She was seen in the ED with a temperature of 39.1°C. On physical exam, the only abnormality noted was that both TMs were red and bulging. A sepsis work-up was performed because of persistent lethargy, and the patient was hospitalized for evaluation. All cultures were negative; neurologic exam failed to identify an obvious cause of the seizures. The infant was discharged after 2 days with the diagnoses of febrile seizures and bilateral otitis media, for which she was prescribed a 10-day course of amoxicillin.

PMH
Minimal prenatal care, but delivered at 36 weeks' gestation via uncomplicated vaginal delivery; birth weight 3300 g; discharged with mother on day

3 of life. Mother states that her child has had only one or two "colds," no other illnesses, and has not required any medical care. No contact with the medical system until the ED visit and hospitalization 3 weeks ago. No immunizations except hepatitis B vaccine given at birth.

FH
No history of seizures among immediate family members. Maternal grandmother has diabetes mellitus and a seizure disorder secondary to head trauma sustained in an automobile accident. No history of CHD or cancer in family members.

SH
Mother age 19, father age 20, brother age 26 months. Mother stays at home, father works intermittently for a temporary agency as a laborer. They live in a government-subsidized, 2-bedroom apartment. Also living with them are maternal grandparents, mother's 20 yo sister and her 17-month-old child. No recent illness among household contacts. No pets at home, and one smoker in house (grandfather). The family receives food stamps but is not enrolled in the Women-Infants-Children (WIC) program. Jennifer's diet consists of whole milk, cereal, and some table foods.

Meds
None, since amoxicillin course was completed about a week and a half ago. No recent OTC medication use.

All
NKDA

ROS
Negative

PE

Gen
Alert, happy, relatively small, appropriately developed 6-month-old infant in NAD. Wt 14 lb (< 25 percentile), length 24.5 in (50 percentile), FOC 43 cm (50 percentile)

VS
BP 110/66, P 130, RR 28, T 36.8°C (axillary)

HEENT
AF open, flat; PERRL; funduscopic exam not performed; ears clear; normal looking TMs, landmarks visualized, no effusion present; nose clear; throat normal

CV
RRR, no murmurs

Lungs
Clear bilaterally

Abd
Soft, non-tender, no masses or organomegaly

GU
Normal external genitalia

GI
Normal bowel sounds; rectal exam deferred, no fissures noted

Ext
Pale nail beds, skin dry and cool; capillary refill < 2 seconds

Neuro
Alert; normal DTRs bilaterally

Labs
Hgb 10.1 g/dL; Hct 32.4%; no other labs obtained

Assessment
Normal-appearing infant, with resolved otitis media, 3 weeks s/p febrile convulsion, in need of immunizations and social service assistance.

▶ Questions

Problem Identification

1. *Create a list of the patient's drug-related problems.*

Desired Outcome

2. *What immediate and long-term goals are reasonable in this case?*

Therapeutic Alternatives

3. *What vaccines should be administered to this child today? (Helpful hint: The following Web sites may be useful in answering this and other questions: www.cdc.gov/nip and www.aap.org)*

Optimal Plan

4. a. *What immunization schedule should be followed for this patient?*
   b. *In addition to vaccination, what additional therapy is warranted in this case, considering the patient's dietary history and laboratory values?*

Outcome Evaluation

5. *How should the response to the pharmacotherapeutic plan be assessed?*

Patient Counseling

6. *What important information about vaccination needs to be explained to this infant's mother?*

▶ Self-study Assignments

1. The routine schedule for immunizing infants and children in the United States is updated by the American Academy of Pediatrics and the CDC each year, in their respective official publications. Review the most current recommendations and provide a summary of how your recommendations for this case would be different if a 6.5-month-old patient in need of immunizations came into your clinic today.

2. Surf the Internet for immunization-related Web sites; then use *www.immunofacts.com* to find the National Immunization Program's home page, and review at least two vaccine information pamphlets (VIPs).

3. Develop a list of diseases and medications that should be considered contraindications to administration of live virus vaccines.

▶ Clinical Pearl

There is no need to restart an immunization series (e.g., DTaP) if the interval between doses is longer than what is recommended in the routine schedule for immunizing infants and children. Instead of starting over, merely count the doses administered (provided that they were given at an appropriate age and with an acceptable minimum interval) and complete the series.

Reference

1. American Academy of Pediatrics. Active and passive immunization. In: Red Book—Report of the Committee on Infectious Diseases, 24th ed. Elk Grove Village, IL, American Academy of Pediatrics, 1997:1–71.

116 CYTOMEGALOVIRUS (CMV) RETINITIS

▶ The Case for Compliance   (Level II)

Winnie M. Yu, PharmD, BCPS

▶ After completing this case study, students should be able to:

- Recognize the common signs and symptoms of CMV retinitis.

- Discuss the risks and benefits of the therapeutic alternatives used for the treatment of CMV retinitis.

- Develop a patient-specific therapeutic plan for the management of CMV retinitis.

- Counsel patients about the medications that are commonly used to manage CMV retinitis.

☀ PATIENT PRESENTATION

Chief Complaint
"I have been seeing floaters in my right eye for the past week."

HPI

Donald Baker is a 27 yo man who first presented to the clinic 2 years ago with fever, lymphadenopathy, and night sweats. He was found to have a CD4 count of 89 cells/mm^3 and was diagnosed with AIDS. At that time, he was started on antiretroviral treatment with indinavir, zidovudine, and lamivudine. Two months ago his regimen was changed to ritonavir, saquinavir, stavudine, and lamivudine. He has been non-adherent with his clinic visits and medications. He was last seen at the clinic 3 months ago complaining of poor appetite, weight loss, and social withdrawal. He was referred to the psychiatrist and was started on medication for depression. Today, he presents complaining of blurred vision and occasional "floaters" in the right eye for the past week. He also reports that he has not been taking his medications for 2 months because he does not believe that they are helpful. He states that his appetite has worsened since he was started on the medication for depression.

PMH

AIDS × 2 years
Oral thrush diagnosed 3 months ago, treated with fluconazole
Syphilis 5 years ago treated with ceftriaxone
Depression × 3 months

FH
Parents deceased 5 years ago secondary to MVA; sister has asthma.

SH
Currently unemployed; homosexual (anal and oral sex) and lives with partner who is HIV (+); has smoked 1 pack per week for 12 years; 5-year history of IVDU, none for 2 years.

ROS
Denies fever, chills, diarrhea, abdominal pain, sore throat, dizziness, or headache.

Meds

Ritonavir 600 mg po BID
Saquinavir soft gel capsules 400 mg po BID
Lamivudine 150 mg po BID
Stavudine 40 mg po BID
Trimethoprim-sulfamethoxazole 1 DS tablet po QD
Azithromycin 1200 mg po every Sunday
Fluconazole 50 mg po QD
Paroxetine 20 mg po QD

All
Penicillin (rash)

PE

Gen
Thin, cachectic male in NAD

VS
BP 134/78, P 83, RR 16, T 36.8°C; Ht 68″, Wt 53 kg

Skin
Soft, intact, warm, and dry

HEENT

NC/AT; PERRLA; EOMI; visual acuity is 20/200 OD and 20/20 OS by the Snellen chart; funduscopic exam reveals white, fluffy lesions with focal hemorrhages on retina of the right eye, consistent with CMV retinitis; external eye structures are normal. There are white flaky plaques throughout the oral cavity; none in the throat.

Neck/LN

Thyroid normal, no lymphadenopathy

Lungs/Chest

Normal breath sounds, chest CTA

CV

RRR, normal S_1 and S_2, no m/r/g

Abd

Soft, NT/ND, no HSM, (+) BS

GU/Rect

Normal male genitalia; rectal exam normal, guaiac (−) stool

MS/Ext

Pulses 2+, no CCE; full ROM

Neuro

A & O × 3, normal DTRs, CNs intact

Labs

See Tables 116–1 and 116–2.

Blood

CMV antibody (+); CMV antigen (−)

Assessment

27 yo HIV-infected man with new onset CMV retinitis in the right eye.

TABLE 116–1. Laboratory Test Results

Two Months Ago			Today		
Na 138 mEq/L	Hgb 11.1 g/dL	AST 90 IU/L	Na 142 mEq/L	Hgb 12.3 g/dL	AST 65 IU/L
K 3.9 mEq/L	Hct 33.3%	ALT 107 IU/L	K 4.6 mEq/L	Hct 36.9%	ALT 79 IU/L
Cl 105 mEq/L	MCV 110 μm³	GGT 185 IU/L	Cl 113 mEq/L	MCV 107 μm³	GGT 112 IU/L
CO_2 22 mEq/L	Plt 107 × 10³/mm³	Alk phos 78 IU/L	CO_2 23 mEq/L	Plt 121 × 10³/mm³	Alk phos 32 IU/L
BUN 12 mg/dL	WBC 4.4 × 10³/mm³	T. bili 2.1 mg/dL	BUN 16 mg/dL	WBC 3.8 × 10³/mm³	T. bili 1.9 mg/dL
SCr 0.9 mg/dL	59% Neutros		SCr 1.0 mg/dL	61% Neutros	
Glu 95 mg/dL	6% Bands		Glu 98 mg/dL	2% Bands	

TABLE 116–2. Surrogate Markers for HIV Infection From 24 Months Ago to 2 Months Ago

Surrogate HIV Markers	(Months Prior)					
	24	21	17	13	8	2
HIV RNA (copies/mL)	277,250	93,740	1032	Undetectable	8488	128,860
CD4 Count (cells/mm³)	89	102	135	114	98	15

▶ Questions

Problem Identification

1. a. *Create a list of this patient's drug-related problems.*
   b. *What are the signs and symptoms of CMV retinitis in this patient?*
   c. *What are the risk factors for CMV retinitis in this patient?*

Desired Outcome

2. *What are the goals of therapy for CMV retinitis in this patient?*

Therapeutic Alternatives

3. *What feasible pharmacotherapeutic alternatives are available for treatment of CMV retinitis in this patient?*

Optimal Plan

4. *Which agent and regimen would you recommend for management of this patient's CMV retinitis?*

Outcome Evaluation

5. *What clinical and laboratory parameters are necessary to evaluate the therapy for achievement of the desired therapeutic outcome and to detect adverse effects?*

Patient Counseling

6. *What information should be provided to the patient to ensure successful therapy?*

▶ Follow-up Questions

1. *Do you agree with the changes that were made in his HIV therapy 2 months ago? Provide a rationale for your answer.*
2. *If the patient received the ganciclovir ocular insert as treatment for his CMV retinitis, how would you manage the disease if he developed extraocular CMV disease 6 months after the implantation?*

▶ Self-study Assignments

1. What is the role of oral ganciclovir in the primary prevention of CMV disease in HIV-infected patients who have CD4 counts < 50 cells/mm^3?
2. List five clinical parameters that you will monitor in a patient who is receiving foscarnet for disseminated CMV infection.

▶ Clinical Pearl

CMV retinitis is the most common form of CMV end-organ disease in HIV-infected patients; retinal detachment occurs in up to 30% of CMV retinitis cases.

References

1. Jacobson MA. Treatment of cytomegalovirus retinitis in patients with the acquired immunodeficiency syndrome. N Engl J Med 1997;337:105–114.
2. Mortality in patients with the acquired immunodeficiency syndrome treated with either foscarnet or ganciclovir for cytomegalovirus retinitis. Studies of Ocular Complications of AIDS Research Group, in collaboration with the AIDS Clinical Trials Group. N Engl J Med 1992;326:213–220.
3. Drew WL, Ives D, Lalezari JP, et al. Oral ganciclovir as maintenance treatment for cytomegalovirus retinitis in patients with AIDS. N Engl J Med 1995;333:615–620.
4. Musch DC, Martin DF, Gordon JF, et al. Treatment of cytomegalovirus retinitis with a sustained-release ganciclovir implant. N Engl J Med 1997;337:83–90.
5. Parenteral cidofovir for cytomegalovirus retinitis in patients with AIDS: The HPMPC peripheral cytomegalovirus retinitis trial. A randomized, controlled trial. Studies of Ocular Complications of AIDS Research Group in Collaboration With the AIDS Clinical Trials Group. Ann Intern Med 1997;126:264–274.

117 TREATMENT OF HIV INFECTION

▶ The Antiretroviral-naive Patient (Level II)

Susan Chuck, PharmD
Keith A. Rodvold, PharmD, FCCP, BCPS

▶ After completing this case study, students should be able to:

- Describe situations in which antiretroviral therapy should be initiated in patients with HIV infection and determine the desired outcome of such therapy.
- Recommend appropriate first-line antiretroviral therapies for the antiretroviral-naive person.
- Provide patient counseling on the proper dose, administration, and adverse effects of antiretroviral agents.

☼ PATIENT PRESENTATION

Chief Complaint
"I am interested in starting HIV meds."

HPI
Raymond Washington is a 41 yo man who has been infected with HIV for 2 years. He comes to the HIV Clinic at regular 2–3 month intervals for routine follow-up, most recently 2 weeks ago. At that time, we had a lengthy discussion about starting antiretroviral therapy, and blood was drawn for baseline surrogate markers.

PMH
HIV infection × 2 years; diagnosed during incarceration
Large cell lymphoma diagnosed 2 years ago; treated with 4 cycles of CHOP with excellent response
Seroconverted to PPD (+) 6 years ago; treated with 12 months of INH

FH
Non-contributory

SH
History of IVDU. Sells miscellaneous items (e.g., purses, T-shirts, sweat shirts, belts) on the street and volunteers time at the half-way house located across from the HIV Clinic.

ROS
The patient voices no complaints. He has had no recent weight loss, fever, night sweats, cough, nausea, vomiting, or diarrhea.

Meds
None

All
ASA → "swelling of face"

PE

Gen
Well-developed man in NAD

VS
BP 112/76, P 80, RR 16, T 97.8°F; Wt 107 kg, Ht 5'11"

Skin
Warm and dry without lesions

HEENT
Oral cavity without thrush/erythema; sinuses nontender; PERRLA; ears and nose clear; funduscopic exam deferred

TABLE 117–1. Laboratory Values for the Previous Visit and for Subsequent Visits

Parameter (units)	2 Weeks Ago	This Visit	1 Month Later	4 Months Later
General				
Weight (kg)	110	107	110	110
Hematology				
Hgb (g/dL)	12.2	12.9	12.4	12.6
Hct (%)	37.9	39.0	38.5	38.4
Plt ($\times 10^3$/mm^3)	220	114	145	161
WBC ($\times 10^3$/mm^3)	2.4	3.3	3.1	3.3
Lymphs (%)	34.6	40.5	40.8	46.1
Monos (%)	21.6	13.0	12.4	16.5
Eos (%)	11.6	8.8	6.5	4.2
Basos (%)	0.7	0.9	1.3	1.0
Neutros (%)	31.5	36.8	39.0	32.2
ANC ($\times 10^3$/mm^3)	1.0	1.2	1.2	1.1
Chemistry				
BUN (mg/dL)	14	17	16	10
SCr (mg/dL)	0.9	1.1	1.1	1.0
T. bili (mg/dL)	—	0.6	—	0.6
Alb (g/dL)	—	4.4	—	4.4
LDH (IU/L)	206	210	186	347
AST (IU/L)	31	34	29	34
ALT (IU/L)	19	20	18	32
Surrogate Markers				
CD4 (%)	18	16	19	20
CD4 (cells/mm^3)	234	240	320	360
CD8 (%)	54	49	52	51
HIV RNA (RT-PCR)[a] (copies/mL)	Detectable 33,995	Detectable 36,873	Non-detectable < 500	Detectable 538

[a] Reverse transcriptase polymerase chain reaction assay.

Neck/LN
No lymphadenopathy

Chest
Clear, normal breath sounds, no rales or rhonchi

CV
RRR; normal S_1 and S_2 without murmurs

Abd
(+) BS, soft without HSM, no pain or tenderness

Genit/Rect
Deferred

MS/Ext
No wasting, full ROM

Neuro
A & O $\times$ 3, no cranial nerve abnormalities noted

Baseline Labs
RPR nonreactive; toxoplasma IgG (−); hepatitis serology (−)

Other Labs
See Table 117–1.

Assessment
HIV-infected man, antiretroviral-naive.

► Questions

Problem Identification

1. a. What information (signs, symptoms, laboratory values) indi-
cates the severity of HIV disease? Provide an assessment of this patient's HIV disease at this visit and his risk of progression to AIDS.

b. Is it rational to begin antiretroviral therapy in this patient?

c. Is prophylactic therapy for any HIV-associated opportunistic pathogen indicated in this patient?

Desired Outcome

2. *What are the goals of pharmacotherapy in this case?*

Therapeutic Alternatives

3. a. *What therapeutic options are available for the treatment of this antiretroviral-naive man?*

   b. *What economic, psychosocial, racial, and ethical considerations are applicable to this patient?*

Optimal Plan

4. a. *Design an individualized antiretroviral regimen for this man. State the drug name, dosage form, dose, schedule, and duration of therapy for the regimen you choose.*

   b. *Design an antiretroviral regimen that would be appropriate if the patient informs you that he has difficulty swallowing large pills.*

   c. *Design an antiretroviral regimen that would be appropriate if the patient states that medicines often upset his bowels, and he prefers to avoid anything that may cause him trouble.*

Outcome Evaluation

5. *What parameters should you select to monitor the clinical efficacy and toxicity of the pharmacotherapeutic regimen? Specify the frequency with which you would monitor these parameters. For laboratory parameters, state the range of values or significant change in values (i.e., log change, x-fold change, and specific HIV RNA values) that would indicate that the desired therapeutic outcome has been achieved.*

Patient Counseling

6. a. *What important information would you provide to this patient about his therapy?*

   b. *Explain in non-technical terms the surrogate markers and their use in monitoring HIV disease.*

   c. *If this man changed his mind about starting antiretrovirals, what questions would you ask him? Explain in non-technical terms when therapy is indicated and what the potential benefits are.*

▶ Clinical Course

Your recommendations on the antiretroviral regimen were accepted. The patient returns to the HIV clinic for his 1-month and 3-month follow-up visits. After each visit the laboratory results are faxed to you.

Parameter	1 Month Later	4 Months Later
Duration of HIV infection	2 years+	2 years+
Current or past history of opportunistic infections	None	None
HIV RNA (RT-PCR)	Non-detectable (< 500 copies/mL)	Detectable (538 copies/mL)
CD4 lymphocyte count	320 cells/mm³	360 cells/mm³
Symptoms of HIV infection	Asymptomatic	Asymptomatic

▶ Follow-up Questions

1. *Considering this new information, provide an assessment of the patient's HIV disease status at each of the two visits.*

2. *Provide an assessment of the antiretroviral regimen efficacy at each follow-up visit.*

▶ Self-study Assignments

1. Review the current literature regarding recommended therapy for the antiretroviral-naive and treatment-experienced individuals. What is the recommended first-line therapy, and what are the indications to change to alternative therapy? What is known about therapy of HIV and survival?

2. Review the current literature regarding the development of HIV resistance to antiretroviral agents and strategies for the prevention and management of resistance.

▶ Clinical Pearl

According to current guidelines, antiretroviral therapy is indicated in 3 groups of HIV-infected individuals: 1) all persons with HIV-related symptoms; 2) a CD4 lymphocyte count below 500 cells/mm³; or 3) HIV RNA > 5000 to 10,000 copies/mL (regardless of the CD4 lymphocyte count).

References

1. Report of the NIH panel to define principles of therapy of HIV infection and guidelines for the use of antiretroviral agents in HIV-infected adults and adolescents. MMWR 1998;47(RR-05):1–82.
2. Drugs for HIV infection. Med Lett 1997;39:111–116.
3. Carpenter CC, Fischl MA, Hammer SM, et al. Antiretroviral therapy for HIV infection in 1997. Updated recommendations of the International AIDS Society—USA Panel. JAMA 1997;277:1962–1969.
4. 1993 AIDS surveillance case definition for adolescents and adults. MMWR 1992;41(RR-17):1–9.
5. CDC 1997 USPHS/IDSA guidelines for the prevention of opportunistic infections in persons infected with HIV. MMWR 1997;46(RR-12):1–46.
6. Carpenter CC, Fischl MA, Hammer SM, et al. Antiretroviral therapy for HIV infection in 1998: Updated recommendations of the International AIDS Society—USA Panel. JAMA 1998;280:78–86.

118 HIV INFECTION AND PCP PNEUMONIA

▶ A Treatment-experienced Patient (Level III)

Linda M. Page, PharmD
Peter L. Anderson, PharmD
Courtney V. Fletcher, PharmD

▶ After completing this case study, students should be able to:

• Identify when changes in antiretroviral therapy are warranted.

- Identify appropriate alternative antiretroviral therapies for the antiretroviral-experienced person.
- Identify and monitor a common opportunistic infection.
- Provide patient counseling on the proper dose, administration, and adverse effects of antiretroviral and other agents used for the HIV-infected person.

☀ PATIENT PRESENTATION

Chief Complaint
"I have been short of breath and having fevers for the past few weeks."

HPI
Charles McDonald is a 31 yo man known to be infected with HIV for at least 2 years. He returns to the HIV Clinic at various intervals for routine follow-up. He has been on stable antiretroviral therapy for the past year consisting of didanosine, stavudine, and indinavir. He received no prior antiretroviral therapy.

PMH
HIV infection, precise duration unknown
Oral thrush, 2 episodes during the last 6 months

FH
Non-contributory

SH
Previously worked 30 hours/week as a tour guide in the mountains. Currently is unemployed. Smoked 3 ppd × 15 years until quitting about 3 months ago. Past history of alcohol abuse.

Meds
Didanosine 200 mg po BID
Stavudine 40 mg po BID
Indinavir 800 mg po Q 8 H
Dapsone 50 mg po QD
Fluconazole 100 mg po QD

All
TMP-SMX → bright red rash that covered his torso and face, reportedly with fever.

Immunizations
Patient unsure about immunization status, thinks he got them as a child.

ROS
(+) SOB, persistent nonproductive cough, feels run-down, (+) fever

PE

Gen
Thin, anxious, acutely ill-appearing, young Caucasian man with tachypnea

VS
BP 126/86, P 92, RR 28, T 39°C; Wt 70.3 kg, Ht 6'0"

Skin
No visible lesions, warm and dry

HEENT
PERRLA; no papilledema; fundi normal; ears and nose clear; oral cavity without inflammation or exudate

Neck/LN
Slight cervical lymphadenopathy, thyroid normal

Lungs/Thorax
CTA, slight axillary lymphadenopathy

CV
NSR, normal S_1 and S_2, no rubs, murmurs, or gallops

Abd
No pain or tenderness, no hepatosplenomegaly, BS (+), slight inguinal lymphadenopathy

Genit/Rect
Guaiac (−) stool, no visible genital or anal lesions, prostate exam not performed

MS/Ext
Pedal pulses 2+, no edema, nails normal, normal ROM

Neuro
A & O × 3, Babinski (−), CN II–XII intact, no other focal neurologic signs

Labs
See Table 118–1.

Chest X-ray
Bilateral subtle infiltrates

Bronchoscopy with BAL
Positive for *Pneumocystis carinii*

Assessment
Breakthrough opportunistic infection.

Plan
1. R/O patient non-compliance with drug regimens, possible drug–drug interactions, and inadequate suppression of HIV replication.
2. Admit patient to the hospital for treatment of acute PCP.

TABLE 118–1. Serial Laboratory Values Beginning One Year Prior to the Present Visit

Parameter (units)	1 Year Ago	6 Months Ago	This Visit	Day 20 of Therapy
General				
Weight (kg)	69.0	72.1	70.3	72
BP (mm Hg)	114/57	120/72	126/86	115/59
Hematology				
Hgb (g/dL)	12.0	10.5	11.9	8.2
Hct (%)	34.9	31.7	34.9	24
Plt ($\times 10^3$/mm^3)	276	390	260	362
WBC count ($\times 10^3$/mm^3)	3.8	4.1	3.3	3.8
Lymphs (%)	23.7	31	17.2	35.4
Monos (%)	13.5	13.1	10.4	10.2
Eos (%)	2.5	2.4	1.5	3.7
Basos (%)	1.0	0.6	1.1	1
Neutros (%)	59.3	52.9	69.8	49.7
CD4 cells (%) [total]	17 [153]	27 [343]	21 [119]	NE
CD8 cells (%) [total]	33 [297]	37 [470]	36 [204]	NE
HIV RNA (copies/mL) by bDNA method	> 750,000	< 500	17,500	NE
Chemistry				
Na (mEq/L)	140	139	136	132
K (mEq/L)	4.1	3.9	4.2	3.1
Cl (mEq/L)	106	106	108	102
BUN (mg/dL)	6	7	9	6
SCr (mg/dL)	0.8	0.8	0.8	0.6
Glu (mg/dL)	85	110	104	209
T. bili (mg/dL)	0.4	0.5	0.4	1.1
Alb (g/dL)	3.2	2.9	2.7	3.0
LDH (IU/L)	591	742	1068	485
AST (IU/L)	55	50	113	87
ALT (IU/L)	70	65	101	89
Ca (mg/dL)	8.7	8.5	8.9	7.8
Phos (mg/dL)	3.5	3.0	3.5	2.7
Mg (mg/dL)	1.6	1.7	1.5	1.3

NE, not evaluated.

► Questions

Problem Identification

1. a. Create a list of the patient's drug-related problems.
   b. What information (signs, symptoms, laboratory values) indicates the presence or severity of the PCP and HIV disease progression?
   c. Could any of the patient's problems have been caused by drug therapy?
   d. Are any of the patient's problems amenable to pharmacotherapy?
   e. What additional information is needed to satisfactorily assess this patient?

Desired Outcome

2. What are the desired goals of pharmacotherapy in this case?

Therapeutic Alternatives

3. a. What non-drug therapies might be useful for this patient?
   b. What feasible pharmacotherapeutic alternatives are available for treatment of PCP and HIV infection in this patient?

Optimal Plan

4. *What drug, dosage form, schedule, and duration of therapy are best for treating this patient's PCP and HIV infections?*

Outcome Evaluation

5. *What clinical and laboratory parameters are necessary to evaluate the PCP and HIV therapy for achievement of the desired therapeutic outcome and to detect or prevent adverse effects?*

Patient Counseling

6. *What information should be provided to the patient to enhance compliance, ensure successful therapy, and minimize adverse effects?*

► Clinical Course

The patient continued to show clinical improvement with treatment. On day 19, he felt dizzy while receiving the pentamidine infusion. He was noted to have frequent 4 to 5 beat runs of ventricular tachycardia with *torsades de pointes*. He was treated with a single IV lidocaine bolus of 100 mg without recurrence. He remained hemodynamically stable throughout this episode. Labs: Na 138 mEq/L, K 3.3 mEq/L, Cl 101 mEq/L, CO_2 25 mEq/L, glucose 88 mg/dL, SCr 1.1 mg/dL, Ca 8.9 mg/dL, Mg 1.3 mg/dL.

► Follow-up Questions

1. *How would you assess the patient's cardiac event? What is the most likely cause?*
2. *Considering this new information, what pharmacotherapeutic recommendation would you make?*

► Self-study Assignments

1. Review the current literature regarding the use of combination therapy, especially with regard to new agents and potential drug interactions.
2. Review the current literature regarding the use of HIV-RNA as a monitoring parameter.
3. Review the current literature regarding recommended therapy for antiretroviral-experienced individuals.
4. Review the current guidelines for prevention and treatment of opportunistic infections.

► Clinical Pearl

A final consideration in the decision to change antiretroviral therapy is the recognition of the still limited choice of available agents and the knowledge that a decision to change may reduce future treatment options for the patient.

References

1. NIH Panel to Define Principles of Therapy of HIV Infection. Report of the NIH panel to define principles of therapy of HIV infection. MMWR 1998;47(RR-5): 1–42.
2. Santamauro JT, Stover DE. Pneumocystis carinii pneumonia. Med Clin North Am 1997;81:299–318.
3. Panel on Clinical Practices for Treatment of HIV Infection. Guidelines for the use of antiretroviral agents in HIV-infected adults and adolescents. MMWR 1998; 47(RR-5): 43–83.
4. Drug Information for the Health Care Professional. USP-DI, 18th ed. Taunton, MA, 1998.
5. Eisenhauer MD, Eliasson AH, Taylor AJ, et al. Incidence of cardiac arrhythmias during intravenous pentamidine therapy in HIV-infected patients. Chest 1994; 105:389–395.

119   BREAST CANCER

▶ **The Role of Neoadjuvant
Chemotherapy**   **(Level II)**

Laura Boehnke Michaud, PharmD

▶ After completing this case study, students should be able to:

- Explain the importance of regular breast self-examinations, screening mammograms, and professional breast exams for women.

- Design appropriate monitoring parameters to detect and prevent adverse effects associated with the chemotherapy regimens used for breast cancer.

- Counsel patients on the most likely adverse effects of chemotherapy and the actions they should take if they occur.

- Provide patient counseling on the proper dosing, administration, and adverse effects of anastrozole therapy.

☀ PATIENT PRESENTATION

Chief Complaint

"I have pain in my breast and under my arm."

HPI

Sara Gleason is a 69 yo woman whose history dates back to 3 to 4 weeks ago when she noted a painful lump in the upper outer quadrant of her left breast, including the axillary area. A mammogram was done that was suggestive of malignancy. She had not had regular mammograms previously.

PMH

CAD; s/p angioplasty 5–6 years ago; denies any chest pain since
HTN; does not remember how long; she states "for years"
S/P cholecystectomy
TAH/BSO at age 45
S/P appendicitis

FH

No known family history of cancer.

SH

Previous smoker, quit 8 years ago. She denies tobacco or drug use.

Endo Hx

Menarche age 12; menopause age 45 (surgical); first child age 17; $G_5P_5A_0$. Last Pap smear 10 years ago. HRT stopped 3 to 4 weeks ago when she found the lump.

Meds

Procardia XL 90 mg po QD
Zestril 20 mg po QD
Paxil 30 mg po QD
Tylenol #3, 2 tablets QD PRN back pain

All

None

ROS

Negative except for complaints noted above.

PE

Gen
Moderately obese 68 yo African-American woman who appears her stated age. Awake, alert, in NAD.

VS
BP 130/84, P 74, RR 88, T 98.7°F; Ht 66″, Wt 78 kg

HEENT
NC/AT; PERRLA; EOMI; ears, nose, and throat are clear.

Neck/LN
Supple. No lymphadenopathy, thyromegaly, or masses. No supraclavicular or infraclavicular adenopathy.

Breasts
Left: skin retraction with arms elevated; no nipple retraction or discharge expressible; edema of the skin in left upper outer quadrant without associated erythema; hard 5 × 5-cm mass in upper outer quadrant, not fixed to skin, no ulceration; 2-cm, firm, tender palpable mass in axilla. Right: without mass or lymphadenopathy.

Lungs
CTA and percussion

CV
RRR; no murmurs, rubs or gallops

Abd
Moderately obese; soft, nondistended, nontender; no HSM; bowel sounds normal. Cholecystectomy scar noted

Spine
No tenderness to percussion

Ext
No CCE

Neuro
No significant deficits noted

Labs

Na 137 mEq/L	Hgb 10.8 g/dL	WBC $7.0 \times 10^3/mm^3$	AST 37 IU/L
K 4.2 mEq/L	Hct 31.8%	34% Neutros	Alk Phos 97 IU/L
Cl 96 mEq/L	RBC $3.42 \times 10^6/mm^3$	42% Lymphs	LDH 547 IU/L
CO_2 24 mEq/L	Plt $313 \times 10^3/mm^3$	10% Monos	T. bili 0.3 mg/dL
BUN 8 mg/dL	PT 11.4 sec	14% Eos	CA 27.29 21.5 U/mL
SCr 1.4 mg/dL	INR 0.9		CEA 2.4 ng/mL
Glu 90 mg/dL	aPTT 23.5 sec		

Chest X-ray
Lungs are clear

Other
Diagnostic bilateral mammogram (see Figure 119–1):
1. American College of Radiology Category V report highly suspicious for malignancy in left breast with evidence for advanced carcinoma with associated diffuse skin thickening, skin retraction. Spiculated mass with extensive infiltration of the surrounding fatty tissue. Overlying skin looks retracted and there is diffuse skin thickening both laterally and medially when compared to the other side. Associated lymphadenopathy with an enlarged lymph node approximately 2 cm in diameter that is suspicious for a metastatic node.
2. Size of the malignancy in left breast measures approximately 8 × 9 × 7 cm. Associated with interductal calcifications extending toward the nipple, indicating that at least a portion of this has a ductal cell origin. There may be extension to the pectoral muscle.
3. The right breast shows no abnormality.

Unilateral ultrasound left breast and left axilla with biopsy:
1. Solid-appearing mass favoring malignancy in left upper outer quadrant. Ill-defined mass that is hypoechoic and has abnormal vascularity demonstrated by color Doppler ultrasound and with cystic shadowing. This mass measures 4.3 × 2.8 × 2 cm in dimension. There is skin thickening and some suggestion of soft tissue edema associated with it. Fine-needle aspiration (FNA) was performed with 2 passes with preliminary cytologic evaluation suggestive of malignancy.
2. Abnormal axillary adenopathy. Within the left axilla are at least 3 lymph nodes that are abnormal in appearance. The node that measures 1.1 × 1.0 × 0.8 cm was sampled with FNA using a 20-gauge needle with 2 passes without complication. Preliminary cytologic evaluation suggested malignancy.

Fine-needle aspiration of left breast mass and left axillary mass:
1. Left breast 2 o'clock: breast carcinoma, ductal type, Black's nuclear grade III (poorly differentiated), ER 54 fm, PR 34 fm.
2. Left axillary lymph node: metastatic adenocarcinoma; the cytomorphology of the malignant cells in the lymph node aspiration is similar to that seen in the breast aspiration material.

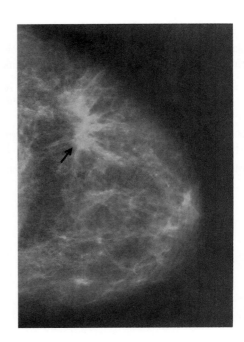

Figure 119–1. Mammogram of left breast. Arrow indicates area of abnormality highly suspicious for malignancy.

Ultrasound liver:
1. No lesions suggestive of metastases were identified in the liver. A 0.6 × 0.7 cm faintly visible hyperechoic area was suspected to the left side and slightly cephalad aspect of the ligamentum venosum. The appearance is more compatible with hemangioma than with metastases.

Bone scan:
1. No definite evidence of active osseous metastases.
2. Significant degenerative changes involving the lower lumbar spine and multiple peripheral joints. Increased tracer uptake in the lower lumbar spine, moderate increased uptake in the shoulders, elbows, wrists, knees, and small joints of both feet is noted. These findings are consistent with degenerative joint disease.

▶ Questions

Problem Identification

1. a. *Identify all of the patient's drug-related problems.*
   b. *Given the above clinical information, what is this patient's current clinical stage of cancer?*

Desired Outcome

2. a. *What is the goal of therapy for this patient?*
   b. *What is the prognosis for this patient based on tumor size and nodal status?*
   c. *In addition to stage of disease, what other factors may be helpful in determining the prognosis for breast cancer?*

Therapeutic Alternatives

3. *List the general types of treatment options that are available for the patient at this time, and briefly discuss their advantages and limitations.*

Optimal Plan

4. *Outline the optimal treatment plan for this patient that includes both pharmacologic and non-pharmacologic measures. If antineoplastic chemotherapy is part of your plan, identify the specific regimen you would use and provide your rationale.*

▶ Clinical Course

The patient does well with the standard therapeutic plan you outlined. Nine months after completion of therapy, she returns to the clinic complaining of bone pain in her lower back and left hip. She is still taking hormonal therapy. Restaging is performed that includes a bone scan, chest x-ray, CT scan of the abdomen, and additional laboratory tests. The bone scan reveals metastases to the lumbar spine and left acetabulum, without impending fracture or spinal cord compression. The chest x-ray shows two small nodules in the lower lobe of the left lung. The physician's assessment is that she has developed bone and lung metastases. The plan is to begin chemotherapy with docetaxel and discontinue the tamoxifen.

Outcome Evaluation

5. a. *What adverse effects can be anticipated with this regimen?*
   b. *What information is needed before calculating an appropriate dose of docetaxel for this patient? What dose would you recommend for this patient?*

Patient Counseling

6. *What information should the patient be given about the general effects she should expect to experience after this treatment?*

▶ Clinical Course

Ms. Gleason responds well to the docetaxel therapy and has received 6 courses. Her lung nodules are no longer detectable. She has 2+ pitting edema in her feet and ankles. Her weight has increased by 3 kg since beginning docetaxel. The physician decides to stop chemotherapy and observe the patient off therapy.

Eighteen months later, the patient complains of new pain in the right hip and left rib cage. A staging work-up reveals bone metastases in the right hip and left 6th and 7th ribs posteriorly. Laboratory values were within normal limits with the exception of the following: LDH 932 IU/L, Hgb 9.0 g/dL, Hct 28.0%, MCV 78 μm³. The patient has been taking acetaminophen 1000 mg every 4 hours with little relief of her pain and is experiencing a great deal of fatigue.

▶ Follow-up Questions

1. *What are the patient's drug-related problems at this time?*
2. *What are the treatment goals at this time?*
3. *What pharmacotherapeutic alternatives are available for each of the patient's current problems?*

▶ Clinical Course

The physician decided to start the patient on anastrozole therapy for her metastatic breast cancer.

▶ Follow-up Question

4. *What important information would you provide to the patient about her new therapy for breast cancer?*

▶ Self-study Assignments

1. Perform a literature search to obtain recent information on clinical trials demonstrating the advantages of bisphosphonates in bone metastases from breast cancer.
2. Perform a literature search to obtain recent information on clinical trials demonstrating the benefits of the new hormonal therapies

anastrozole, letrozole, and toremifene, and the role they play in treating breast cancer.

3. Perform a literature search to obtain information regarding the role of high-dose chemotherapy with peripheral stem cell support as a treatment option for breast cancer.

4. Develop a treatment plan for hand/foot syndrome (palmar plantar erythrodysesthesia) associated with chemotherapy.

5. Develop a treatment plan for chemotherapy-associated anemia.

► Clinical Pearl

Breast cancer in its early stages is a very curable cancer (Stage I has 70% to 90% 5-year disease-free survival), but in advanced stages the spread of disease virtually eliminates the possibility of cure (in Stage IV, up to 10% survive 5 years with minimal disease but are rarely "cured"). This is very strong evidence supporting routine screening and patient education efforts.

References

1. Bonadonna G, Valagussa P. Primary chemotherapy in operable breast cancer. Semin Oncol 1996;23:464–474.
2. Fisher B, Dignam J, Wolmark N, et al. Tamoxifen and chemotherapy for lymph node-negative, estrogen receptor-positive breast cancer. J Natl Cancer Inst 1997;89:1673–1682.
3. Fulton B, Spencer CM. Docetaxel: A review of its pharmacodynamic and pharmacokinetic properties and therapeutic efficacy in the management of metastatic breast cancer. Drugs 1996;51:1075–1092.
4. Buzdar A, Jonat W, Howell A, et al. Anastrozole, a potent and selective aromatase inhibitor, versus megestrol acetate in postmenopausal women with advanced breast cancer: Results of overview analysis of two phase III trials. Arimidex Study Group. J Clin Oncol 1996;14:2000–2011.

120   NON–SMALL CELL LUNG CANCER

► Remember the Surgeon General's Warning   (Level II)

Kimberly Heying, PharmD
Jane M. Pruemer, PharmD, FASHP

► After completing this case study, students should be able to:

- Identify the most common symptoms of non–small cell lung cancer (NSCLC).
- Monitor cisplatin and etoposide therapy.
- Identify potential complications associated with NSCLC.
- Design a pharmacotherapeutic plan for the treatment of hypercalcemia.
- Counsel patients on the anticipated side effects of cisplatin, etoposide, and radiation therapy.

☼ PATIENT PRESENTATION

Chief Complaint
"I have been coughing up blood."

HPI
This 58 yo woman presents to the ED with complaints of a dry, non-productive cough for 2 months, dyspnea on exertion, and hemoptysis for 1 week.

PMH
HTN
Hyperlipidemia
Anemia of unknown etiology × 1 year
Aortic insufficiency
Hysterectomy
PPD (−)

FH
No history of cancer, heart disease, or stroke.

SH
Divorced, lives with daughter; 40 pack-year cigarette smoking history (approximately 1 ppd × 40 years); no EtOH use; no known recent exposure to TB.

Meds
Folic acid 1 mg po QD
$FeSO_4$ 325 mg po TID
Premarin 0.625 mg po QD
Cardizem CD 240 mg po QD
HCTZ 25 mg po QD
Zocor 20 mg po QD
Axid 150 mg po BID
Trinalin 1 tablet po Q 6 H PRN

All
NKDA

ROS
(+) for pulmonary symptoms as in noted in HPI; no headaches, dizziness, or blurred vision.

PE

Gen
Mildly overweight African-American woman in slight distress

VS
BP 120/65, P 90, RR 30, T 99°F; Ht 63″, Wt 154 lb

Skin
Patches of dry skin; no lesions

HEENT
PERRLA; EOMI; fundi benign; TMs intact

Neck/LN

No lymphadenopathy; neck supple

Breasts

No masses, no discharge

Lungs

Wheezing in RUL; remainder of lung fields are clear

Heart

RRR; slight systolic murmur on left lateral side; normal S_1, S_2

Abd

Soft, non-tender; no splenomegaly or hepatomegaly

GU/Rect

Normal female genitalia; guaiac (−) stool

Neuro

A & O × 3; sensory and motor intact, +5 upper, +4 lower; CN II–XII intact; (−) Babinski

Labs

Na 138 mEq/L	Hgb 11.9 g/dL	Ca 8.7 mg/dL
K 3.1 mEq/L	Hct 36.8%	Mg 2.0 mg/dL
Cl 99 mEq/L	Plt $267 \times 10^3/mm^3$	
CO_2 23 mEq/L	WBC $9.4 \times 10^3/mm^3$	
BUN 13 mg/dL		
SCr 1.0 mg/dL		
Glu 118 mg/dL		

Chest X-ray

PA and lateral views reveal a possible mass in right upper lobe (see Figure 120–1).

Assessment

1. Hemoptysis; R/O malignancy vs. TB vs. other types of infection
2. Anemia; on iron and folate supplementation
3. Hyperlipidemia; receiving Zocor
4. HTN; controlled on Cardizem CD and HCTZ
5. Hypokalemia, possibly due to HCTZ; will provide K+ supplementation

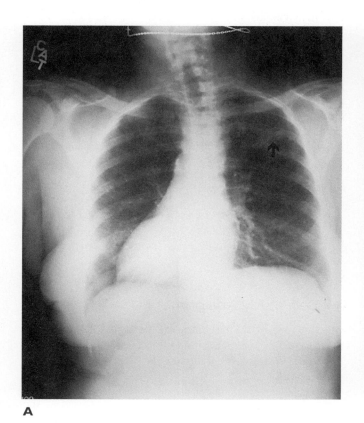

A

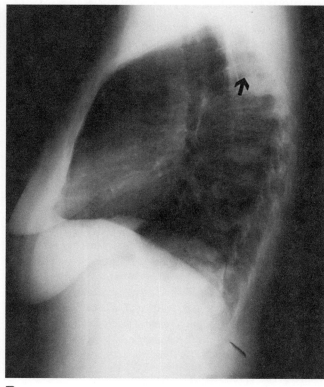

B

Figure 120–1. Chest x-ray with PA **(A)** and lateral **(B)** views showing a possible mass in the right upper lobe (arrows).

► Clinical Course

The patient was further evaluated for lung cancer on an outpatient basis. A bronchoscopy was performed that identified squamous cell carcinoma. The chest CT scan revealed a 2.5 cm × 2 cm right lung mass (see Figure 120–2.) A mediastinoscopy was performed to determine the resectability of the tumor. The mediastinoscopy and biopsy revealed unresectable Stage IIIB NSCLC with metastasis to the contralateral mediastinal nodes. PFTs included FEV_1 1.49 L, FVC 1.9 L. An echocardiogram showed mild LVH with an LVEF of 55%.

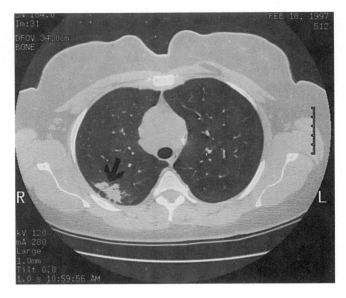

Figure 120–2. CT scan of the chest revealing a 2.5 cm × 2 cm right lung mass (arrow).

► Questions

Problem Identification

1. a. Identify the patient's drug-related problems.
   b. What signs, symptoms, and other information indicate the presence of NSCLC in this patient?

Desired Outcome

2. What is the desired goal for this patient, and what is the likelihood of it being achieved?

Therapeutic Alternatives

3. a. What chemotherapeutic regimens may be considered for NSCLC?
   b. What non-drug therapies may be used for NSCLC?

Optimal Plan

4. a. Design a specific chemotherapeutic regimen to treat this patient, and explain why you chose this regimen.
   b. What additional measures should be taken to ensure the tolerability of the regimen and to prevent adverse effects?
   c. What additional laboratory and clinical information is needed prior to administration of the chemotherapy?
   d. Calculate the patient's BSA and the amount of each drug to be administered based on the regimen chosen.

Outcome Evaluation

5. What clinical and laboratory parameters are necessary to evaluate the therapy for achievement of the desired therapeutic outcome and the occurrence of adverse effects?

Patient Counseling

6. What information should be provided to the patient to optimize therapy and minimize adverse effects?

► Clinical Course

The patient's subsequent courses were further complicated by the occurrence of DVT, CVA, renal insufficiency, electrolyte abnormalities, weight loss, anemia, nausea/vomiting, and infections. At one point, the patient presented with a serum calcium level of 11.5 mg/dL and an albumin of 2.0 g/dL with symptoms of weakness, confusion, nausea, and vomiting.

► Follow-up Questions

1. Calculate the patient's corrected calcium level and provide an interpretation of that value.
2. What treatment modalities may be used to correct hypercalcemia?

► Self-study Assignments

Carboplatin is dosed based on glomerular filtration rate (GFR) and the target area under the curve (AUC) desired. This equation individualizes the dose to prevent underdosing or overdosing to promote an optimal therapeutic response.

1. Define the Calvert formula for dosing carboplatin.
2. Read the background literature for dosing carboplatin using AUC and write a two-page summary on the advantages and limitations of this approach.
3. Suppose that the physician decides to substitute carboplatin for cis-

platin in a patient's regimen. Calculate this patient's carboplatin dose for a desired target AUC of 6 mg/mL × min.

Lung cancer is the leading cause of cancer death in both men and women.

References

1. Clinical practice guidelines for the treatment of unresectable non-small cell lung cancer. Adopted on May 16, 1997 by the American Society of Clinical Oncology. J Clin Oncol 1997;15:2996–3018.
2. Pritchard RS, Anthony SP. Chemotherapy plus radiotherapy compared with radiotherapy alone in the treatment of locally advanced, unresectable, non-small-cell lung cancer. A meta-analysis. Ann Intern Med 1996;125:723–729.

121   COLON CANCER

► **The Editor**   (Level I)

Daniel Sageser, PharmD

► After completing this case study, students should be able to:

- Discuss the therapeutic alternatives for treating colon cancer.
- Describe the treatment for side effects associated with colon cancer therapy.
- Develop an optimal chemotherapy treatment plan for patients with colorectal cancer.
- Discuss important issues about chemotherapy regimens for colorectal cancer with patients.

☼ PATIENT PRESENTATION

Chief Complaint
"I'm back in for more chemotherapy."

HPI
Edmund Keller is a 54 yo man diagnosed with colon cancer 10 months ago. He had been asymptomatic until the onset of RLQ discomfort. Two days after the initial symptom onset, he experienced extreme abdominal pain and presented to the ED. An abdominal CT scan showed a large tumor in the LLQ involving the colon. A 15-cm tumor was subsequently resected, and all gross disease was removed. A diverting colostomy was performed at that time. The liver was clear on CT scan and examination by surgeons. The pathology report on the colon tumor was consistent with mucinous adenocarcinoma. Final staging was Duke's stage C, (T4b, N1 M0). The patient underwent 9 months of fluorouracil 450 mg/m² weekly with lev-

amisole 50 mg po TID for 3 days repeated every 2 weeks. Last month, his serum CEA began to rise sharply, and exploratory laparotomy revealed recurrent disease in the pelvis and terminal ileum, as well as 2 implants in the bowel; all areas of tumor were resected.

PMH
Appendectomy 12 years ago
S/P nasal septum surgery to relieve an obstruction on the right nostril
Radial keratotomy 3 years ago
Sleep apnea recently diagnosed, uses C-PAP machine at home PRN
Type 2 DM × 2 years

FH
Father age 81 alive and well, mother age 76 has type 2 DM but is otherwise in good health. Patient has 5 siblings, 2 with hypertension. No family history of cancer. He is married and has 3 children, all alive and well.

SH
Worked at local newspaper as editor throughout his working life. He smoked 1 to 1½ ppd for 30 years until he quit 10 years ago; drinks 3–4 beers/week.

All
Allopurinol → generalized maculopapular rash

ROS
Sweats occasionally at night but has done so for years. Has recently lost weight. Is finally getting his strength back after second surgery. No chest pain, palpitations, SOB, DOE, or wheezing. Complains of mild irritation around the colostomy site but states that the colostomy is working well, with no current malodorous problems. Has had some diarrhea on 5-FU/levamisole therapy. Has a few aches and pains, which are normal for him. Complains of occasional dizziness, which was diagnosed as an inner ear problem.

Meds
Metformin 500 mg po BID
Diphenhydramine 25 mg, 2 caps po BID PRN
Temazepam 15 mg po Q HS PRN sleep
Prochlorperazine 5 mg, 1–2 tablets po Q 6 H PRN nausea/vomiting
Loperamide 2 mg po PRN diarrhea

PE

Gen
Well-developed, muscular, middle aged man in NAD

VS
BP 120/70, P 84 and regular, RR 18, T 98.4°F; Ht 72," Wt 198 lb, BSA 2.11 m²

HEENT
Nasal septal deviation to the right, evidence of past surgery

Neck/LN
Neck supple; no thyromegaly or palpable lymph nodes

Thorax
No crackles or wheezing

Cardiac
RRR; normal heart sounds; no murmurs or cardiomegaly

Abdomen
Diverting colostomy in RLQ. He is tender at both costal margins. No masses are palpable.

Genital/Rect
Normal male genitalia; heme (−) stool

Ext
Pulses intact; no CCE

Neuro
A & O × 3; CNs intact; reflexes 2+ and symmetrical. No peripheral neurologic deficits secondary to diabetes.

Labs

Na 135 mEq/L	Hgb 13.3 g/dL	AST 15 IU/L
K 3.9 mEq/L	Hct 38.5%	ALT 100 IU/L
Cl 102 mEq/L	RBC 4.41×10^6/mm³	LDH 543 IU/L
CO_2 25 mEq/L	Plt 213×10^3/mm³	Alb 2.5 g/dL
BUN 20 mg/dL	WBC 3.87×10^3/mm³	Ca 7.2 mg/dL
SCr 1.2 mg/dL	ANC 2.14×10^3/mm³	Phos 2.1 mg/dL
Glu 187 mg/dL	CEA 19.3 ng/mL	Uric acid 2.2 mg/dL

Assessment
Patient with recurrence of mucinous adenocarcinoma of the colon who has tolerated 5-FU/levamisole therapy well for a 9-month course. Progression of malignancy was evident and all known masses have been surgically resected. Patient has presented to Cancer Center for chemotherapy. Since patient is 54 years old, has tolerated chemotherapy in the past, and has had resection of all bulky disease, aggressive treatment is warranted. Patient states QOL has been good even during 5-FU/levamisole therapy, and he is eager to try a new regimen.

▶ Questions

Problem Identification

1. Create a list of the patient's drug-related problems.

Desired Outcome

2. What is the desired outcome for chemotherapy in this patient?

Therapeutic Alternatives

3. What chemotherapeutic options are available for this patient?

Optimal Plan

4. Design a chemotherapy regimen for treating this patient's recurrent colon carcinoma.

Outcome Evaluation

5. What parameters should be monitored to evaluate the efficacy and adverse effects of the regimen you recommended?

Patient Counseling

6. What information should be provided to the patient to ensure the safety and efficacy of your regimen?

▶ Self-study Assignments

1. Develop standardized, written, patient counseling information on the treatment of chemotherapy-induced diarrhea for regimens containing 5-FU or irinotecan.
2. All of the chemotherapeutic regimens in this case can cause anorexia. Develop a plan for managing this side effect if it occurs. Include both non-pharmacologic and pharmaceutical options.

▶ Clinical Pearl

Always reinforce the use of loperamide at the first signs of diarrhea during irinotecan therapy. Specific patient counseling is required because the loperamide dosage regimen used is above the maximum recommended dose.

References

1. Kawato Y, Aonuma M, Hirota Y, et al. Intracellular roles of SN-38, a metabolite of the camptothecin derivative CPT-11, in the antitumor effect of CPT-11. Cancer Res 1991;51:4187–4191.
2. Rothenberg ML, Eckardt JR, Kuhn JG, et al. Phase II trial of irinotecan in patients with progressive or rapidly recurrent colorectal cancer. J Clin Oncol 1996;14:1128–1135.
3. Camptosar package insert. Kalamazoo, MI, Pharmacia & Upjohn, 1997.
4. Abigerges D, Armand JP, Chabot GG, et al: Irinotecan (CPT-11) high-dose escalation using intensive high-dose loperamide to control diarrhea. J Natl Cancer Inst 1994;86:446–449.

122 PROSTATE CANCER

▶ For Men Only   (Level II)

Judith A. Smith, PharmD
Barry R. Goldspiel, PharmD, FASHP

▶ After completing this case study, students should be able to:

- Describe the typical symptoms associated with prostate cancer at initial diagnosis and at disease progression.

- Recommend a pharmacotherapeutic plan for patients with hormone-refractory Stage D prostate cancer.

- Counsel patients about the common toxicities associated with the hormonal and chemotherapeutic agents used in prostate cancer treatment.

☀ PATIENT PRESENTATION

Chief Complaint

"I'm having more pain in my lower back, some pain in my shoulder, and I don't have any energy. My doctor said I should come here so you can put me on a research study."

HPI

Ralph Crowden is a 69 yo man with Stage D prostate cancer who has been complaining over the past year of an increasing frequency and intensity of pain in his lower back. He takes naproxen and Darvocet-N 100 for this pain and has been taking increasing doses because of the new shoulder pain. His local physician noted a steady increase in his PSA to 49 ng/mL, and his bicalutamide was discontinued 1 week ago.

PMH

Stage D_2 prostate cancer diagnosed 3 years ago; originally treated with goserelin acetate implant 10.8 mg SC Q 3 months plus bicalutamide 50 mg po QD.
Type 2 DM
GERD
PUD
Mild arthritis involving the hands and knees
Anemia of chronic disease

FH

Father died from prostate cancer at age 77; mother died of "natural causes" at age 87.

SH

Retired farmer from the Midwest. He is married with 3 sons all in good health. His wife recently underwent triple bypass surgery. He has 2 brothers, both alive and well. He denies any history of tobacco or alcohol use.

ROS

Patient states that his shoulder started hurting a week ago and that he has problems when he goes to the bathroom. He says it takes him a long time to start to urinate and then dribbles come out. He states that this seems to have gotten worse over the past year. The patient noted shortness of breath while working on his farm. Also, he has experienced mild rib pain. The stiffness and pain in his knees has worsened significantly, and he now requires a cane or wheelchair when traveling.

Meds

Goserelin acetate implant 10.8 mg SC Q 3 months
Humulin Insulin NPH 10 units SC Q AM
Humulin Insulin Regular per sliding scale
Metformin 500 mg po BID
Glyburide 5 mg po BID
Darvocet-N 100 1 tablet po Q HS and Q 4 H PRN

Naproxen 500 mg po TID
Misoprostol 200 μg po TID
Docusate sodium 100 mg po TID
Ferrous sulfate 325 mg po BID
Acetaminophen 500 mg po Q 4 H PRN

All

Aspirin → diarrhea

PE

Gen

The patient is an elderly, mildly obese, Caucasian man in considerable pain and discomfort

VS

BP 132/80, P 78, RR 20, T 36.9°C; Ht 60.5″, Wt 89.3 kg, BSA 2.08 m²

Skin

Non-abraded, dry

HEENT

PEERLA, EOMI, disks flat, TMs intact, no hemorrhages or exudates

Neck/LN

Supple, no nodes palpated

Chest

Clear, good breath sounds

CV

RRR, normal S_1 and S_2, mild S_3 gallop

Abd

Soft, non-tender, bowel sounds present in all quadrants, no hepato-splenomegaly

Genit/Rect

Normal male genitalia; enlarged boggy prostate on rectal exam with firm nodule in the posterior lobe

MS/Ext

Extreme pain noted when lower back examined and mild pain on shoulder exam. Limited ROM in right shoulder and bilateral knee joints. Pulses 2+

Neuro

A & O × 3, CN II–XII intact, sensory and motor levels intact, Babinski (−), DTRs 2+

Labs

Na 137 mEq/L	Hgb 8.9 g/dL	AST 37 IU/L	Ferritin 1818 μg/dL
K 4.6 mEq/L	Hct 31%	ALT 10 IU/L	Iron 97 μg/dL
Cl 104 mEq/L	Plt 129 × 10³/mm³	Alk Phos 1465 IU/L	Transferrin 183 mg/dL
CO₂ 22 mEq/L	WBC 4.2 × 10³/mm³	T. bili 0.4 mg/dL	Transferrin sat 38%
BUN 24 mg/dL	38% PMNs	Pt 12.3 sec	Vit B₁₂ 376 pg/mL
SCr 1.0 mg/dL	51% Lymphs	aPTT 23.2 sec	PSA 225 ng/mL
Glu 198 mg/dL	6% Monos		Testosterone 2.5 ng/dL
	2% Eos		
	3% Basos		

Bone Scan

Increased uptake in the rib cage, lower spine, pelvis, and left shoulder (see Figure 122–1).

Ultrasound-guided Transrectal Prostate Biopsy

Positive for adenocarcinoma, Gleason score $4 + 4 = 8$.

Assessment

69 yo man with progressive metastatic prostate cancer here for consideration of experimental therapy. New metastatic sites include ribs, left shoulder, and pelvis.

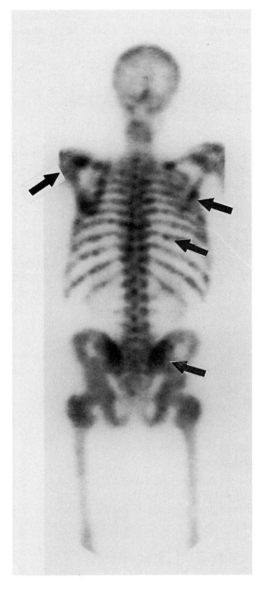

Figure 122–1. Bone scan showing increased uptake in the rib cage, lower spine, pelvis, and left shoulder (arrows) indicating sites of probable new metastatic disease.

► Questions

Problem Identification

1. a. *Create a list of this patient's drug-related problems.*
   b. *What signs, symptoms, and other information are consistent with progressive prostate cancer in this case?*
   c. *What is your assessment of the appropriateness of the initial therapy (goserelin plus bicalutamide) that this patient received for Stage D_2 prostate cancer?*
   d. *Would you consider this patient an appropriate candidate for a clinical research trial?*

Desired Outcome

2. *Considering this patient's disease stage and treatment history, what are the reasonable therapeutic goals?*

Therapeutic Alternatives

3. *What pharmacotherapeutic options are available for the treatment of this patient?*

Optimal Plan

4. *Design an optimal pharmacotherapeutic plan for this patient, considering that he is not eligible for a clinical research study at this time and wants to receive some chemotherapy in addition to adjusting his pain control medications.*

Outcome Evaluation

5. *How should the therapy you recommended be monitored for efficacy and adverse effects?*

Patient Counseling

6. *What information should be provided to the patient about his new therapy?*

▶ Clinical Course

During his second cycle of chemotherapy, the patient became progressively weaker and remained in bed most of the day. The pain in his back and shoulder worsened, and he also developed significant hip and rib pain. His PSA rose to 500 ng/mL. He subsequently developed a fever while his ANC was $0.400 \times 10^3/\text{mm}^3$. He was admitted to the hospital and treated with IV ceftazidime. His chemotherapy was discontinued, his fever eventually resolved, his ANC rose to $1.5 \times 10^3/\text{mm}^3$, and antibiotics were then discontinued. His pain medications were adjusted, but he is still experiencing considerable pain whenever he tries to get up out of bed. His physician feels that the patient is not benefiting from the chemotherapy. The patient stated that he does not want any more chemotherapy and "just wants to be left alone."

▶ Follow-up Question

1. *Given the patient's wish to not receive any chemotherapy agents and his probable ineligibility for clinical trials (based on his poor performance status), what therapeutic options are available for him at this time?*

▶ Self-study Assignments

1. Outline the effective treatment options for localized prostate cancer.
2. Provide the rationale for and identify patients who are appropriate candidates for neoadjuvant androgen ablative therapy prior to surgery or radiation for locally advanced prostate cancer.
3. Locate information resources that are available to prostate cancer patients and their families.
4. Identify information sources you can use to find clinical studies that are available for patients with prostate cancer.

▶ Clinical Pearl

The radionuclides strontium 89 or samarium 153 lexidronam may relieve pain in prostate cancer patients with osteoblastic metastases.

References

1. Roach M, Small EJ. Using the serum prostate specific antigen (PSA) to screen for and manage prostate cancer. Princ Pract Oncol Updates 1997;11:1–14.
2. Garnick MB. Hormonal therapy in the management of prostate cancer: From Huggins to the present. Urology 1997;49(3A suppl):5–15.
3. Millikan R, Logothetis C. Update of the NCCN guidelines for treatment of prostate cancer. Oncology (Huntingt) 1997;11(11A):180–193.
4. Kelly WK, Slovin S, Scher HI. Steroid hormone withdrawal syndromes. Pathophysiology and clinical significance. Urol Clin North Am 1997;24:421–431.
5. Sartor O, Cooper M, Weinberger M, et al. Surprising activity of flutamide withdrawal, when combined with aminoglutethimide, in treatment of "hormone-refractory" prostate cancer. J Natl Cancer Inst 1994;86:222–227.
6. Hudes G. Estramustine-based chemotherapy. Semin Urol Oncol 1997;15:13–19.
7. Tannock IF, Osoba D, Stockler MR, et al. Chemotherapy with mitoxantrone plus prednisone or prednisone alone for symptomatic hormone-resistant prostate cancer: A Canadian randomized trial with palliative end points. J Clin Oncol 1996;14:1756–1764.
8. Hudes GR, Greenberg R, Krigel RL, et al. Phase II study of estramustine and vinblastine, two microtubule inhibitors, in hormone-refractory prostate cancer. J Clin Oncol 1992;10:1754–1761.

123 MALIGNANT LYMPHOMA

▶ The French Chef   (Level I)

Krista M. King, PharmD, BCOP

▶ After completing this case study, students should be able to:

- Identify and describe the components of the staging work-up and the corresponding staging and classification systems for non-Hodgkin's lymphoma (NHL).
- Describe the pharmacotherapeutic treatment of choice and the alternatives available for the treatment of NHL.
- Identify acute and chronic toxicities associated with the drugs used to treat NHL and the measures used to prevent or treat these toxicities.
- Identify monitoring parameters for response and toxicity in patients with NHL.
- Provide detailed patient counseling corresponding to the chemotherapeutic regimen.

☀ PATIENT PRESENTATION

Chief Complaint
"I'm here to find out the best way to treat my lymphoma."

HPI
Michael Donato is a 68 yo man who presents for recommendations about treatment of a newly diagnosed gastric large cell lymphoma. He had been well until approximately 2 months ago when he began to experience epigastric pain, most notable after eating. He had a remote history of duodenal ulcers 12 years ago. Therefore, the patient thought that he had an ulcer recurrence. He saw his physician who recommended omeprazole. The patient took omeprazole for about 6 weeks without resolution of his symp-

toms. His pain worsened and he experienced marked weight loss. He became so ill that he was eventually admitted to the hospital where he was noted to be febrile with guaiac (+) stools. A thorough GI work-up including an endoscopy revealed large gastric ulcers, which were biopsied and found to be malignant. The patient was then referred to an oncologist for further evaluation and treatment recommendations.

PMH

Duodenal ulcers 12 years ago
HTN × 20 years
CRI secondary to hypertension
Right inguinal hernia
Type 2 DM recently diagnosed

FH

The patient has 3 sisters, all in good health. He has 2 daughters, both in good health. None of his relatives have any history of malignancy.

SH

The patient is a French chef and restaurant owner. He smoked 2 packs of cigarettes/day for 40 years but has recently decreased to 5 cigarettes/day. He drinks about 2 glasses of alcoholic beverages/day. He does not use street drugs. The patient is married and was accompanied to the clinic by his wife, who appears to be very supportive.

ROS

The patient reports pain in his stomach, indigestion-like pain when he eats, and early satiety. Over the last several months, he reports fatigue necessitating frequent naps and abbreviated workdays. He describes fevers, night sweats, and weight loss of about 20 pounds over the past 2 months. He denies headaches, changes in vision, or fainting episodes. He reports no lesions in his mouth, difficulty swallowing, or nosebleeds. He denies chest pain, tachycardia, or swelling in the extremities. The patient denies wheezing, shortness of breath, or cough. He also denies burning on urination, frequency, dribbling, or blood in the urine. He has not noticed any bleeding or bruising. He has not received any prior transfusions.

Meds

Omeprazole 20 mg po QD
Captopril 25 mg po QD
Zolpidem 10 mg po HS PRN sleep
Oxycodone/acetaminophen 1 tablet po Q 4–6 H PRN pain
Glipizide 2.5 mg po QD

All

NKDA

PE

Gen

The patient is an elderly man who is slightly anxious, but not in any acute distress

VS

BP 150/100, P 80, RR 18, T 37°C; Ht 69″, Wt 71 kg

Skin

No rashes or moles noted

HEENT

Male pattern baldness is noted. TMs are clear. Examination of the oral cavity reveals no masses in the tonsils, palate, or floor of the mouth; there are no ulcers in the mucosa. There are several teeth with caries, but no gingival inflammation is noted. The funduscopic examination is significant for a cataract in the left lens and the right is significant for cotton wool exudates. The optic disks appear normal.

Neck

Supple, no masses noted

Chest

Lungs are CTA & P

CV

RRR with S_4 noted

Abd

Soft and non-tender. There is a palpable epigastric mass measuring about 10–12 cm in diameter that is tender to palpation. There is no hepatosplenomegaly. Bowel sounds are normoactive.

GU/Rect

Normal male genitalia; stool is guaiac (+)

Ext

Without edema

Neuro

Symmetrical cranial nerve function. Symmetric facial muscle movement, and the tongue is midline. The palate is symmetric. Balance and coordination of the upper extremities are intact with no evidence of tremor. There is symmetric coordination of rapidly alternating movements. Motor strength in the upper and lower extremities is normal and symmetric.

LN Survey

The lymph node survey is negative for any palpable peripheral nodes in the preauricular, postauricular, cervical, supraclavicular, infraclavicular, axillary, inguinal, or femoral areas. There is a small cystic subcutaneous nodule in the right occipital region.

Labs

Na 141 mEq/L	Hgb 10.2 g/dL	ALT 27 IU/L	PT 12.2 sec
K 5.9 mEq/L	Hct 30.5%	Alk phos 75 IU/L	aPTT 21.7 sec
Cl 102 mEq/L	Plt 254 × 10³/mm³	LDH 939 IU/L	Phos 4.0 mg/dL
CO_2 30 mEq/L	WBC 9.2 × 10³/mm³	T. bili 0.6 mg/dL	Uric acid 8.0 mg/dL
BUN 20 mg/dL	70% Neutros	T. prot 6.3 g/dL	β-2 microglob 4.8 mg/dL
SCr 1.8 mg/dL	2% Bands	Alb 3.7 g/dL	
Glu 150 mg/dL	18% Lymphs		
	9% Monos		
	1% Eos		

UGI Endoscopy

Extensive tumor ulceration in the antrum of the stomach.

CT abd

Thickened stomach wall with perigastric adenopathy. There are no apparent lesions in the liver or spleen.

Chest X-ray
No adenopathy in the hilum or mediastinum.

Tumor Pathology
Diffuse large cell lymphoma, B-cell type; *Helicobacter pylori* negative.

Initial Assessment
Bulky primary gastric large cell lymphoma. Further staging will include bilateral BM biopsies, gallium scan, HIV test, CT of the pelvis and chest, and a baseline cardiac assessment in light of the patient's HTN history.

▶ Clinical Course

- Bone marrow biopsies are negative for lymphoma.
- Gallium scan reveals a gallium-avid lesion in the mid-upper ante-

rior abdomen inferior to the left lobe of the liver consistent with the patient's history of active lymphoma. Questionable tracer activity is noted in the left iliac area that represents bowel activity versus lymphomatous involvement.

- HIV test is negative.
- CT of the pelvis reveals no evidence of pelvic adenopathy.
- CT of the chest shows slightly enlarged lymph nodes in the left axilla representing hyperplastic changes. Mediastinal adenopathy is not noted.
- MUGA scan reveals a LVEF of 48% with moderate septal left ventricular hypokinesis.

Assessment
Primary gastric large cell lymphoma, stage IEB

▶ Questions

Problem Identification

1. a. *Identify all of the drug-related problems of this patient.*
   b. *What clinical and other information is consistent with the diagnosis of non-Hodgkin's lymphoma?*
   c. *Explain what system of staging was used and how his stage of disease was determined.*
   d. *What laboratory and clinical features does this patient have that may affect his prognosis?*

Desired Outcome

2. *What are the goals of therapy in this case?*

Therapeutic Alternatives

3. *What alternative drug therapies are available for the treatment of this non-Hodgkin's lymphoma?*

Optimal Plan

4. a. *What drug, dosage form, schedule, and duration of therapy are best for treating this patient's non-Hodgkin's lymphoma?*
   b. *What other interventions should be made to maintain control of the patient's other concurrent diseases?*
   c. *What non-drug therapies might be useful for this patient?*

Outcome Evaluation

5. a. *How is the response to the treatment regimen for the non-Hodgkin's lymphoma assessed?*
   b. *What acute adverse effects are associated with the chemotherapy regimen, and what parameters should be monitored?*
   c. *What pharmacologic measures should be instituted to treat or prevent the acute toxicities associated with the chemotherapy regimen?*
   d. *What are potential late complications of the chemotherapy regimen, and how can they be detected and prevented?*

Patient Counseling

6. *What information would you provide to the patient about the chemotherapy agents?*

▶ Clinical Course

The patient tolerated cycle 1 of chemotherapy very well without nausea or vomiting. His hypertensive medication was changed to an extended release diltiazem product with average systolic BPs in the 130s and average diastolic BPs in the 80s. The serum potassium decreased after the captopril was discontinued. During the chemotherapy infusion, the patient had a positive fluid balance for 2 days with 2+ pedal edema requiring diuresis with furosemide. Renal function remained stable and tumor lysis syndrome was not observed. Elevated blood glucose levels were problematic and the patient was covered with sliding scale insulin. No signs of acute GI bleeding or perforation were seen. One week after cycle 1 of chemotherapy, the patient experienced severe epigastric pain. He also complained of poor food tolerance and discomfort with eating. He returned to the clinic for evaluation.

▶ Follow-up Question

1. *What could be the possible causes of the epigastric pain experienced by the patient?*

▶ Clinical Course

The cause of the pain was investigated. An abdominal series to rule out perforation was negative. An endoscopy found no definitive etiology for the patient's abdominal pain. Diffuse involvement of malignancy throughout the gastric wall was noted. The pain was thought to be due to tumor necrosis.

▶ Self-study Assignments

1. What is the role of bone marrow or stem cell transplantation for aggressive non-Hodgkin's lymphoma?

2. What is the role of dexrazoxane, an anthracycline cardioprotector, in the treatment of malignancy?

3. Do any of the patient's medications need to be dose-adjusted for renal insufficiency?

▶ Clinical Pearl

The diagnosis of non-Hodgkin's lymphoma must be established by an appropriate biopsy to provide tissue for pathologic review. The prognosis and treatment of non-Hodgkin's lymphoma is dependent on the histologic type and the presence of certain adverse clinical features.

References

1. The International Non-Hodgkin's Lymphoma Prognostic Factors Project. A predictive model for aggressive non-Hodgkin's lymphoma. N Engl J Med 1993;329: 987–994.

2. Rodriguez J, Cabanillas F, McLaughlin P, et al. A proposal for a simple staging system for intermediate grade lymphoma and immunoblastic lymphoma based on the "tumor score." Ann Oncol 1992;3:711–717.

3. Fisher RI, Gaynor ER, Dahlberg S, et al. Comparison of a standard regimen (CHOP) with three intensive chemotherapy regimens for advanced non-Hodgkin's lymphoma. N Engl J Med 1993;328:1002–1006.

4. Doroshow JH. Anthracyclines and anthracenediones. In: Chabner BA, Longo DL, eds. Cancer Chemotherapy and Biotherapy, 2nd ed. Philadelphia, Lippincott-Raven, 1996:409–429.

5. Steinherz LJ, Yahalom J. Cardiac complications of cancer therapy. In: DeVita VT Jr., Hellman S, Rosenberg ST, eds. Cancer: Principles & Practice of Oncology, 4th ed. Philadelphia, JB Lippincott, 1993:2370–2385.

6. Carlson RW. Reducing the cardiotoxicity of the anthracyclines. Oncology (Huntingt) 1992;6:95.

7. Basser RL, Green MD. Strategies for prevention of anthracycline cardiotoxicity. Cancer Treat Rev 1993;19:57–77.

8. Ganz WI, Sridhar KS, Ganz SS, et al. Review of tests for monitoring doxorubicin-induced cardiomyopathy. Oncology 1996;53:461–470.

124 OVARIAN CANCER

▶ Dorothy Walker's Ordeal (Level II)

William C. Zamboni, PharmD
James A. Trovato, PharmD

▶ After completing this case study, students should be able to:

- Recognize the signs and symptoms of ovarian cancer.

- Describe the significance of stage of disease at initial presentation and the amount of residual disease after primary cytoreduction surgery as a function of survival in patients with ovarian cancer.

- Recommend a pharmacotherapeutic plan for the chemotherapeutic treatment of newly diagnosed and relapsed ovarian cancer.

- Recognize the dose-limiting and most common toxicities of the chemotherapeutic agents used in the treatment of ovarian cancer.

☼ PATIENT PRESENTATION

Chief Complaint
"I'm a little nervous about getting my chemotherapy today."

HPI
Dorothy Walker is a 46 yo woman who presented to the ED 8 weeks ago with a 3-day history of acute abdominal pain. She also reported a weight gain of about 20 pounds. CT scans of the abdomen and pelvis showed a large, soft-tissue pelvic mass. Exploratory laparotomy revealed a 20 × 10 cm tumor mass on the left ovary, positive microscopic disease in the omentum, and positive bilateral external iliac nodes. A 3-cm tumor mass was also found in the liver. A total abdominal hysterectomy and left oophorectomy were performed at that time. Tumor biopsies from the ovary and liver were positive for epithelial ovarian cancer. Bulky residual disease persists in the mesenteric lymph nodes, pre-sacral spine (1.5 cm), and para-aortic region (2.2 cm). She is now admitted to undergo her first cycle of consolidative chemotherapy.

PMH
Right sided oophorectomy for ruptured ectopic pregnancy 12 years ago
Type 2 DM × 10 years
HTN × 5 years
Bilateral numbness in feet

FH
Divorced with no children; mother, maternal aunt, and cousin all have ovarian cancer. Father is alive and well.

SH
Smokes 2 packs/week; denies alcohol use; denies current IVDU, although she last snorted heroin 1 year ago.

Meds
Prempro (conjugated estrogens 0.625 mg/medroxyprogesterone acetate 2.5 mg) 1 tablet po QD
Procardia XL 60 mg po QD
Glucotrol 10 mg po QD

All
Penicillin → seizures
Aspirin → stomach cramps

ROS
Stomach area feels heavy and painful. Sometimes feels nauseated.

PE

Gen
The patient is a pleasant but anxious-appearing woman in NAD

VS
BP 181/130, P 110, RR 22, T 99.6°F; Wt 86 kg, Ht 64″

Skin
No erythema, rash, ecchymoses, petechiae, or breakdown

LN
No cervical or axillary lymphadenopathy

HEENT
PERRLA; EOMI; TM's intact; fundi benign; OP with dry mucus membranes

Breasts
Without masses, discharge, or adenopathy. No nipple or skin changes.

CV
RRR; no m/r/g

Pulm
Lungs are clear to auscultation with a slight decrease at the left base; mainly resonant throughout all lung fields by percussion.

Abd
Soft, non-tender, without hepatosplenomegaly

GU/Rect
Heme (−) dark brown stool; no rectal wall tenderness or masses. Normal female genitalia.

Ext
No c/c/e

Neuro
No dysarthria noted, speech rate normal. CN II–XII intact. Normal motor strength throughout; muscle tone normal. Sensation decreased to light touch and pinprick below the knees bilaterally. Vibration sense diminished at the great toes bilaterally. Reflexes 2+ and symmetric throughout. Babinski (−) bilaterally. Cerebellar intact; finger-to-nose and heel-to-shin are without dysmetria. Rapid alternating movements and gross and fine motor coordination are normal. Good sitting and standing balance without an assistive device. Gait normal in speed and step length; able to toe and tandem walk without difficulty. A & O × 3. Able to do serial 7s. Able to abstract. Short- and long-term memories are intact.

Labs

Na 137 mEq/L	Hgb 13.6 g/dL	WBC $5.2 \times 10^3/mm^3$	AST 21 IU/L
K 3.1 mEq/L	Hct 38 %	60% PMNs	ALT 24 IU/L
Cl 99 mEq/L	Plt $150 \times 10^3/mm^3$	3% Bands	T. bili 0.8 mg/dL
CO_2 22 mEq/L		30% Lymphs	Amylase 129 IU/L
BUN 20 mg/dL		5% Monos	Lipase 62 IU/L
SCr 1.5 mg/dL		1% Eos	CA-125 165 IU/mL
Glu 180 mg/dL		1% Basos	

UA
WBC 5–10/hpf, RBC 0–2/hpf, 1+ ketones, 1+ protein, pH 5.0

▶ Questions

Problem Identification

1. a. *What are the patient's drug-related problems?*
   b. *What clinical and other information indicates the presence and severity of ovarian cancer?*
   c. *What stage of ovarian cancer does this patient have, and how does the stage of disease affect the choice of therapy?*
   d. *What is the significance of the size of residual tumor after primary cytoreductive surgery?*

Desired Outcome

2. *What are the goals of therapy for this patient?*

Therapeutic Alternatives

3. *What consolidative chemotherapy options are available for this patient?*

Optimal Plan

4. *Which consolidative chemotherapy regimen and ancillary treatment measures would you recommend for this patient?*

Outcome Evaluation

5. *How would you monitor the therapy for efficacy and adverse effects?*

Patient Counseling

6. *What information would you provide to the patient about this therapy?*

▶ Clinical Course

The patient completed her first 3 cycles of cisplatin and paclitaxel without any problems except for moderate nausea and vomiting. Her tumor continued to respond to therapy. Serum CA-125 at this time was 88 IU/mL. Two weeks prior to the start of her next cycle of chemotherapy, she started complaining of intermittent numbness in her toes. She was also noted to have an increased BUN (40 mg/dL) and serum creatinine (2.0 mg/dL).

▶ Follow-up Questions

1. *What chemotherapeutic regimen would you recommend for this patient for her next cycle? Provide the rationale for your answer.*
2. *Describe how you would calculate a carboplatin dose for this patient based on a target AUC.*

▶ Clinical Course

The patient's fourth cycle of chemotherapy was changed to the regimen you recommended. She completed 3 cycles without further complications. The numbness in her toes subsided approximately 2 months after the last cycle of the initial regimen containing cisplatin. Her serum CA-125 level continued to decline and was reported to be 32 IU/mL 2 weeks after her 6th and final cycle of chemotherapy. Based on her CA-125 levels and negative CT scans, the patient was defined as having achieved a clinical complete response.

Eight months after receiving her last chemotherapy cycle, she presented to the ED with a 1-day history of sharp abdominal pain and vomiting. She reported that the onset of pain had awakened her from sleep. The pain was described as starting in the lower abdomen and traveling upward. She also experienced nausea and vomiting that was productive of a dark brown material. She reported a 2-month history of constipation and straining with bowel movements, which she attributed to her diet. Laboratory data were normal except for a serum CA-125 of 247 IU/mL. Radiographic imaging of the abdomen and pelvis revealed a mass (5 cm × 6 cm × 6 cm) arising from the retroperitoneum and a 2-cm mass in the head of the pancreas. Biopsies of the pancreas and abdominal/pelvic mass were positive for recurrent epithelial ovarian cancer. She underwent cytoreductive surgery and is now admitted for her first cycle of chemotherapy.

▶ Follow-up Questions

1. *What chemotherapeutic options are available for this patient's relapsed ovarian cancer?*
3. *Which of the chemotherapeutic regimens would you suggest for the patient's locally relapsed ovarian cancer and why?*

▶ Clinical Course

After 2 cycles of salvage regimen (paclitaxel and carboplatin), CA-125 levels did not decline and radiographic findings showed progression of disease. Considering the poor prognosis and aggressive nature of her disease, it was decided to enter her on a phase I trial of docetaxel and topotecan. Even though docetaxel and topotecan are approved for use in humans, the combination has not been evaluated in patients. Thus, a phase I trial of the combination was developed to determine the maximum tolerated dose of docetaxel in combination with a fixed dose of topotecan. Her treatment was ongoing at the time of this writing.

▶ Self-study Assignments

1. Calculate the carboplatin dose required for this patient using an equation based on a target AUC of 7.5 mg/mL·min.
2. What is the probable cause of paclitaxel hypersensitivity reactions?
3. What are the theoretical advantages of intraperitoneal (IP) therapy?

▶ Clinical Pearl

The objective of phase I clinical trials is to determine the maximum tolerated dose and dose-limiting toxicities. In phase I trials, the dose of a chemotherapeutic agent is increased in cohorts of patients until dose-limiting toxicity is achieved.

References

1. Cannistra SA. Cancer of the ovary. N Engl J Med 1993;329:1550–1559.
2. Alberts DS, Green S, Hannigan EV, et al. Improved therapeutic index of carboplatin plus cyclophosphamide versus cisplatin plus cyclophosphamide: final report by the Southwest Oncology Group of a phase III randomized trial in stages III and IV ovarian cancer. J Clin Oncol 1992;10:706–717.
3. McGuire WP, Hoskins WJ, Brady MF, et al. Cyclophosphamide and cisplatin compared with paclitaxel and cisplatin in patients with stage III and stage IV ovarian cancer. N Engl J Med 1996;334:1–6.
4. Morgan RJ Jr, Copeland L, Gershenson D, et al. NCCN Ovarian cancer practice guidelines. The National Comprehensive Cancer Network. Oncology (Huntingt) 1996;10 (11 suppl):293–310.
5. Alberts DS, Liu PY, Hannigan EV, et al. Intraperitoneal cisplatin plus intravenous cyclophosphamide versus intravenous cisplatin plus intravenous cyclophosphamide for stage III ovarian cancer. N Engl J Med 1996;335:1950–1955.

125 ACUTE LYMPHOCYTIC LEUKEMIA

▶ Jenny's Long Battle   (Level II)

Mark T. Holdsworth, PharmD, BCPS

▶ After completing this case study, students should be able to:

- Identify common drug-induced diseases in children with acute lymphocytic leukemia (ALL) during induction therapy.
- Provide adequate initial pharmacotherapy for these common drug-induced diseases in ALL.
- Interpret the laboratory values that signify the response of ALL to chemotherapy.
- Discuss key items that should be presented to a patient's family when educating them about the chemotherapy agents used during induction therapy.
- Describe the ancillary medications and supportive care measures that are necessary when administering intermediate-dose methotrexate.

☀ PATIENT PRESENTATION

Chief Complaint
Fatigue and low-grade temperature.

HPI
Jenny Martinez is a 3 yo girl brought to the pediatric clinic by her parents who report that for the past week she has been quite fatigued and has had fevers, easy bruising, and puffiness of the extremities.

PMH
Up-to-date on immunizations; no prior surgeries or serious medical problems

FH
Noncontributory

SH
Not applicable

ROS
Noncontributory

Meds
None

All
NKDA

PE

Gen
Alert, interactive, well developed but ill appearing child

VS
BP 130/83, P 95, RR 34, T 36.8°C; Ht 38″, Wt 17.3 kg, BSA 0.6 m²

Skin
Diffuse pallor; random tan macular bruises just inferior to the hairline, face, and over the proximal upper extremity, with a petechial-appearing rash over the buttocks and lower left flank.

HEENT
Head is NC/AT, PERRLA, EOMI, nares are clear bilaterally, throat shows no erythema. Question of petechial hemorrhage of mucous membranes.

Neck/LN
Neck is supple and non-tender with shotty cervical and submandibular lymphadenopathy

Lungs/Thorax
CTA bilaterally without wheezes or crackles, and there is good air movement throughout

Breasts
Undeveloped

CV
Heart has RRR without murmur

Abd
Soft and non-tender, without distention. There are good bowel sounds and no masses present. Hepatosplenomegaly is noted.

Genit/Rect
No tenderness, bruising, or blood observed

MS/Ext
Shotty lymphadenopathy in the inguinal area; femoral pulses are 2+ bilaterally. Extremities display no CCE, and there is no bone pain elicited with palpation.

Neuro
Without dysmorphic features or deformities. Frequent rapid eye blinking (R > L); eyes seemed briefly dysconjugate when asked to focus. Fixes and follows well with conjugate eye movements. Hearing appears intact. Motor exam shows normal muscle tone and bulk. Gait is essentially normal. DTRs are normal. General muscle strength is symmetric and normal. Facial strength appears symmetric and normal.

Labs

Hgb 5.7 g/dL	AST 93 IU/L	PT 12 sec
Hct 17.2%	ALT 60 IU/L	aPTT 24 sec
WBC 12.5 × 10³/mm³	LDH 1275 IU/L	Varicella titer (+)
2% Segs	T. bili 0.7 mg/dL	Anti-HAV (−)
0% Bands	T. prot 6.9 g/dL	HBsAg (−)
85% Lymphs	Alb 3.5 g/dL	Anti-HBs (−)
4% Monos	Ca 9.3 mg/dL	Anti-HCV (−)
1% Myelos	Phos 4.1 mg/dL	
8% Blasts	Uric acid 4.1 mg/dL	

BM Aspirate
90% blasts, 3% erythroid precursors, 2% lymphocytes, 2% metamyelocytes, 1% promyelocytes, 2% myelocytes. DNA index 1.0. Early pre-B cell ALL with L1 morphology. RT-PCR positive for TEL-AML 1 fusion transcript and negative for E2A-PBX1.

Chest X-ray
Normal with no mediastinal mass noted

LP
Glucose 55 mg/dL, T. protein 15 mg/dL, no blasts present

Assessment
Acute lymphocytic leukemia with pancytopenia and replacement of normal bone marrow elements.

▶ Clinical Course

The patient was admitted to the pediatric subacute care unit. Medications and treatments upon admission included the following:

Day 1 (day of admission):

- 1 unit of irradiated/filtered platelets
- 1 unit PRBCs
- D_5 0.9% NS IV with $NaHCO_3$ 30 mEq/L at 2000 mL/m²/day
- Allopurinol 150 mg po QD

Day 2 induction chemotherapy orders:

- Vincristine 1 mg IV Q week × 4
- Prednisone 10 mg po TID × 28 days
- Asparaginase 4100 units IM on chemotherapy days 2, 5, 8, 12, 15, 19
- Triple intrathecal therapy (TIT) on chemotherapy days 2 and 16: methotrexate 12 mg + hydrocortisone 12 mg + cytarabine 24 mg

On day 1 of admission, the patient developed a fever of 38.5°C. Four hours after the LP on day 2, she developed moderate nausea and vomiting with 4 vomiting episodes. The patient remained in the hospital for the first 5 days. During week 2, the parents notify the clinic that Jenny has not had a bowel movement in 4 days and appears to be having abdominal pain. Examples of hematology tests obtained during the remainder of induction therapy included the following:

Parameter (units)	Week 2 (Day 7)	Week 3 (Day 18)	Week 4 (Day 28)
Hgb (g/dL)	8.7	11.7	12.8
Hct (%)	25.1	35.3	38.2
Plt (× 10³/mm³)	22.0	70.0	326.0
WBC (× 10³/mm³)	0.670	2.35	11.0
Segs (%)	5	18	86
Bands (%)	0	0	0
Lymphs (%)	92	68	10
Monos (%)	1	12	4
Myelos (%)	0	2	0
Blasts (%)	2	0	0

On day 15 of chemotherapy another BM aspirate revealed: 1% blasts, 4% promyelocytes, 2% myelocytes, 4% metamyelocytes, 63% erythroblasts and other erythroid precursors, 9% lymphocytes, 4% plasma cells, 10% bands, 1% neutrophils, 0% eosinophils, 0% basophils, 1% reticulum cells, and 1% monocytes. Day 15 LP showed CSF glucose 47 mg/dL, T. prot 14 mg/dL, no blasts present. On day 29 of chemotherapy (end of induction), the BM aspirate results were: 2% blasts, 3% promyelocytes, 5% myelocytes, 7% metamyelocytes, 8% bands, 8% neutrophils, 56% erythroblasts and other erythroid precursors, 5% lymphocytes, 1% monocytes, and 5% eosinophils and precursors. After completion of induction therapy, she entered a consolidation phase (weeks 5 through 24), which consisted of the following.

- Mercaptopurine 50 mg/m^2 po daily
- Methotrexate 1 g/m^2 IV × 1 dose on weeks 7, 10, 13, 16, 19, and 22
- Vincristine 2 mg/m^2 IV × 1 dose on weeks 8, 9, 17, and 18
- Prednisone 10 mg po TID × 7 days on weeks 8 and 17
- TIT (using the same regimen as on day 2 of induction) × 1 dose on weeks 5, 6, 9, 12, 15, and 18

After completing the consolidation phase, the plan is for her to receive maintenance therapy for 2.5 years with the following.

- Mercaptopurine 50 mg/m^2 po daily
- Methotrexate 20 mg/m^2 IM × 1 dose weekly
- Vincristine 2 mg/m^2 IV × 1 every 15 weeks
- Prednisone 50 mg/m^2 po × 7 days, every 15 weeks
- TIT (using the same regimen as on day 2 of induction) × 1 dose every 8 weeks

▶ Questions

Problem Identification

1. a. Identify the patient's drug- and disease-related problems upon initial presentation to the hospital.
   b. What drug-related problems developed during her initial hospitalization, and which of these could have been prevented by pharmacotherapy?
   c. If vincristine and the TIT are to be administered on the same day, what precautions must be observed to avoid severe drug toxicity?

Desired Outcome

2. a. What are the initial goals of pharmacotherapy in this patient, and were they achieved?
   b. What are the long-term treatment goals, and what indicators of achieving these goals exist in this patient?

Therapeutic Alternatives

3. List the therapeutic alternatives for this patient's drug- and disease-related problems that developed during induction therapy (see question 1.b.) and discuss the risks and benefits of these therapies.

Optimal Plan

4. Outline the optimal treatment schedule and duration for each of the drug-related problems described in the previous answer. What therapeutic alternatives should be considered if initial therapy fails?

Outcome Evaluation

5. Which key laboratory parameters are indicative of an adequate response at the end of induction therapy?

Patient Counseling

6. What information should be provided to the patient's parents about the potential beneficial and adverse effects from the chemotherapy agents used during induction therapy?

▶ Follow-up Questions

1. During week 7 of consolidation, Jenny is scheduled to receive her first course of intermediate dose methotrexate (1 g/m^2). Which additional medications and supportive measures will be necessary for administration of this dose of methotrexate?
2. What laboratory tests and examinations must be performed prior to the methotrexate administration?
3. After the methotrexate administration, the 24-hour peak concentration is 8.7 μmol. The 48-hour concentration is undetectable (< 0.1 μmol). What is the significance of these findings, and what additional changes in therapy should be made based on these concentrations?
4. It is now week 63, and Jenny is receiving the maintenance phase of her chemotherapy protocol. Which laboratory test is closely monitored to gauge the adequacy of her chemotherapy doses?
5. What is the target value for this laboratory measurement, and how will the chemotherapy doses be changed if the laboratory test(s) is above the target range?

▶ Self-study Assignments

1. Provide the current antiemetic recommendations for both moderately and severely emetogenic chemotherapy in children. Include a brief summary of common moderate and severely emetogenic chemotherapy regimens in children.
2. Provide evidence to support the value of maintaining adequate dose intensity in the maintenance phase of ALL therapy (focus on trials that report the actual received-dose intensity).
3. Provide the current recommendations regarding the site of treatment (i.e., home versus inpatient unit) for treating febrile neutropenia in children. What patient characteristics might make outpatient treatment possible?

Clinical Pearl

Although a DNA index = 1.0 generally is a high risk feature for childhood ALL, the TEL-AML 1 fusion transcript [associated with t(12;21)] in this patient indicates a good prognosis case of B-ALL, resulting in a less intensive chemotherapy protocol than would otherwise be indicated.[9]

References

1. Holdsworth MT, Raisch DW, Winter SS, et al. Assessment of the emetogenic potential of intrathecal chemotherapy and response to prophylactic treatment with ondansetron. Support Care Cancer 1998;6:132–138.
2. Reiter A, Schrappe M, Ludwig WD, et al. Chemotherapy in 998 unselected childhood acute lymphoblastic leukemia patients. Results and conclusions of the multicenter trial ALL-BFM 86. Blood 1994;84:3122–3133.
3. Cordonnier C, Herbrecht R, Pico JL, et al. Cefepime/amikacin versus ceftazidime/amikacin as empirical therapy for febrile episodes in neutropenic patients: A comparative study. Clin Infect Dis 1997;24:41–51.
4. Pizzo PA. Management of fever in patients with cancer and treatment-induced neutropenia. N Engl J Med 1993;328:1323–1332.
5. Rubenstein EB, Rolston K. Outpatient management of febrile episodes in neutropenic cancer patients. Support Care Cancer 1994;2:369–373.
6. Mitchell PL, Morland B, Stevens MC, et al. Granulocyte colony-stimulating factor in established febrile neutropenia: A randomized study of pediatric patients. J Clin Oncol 1997;15:1163–1170.
7. Pui CH, Boyett JM, Hughes WT, et al. Human granulocyte colony-stimulating factor after induction chemotherapy in children with acute lymphoblastic leukemia. N Engl J Med 1997;336:1781–1787.
8. Pearson AD, Amineddine HA, Yule M, et al. The influence of serum methotrexate concentrations and drug dosage on outcome in childhood acute lymphoblastic leukaemia. Br J Cancer 1991;64:169–173.
9. Shurtleff SA, Buijs A, Behm FG, et al. TEL/AML1 fusion resulting from a cryptic t(12;21) is the most common genetic lesion in pediatric ALL and defines a subgroup of patients with an excellent prognosis. Leukemia 1995;9:1985–1989.

126 CHRONIC MYELOGENOUS LEUKEMIA

▶ A Long Arm Translocation   (Level II)

Terri G. Davidson, PharmD
Catherine A. Smith, PharmD

▶ After completing this case study, students should be able to:

- Identify the presenting signs and symptoms of chronic myelogenous leukemia (CML).
- Identify important prognostic indicators for CML.
- Construct chemotherapy treatment options for CML.
- List appropriate parameters to monitor for potential adverse effects of treatment for CML.
- Educate patients on treatment complications and the most common side effects of current chemotherapy regimens used to treat CML.

☀ PATIENT PRESENTATION

Chief Complaint
"I've been really tired lately."

HPI
John Pella is a 51 yo man who complains of shortness of breath on exertion, an unintentional weight loss of 14 pounds, and fatigue beginning 4 months ago. He also notes fullness in his left upper quadrant and early satiety.

PMH
Appendectomy (1955) complicated with infection
Tonsillectomy (1958)
Hernia repair (1992)

FH
Father died of pulmonary embolism at age 54. Mother is 73 yo with type 2 diabetes. His 47 yo sister and 23 yo old son are in good health. Grandparents may have had CAD. No history of cancer.

SH
Married and lives with his wife of 30 years. He works full-time in the maintenance department of a local packaging company. Smoked 1/2 to 3/4 pack of cigarettes/day for over 20 years until he quit 4 years ago. Denies alcohol consumption.

ROS
Increased weakness and tiredness. Occasional fever, chills, and night sweats; shortness of breath on exertion. Denies bleeding, headaches, nausea, vomiting, chest pain, or urinary symptoms.

Meds
None

All
Penicillin → skin rash (35 years ago)

PE

Gen
WDWN Caucasian man in NAD who appears his stated age

VS
BP 120/88, P 84, RR 18, T 98.6°F, actual weight 90.9 kg, Ht 73 1/4"

Skin
Warm, dry, with good turgor. No evidence of rash, ecchymoses, petechiae, or cyanosis.

HEENT
PERRLA, EOMI, sclerae anicteric, TMs clear. No sinus discharge or tenderness. Oral mucosa moist and intact

Neck

Supple without masses. No carotid bruits auscultated. No thyromegaly appreciated

LN

Approximately 1-cm, non-tender palpable node in right inguinal area. No other lymphadenopathy noted

Chest

CTA, no rales or rhonchi

CV

NSR; normal S_1 and S_2 without murmur

Abd

Soft, symmetrical, and non-tender. Spleen palpable 8 cm below costal margin. Normoactive bowel sounds. No hepatomegaly noted. Well-approximated abdominal surgical scar noted.

Rect

Deferred

MS/Ext

No joint deformities or peripheral edema. ROM and muscle strength symmetrical throughout

Neuro

CN II–XII intact. DTRs 1+ throughout. Gait steady. A & O × 3

Labs

Na 143 mEq/L	Hgb 12.1 g/dL	AST 30 IU/L	Ca 8.9 mg/dL
K 4.4 mEq/L	Hct 32%	ALT 86 IU/L	Mg 3.0 mEq/L
Cl 109 mEq/L	Plt $456 \times 10^3/mm^3$	Alk phos 29 IU/L	Phos 4.8 mg/dL
CO_2 24 mEq/L	WBC $97.0 \times 10^3/mm^3$	LDH 325 IU/L	Uric acid 0.9 mg/dL
BUN 50 mg/dL	24% Segs	T. bili 4.9 mg/dL	LAP absent
SCr 0.7 mg/dL	8% Bands	T. prot 2.9 g/dL	
Glu 148 mg/dL	64% Lymphs	Alb 1.6 g/dL	
Retic 2.3%	3% Myelos	INR 1.64	
	1% Monos	aPTT 50.8 sec	

► Clinical Course

Cytogenetic studies performed on a bone marrow biopsy revealed a translocation involving the long arms of chromosomes 9 and 22 [t(9q;22q)]. The marrow was hypercellular and consisted of 2% to 3% myeloblasts but showed no other blastic abnormalities. This information is consistent with the characteristics of CML in chronic phase (CML-CP).

► Questions

Problem Identification

1. a. *What information in the patient's history is consistent with a diagnosis of CML-CP (see Figure 126–1)?*
   b. *Describe the natural progression of CML.*
   c. *List factors that signal a poor prognosis for CML patients in chronic phase.*

Desired Outcome

2. *What are long-term therapy goals for this patient?*

Therapeutic Alternatives

3. *What pharmacologic and/or non-pharmacologic alternatives should be considered for this patient?*

Optimal Plan

4. *Considering all patient factors, describe the optimal initial treatment plan for this patient.*

Outcome Evaluation

5. *Describe parameters for monitoring disease response and toxicity for the treatment option you recommended.*

Patient Counseling

6. *What information should be given to the patient prior to treatment?*

► Clinical Course

The regimen you recommended was initiated. At the 4-week follow-up visit, the patient's WBC count was $70 \times 10^3/mm^3$. Hydroxyurea 2 g/d was added.

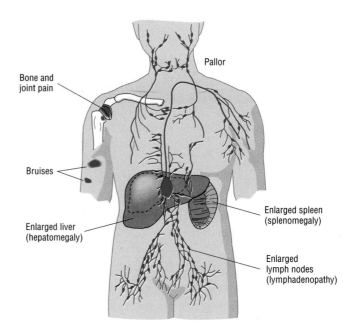

Figure 126–1. Common signs and symptoms of leukemia.

At the 3-month follow-up visit, his WBC count had decreased to $20 \times 10^3/mm^3$. After 6 months of treatment, his WBC count rose to $124 \times 10^3/mm^3$, and a bone marrow biopsy revealed no cytogenetic response. The patient discussed further treatment options with his physician. An allogeneic BMT from a matched-related sibling was chosen, using busulfan (4 mg/kg/d) for 4 days followed by cyclophosphamide (50 mg/kg/d) for 2 days as the BMT preparative regimen.

▶ Follow-up Questions

1. What is the rationale for adding hydroxyurea, cytarabine, or hydroxyurea plus cytarabine in this patient at the 4-week follow-up visit? What outcomes would be expected from using this combination therapy?
2. What is the goal of therapy for allogeneic BMT in the management of CML-CP?
3. Is this CML patient an optimal candidate for a BMT? Why or why not?
4. List common complications of allogeneic BMT and this preparative regimen.
5. Identify important laboratory/clinical values to monitor during the BMT course.
6. When the patient is discharged after BMT, what important information should be relayed to him?
7. If relapse occurs after allogeneic BMT, what treatment alternatives remain for this patient?
8. If the patient progresses to CML-blast crisis despite BMT, what is the best treatment option for him?

▶ Self-study Assignments

1. Describe the response criteria (complete, partial, minor, and no response) for interferon therapy in patients with CML, including WBC count, splenomegaly, and percent of Ph+ marrow cells.
2. How does the treatment of a Ph− CML patient differ from Ph+ disease?
3. Discuss the role of chlorambucil, melphalan, 6-mercaptopurine, cyclophosphamide, L-phenylalanine mustard, homoharringtonine, and radioactive phosphorous in the treatment of CML-CP.

▶ Clinical Pearl

- Interferon alfa has the potential to produce cytogenetic remission in 20% to 40% of CML patients.

References

1. Hehlmann R, Heimpel H, Hasford J, et al. Randomized comparison of busulfan and hydroxyurea in chronic myelogenous leukemia: Prolongation of survival by hydroxyurea. Blood 1993;82:398–407.
2. Kantarjian HM, O'Brien S, Anderlini P, et al. Treatment of myelogenous leukemia: Current status and investigational options. Blood 1996;87:3069–3081.
3. Devergie A, Apperley JF, Labopin M, et al. European results of matched unrelated donor bone marrow transplantation for chronic myeloid leukemia. Impact of HLA class II matching. Bone Marrow Transplant 1997;20:11–19.
4. Chronic Myeloid Leukemia Trialists' Collaboration Group. Interferon alfa versus chemotherapy for chronic myeloid leukemia: A meta-analysis of seven randomized trials. J Natl Cancer Inst 1997;89:1616–1620.
5. Kurzrock R, Talpaz M, Kantarjian H, et al. Therapy of chronic myelogenous leukemia with recombinant interferon-gamma. Blood 1987;70:943–947.
6. Kantarjian HM, Keating MJ, Estey EH, et al. Treatment of advanced stages of Philadelphia chromosome-positive chronic myelogenous leukemia with interferon-alpha and low-dose cytarabine. J Clin Oncol 1992;10:772–778.
7. Guilhot F, Chastang C, Michallet M, et al. Interferon alfa-2b combined with cytarabine versus interferon alone in chronic myelogenous leukemia. N Engl J Med 1997;337:223–229.

127 MELANOMA

▶ **Remember Your ABCDE's**   (Level I)

Jennifer A. Torma, PharmD
Rowena N. Schwartz, PharmD

▶ After completion of this case study, students should be able to:

- Identify risk factors for the development of melanoma.
- Outline the therapeutic approach to a patient with melanoma.
- Counsel patients with the diagnosis of melanoma on the adverse effects of alfa-interferon.
- Identify chemotherapy agents used in the treatment of metastatic melanoma.

☀ PATIENT PRESENTATION

Chief Complaint
"I'm here for my interferon treatment"

HPI
Samuel Neilson is a 38 yo Caucasian man who was referred to the dermatology clinic by his PCP after discovering a suspicious-looking mole on his left scapula (see Figure 127–1). An excisional biopsy of the mole resulted in the diagnosis of superficial spreading melanoma. The patient underwent wide excision of the primary tumor and regional lymph node dissection. CT scans of the lungs, abdomen, and pelvis were unremarkable. Based on the tumor thickness of 3.6 mm and metastatic local lymph node involvement measuring 2.1 cm, his melanoma was clinically and pathologically classified as Stage III. He presents to the clinic today for the first day of interferon alfa-2b (IFNα-2b).

PMH
Seasonal allergic rhinitis

FH
Mother alive and healthy at age 62; father with h/o CAD, ↓ at age 58 secondary to AMI; sister alive and healthy at age 42; no known family history

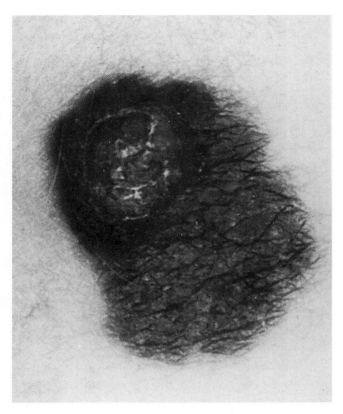

Figure 127–1. Superficial spreading melanoma developing in contiguity with a dysplastic nevus. *(Reprinted with permission from Lejeune FJ, Chaudhuri PK, Das Gupta TK, eds.* Malignant Melanoma: Medical and Surgical Management. *New York, McGraw-Hill, 1994.)*

of cancer, familial atypical multiple mole syndrome, or hereditary dysplastic nevus syndrome.

SH
Works as a sixth grade school teacher. Lives with wife, who is also a school teacher, and two sons, ages 7 and 10 years old. One year ago he relocated to Pittsburgh from Colorado, where he had lived for 37 years. History of severe blistering sunburns during summers as a child. Eight pack-year history of smoking, quit 4 years ago. Drinks 2 to 3 beers on weekends.

ROS
No changes in vision or hearing; no headaches, cough, fevers, chills, night sweats, nausea, or vomiting; no changes in bowel or bladder habits

All
Penicillin caused rash and diarrhea when given as a child

Meds
No chronic medications; uses an OTC antihistamine in the spring and summer (April through August) for seasonal allergic rhinitis

PE

Gen
WDWN Caucasian man, appearing anxious

VS
BP 130/72, P 82, RR 18, T 37.1°C; Ht 5′9″, Wt 83.2 kg

Skin
Slightly diaphoretic, fair in complexion, left scapula wound apparent, scattered multiple nevi

HEENT
PERRLA, EOMI; sclera anicteric; throat without lesions or erythema

Neck/LN
Supple, no lymphadenopathy, thyroid without masses

Lungs
CTA bilaterally without wheezes, rales, or rhonchi

CV
RRR; S_1, S_2 normal; no m/r/g; no JVD

Abd
Soft, non-tender; (+) BS; no rebound, guarding, or distention; no HSM

Rect
Normal sphincter tone, heme (−), prostate normal size without nodules

Ext
No CCE, distal pulses 2+ bilaterally

Neuro
A & O × 3, CN II–XII intact, DTRs 2+ and symmetrical throughout, cerebellar function intact, sensory levels grossly intact, 5/5 motor strength throughout, Babinski downgoing bilaterally

Labs

Na 143 mEq/L	Hgb 14.8 g/dL	Ca 8.2 mg/dL
K 4.2 mEq/L	Hct 42%	Mg 1.9 mg/dL
Cl 98 mEq/L	Plt 209 × 10³/mm³	PO₄ 3.9 mg/dL
CO₂ 23 mEq/L	WBC 9.2 × 10³/mm³	AST 30 IU/L
BUN 9 mg/dL	PMNs 66%	ALT 28 IU/L
Scr 0.8 mg/dL	Bands 4%	Alk phos 103 IU/L
Glu 96 mg/dL	Eos 3%	LDH 168 IU/L
	Basos 1%	T. bili 0.9 mg/dL
	Lymphs 22%	T. prot 6.8 g/dL
	Monos 4%	Alb 4.0 g/dL

Assessment
38 yo man with newly diagnosed melanoma s/p excision presenting to the clinic to begin high-dose phase of adjuvant IFNα-2b therapy

► Questions

Problem Identification

1. a. Create a list of the patient's drug-related problems.
   b. What risk factor(s) does this patient have for the development of melanoma?
   c. What are the characteristics of Stage III melanoma, in terms of tumor size/thickness, nodal involvement, and metastases?

Desired Outcome

2. What are the goals of using adjuvant IFNα-2b in this patient?

Therapeutic Alternatives

3. If IFNα-2b therapy was not chosen for this patient, are other feasible pharmacotherapeutic options available?

Optimal Plan

4. a. As the first step in developing a treatment plan for adjuvant treatment with IFNα-2b for this patient, calculate his body surface area.
   b. Determine dose of interferon for high-dose intravenous therapy and describe how the dose should be prepared for administration.
   c. Determine dose of interferon for the subcutaneous 48-week phase.
   d. What supportive measures may be used to minimize adverse effects of the IFNα-2b therapy?

Outcome Evaluation

5. a. What parameters will you monitor to assess interferon efficacy?
   b. What parameters will you monitor for adverse effects of interferon during the high-dose phase?
   c. What parameters will you monitor for adverse effects of interferon during the low-dose maintenance phase?

Patient Counseling

6. a. What information should the patient receive prior to his high-dose phase?
   b. What information should the patient receive prior to initiating the low-dose phase of the regimen?
   c. What information would you give to the patient regarding sun exposure?

► Clinical Course

During the third week of high-dose IV interferon therapy, Mr. Neilson's laboratory test results reveal AST 201 IU/L, ALT 284 IU/L, and SCr 1.4 mg/dL. His weight is 77.5 kg upon presentation to the clinic.

► Follow-up Questions

1. Given this new information, what changes, if any, should be made in the patient's interferon therapy?

► Clinical Course

Seven months after initiation of maintenance IFNα-2b, Mr. Neilson is brought to the ED by his wife. She reports that he has been getting increasingly lethargic and confused at times over the past few days. He is hospitalized because of acute mental status changes.

2. What information is needed to fully assess the patient's acute mental status changes?
3. What possible complications resulting from the interferon therapy might account for his acute mental status changes?
4. Should any changes be made in the patient's interferon therapy at this point?
5. If the patient develops metastatic disease, what pharmacotherapeutic options are available?

► Self-study Assignments

1. Outline the chemotherapy and other options available to patients for the treatment of melanoma.
2. List expected or possible adverse effects associated with the chemotherapy used to treat melanoma.
3. Perform a literature search using MedLine and the Internet. Outline other treatment approaches that are currently being investigated for the treatment of melanoma.

► Clinical Pearl

Clinical features of pigmented lesions that suggest melanoma include Asymmetry, Border irregularity, Color variegation, Diameter >6 inches, and Evolution of the mole (the ABCDE's of melanoma).

References

1. Kirkwood JM, Strawderman MH, Ernstoff MS, et al. Interferon alfa-2b adjuvant therapy of high-risk resected cutaneous melanoma: The Eastern Cooperative Oncology Group Trial EST 1684. J Clin Oncol 1996;14:7–17.
2. Cole BF, Gelber RD, Kirkwood JM, et al. Quality-of-life-adjusted survival analysis of interferon alfa-2b adjuvant treatment of high-risk resected cutaneous melanoma: An Eastern Cooperative Oncology Group study. J Clin Oncol 1996;14:2666–2673.
3. Cocconi G, Bella M, Calabresi F, et al. Treatment of metastatic malignant melanoma with dacarbazine plus tamoxifen. N Engl J Med 1992;327:516–523.

128 BONE MARROW TRANSPLANTATION

► A Dilemma in Antibiotic Therapy   (Level II)

Simon Cronin, PharmD, MS

► After completing this case study, students should be able to:

• Understand the difference between autologous and allogeneic bone marrow transplantation (BMT).

- Differentiate peripheral stem cell transplantation (PSCT) from BMT.
- Discuss the therapy of vancomycin-resistant enterococcal (VRE) infection with special emphasis on the BMT arena.
- Provide drug information to patients being treated for VRE.

☀ PATIENT PRESENTATION

Chief Complaint
"I have a fever, I am unable to swallow without severe pain, and my mouth is very sore."

HPI
Keith Jameson is a 23 yo man admitted for an autologous PSCT for NHL Stage IIB. His preparative regimen consisted of high dose cyclophosphamide (1800 mg/m^2/day × 4 days) plus mesna and etoposide (200 mg/m^2 Q 12 H × 4 days). The cyclophosphamide and the etoposide were administered on the same days. The fifth day of chemotherapy consisted of a single dose of carmustine (450 mg/m^2).

The patient was already febrile (101°F) on the day of admission, and a chest x-ray was suspicious for a LLL pneumonia. The ANC was 5.7 × 10^3/mm^3. Antibiotics were initiated on the next day (ceftazidime 2 g Q 8 H + vancomycin 1 g Q 12 H). The patient also received antifungal prophylaxis with fluconazole 100 mg po QD. After 72 hours of IV antibiotics, vancomycin was discontinued because of negative cultures. The patient required continuous narcotic analgesia for severe esophagitis/mucositis.

Because of unrelenting fevers, levofloxacin 500 mg IV QD was added on the sixth day of the hospital admission (the day of the PSCT), and clindamycin 900 mg IV Q 8 H was added on the seventh day. Antibiotic therapy was modified 6 days later because of new blood culture information.

PMH
NHL initially diagnosed 2 years ago after he presented with a lump in the left neck that was biopsied and found to be consistent with large-cell NHL. A CT scan revealed mediastinal lymph node involvement (Stage IIB). Despite multiple courses of chemotherapy and radiation, cervical and mediastinal disease were still evident by CT scan prior to this hospital admission. Nevertheless, he was given high-dose cyclophosphamide followed by G-CSF in order to boost the PSC numbers. The PSCs were then harvested by apheresis and stored in liquid nitrogen containing dimethyl-sulfoxide in readiness for the transplant.
Hx several episodes of sepsis necessitating IV antibiotics.
S/P DVT 6 months PTA.
Hx severe back pain (related to NHL).

FH
Married with 1 child. Both parents are alive and well, although his father has prostate cancer that is currently in remission.

Meds
Fluconazole 100 mg IV QD
Acyclovir 450 mg IV Q 8 H
Famotidine 20 mg IV Q 12 H
Fentanyl patch 50 μg Q 3 days
Clindamycin 900 mg IV Q 8 H
Ceftazidime 2 g IV Q 8 H
Levofloxacin 500 mg IV QD

All
Morphine → intense pruritus
IV contrast dye → body rash

ROS
No c/o dysuria, abdominal pain, diarrhea, or SOB; (+) productive cough

PE

Gen
Patient is a WDWN African-American man in NAD

VS
BP 115/68, P 86, RR 18, T 101°F, Wt 97 kg (admission wt 95.6 kg), Ht 68"

HEENT
Face edematous, grade II–III oral/esophageal mucositis

Skin
Warm, dry; no rash

Neck/LN
Supple; no thyromegaly; a left cervical LN was palpable but was smaller than before the high-dose cyclophosphamide

Lungs
Some decreased breath sounds on left

Heart
RRR; no murmurs, rubs, or gallops; normal heart sounds

Abd
Slight distention, RUQ tenderness, mild hepatomegaly

Ext
Bilateral edema grade I–II in both LE

Neuro
A & O × 3; CN II–XII intact; sensory and motor levels intact; Babinski (−)

Labs
Na 136 mEq/L	Hgb 8.6 g/dL	AST 22 IU/L
K 4.2 mEq/L	Hct 25%	ALT 29 IU/L
BUN 4.0 mg/dL	Plt 9.0 × 10^3/mm^3	Alk Phos 141 IU/L
SCr 0.5 mg/dL	WBC 0.200 × 10^3/mm^3	LDH 138 IU/L
Glu 98 mg/dL		T. bili 2.1 mg/dL

Blood Cultures
E. faecium (2/2 containers)
E. faecium (2/2 containers)

MICs
ampicillin > 64 μg/mL, gentamicin > 500 μg/mL, imipenem > 16 μg/mL, erythromycin > 8 μg/mL, levofloxacin > 8 μg/mL, ciprofloxacin

> 4 µg/mL, doxycycline < 4 µg/mL, vancomycin > 16 µg/mL, quin-upristin/dalfopristin (investigational) < 1.0 µg/mL

Other Cultures

All other culture sites (stool, urine, sputum, central venous catheter) are negative.

Assessment

New bacteremia with vancomycin-resistant enterococci (VRE) in a neutropenic host who is day +8 post-autologous PSCT for NHL. Patient is hemodynamically stable.

▶ Questions

Problem Identification

1. a. *What risk factors did this patient have for developing VRE sepsis?*
   b. *What other potential drug-related problems does this patient have?*

Desired Outcome

2. *What are the therapeutic goals in this patient?*

Therapeutic Alternatives

3. *What alternative antibiotic(s) would effectively treat the VRE infection in this patient?*

Optimal Plan

4. a. *Outline an appropriate antibiotic regimen for treating this patient's VRE infection.*
   b. *What other pharmacotherapeutic measures should be implemented to enhance the patient's defense mechanisms against infection and to prevent other types of infection?*

Outcome Evaluation

5. *What parameters should you monitor to assess the response to therapy and to detect adverse effects?*

Patient Counseling

6. *How will you explain to the patient that he has an antibiotic-resistant infection?*

▶ Clinical Course

The antibiotic regimen you suggested was initiated. The patient continued to have low-grade fevers without chills and was hemodynamically stable. By day +11 post-transplant, he was afebrile, facial swelling was still evident, and there were new findings of LUQ abdominal tenderness and a 2-kg weight gain. At this time, the patient did not show signs of engraftment (WBC $0.2 \times 10^3/mm^3$), and other labs included Hgb 8.8 g/dL, BUN 5 mg/dL, SCr 0.5 mg/dL, T. bili 3.9 mg/dL, AST 32 IU/L, ALT 16 IU/L, LDH 138 IU/L, and alk phos 144 IU/L.

By day +14, the facial swelling and oral mucositis had dramatically improved, the WBC was $1.6 \times 10^3/mm^3$, and all blood cultures since the change in antibiotic therapy were negative for bacterial growth. On day +15, the bilirubin was 2.0 mg/dL and the alk phos was 130 IU/L. He continued to remain afebrile with negative cultures.

All remaining antibiotics were discontinued on day +18, and the patient was discharged from the hospital on day +19 on a fentanyl patch 50 µg Q 3 days (for pain), and omeprazole 20 mg/day (for complaints of burning in his stomach).

▶ Follow-up Questions

1. *Review the clinical and laboratory data on day +11 and suggest a possible reason for the change in liver function tests.*
2. *Assume that the LFT changes are not related to infection. Outline a therapeutic plan aimed at treating this new problem, should it progress.*

▶ Self-study Assignments

1. What is the difference between autologous bone marrow versus peripheral stem cell (PSC) transplantation, and what is the significance of the cell count in the transplanted PSCs?
2. Aside from the complications reviewed in this case, derive a list of potential problems that could occur after an allogeneic marrow transplant.

▶ Clinical Pearl

Decreasing the duration of neutropenia reduces the risk of post-transplant fever and infection and therefore reduces the duration of antibiotic therapy.

References

1. Murray BE. Vancomycin-resistant enterococci. Am J Med 1997;102:284–293.
2. Jones RJ, Lee KSK, Beschorner WL, et al. Venoocclusive disease of the liver following bone marrow transplantation. Transplantation 1987;44:778–783.
3. Terra S, Spitzer TR, Tsunoda SM. A review of tissue plasminogen activator in the treatment of veno-occlusive disease after bone marrow transplantation. Pharmacotherapy 1997;17:929–937.
4. Bianco JA, Applebaum FR, Nemunaitis J, et al. Phase I-II trial of pentoxifylline for the prevention of transplantation related toxicities following bone marrow transplantation. Blood 1991;78:1205–1211.

Nutrition and Nutritional Disorders

Gary R. Matzke, PharmD, FCP, FCCP, Section Editor

129 PARENTERAL NUTRITION

▶ **To Diet in Vein**   **(Level III)**

Douglas D. Janson, PharmD, BCNSP

▶ After completing this case study, students should be able to:

- Describe how an acute illness with a systemic physiologic stress response causes malnutrition.

- Define how to objectively categorize adult obesity.

- Design a patient-specific total parenteral nutrition (TPN) prescription after assessing the clinical and laboratory data.

- Construct and evaluate appropriate monitoring parameters for a hospitalized patient receiving TPN.

☀ PATIENT PRESENTATION

Chief Complaint
"My belly hurts and it's getting harder to breathe."

HPI
Stephen Carter is a 28 yo man diagnosed with acute gallstone pancreatitis and respiratory distress. The patient was transferred from an outside hospital to the university hospital's SICU for further management. He presented to his local hospital 4 days ago after experiencing 3 days of constant mid-epigastric abdominal pain with sharp and shooting episodes radiating to his back. He also reported N/V, fever, and chills at home. Admission laboratory results from the outside hospital included WBC $14.4 \times 10^3/mm^3$, T. bili 8.2 mg/dL, and lipase 2,184 IU/L. Imaging results from the outside hospital revealed cholelithiasis, CBD dilatation and perihepatic fluid, and evidence of acute pancreatitis. An ERCP revealed mild dilation of the CBD with no stones or filling defects; a papillotomy was not performed. A CXR revealed elevated diaphragms bilaterally with a left pleural effusion. Prior to transfer the patient had an episode of respiratory compromise with oxygen desaturation and tachycardia.

PMH
5 episodes over the last year of "sharp and shooting" mid-epigastric pain, thought to be related to spicy food; all resolved within 24 hours and no medical attention was sought.

PSH
Appendectomy 10 years ago

FH
Non-contributory

SH
Reports drinking 2 to 3 6-packs of beer 3 times/week; no tobacco use. Married × 2 years and employed as a driver for a hospice.

ROS
Describes a painful burning abdominal sensation rated as 7 on a scale of 1–10; denies N/V presently; denies color change in skin or sclerae.

Meds
Furosemide 20 mg IV × 1
Ticarcillin/clavulanic acid 3.0 g/0.1 g IV Q 6 H

Famotidine 20 mg IV BID
Heparin 5000 units SQ BID
Meperidine 50–75 mg IV Q 4 H PRN pain
Prochlorperazine 10 mg IV Q 6 H PRN N/V
Acetaminophen 650 mg pr Q 4 H PRN fever
5% dextrose in 0.9% NaCl with 20 mEq KCl/L @ 125 mL/hour

All

NKDA

PE

Gen

Obese, tall, Caucasian young man in mild respiratory distress; speaks in short phrases with rapid and shallow breathing

VS

BP 170/95, P 136, RR 38, T 37.6°C; Ht 6'6", Wt 130 kg

Skin

Warm, moist, diaphoretic; (−) jaundice

HEENT

PERRLA, EOMI, sclerae mildly icteric

Neck/LN

Supple, no cervical lymphadenopathy or thyromegaly

Lungs/Thorax

Bronchial breath sounds with fine rhonchi and bilateral expiratory wheezes, greater on right than left; spontaneously breathing on 40% Fio_2 by FM with airway patent; Sao_2 89% to 93%; right subclavian triple lumen central venous catheter intact/patent.

CV

Normal S_1 and S_2, no S_3 or S_4; 2+ carotid, radial, and dorsalis pedis pulses bilaterally

Abd

Distended; tenderness to palpation in RUQ with some epigastric tenderness; soft, hypoactive bowel sounds; NG tube in right nostril to low continuous suction

Genit/Rect

Foley catheter intact/patent for yellow urine; normal rectal exam with brown, heme (−) stool

MS/Ext

No CCE

Neuro

A & O × 3; CN II–XII intact; motor strength 5+ throughout; sensation intact and reflexes symmetric with downgoing toes

Labs

Na 141 mEq/L	Hgb 14.1 g/dL	AST 50 IU/L	Ca 8.9 mg/dL
K 3.6 mEq/L	Hct 41.9%	ALT 103 IU/L	Mg 2.0 mEq/L
Cl 101 mEq/L	Plt 183 × 10³/mm³	Alk Phos 114 IU/L	Phos 2.7 mg/dL
CO_2 28 mEq/L	WBC 19.7 × 10³/mm³	GGT 216 IU/L	PT 12.1 sec
BUN 10 mg/dL	68% Neutros	T. bili 1.8 mg/dL	INR 0.9
SCr 0.7 mg/dL	16% Bands	Amylase 36 IU/L	
Glu 159 mg/dL	11% Lymphs	Lipase 209 IU/L	
	4% Monos		
	1% Metas		

ECG

Sinus tachycardia without ectopy

ABG

pH 7.4, $Paco_2$ 45 mm Hg, Pao_2 72 mm Hg, HCO_3 27 mEq/L, BE 3 mEq/L, Sao_2 93

Intake/Output

3700 mL/4535 mL (with 2285 mL urine output and 2250 mL NG tube output)

Chest X-ray

Large left and small right pleural effusions; LLL atelectasis and pneumonitis

Abd CT

Edematous pancreas with extensive peripancreatic inflammatory changes consistent with acute pancreatitis. Regions of nonenhancement in the pancreatic head and body are consistent with pancreatic necrosis. Dilated small bowel loops without definite transition zone are probably secondary to ileus.

Assessment

Acute necrotizing pancreatitis secondary to cholelithiasis in a young, moderately obese male with a history of EtOH use, now exhibiting signs and symptoms of respiratory compromise from large left pleural effusion and/or pulmonary edema.

▶ Questions

Problem Identification

1. a. Create a list of this patient's problems related to nutrition, fluid, and electrolytes.
   b. What is acute pancreatitis and what are the common causes?
   c. What are the clinical, laboratory, and radiologic characteristics of acute pancreatitis in this patient?
   d. What clinical, laboratory, and radiologic characteristics indicate that this patient has severe (or complicated) acute pancreatitis?
   e. Describe why this patient is at nutrition risk and characterize the type of malnutrition he will likely develop.

f. What additional nutritional assessment data should you request and why?

Desired Outcome

2. *What are the goals of specialized nutrition support in this patient?*

Therapeutic Alternatives

3. *What are the therapeutic options for specialized nutrition intervention in this patient?*

Optimal Plan

4. a. *What method is used to classify this patient as obese?*
   b. *What body weight would be used to estimate the nutrient requirements in this obese man?*
   c. *What are the ranges of estimated daily goals for calories (kcal/kg/day), protein (g/kg/day), and hydration (mL/kg/day) for this patient?*
   d. *Design a TPN formulation for the first day of treatment that includes the volume and rate (mL/hour), final amino acids (g/L), dextrose (g/L), lipid emulsion (g/L), electrolytes (mEq/day or mmol/day), vitamins, trace elements, and other additives.*
   e. *What other order(s) would you suggest at the initiation of the TPN?*

Outcome Evaluation

5. a. *What monitoring parameters and frequency are required for monitoring the TPN regimen?*
   b. *Within the first week of TPN, a nitrogen balance study was performed with the following results: 19.5 grams of urine urea nitrogen (UUN) measured from a 24-hour urine collection. Why is a nitrogen balance study done during specialized nutrition support?*
   c. *Interpret the aforementioned data to calculate the nitrogen balance. Hint: refer to the section "Assessment of Nutrient Requirements" in textbook Chapter 126 for this information.*

► Clinical Course

The patient was given the supportive care you recommended and stabilized during the first week of hospitalization. All cultures, including drainage fluid tapped from his left pleural effusion, were negative. On hospital days 4 through 6, attempts were made to initiate enteral nutrition via a fluoroscopically placed nasojejunal feeding tube. However, the tube was discontinued because of persistent hiccoughs, nausea, abdominal distension, and increased pain, despite the use of antiemetics and narcotic analgesics. Consequently, the patient continued on TPN.

On hospital day 8, the patient underwent a surgical cholecystectomy. Postoperatively, he had intermittent fevers despite empiric antimicrobial therapy; a repeat abdominal CT showed persistent peripancreatic fluid collections. Infected necrotizing pancreatitis was diagnosed after the fluid cultures aspirated from the collections grew vancomycin-sensitive *Enterococcus*. On hospital day 13, he underwent an exploratory laparotomy, debridement of necrotic pancreas, drainage of peripancreatic abscess, and placement of a transgastric jejunostomy tube. Two days later, the patient

underwent another exploratory laparotomy for further debridement of necrotic pancreas. The following day, an enteral feeding formula was initiated at a slow rate through the jejunostomy port of the transgastric jejunostomy. Over the next 2 to 3 days, enteral feedings were titrated to the full goal rate, meeting the daily calorie and protein requirements with weaning off of the TPN.[6]

Patient Counseling

6. a. *What information should be provided to the patient and family during his hospitalization regarding the parenteral and enteral nutrition therapy?*
   b. *Explain to the patient the transition from parenteral to enteral nutrition through use of the jejunostomy port of the transgastric jejunostomy tube.*
   c. *Explain the anticipated course for enteral nutrition and the transition back to oral food ingestion.*

► Self-study Assignments

1. Will this patient have diabetes mellitus after recovery from his illness, or is this a case of disease-limited glucose intolerance from the acute pancreatitis?
2. Explain how hypochloremic metabolic alkalosis can develop if insufficient replacement of IV fluid occurs during chronic gastric suctioning with an NG tube.
3. Describe the rationale for the addition of folic acid and thiamine for a patient admitted with a history of active alcohol abuse.

► Clinical Pearl

Glycemic control in the range of 100 to 200 mg/dL is acceptable during TPN infusion. During a constant delivery of dextrose through TPN, the dose of regular insulin to be added to the next day's TPN prescription can be determined by assessing the amount of sliding-scale insulin used in the previous 24 hours. Adding about two-thirds of this insulin to the TPN bag is reasonable with continued glycemic monitoring. This avoids therapy-related hypoglycemia and prevents the need to discard the TPN bag.

References

1. Steinberg W, Tenner S. Acute pancreatitis. N Engl J Med 1994;330:1198–1210.
2. Kusske AM, Katona DR, Reber HA. Nutritional support in pancreatic disease. In: Rombeau JL, Rolandelli RH, eds. Clinical Nutrition: Enteral and Tube Feeding, 3rd ed. Philadelphia, Saunders, 1997:429–438.
3. Marulendra S, Kirby DF. Nutrition support in pancreatitis. Nutri Clin Pract 1995;10:45–53.
4. National Institutes of Health. Clinical guidelines on the identification, evaluation, and treatment of overweight and obesity in adults—the evidence report. Obes Res 1998(6 suppl 2):51S–209S.
5. National Advisory Group on Standards and Practice Guidelines for Parenteral Nutrition. Safe practices for parenteral nutrition formulations. J Parenter Enteral Nutr 1998;22:49–66.
6. De Beaux AC, Plester C, Fearon KCH. Flexible approach to nutritional support in severe acute pancreatitis. Nutrition 1994;10:246–249.

130 ADULT ENTERAL NUTRITION

▶ **Down the Tube**   (Level III)

Carol J. Rollins, MS, RD, PharmD, BCNSP

▶ After completing this case study, students should be able to:

- Calculate the protein, calorie, and fluid requirements for a patient who is to receive enteral nutrition therapy.
- Recommend an appropriate enteral formula and feeding route.
- Implement an appropriate monitoring plan to achieve the desired nutritional endpoints and avoid complications.
- Design an appropriate regimen for administering medications via a

feeding tube, including recommending alternate dosage forms for medications that cannot be crushed.

☀ PATIENT PRESENTATION

Miguel Ramirez is a 68 yo Hispanic man referred to your home health care company for initiation of tube feedings. During your conversation with him, he states to you, "I've lost a lot of weight since I started chemo." The physician's orders read: "Standard 1 kcal/cc formula, 2300–2400 kcal/day via enteral pump. Receiving cycle 2 of Taxol plus 5-FU today for gastric/esophageal cancer. The dose was decreased 25% today due to grade III mucositis with the first cycle." The patient has insurance coverage through Medicare, Parts A and B.

▶ Questions

Problem Identification

1. a. What other information is necessary or would be helpful to evaluate the orders and provide recommendations for a feeding plan?
   b. How can you obtain this information for your home health care company, which is located across town from the clinic and hospital?
   c. Is insurance coverage an issue in this situation?

▶ Clinical Course

After following appropriate procedures, you obtain the following additional information about the patient.

HPI

Mr. Ramirez saw his PCP 6 months ago for LUQ pain of 2 to 3 months duration. Weight at that time was 74 kg and height was 71 inches. He was slightly anemic (Hgb 11.9 g/dL). Famotidine was initiated for PUD. A GI consult was requested because several stools were positive for occult blood. Colonoscopy was negative. Four weeks later, the Hgb was 10.3 g/dL. An upper GI endoscopy resulted in the diagnosis of a tumor in the cardia of the stomach. CT scans of the chest, abdomen, and pelvis revealed the gastric mass and gastrohepatic adenopathy.

Surgery was performed 3 weeks later that included a near-total gastrectomy with distal pancreatectomy, splenectomy, and partial esophagectomy with a gastroesophageal anastamosis in the right chest and placement of a feeding jejunostomy. Pathology revealed a poorly differentiated gastric adenocarcinoma with transmural invasion and tumor present on the serosal margin. There was involvement of the esophageal wall and continuous spread to the peripancreatic soft tissue including neural invasion. Ten of 16 lymph nodes were positive for metastasis.

Three cycles of Taxol plus cisplatin were given, with the third cycle reduced by 25% because of nausea, vomiting, and dehydration associated with

previous courses. Therapy was also complicated by anorexia and severe hypomagnesemia requiring IV replacement and continued oral magnesium supplementation. Dietary education for anorexia was provided. Chemotherapy with Taxol plus 5-FU was started with 3 cycles to be given, followed by radiotherapy.

PMH
Superior vena cava syndrome
DVT
PUD

FH
Adopted, no family history available.

SH
Married, no children; clerical worker; 30 pack-year tobacco use, quit 8 years ago; occasional alcohol use, average of 2 beers/week

ROS
From clinic visit today.
Constitutional: Moderate fatigue, weakness, poor appetite, dysphagia
ENT: Vision satisfactory, no eye pain. No tinnitus or ear pain. No throat pain, but difficulty swallowing the past 2 weeks with poor tolerance to solid foods and difficulty taking large tablets.
CV: No SOB, DOE, chest pain
Resp: No cough or sputum production
GI: Continued persistent abdominal and back pain; gradually improving with increased morphine dose and more frequent cyclobenzaprine use. No emesis or diarrhea; complains of intermittent nausea and mild/moderate constipation.
GU: No urinary frequency, nocturia, dysuria or hematuria
MS: (+) abdominal and back pain; no other muscle aches or bone pain
Skin: No rashes, nodules, or itching
Neuro: No headaches, dizziness, unsteady gait, or seizures
Endo: No thyroid problems
Heme/LN: No recent blood transfusions or swollen glands

Meds

Morphine sulfate sustained release tablet, 60 mg po TID
Morphine sulfate solution (20 mg/5 mL), 20 mg po Q 4–6 H PRN pain
Pepcid 40 mg po Q HS
Megestrol acetate 40 mg, 5 tablets po QID
Magnesium oxide 400 mg po TID
Coumadin 7.5 mg po QD
Docusate sodium 100 mg po QID
Cyclobenzaprine HCl 10 mg po TID PRN back spasms
Cephalexin 500 mg po QID × 10 days (completed today)

All

NKDA; food allergy to hazelnuts and tofu (hives, wheezing)

PE

Gen
Thin, pale-appearing Hispanic man; alert and conversant

VS
BP 122/71, P 88, RR 16; W 52.5 kg

Skin
No nodules, masses, or rash; no ecchymoses or petechiae; stage I pressure ulcer, 2 cm, right buttocks. Redness at edges of implantable venous access device that is very prominent on upper left chest wall.

HEENT
PERRLA; EOM's intact. Eyes anicteric. No mouth lesions; tongue normal size.

Neck
Neck supple but thin; no thyromegaly or masses

LN
No cervical, supraclavicular, axillary or inguinal adenopathy

Heart
RRR with no gallop, rubs, or murmur

Lungs
Basilar crackling rales, which improved after coughing. A well-healed surgical incision is visible on the left posterior chest wall.

Abd
Abdomen flat. Jejunostomy tube with slight erythema around the exit site, no drainage. A well-healed midline and RUQ incision with mild tenderness in the RUQ and epigastric area. No masses palpable.

Genit/Rectal
Normal male genitalia; non-distended bladder; hard stool in rectal vault

MS/Ext
No clubbing or cyanosis; moderate ankle to mid-calf edema; no spine or CVA tenderness

Neuro
CNs intact; DTRs active and equal

Endoscopy Report
From 2 days ago. Endoscope inserted to distal esophagus; stopped short of anastamosis by stricture. Biopsies from site of stricture were negative for adenocarcinoma. Tissue friable; stricture dilation not attempted due to risk of perforation.

Labs

Na 131 mEq/L	Hgb 9.9 g/dL	WBC $10.1 \times 10^3/mm^3$	AST 16 IU/L	Alb 2.3 g/dL
K 3.6 mEq/L	Hct 28.4%	66% Segs	ALT 21 IU/L	T. chol 160 mg/dL
Cl 104 mEq/L	RBC $2.75 \times 10^6/mm^3$	9% Bands	Alk phos 50 IU/L	Trig 350 mg/dL
CO_2 26 mEq/L	Platelets $100 \times 10^3/mm^3$	18% Lymphs	LDH 100 IU/L	Ca 7.8 mg/dL
BUN 23 mg/dL	MCV 105 μm^3	7% Monos	T. bili 0.9 mg/dL	Mg 2.8 mg/dL
SCr 1.0 mg/dL			D. bili 0.3 mg/dL	Phos 3.8 mg/dL
Glu 105 mg/dL			T. prot 4.2 g/dL	

Other
Peripheral blood smear: anisocytosis 2+, poikilocytosis 2+, macrocytosis 2+.

Assessment
Continued weight loss related to esophageal stricture and chemotherapy with no evidence of cancer recurrence at the stricture.

▶ Questions (continued)

    d. Create a drug-related problem list for this patient.
    e. What information indicates the presence or severity of malnutrition?
    f. What type and degree of malnutrition does this patient exhibit? What evidence supports your assessment?

Desired Outcome

  2. *a. What are the goals of nutrition support in this patient?*

    b. What outcomes should be considered for the patient's other medical problems?

Therapeutic Alternatives

  3. *a. What are the potential alternatives for improving nutritional status in this patient other than initiating specialized nutrition support?*

    b. What are the potential routes for specialized nutrition support and the reason(s) why each is or is not appropriate for this patient?

    c. A major economic issue is Medicare coverage for home enteral therapy. Based on the information now available to you, does this patient meet the necessary criteria?

Optimal Plan

4. a. *Estimate the protein, calorie, and fluid requirements for this patient.*

   b. *What type of formula (e.g., polymeric, monomeric) is most appropriate for this patient?*

   c. *What administration regimen should be used for tube feedings?*

   d. *Assuming that the patient is to continue his current medications during tube feedings, how should each of these be administered?*

Outcome Evaluation

5. *What clinical and laboratory parameters are necessary to evaluate the therapy for detection and/or prevention of adverse effects and to evaluate achievement of the desired response?*

Patient Counseling

6. *What information should be provided to the patient or his caregiver to enhance compliance, ensure successful therapy, and minimize adverse effects of enteral nutrition therapy?*

► Clinical Course

Feeding was initiated about 24 hours after the initial orders were sent to your home infusion company. A 1.06 calorie/mL, 0.034 gram protein/mL, 290 mOsm/kg polymeric formula was started using an enteral infusion pump via jejunostomy tube at 40 mL/hr for 18 hours/day with plans for laboratory evaluation on day 3. Feedings would be advanced to 65 mL/hr on day 4 if electrolytes and fluid status were acceptable. Serum electrolytes drawn on day 3 revealed K 3.2 mEq/L, phos 2.1 mg/dL, and Mg 1.9 mg/dL. The WBC count was $1.5 \times 10^3/mm^3$ with 33% neutrophils. The doctor was notified of the laboratory results. Because the patient had a temperature of 102°F during the night, the doctor decided to admit him to the hospital with neutropenic fever as the admitting diagnosis. Electrolytes were monitored daily during the 7 days of hospitalization and replaced IV as needed. Tube feedings were advanced to 65 mL/hr after 24 hours of hospitalization, then to the goal of 95 mL/hr by continuous infusion in another 12 hours. No further electrolyte replacement was needed after day 5 of hospitalization. The patient was changed to an 18-hour infusion of tube feeding at 130 mL/hr on hospital day 6, and then discharged home on day 7. He has done well at home, gaining 10 kg over the past 3 months. There have been no further electrolyte abnormalities despite chemotherapy and radiotherapy.

► Self-study Assignments

1. Select a current patient you are following and design an appropriate regimen for administering medications via a feeding tube, including alternate dosage forms for medications that cannot be crushed and proper dosage adjustments for different forms where necessary.

2. Educate an actual patient or do a mock education with a classmate about medication administration through a feeding tube.

3. Determine the potential for various enteral formulas to interfere with anticoagulation using warfarin sodium.

4. Identify the metabolic changes associated with refeeding syndrome and the characteristics that increase the risk of this complication.

► Clinical Pearl

Medications administered through a feeding tube frequently clog the tube; therefore, a pharmacist should evaluate the medication regimen for alternate dosage forms that do not require crushing or administration through the tube.

References

1. ASPEN Board of Directors. Guidelines for the use of parenteral and enteral nutrition in adult and pediatric patients. JPEN 1993;17(suppl 4):1SA–52SA.

131   OBESITY

► Stomach Staples and a Tummy Tuck?   (Level II)

Dannielle C. O'Donnell, PharmD, BCPS

► After completing this case study, students should be able to:

- Calculate a body mass index (BMI) and waist:hip ratio (WHR) and determine their significance with respect to risk of morbidity and mortality from obesity.

- Develop a pharmacotherapeutic plan and treatment strategy for obese patients.

- Identify common obesity-related comorbidities.

- Provide patient counseling on the expected benefits, possible adverse effects, and drug interactions with anorectic therapy.

☼ PATIENT PRESENTATION

Chief Complaint
"I'm starving myself but I just can't seem to lose any weight. I want stomach staples and a tummy tuck!"

HPI
Elizabeth Notlesh is a 55 yo woman who states that she had maintained her ideal weight until her total hysterectomy at the age of 35. She says that the "hormones" she took for the first year after her hysterectomy caused her to gain weight and that the weight gain continued after stopping the hormones. She has previously tried OTC diet pills, a list of fad diets, "water pills," and most recently "herbal fen-phen" with initial modest success followed by weight regain. She is tearful as she talks about her weight struggles, attributing physical and marital problems to her weight.

PMH
Hypercholesterolemia × 12 years

Gallstones 4 years ago treated with lithotripsy and 2 years of ursodeoxy-
cholic acid
Hypothyroidism × 8 years
DJD of the knees bilaterally
Depression

PSH

TAH 20 years ago
Hernia repair 15 years ago
Trigger finger release bilaterally last year

FH

Mother had an MI at the age of 64; father died in an MVA at the age of 67.
Maternal grandmother died at age 72 with diabetes. She states that her
mother was "slightly overweight but not obese." No other family members
have significant medical history, including obesity.

SH

She is a married housewife who cares for her mother-in-law and has one
son who lives out of state. She has never smoked and denies IVDA. She previously enjoyed walking for exercise, but this is now limited by her knee
pain and need to supervise her mother-in-law.

Diet

She had instruction on a low-fat, low-cholesterol diet several years ago, to
which she is adhering, although she states that she is somewhat "bored"
with her current food plan. In her attempt to lose weight, she has cut down
her number of meals to one daily each evening that includes larger portion
sizes and a dessert she generally bakes. Upon further probing, she does admit to regular snacking throughout the evening.

Meds

Levothyroxine 0.15 mcg po QD
Calcium carbonate 500 mg po TID
Simvastatin 20 mg po Q HS
Acetaminophen 500 mg po PRN knee pain
Intra-articular cortisone injection, left knee 3 months ago

All

Adhesive tape → rash

ROS

She complains of general fatigue, "feeling blue," chronic bilateral knee
pain, and a constant gnawing in her stomach and preoccupation with food
and her weight. She denies symptoms of cold or heat intolerance; changes in

skin, hair, or nails; nervousness; irritability; lethargy; muscle weakness; palpitations; diarrhea or constipation; polyuria; polydipsia; chest pain; shortness
of breath; recent head trauma; or thoughts of harming herself or others.

PE

Gen

The patient is a pleasant, but tearful, obese Caucasian woman in NAD

VS

BP 138/84, P 80, RR 16, T 36.4°C; Ht 162 cm, Wt 80 kg, waist 102 cm,
hip 112 cm

Skin

Warm, with normal distribution of body hair. No significant lesions or
discolorations

HEENT

NC/AT; PERRLA; EOMI; TMs intact

CV

RRR, S_1 and S_2 normal; no murmurs, rubs, or gallops

Pulm

CTA & P bilaterally

Abd

Obese with multiple striae, NT, ND, (+) BS, no palpable masses, hysterectomy and hernia scars present and well healed

GU/Rect

Pelvic and rectal exams deferred

Ext

LE varicosities present. Palpation of knees reveals bony hypertrophy, and
limited ROM elicits bony crepitus and patient discomfort bilaterally.
Pedal pulses 2+ bilaterally

Neuro

A & O × 3; CN II–XII intact; Romberg test (−); sensory and motor levels
intact; 2+ triceps tendons and DTR; Babinski (−)

Labs (Fasting)

Na 138 mEq/L	AST 28 IU/L
K 3.9 mEq/L	T. chol 271 mg/dL
Cl 96 mEq/L	LDL-C 163 mg/dL
CO_2 26 mEq/L	HDL-C 41 mg/dL
BUN 13 mg/dL	Trig 334 mg/dL
SCr 1.0 mg/dL	TSH 0.9 μIU/mL
Glu 130 mg/dL	

► Questions

Problem Identification

1. a. Create a drug-related problem list for this patient.
   b. Calculate the patient's BMI and WHR and contrast with weight

*the clinical implications of these values on defining obesity
and on stratifying mortality risk.*
   c. *What information (signs, symptoms, laboratory values) indicates the presence or severity of obesity?*
   d. *Could any of the patient's problems have been caused by
drug therapy?*

e. *What other medical conditions should be considered to exclude primary causes of her obesity?*

Desired Outcome

2. *What are the goals of pharmacotherapy for the patient's obesity?*

Therapeutic Alternatives

3. a. *What non-drug therapies might be useful for this patient?*
   b. *What pharmacotherapeutic alternatives are available for this patient's obesity?*

Optimal Plan

4. a. *What drug(s), dosage form(s), dose(s), schedule(s), and duration are appropriate to treat this patient's obesity and why?*
   b. *What alternatives would be appropriate if initial therapy fails?*

Outcome Evaluation

5. *What clinical and laboratory parameters are necessary to evaluate the therapy for achievement of the desired therapeutic outcome and to detect or prevent adverse effects?*

Patient Counseling

6. *What general and medication-specific information should be provided to the patient to enhance adherence, ensure successful therapy, and minimize adverse effects?*

▶ Clinical Course

Ms. Notlesh has joined the YWCA and shows progress at each of her 2-week weigh-ins, averaging a 2-kg weight loss at each visit through the end of week 8. Her blood pressure is stable, and she denies any adverse effects of her medication. However, at her 10-week visit she had lost only 1 additional kg; today at her 12-week visit, she has lost an additional 0.5 kg. Her FBG is now 108 mg/dL and her lipid profile includes total cholesterol 242 mg/dL, LDL-C 127 mg/dL, HDL-C 62 mg/dL, and triglycerides 265 mg/dL. She states that she is as compliant with her lifestyle modifications as in previous weeks and overall is in "much better spirits," but she is starting to become frustrated again. Although she is pleased with the improvement in her blood glucose and lipids, she continues to complain of knee pain while taking her acetaminophen on a PRN basis and wonders if she should have something stronger.

▶ Follow-up Questions

1. *What changes, if any, should be made in her weight loss regimen?*
2. *What, if anything, would you suggest to improve her knee symptoms?*

▶ Self-study Assignments

1. List the limitations of height-weight charts or BMI determinations. What are the most accurate methods for quantifying body fat, and why are they not routinely employed?
2. Assume that you are a member of a pharmacy and therapeutics committee for a managed care corporation. Justify whether anti-obesity drugs should be a covered benefit, and if so, which specific agent(s) should be added to the formulary.
3. Compile a compendium of common herbal and dietary supplements that claim weight loss benefits, and make a list of the evidence for their safety and efficacy.

▶ Clinical Pearl

Intermittent use of anorectic agents (i.e., for 4 weeks every few months, over the holidays, during vacations, or during periods of stress) may be effective in preventing weight regain in the later maintenance phase.

References

1. Rosenbaum M, Leibel RL, Hirsch J. Obesity. N Engl J Med 1997;337:396–407.
2. Pi-Sunyer, FX. A review of long-term studies evaluating the efficacy of weight loss in ameliorating disorders associated with obesity. Clin Ther 1996;18:1006–1035.
3. Popovich NG, Wood OB. Drug therapy for obesity: An update. J Am Pharm Assoc 1997;NS37:31–39, 56.
4. Weiser M, Frishman WH, Michaelson MD, et al. The pharmacologic approach to the treatment of obesity. J Clin Pharmacol 1997;37:453–473.
5. Long-term pharmacotherapy in the management of obesity. National Task Force on the Prevention and Treatment of Obesity. JAMA 1996;276:1907–1915.
6. Anchors JM. Safer than Phen-fen. Rocklin, CA, Prima Publishing, 1997.
7. Bostwick JM, Brown TM. A toxic reaction from combining fluoxetine and phentermine. J Clin Psychopharmacol 1996;168:189–190. Letter.

APPENDIX A
COMMON LABORATORY TESTS

The following table is an alphabetical listing of common laboratory tests and their reference ranges for adults as measured in plasma or serum (unless otherwise indicated). Reference values differ among laboratories, so readers should refer to the published reference ranges used in each institution. Values are reported in traditional units only.

Laboratory Test	Reference Range for Adults
Acid phosphatase	0 to 0.8 IU/L
Activated partial thromboplastin time (APTT)	25 to 40 sec
Adrenocorticotropic hormone (ACTH)	15 to 80 pg/mL
Alanine aminotransferase (ALT)	5 to 35 IU/L
Albumin	3.5 to 5.0 g/dL
Alkaline phosphatase	30 to 120 IU/L
Alpha-fetoprotein (AFP)	0 to 20 ng/mL
Amikacin, therapeutic	15 to 30 mg/L peak; $\leq$ 8 mg/L trough
Ammonia	15 to 45 μg/dL
Amylase	0 to 130 IU/L
Anion gap	8 to 16 mEq/L
Anti-double–stranded DNA (anti-ds DNA)	Negative
Anti-HAV	Negative
Anti-HBc	Negative
Anti-HBs	Negative
Anti-HCV	Negative
Anti-Sm antibody	Negative
Antinuclear antibody (ANA)	Negative at 1:20 dilution
Aspartate aminotransferase (AST)	5 to 40 IU/L
β_2-microglobulin	0.6 to 2.0 mg/dL
Bilirubin, direct	0.1 to 0.3 mg/dL
Bilirubin, indirect	0.1 to 1.0 mg/dL
Bilirubin, total	0.1 to 1.2 mg/dL
Bleeding time	3 to 7 min
Blood gases, arterial (ABG)	
pH	7.35 to 7.45
p_{CO_2}	35 to 45 mm Hg
p_{O_2}	80 to 100 mm Hg
HCO_3	22 to 26 mEq/L
O_2 saturation (Sa_{O_2})	$\geq$ 95%
Blood urea nitrogen (BUN)	5 to 25 mg/dL
BUN-to-creatinine ratio	10:1 to 20:1

Laboratory Test	Reference Range for Adults
C-reactive protein	0.0 to 0.8 mg/dL
CA-125	< 35 IU/mL
CA 15-3	< 22 U/mL
CA 27.29	< 38 U/mL
Calcium, ionized	4.4 to 5.9 mg/dL; 2.2 to 2.5 mEq/L
Calcium, total	9 to 11 mg/dL; 4.5 to 5.5 mEq/L
Carbamazepine, therapeutic	4 to 12 mg/L
Carboxyhemoglobin	< 3%
Carcinoembryonic antigen (CEA)	< 3 ng/mL non-smokers; 0 to 6 ng/mL smokers
CD4 lymphocyte count	31 to 61% of total lymphocytes
CD8 lymphocyte count	18 to 39% of total lymphocytes
Cerebrospinal fluid (CSF)	
Pressure	75 to 175 mm H_2O
Glucose	30 to 80 mg/dL
Protein	15 to 45 mg/dL
WBC	< 10/mm^3
Chloride	95 to 105 mEq/L
Cholesterol, HDL	≥ 35 mg/dL desirable
Cholesterol, LDL	< 130 mg/dL desirable
	130 to 159 mg/dL borderline high
	≥ 160 mg/dL high risk
Cholesterol, total	< 200 mg/dL desirable
	200 to 239 mg/dL borderline high
	≥ 240 mg/dL high
CO_2 content	22 to 30 mEq/L
Complement component 3 (C3)	70 to 160 mg/dL
Complement component 4 (C4)	20 to 40 mg/dL
Copper	70 to 150 μg/dL
Cortisol (serum)	
8:00 A.M. to 10:00 A.M.	5 to 23 μg/dL
4:00 P.M. to 6:00 P.M.	3 to 13 μg/dL
Cortisol, free (urine)	10 to 110 μg/24 h
Creatine (phospho)kinase (CPK, CK)	30 to 180 IU/L
CK-MB	> 5% in myocardial infarction
Creatinine clearance (CLcr, urine)	85 to 135 mL/min
Creatinine, serum	0.5 to 1.5 mg/dL
Cryptococcal antigen	< 1:8
D-dimers	< 200 ng/mL
Dexamethasone suppression test	8:00 A.M. cortisol < 10 μg/dL
DHEAS	1 to 12 μmol/L
Digoxin, therapeutic	> 0.8 ng/mL
Erythrocyte sedimentation rate (ESR)	
Westergren	0 to 20 mm/h men; 0 to 30 mm/h women
Wintrobe	0 to 9 mm/h men; 0 to 15 mm/h women
Erythropoietin	2 to 25 IU/L; 2 to 25 mIU/mL
Ethanol, legal intoxication	≥ 50 to 100 mg/dL; ≥ 0.05 to 0.1%
Ethosuccimide, therapeutic	40 to 100 mg/L
Ferritin	2 to 20 μg/dL; 20 to 200 ng/mL
Fibrin degradation products (FDP)	2 to 10 mg/L
Fibrinogen	200 to 400 mg/dL

Laboratory Test	Reference Range for Adults
Folic acid	0.2 to 1.0 µg/dL; 2 to 10 ng/mL
Folic acid (RBC)	165 to 760 ng/mL
Follicle-stimulating hormone (FSH)	30 to 100 mIU/mL (postmenopausal women)
	5 to 22 mIU/mL (women, midcycle)
Free thyroxine index (FT$_4$I)	6.5 to 12.5
Gamma glutamyl transferase (GGT)	0 to 30 IU/L
Gentamicin, therapeutic	4 to 10 mg/L peak; $\leq$ 2 mg/L trough
Globulin	2.3 to 3.5 g/dL
Glucose, fasting (FBG)	70 to 110 mg/dL
Glucose, two-hour postprandial blood (PPBG)	< 140 mg/dL
Haptoglobin	60 to 270 mg/dL
HBeAg	Negative
HBsAg	Negative
HBV DNA	Negative
Hematocrit	40 to 54% men
	36 to 46% women
Hemoglobin	13.5 to 17.5 g/dL men
	12 to 16 g/dL women
Hemoglobin A$_{1c}$ (HbA$_{1c}$)	3.8 to 6.4%
Imipramine, therapeutic	100 to 300 ng/mL
International normalized ratio (INR), therapeutic	2.0 to 3.0 (2.5 to 3.5 for mechanical prosthetic heart valves and to prevent reinfarction, stroke, and death after acute MI)
Iron, serum	50 to 160 µg/dL men
	40 to 150 µg/dL women
Lactate	0.5 to 1.5 mEq/L
Lactate dehydrogenase (LDH)	100 to 190 IU/L
Lidocaine, therapeutic	1.5 to 6.0 mg/L
Lipase	20 to 180 IU/L
Lithium, therapeutic	0.5 to 1.25 mEq/L
Luteinizing hormone (LH)	24 to 105 mIU/mL (midcycle peak)
Magnesium	1.8 to 3.0 mg/dL; 1.5 to 2.5 mEq/L
Mean corpuscular hemoglobin (MCH)	26 to 34 pg
Mean corpuscular hemoglobin concentration (MCHC)	31 to 37 g/dL
Mean corpuscular volume (MCV)	80 to 100 µm^3
Nortriptyline, therapeutic	50 to 140 ng/mL
Osmolality (serum)	280 to 300 mOsm/kg
Osmolality (urine)	200 to 800 mOsm/kg
Parathyroid hormone (PTH), intact	10 to 65 pg/mL
Parathyroid hormone (PTH), N-terminal	8 to 24 pg/mL
Parathyroid hormone (PTH), C-terminal	50 to 330 pg/mL
Phenobarbital, therapeutic	15 to 40 mg/L
Phenytoin, therapeutic	10 to 20 mg/L
Phosphorus	2.5 to 4.5 mg/dL; 1.7 to 2.6 mEq/L
Platelet count	150,000 to 400,000/mm^3
Potassium	3.5 to 5.0 mEq/L
Prealbumin (transthyretin)	10 to 40 mg/dL
Primidone	5 to 20 mg/L
Procainamide, therapeutic	3 to 14 mg/L

Laboratory Test	Reference Range for Adults
Prolactin	< 20 ng/mL or μg/L
Prostate-specific antigen (PSA)	0 to 4 ng/mL
Protein, total	6.0 to 8.0 g/dL
Prothrombin time (PT)	10 to 12 sec
Quinidine, therapeutic	2 to 6 mg/L
Radioactive iodine uptake (RAIU)	< 6% in 2 hours
Red blood cell (RBC) count, total	4.6 to 6.0 × 10^6/mm³ men
	4.0 to 5.0 × 10^6/mm³ women
Red blood cell (RBC) folic acid	165 to 760 ng/mL
Red cell distribution width (RDW)	11.5 to 14.5%
Reticulocyte count	0.5 to 1.5% of total RBC count
Retinol-binding protein (RBP)	2.7 to 7.6 mg/dL
Rheumatoid factor (RF) titer	< 1:20
Salicylate, therapeutic	150 to 300 mg/L
Sodium	135 to 145 mEq/L
Testosterone, total	3 to 10 ng/mL men
	0.3 to 1.0 ng/mL women
Testosterone, free	> 40 pmol/L men
	2.4 to 12.5 pmol/L women
Theophylline, therapeutic	5 to 20 mg/L
Thrombin time	20 to 24 sec
Thyroid-stimulating hormone (TSH)	0.3 to 5.0 μIU/mL
Thyroid-binding globulin (TBG)	10 to 26 μg/dL
Thyroxine (T_4), free	0.8 to 2.8 ng/dL
Thyroxine (T_4), total	4.5 to 11.5 μg/dL
Thyroxine-binding prealbumin (transthyretin)	10 to 40 mg/dL
Thyroxine index, free (FT_4I)	6.5 to 12.5
Tobramycin, therapeutic	4 to 10 mg/L peak; ≤ 2 mg/L trough
Total iron-binding capacity (TIBC)	250 to 450 μg/dL
Transferrin	200 to 430 mg/dL
Transferrin saturation	30 to 50%
Transthyretin (thyroxine-binding prealbumin)	10 to 40 mg/dL
Triglycerides	< 200 mg/dL normal
	200 to 399 mg/dL borderline-high
	400 to 1000 mg/dL high
	> 1000 mg/dL very high
Triiodothyronine (T_3)	75 to 200 ng/dL
Triiodothyronine (T_3) resin uptake	25 to 35%
Troponin-I (cardiac)	< 1.5 ng/mL
TSH receptor antibodies (TSH Rab)	0 to 1 U/mL
Uric acid	3.5 to 8.0 mg/dL
Urinalysis (urine)	
pH	4.5 to 8.0
Specific gravity	1.005 to 1.030
Protein	Negative
Glucose	Negative
Ketones	Negative
RBC	1 to 2 per low-power field
WBC	3 to 4 per low-power field
Casts	Occasional hyaline

Laboratory Test	Reference Range for Adults
Urobilinogen (urine)	0.5 to 4.0 Ehrlich Units/24 h
Valproic acid, therapeutic	50 to 150 mg/L
Vancomycin, therapeutic	15 to 30 mg/L peak
Vitamin A (retinol)	30 to 95 μg/dL
Vitamin B_{12}	200 to 900 pg/mL
Vitamin D_3, 1,25-dihydroxy	20 to 76 pg/mL
Vitamin D_3, 25-hydroxy	10 to 50 ng/mL
Vitamin E (alpha tocopherol)	5 to 20 mg/L
White blood cell (WBC) count, total	4500 to 10,000/mm^3
WBC differential (peripheral blood)	
Polymorphonuclear neutrophils (PMNs)	50 to 65%
Bands	0 to 5%
Eosinophils	0 to 3%
Basophils	1 to 3%
Lymphocytes	25 to 35%
Monocytes	2 to 6%
WBC differential (bone marrow)	
Polymorphonuclear neutrophils (PMNs)	3 to 11%
Bands	9 to 15%
Metamyelocytes	9 to 25%
Myelocytes	8 to 16%
Promyelocytes	1 to 8%
Myeloblasts	0 to 5%
Eosinophils	1 to 5%
Basophils	0 to 1%
Lymphocytes	11 to 23%
Monocytes	0 to 1%
Zinc	60 to 150 μg/dL

A & O	Alert and oriented	Amp	Ampule
A & P	Auscultation and percussion, anterior and posterior, assessment and plans	ANA	Antinuclear antibody
		ANC	Absolute neutrophil count
A & W	Alive and well	ANLL	Acute non-lymphocytic leukemia
aa	Of each (ana)	AODM	Adult onset diabetes mellitus
AA	Aplastic anemia	AOM	Acute otitis media
AAA	Abdominal aortic aneurysm	AP	Anterior–posterior
AAL	Anterior axillary line	APAP	Acetaminophen (acetyl-p-aminophenol)
AAO	Awake, alert, and oriented	aPTT	Activated partial thromboplastin time
Abd	Abdomen	ARC	AIDS-related complex
ABG	Arterial blood gases	ARDS	Adult respiratory distress syndrome
ABP	Arterial blood pressure	ARF	Acute renal failure
ABW	Actual body weight	AS	Left ear (auris sinistra)
AC	Before meals (ante cibos)	ASA	Aspirin (acetylsalicylic acid)
ACEI	Angiotensin-converting enzyme inhibitor	ASCVD	Arteriosclerotic cardiovascular disease
ACLS	Advanced cardiac life support	ASD	Atrial septal defect
ACT	Activated clotting time	ASH	Asymmetric septal hypertrophy
ACTH	Adrenocorticotropic hormone	ASHD	Arteriosclerotic heart disease
AD	Alzheimer's disease, right ear (auris dextra)	AST	Aspartate aminotransferase
ADA	American Diabetes Association, adenosine deaminase	ATG	Antithymocyte globulin
		ATN	Acute tubular necrosis
ADH	Antidiuretic hormone	AU	Each ear (auris uterque)
ADHD	Attention-deficit hyperactivity disorder	AV	Arteriovenous, atrioventricular
ADL	Activities of daily living	AVM	Arteriovenous malformation
ADR	Adverse drug reaction	AVR	Aortic valve replacement
AED	Antiepileptic drug	AWMI	Anterior wall myocardial infarction
AF	Atrial fibrillation; anterior fontanelle	AWP	Average wholesale price
AFB	Acid-fast bacillus	BAC	Blood alcohol concentration
AFP	Alfa-fetoprotein	BAL	Bronchioalveolar lavage
A/G	Albumin-globulin ratio	BBB	Bundle branch block, blood–brain barrier
AI	Aortic insufficiency	BC	Blood culture
AIDS	Acquired immunodeficiency syndrome	BCG	Bacillus Calmette Guérin
AKA	Above-knee amputation	BCNP	Board Certified Nuclear Pharmacist
ALD	Alcoholic liver disease	BCNSP	Board Certified Nutrition Support Pharmacist
ALL	Acute lymphocytic leukemia, allergies	BCNU	Carmustine
ALP	Alkaline phosphatase	BCOP	Board Certified Oncology Pharmacist
ALS	Amyotrophic lateral sclerosis	BCP	Birth control pill
ALT	Alanine aminotransferase	BCPP	Board Certified Psychiatric Pharmacist
AMA	Against medical advice; American Medical Association	BCPS	Board Certified Pharmacotherapy Specialist
		BE	Barium enema; base excess
AMI	Acute myocardial infarction	BID	Twice daily (bis in die)
AML	Acute myelogenous leukemia		

BKA	Below-knee amputation		CO	Cardiac output, carbon monoxide
BM	Bone marrow, bowel movement		COLD	Chronic obstructive lung disease
BMD	Bone mineral density		COPD	Chronic obstructive pulmonary disease
BMR	Basal metabolic rate		CP	Chest pain, cerebral palsy
BMT	Bone marrow transplantation		CPA	Costophrenic angle
BP	Blood pressure		CPAP	Continuous positive airway pressure
BPH	Benign prostatic hyperplasia		CPK	Creatine phosphokinase
bpm	Beats per minute		CPR	Cardiopulmonary resuscitation
BR	Bedrest		CRF	Chronic renal failure, corticotropin-releasing factor
BRBPR	Bright red blood per rectum		CRI	Chronic renal insufficiency
BRM	Biological response modifier		CRNA	Certified Registered Nurse Anesthetist
BRP	Bathroom privileges		CRNP	Certified Registered Nurse Practitioner
BS	Bowel sounds, breath sounds, blood sugar		CRTT	Certified Respiratory Therapy Technician
BSA	Body surface area		CS	Central Supply, C-section
BSO	Bilateral salpingo-oophorectomy		CSA	Cyclosporine
BTFS	Breast tumor frozen section		CSF	Cerebrospinal fluid, colony-stimulating factor
BUN	Blood urea nitrogen		CT	Computed tomography, chest tube
Bx	Biopsy		CTB	Cease to breathe
C & S	Culture and sensitivity		CTZ	Chemoreceptor trigger zone
CA	Cancer, calcium		CV	Cardiovascular
CABG	Coronary artery bypass graft		CVA	Cerebrovascular accident
CAD	Coronary artery disease		CVAT	Costovertebral angle tenderness
CAH	Chronic active hepatitis		CVP	Central venous pressure
CAPD	Continuous ambulatory peritoneal dialysis		Cx	Culture
CBC	Complete blood count		CXR	Chest x-ray
CBD	Common bile duct		D & C	Dilatation and curettage
CBG	Capillary blood gas		d4T	Stavudine
CC	Chief complaint		D_5W	5% dextrose in water
CCA	Calcium channel antagonist		DBP	Diastolic blood pressure
CCB	Calcium channel blocker		D/C	Discontinue, discharge
CCE	Clubbing, cyanosis, edema		DCC	Direct current cardioversion
CCMS	Clean catch midstream		ddC	Zalcitabine
CCN	Lomustine		ddI	Didanosine
CCPD	Continuous cycling peritoneal dialysis		DES	Diethylstilbestrol
CCU	Coronary care unit		DI	Diabetes insipidus
CEA	Carcinoembryonic antigen		DIC	Disseminated intravascular coagulation
CF	Cystic fibrosis		Diff	Differential
CFU	Colony-forming unit		DIP	Distal interphalangeal
CHD	Coronary heart disease		DJD	Degenerative joint disease
CHF	Congestive heart failure		DKA	Diabetic ketoacidosis
CHO	Carbohydrate		dL	Deciliter
CI	Cardiac index		DM	Diabetes mellitus
CK	Creatine kinase		DMARD	Disease-modifying antirheumatic drug
CLL	Chronic lymphocytic leukemia		DNA	Deoxyribonucleic acid
CM	Costal margin		DNR	Do not resuscitate
CMG	Cystometrogram		DO	Doctor of Osteopathy
CML	Chronic myelogenous leukemia		DOA	Dead on arrival
CMV	Cytomegalovirus		DOB	Date of birth
CN	Cranial nerve		DOE	Dyspnea on exertion
CNS	Central nervous system		DPGN	Diffuse proliferative glomerulonephritis
C/O	Complains of		DRE	Digital rectal examination

DRG	Diagnosis-related group		Fx	Fracture
DST	Dexamethasone suppression test		G	Gravida
DTIC	Dacarbazine		G-CSF	Granulocyte colony-stimulating factor
DTP	Diphtheria–tetanus–pertussis		G6PD	Glucose-6-phosphate dehydrogenase
DTR	Deep tendon reflex		GAD	Generalized anxiety disorder
DU	Duodenal ulcer		GB	Gallbladder
DVT	Deep vein thrombosis		GBS	Group B streptococcus
Dx	Diagnosis		GC	Gonococcus
EBV	Epstein–Barr virus		GE	Gastroesophageal, gastroenterology
EC	Enteric-coated		GERD	Gastroesophageal reflux disease
ECF	Extended care facility		GFR	Glomerular filtration rate
ECG	Electrocardiogram		GGT	Gamma-glutamyl transferase
ECMO	Extracorporeal membrane oxygenator		GGTP	Gamma-glutamyl transpeptidase
ECOG	Eastern Cooperative Oncology Group		GI	Gastrointestinal
ECT	Electroconvulsive therapy		GM-CSF	Granulocyte-macrophage colony-stimulating factor
ED	Emergency Department		GN	Glomerulonephritis, graduate nurse
EEG	Electroencephalogram		gr	Grain
EENT	Eyes, ears, nose, throat		gtt	Drops (guttae)
EF	Ejection fraction		GT	Gastrostomy tube
EGD	Esophagogastroduodenoscopy		GTT	Glucose tolerance test
EKG	Electrocardiogram		GU	Genitourinary; gastric ulcer
EMG	Electromyogram		GVHD	Graft-versus-host disease
EMT	Emergency Medical Technician		GVL	Graft-versus-leukemia
Endo	Endotracheal, endoscopy		Gyn	Gynecology
EOMI	Extraocular movements (or muscles) intact		H & H	Hemoglobin and hematocrit
EPO	Erythropoietin		H & P	History and physical examination
EPS	Extrapyramidal symptoms		H/A	Headache
ERCP	Endoscopic retrograde cholangiopancreatography		HAV	Hepatitis A virus
ERT	Estrogen replacement therapy		Hb, hgb	Hemoglobin
ESR	Erythrocyte sedimentation rate		HbA$_{1c}$	Glycosylated hemoglobin
ESRD	End-stage renal disease		HBIG	Hepatitis B immune globulin
ESWL	Extracorporeal shockwave lithotripsy		HBP	High blood pressure
ET	Endotracheal		HBsAg	Hepatitis B surface antigen
EtOH	Ethanol		HBV	Hepatitis B virus
FB	Finger-breadth, foreign body		HC	Hydrocortisone, home care
FBS	Fasting blood sugar		HCG	Human chorionic gonadotropin
FDA	Food and Drug Administration		HCO$_3$	Bicarbonate
FDP	Fibrin degradation products		Hct	Hematocrit
FEM-POP	Femoral–popliteal		HCTZ	Hydrochlorothiazide
FEV$_1$	Forced expiratory volume in one second		HCV	Hepatitis C virus
FFP	Fresh frozen plasma		HD	Hodgkin's disease
FH	Family history		HDL-C	High-density lipoprotein cholesterol
Fio$_2$	Fraction of inspired oxygen		HEENT	Head, eyes, ears, nose, and throat
FM	Face mask		HEPA	High-efficiency particulate air
FOC	Fronto-occipital circumference		HGH	Human growth hormone
FPG	Fasting plasma glucose		HH	Hiatal hernia
FSH	Follicle-stimulating hormone		Hib	*Haemophilus influenzae* type B
FTA	Fluorescent treponemal antibody		HIV	Human immunodeficiency virus
F/U	Follow-up		HJR	Hepatojugular reflux
FUDR	Floxuridine		HLA	Human leukocyte antigen
FUO	Fever of unknown origin		HMG-CoA	Hydroxy-methylglutaryl coenzyme A

H/O	History of		JRA	Juvenile rheumatoid arthritis
HOB	Head of bed		JVD	Jugular venous distention
HPA	Hypothalamic–pituitary axis		JVP	Jugular venous pressure
hpf	High-power field		kcal	Kilocalorie
HPI	History of present illness		KCL	Potassium chloride
HR	Heart rate		KUB	Kidney, ureters, bladder
HRT	Hormone replacement therapy		KVO	Keep vein open
HS	At bedtime (hora somni)		L	Liter
HSM	Hepatosplenomegaly		LAD	Left anterior descending, left axis deviation
HSV	Herpes simplex virus		LAO	Left anterior oblique
HTN	Hypertension		LAP	Leukocyte alkaline phosphatase
Hx	History		LBBB	Left bundle branch block
I & D	Incision and drainage		LBP	Low back pain
I & O	Intake and output		LCM	Left costal margin
IABP	Intra-arterial balloon pump		LDH	Lactate dehydrogenase
IBD	Inflammatory bowel disease		LDL-C	Low-density lipoprotein cholesterol
IBW	Ideal body weight		LE	Lower extremity
ICP	Intracranial pressure		LES	Lower esophageal sphincter
ICS	Intercostal space		LFT	Liver function test
ICU	Intensive care unit		LH	Luteinizing hormone
ID	Identification, infectious disease		LHRH	Luteinizing hormone-releasing hormone
IDDM	Insulin-dependent diabetes mellitus		LLE	Left lower extremity
IFN	Interferon		LLL	Left lower lobe
IHD	Ischemic heart disease		LLQ	Left lower quadrant
IM	Intramuscular, infectious mononucleosis		LLSB	Left lower sternal border
IMV	Intermittent mandatory ventilation		LMD	Local medical doctor
INH	Isoniazid		LMP	Last menstrual period
INR	International normalized ratio		LOC	Loss of consciousness, laxative of choice
IOP	Intraocular pressure		LOS	Length of stay
IP	Intraperitoneal		LP	Lumbar puncture
IPG	Impedance plethysmography		LPN	Licensed Practical Nurse
IPN	Interstitial pneumonia		LPO	Left posterior oblique
IPPB	Intermittent positive pressure breathing		LPT	Licensed Physical Therapist
IRB	Institutional Review Board		LR	Lactated Ringer's
ISA	Intrinsic sympathomimetic activity		LS	Lumbosacral
ISDN	Isosorbide dinitrate		LSB	Left sternal border
ISH	Isolated systolic hypertension		LTCF	Long-term care facility
ISMN	Isosorbide mononitrate		LUE	Left upper extremity
IT	Intrathecal		LUL	Left upper lobe
ITP	Idiopathic thrombocytopenic purpura		LUQ	Left upper quadrant
IU	International unit		LUSB	Left upper sternal border
IUD	Intrauterine device		LVH	Left ventricular hypertrophy
IV	Intravenous		MAP	Mean arterial pressure
IVC	Inferior vena cava, intravenous cholangiogram		MAR	Medication administration record
IVDA	Intravenous drug abuse		mcg	Microgram
IVDU	Intravenous drug use		MCH	Mean corpuscular hemoglobin
IVF	Intravenous fluids		MCHC	Mean corpuscular hemoglobin concentration
IVIG	Intravenous immunoglobulin		MCL	Midclavicular line
IVP	Intravenous pyelogram, intravenous push		MCP	Metacarpophalangeal
IVSS	Intravenous soluset		MCV	Mean corpuscular volume
IWMI	Inferior wall myocardial infarction		MD	Medical Doctor
JODM	Juvenile-onset diabetes mellitus		MDI	Metered-dose inhaler

MEFR	Maximum expiratory flow rate
mEq	Milliequivalent
mg	Milligram
MHC	Major histocompatibility complex
MI	Myocardial infarction, mitral insufficiency
MIC	Minimum inhibitory concentration
MICU	Medical intensive care unit
mL	Milliliter
MM	Multiple myeloma
MMEFR	Maximal midexpiratory flow rate
MMR	Measles–mumps–rubella
MOM	Milk of magnesia
m/r/g	Murmur/rub/gallop
MRI	Magnetic resonance imaging
MRSA	Methicillin-resistant *Staphylococcus aureus*
MS	Mental status, mitral stenosis, musculoskeletal, multiple sclerosis, morphine sulfate
MSE	Mental status exam
MSW	Master of Social Work
MTD	Maximum tolerated dose
MTP	Metatarsophalangeal
MTX	Methotrexate
MUD	Matched unrelated donor
MUGA	Multiple gated acquisition
MVA	Motor vehicle accident
MVI	Multivitamin
MVR	Mitral valve replacement
N & V	Nausea and vomiting
NAD	No acute (or apparent) distress
N/C	Non-contributory, nasal cannula
NC/AT	Normocephalic, atraumatic
NCEP	National Cholesterol Education Program
NG	Nasogastric
NHL	Non-Hodgkin's lymphoma
NIDDM	Non-insulin–dependent diabetes mellitus
NKA	No known allergies
NKDA	No known drug allergies
NL	Normal
NOS	Not otherwise specified
NPH	Neutral protamine Hagedorn, normal pressure hydrocephalus
NPN	Non-protein nitrogen
NPO	Nothing by mouth (nil per os)
NS	Neurosurgery, normal saline
NSAID	Nonsteroidal anti-inflammatory drug
NSR	Normal sinus rhythm
NSS	Normal saline solution
NSVT	Non-sustained ventricular tachycardia
NTG	Nitroglycerin
NT/ND	Non-tender, non-distended
NVD	Nausea/vomiting/diarrhea, neck vein distention
NYHA	New York Heart Association
O & P	Ova and parasites
OA	Osteoarthritis
OB	Obstetrics
OBS	Organic brain syndrome
OCD	Obsessive-compulsive disorder
OCG	Oral cholecystogram
OD	Right eye (oculus dexter), overdose, Doctor of Optometry
OHTx	Orthotopic heart transplantation
OLTx	Orthotopic liver transplantation
OOB	Out of bed
OP	Oropharynx
OPD	Outpatient department
OPG	Ocular plethysmography
OPV	Oral poliovirus vaccine
OR	Operating room
OS	Left eye (oculus sinister)
OT	Occupational therapy
OTC	Over-the-counter
OU	Oculus uterque (each eye)
P	Pulse, plan, percussion, pressure, para
P & A	Percussion and auscultation
P & T	Peak and trough
PA	Physician Assistant, posterior–anterior, pulmonary artery
PAC	Premature atrial contraction
Paco$_2$	Arterial carbon dioxide tension
Pao$_2$	Arterial oxygen tension
PAT	Paroxysmal atrial tachycardia
PBI	Protein-bound iodine
PBSCT	Peripheral blood stem cell transplantation
PC	After meals (post cibum)
PCA	Patient-controlled analgesia
PCN	Penicillin
PCP	*Pneumocystis carinii* pneumonia, phencyclidine, primary care physician
PCWP	Pulmonary capillary wedge pressure
PDA	Patent ductus arteriosus
PE	Physical examination, pulmonary embolism
PEEP	Positive end-expiratory pressure
PEFR	Peak expiratory flow rate
PEG	Percutaneous endoscopic gastrostomy, polyethylene glycol
PERLA	Pupils equal, react to light and accommodation
PERRLA	Pupils equal, round, and reactive to light and accommodation
PET	Positron emission tomography
PFT	Pulmonary function test
pH	Hydrogen ion concentration
PharmD	Doctor of Pharmacy
PI	Principal investigator
PID	Pelvic inflammatory disease

PIP	Proximal interphalangeal	RCA	Right coronary artery
PKU	Phenylketonuria	RCM	Right costal margin
PMD	Private medical doctor	RDA	Recommended daily allowance
PMDD	Postmenopausal dysphoric disorder	RDP	Random donor platelets
PMH	Past medical history	RDW	Red cell distribution width
PMI	Point of maximal impulse	REM	Rapid eye movement
PMN	Polymorphonuclear leukocyte	RES	Reticuloendothelial system
PMS	Premenstrual syndrome	RF	Rheumatoid factor, renal failure, rheumatic fever
PNC-E	Postnecrotic cirrhosis—ethanol	RHD	Rheumatic heart disease
PND	Paroxysmal nocturnal dyspnea	RLE	Right lower extremity
PNH	Paroxysmal nocturnal hemoglobinuria	RLL	Right lower lobe
po	By mouth (per os)	RLQ	Right lower quadrant
POAG	Primary open-angle glaucoma	RML	Right middle lobe
POD	Postoperative day	RN	Registered nurse
PP	Patient profile	RNA	Ribonucleic acid
PPBG	Postprandial blood glucose	R/O	Rule out
ppd	packs per day	ROM	Range of motion
PPD	Purified protein derivative	ROS	Review of systems
PPI	Proton pump inhibitor	RPGN	Rapidly progressive glomerulonephritis
pr	Per rectum	RPh	Registered Pharmacist
PRA	Panel-reactive antibody, plasma renin activity	RPR	Rapid plasma reagin
PRBC	Packed red blood cells	RR	Respiratory rate, recovery room
PRN	When necessary, as needed (pro re nata)	RRR	Regular rate and rhythm
PSA	Prostate-specific antigen	RRT	Registered Respiratory Therapist
PSCT	Peripheral stem cell transplant	RT	Radiation therapy
PSE	Portal systemic encephalopathy	RTA	Renal tubular acidosis
PSH	Past surgical history	RTC	Return to clinic
PT	Prothrombin time, physical therapy, patient	RUE	Right upper extremity
PTA	Prior to admission	RUL	Right upper lobe
PTCA	Percutaneous transluminal coronary angioplasty	RUQ	Right upper quadrant
PTH	Parathyroid hormone	Rx	Prescribed, prescription
PTSD	Post-traumatic stress disorder	SA	Sino-atrial
PTT	Partial thromboplastin time	SAH	Subarachnoid hemorrhage
PTU	Propylthiouracil	Sao_2	Arterial oxygen percent saturation
PUD	Peptic ulcer disease	SBE	Subacute bacterial endocarditis
PVC	Premature ventricular contraction	SBFT	Small bowel follow-through
PVD	Peripheral vascular disease	SBO	Small bowel obstruction
Q	Every (quaque)	SBP	Systolic blood pressure, spontaneous bacterial peritonitis
QA	Quality assurance		
QD	Every day (quaque die)	SC	Subcutaneous, subclavian
QI	Quality improvement	SCID	Severe combined immunodeficiency
QID	Four times daily (quater in die)	SCLC	Small cell lung cancer
QNS	Quantity not sufficient	SCr	Serum creatinine
QOD	Every other day	SD	Standard deviation
QOL	Quality of life	SDP	Single donor platelets
QS	Quantity sufficient	SEM	Systolic ejection murmur
R & M	Routine and microscopic	SG	Specific gravity
RA	Rheumatoid arthritis, right atrium, room air	SGOT	Serum glutamic oxaloacetic transaminase
RAIU	Radioactive iodine uptake	SGPT	Serum glutamic pyruvic transaminase
RAO	Right anterior oblique	SH	Social history
RBBB	Right bundle branch block	SIADH	Syndrome of inappropriate antidiuretic hormone secretion
RBC	Red blood cell		

SICU	Surgical intensive care unit
SIDS	Sudden infant death syndrome
SIMV	Synchronized intermittent mandatory ventilation
SJS	Stevens–Johnson syndrome
SL	Sublingual
SLE	Systemic lupus erythematosus
SOB	Shortness of breath
S/P	Status post
SPEP	Serum protein electrophoresis
SPF	Sun protection factor
SQ	Subcutaneous
SSI	Supplemental Security Income
SSKI	Saturated solution of potassium iodide
SSRI	Selective serotonin reuptake inhibitor
STAT	Immediately, at once
STD	Sexually transmitted disease
SVC	Superior vena cava
SVRI	Systemic vascular resistance index
SVT	Supraventricular tachycardia
SW	Social worker
Sx	Symptoms
T	Temperature
T & A	Tonsillectomy and adenoidectomy
T & C	Type and crossmatch
TAH	Total abdominal hysterectomy
TB	Tuberculosis
TBG	Thyroid-binding globulin
TBI	Total body irradiation, traumatic brain injury
T/C	To consider
TCA	Tricyclic antidepressant
TCN	Tetracycline
TED	Thromboembolic disease
TEN	Toxic epidermal necrolysis
TENS	Transcutaneous electrical nerve stimulation
TFT	Thyroid function test
TG	Triglyceride
THC	Tetrahydrocannabinol
TIA	Transient ischemic attack
TIBC	Total iron-binding capacity
TID	Three times daily (ter in die)
TKR	Total knee replacement
TLI	Total lymphoid irradiation
TLS	Tumor lysis syndrome
TM	Tympanic membrane
TMJ	Temporomandibular joint
TMP-SMX	Trimethoprim-sulfamethoxazole
TNTC	Too numerous to count
TOD	Target organ damage
TPN	Total parenteral nutrition
TPR	Temperature, pulse, respiration
TSH	Thyroid-stimulating hormone
TSS	Toxic shock syndrome
TTP	Thrombotic thrombocytopenic purpura
TURP	Transurethral resection of the prostate
Tx	Treat, treatment
UA	Urinalysis, uric acid
UC	Ulcerative colitis
UCD	Usual childhood diseases
UE	Upper extremity
UFC	Urinary free cortisol
UGI	Upper gastrointestinal
UOQ	Upper outer quadrant
URI	Upper respiratory infection
USP	United States Pharmacopeia
UTI	Urinary tract infection
UV	Ultraviolet
VA	Veterans' Affairs
VDRL	Venereal Disease Research Laboratory
VF	Ventricular fibrillation
VLDL-C	Very low-density lipoprotein cholesterol
VNA	Visiting Nurses' Association
VO	Verbal order
VOD	Veno-occlusive disease
VP-16	Etoposide
V/Q	Ventilation/perfusion
VRE	Vancomycin-resistant enterococcus
VS	Vital signs
VSS	Vital signs stable
VT	Ventricular tachycardia
WA	While awake
WBC	White blood cell
W/C	Wheelchair
WDWN	Well-developed, well-nourished
WNL	Within normal limits
W/U	Work-up
yo	Year-old
ZDV	Zidovudine

29 PEDIATRIC GASTROENTERITIS

▶ Dihydrogen Monoxide and Other
Critical Elements   (Level II)

William McGhee, PharmD
Basil J. Zitelli, MD, FAAP

A 5-day history of vomiting, diarrhea, and other symptoms causes a young mother to seek medical attention at the ED for her 5-month-old son. The patient has signs of moderate dehydration on physical and laboratory examination. The presumed diagnosis is viral gastroenteritis probably caused by rotavirus. Students should understand that replacement of fluid and electrolyte losses is critical to the effective treatment of acute diarrhea. Oral rehydration therapy with carbohydrate-based solutions is the primary treatment of diarrhea in children with mild to moderate dehydration. Intravenous fluids may be needed for cases of severe dehydration. Early feeding of patients with an age-appropriate diet helps to reduce stool volume after completion of rehydration therapy. Although antidiarrheal products are available, they have limited effectiveness, can cause adverse effects, and may shift attention from appropriate fluid and electrolyte replacement.

▶ Questions

Problem Identification

1. a. Create a list of the patient's drug-related problems.

- This patient has typical viral gastroenteritis, probably rotavirus infection, which is characterized by the acute onset of emesis, progressing to watery diarrhea with diminishing emesis. Rotavirus is the most common cause of pediatric gastroenteritis in the U.S., accounting for 25% of cases. Other common viruses include Norwalk-like viruses and adenovirus.[1] Rotavirus is transmitted by the fecal–oral route. Infection occurs when ingested virus infects enterocytes in the small intestine, leading to cell death and loss of brush border digestive enzymes. Approximately 48 hours after exposure, infected children develop fever, vomiting, and watery diarrhea. Fever and vomiting usually subside in 1 to 2 days, but diarrhea can continue for several days leading to significant dehydration. Approximately 65% of hospitalizations and 85% of diarrhea-related deaths occur in the first year of life.

- The patient has moderate dehydration (acute weight loss of 8%, from 7.1 kg to 6.5 kg) as well as clinical and laboratory evidence of dehydration with metabolic acidosis.

b. What information (signs, symptoms, laboratory values) indicates the presence or severity of gastroenteritis?

- By history, the patient had a 5-day history of fever, vomiting, and diarrhea of acute onset; he had a reported decrease in the number of wet diapers; and his lips appeared to be dry. An actual weight loss of 0.6 kg (8%) was documented.

- He has a social history of day care attendance, where several of his day care mates had similar illnesses recently, as well as a 2-year-old sibling with a recent history of diarrhea for 3 days. This is a typical history in pediatric gastroenteritis.

- On physical exam, his skin turgor was decreased and the capillary refill was increased at 2 to 3 seconds. His tongue was dry with cracked and dry lips. His anterior fontanelle was sunken and he had sunken eyes, and he was tachycardic and tachypneic.

- His labs indicated metabolic acidosis (total CO_2 13 mEq/L and Cl 110 mEq/L) and his urinalysis showed a specific gravity of 1.028 (moderate dehydration). His dehydration was isotonic (defined as serum sodium between 130 and 150 mEq/L).

- See Table 29–1 for clinical assessment guidelines for dehydration.

Desired Outcome

2. What are the goals of pharmacotherapy in this case?

- Replacement of fluid and electrolyte losses is the critical central element of effective treatment of acute diarrhea.[2] This is necessary to prevent excessive water, electrolyte, and acid–base disturbances.

- Other secondary goals may include providing symptomatic relief and treating any curable causes of diarrhea.

Therapeutic Alternatives

3. a. What non-drug therapies might be useful for this patient?

- *Oral rehydration therapy (ORT)* with carbohydrate-based solu-

TABLE 29–1. Clinical Assessment Guidelines for Dehydration in Children of All Ages[2,3]

Parameter	Mild	Moderate	Severe
Weight loss	3–5%	6–9%	≥10%
Body fluid loss	30–50 mL/kg	50–100 mL/kg	>100 mL/kg
Stage of shock	Impending	Compensated	Uncompensated
Heart rate	Normal	Increased	Increased
Blood pressure	Normal	Normal	Normal to reduced
Respiratory rate	Normal	Normal	Increased
Skin turgor	Normal	Decreased	"Tenting"
Anterior fontanelle	Normal	Sunken	Sunken
Capillary refill	<2 seconds	2–3 seconds	>3 seconds
Mucous membranes	Slightly dry	Dry	Dry
Tearing	Normal/absent	Absent	Absent
Eye appearance	Normal	Sunken orbits	Deeply sunken orbits
Mental status	Normal	Normal to listless	Normal to lethargic to comatose
Urine volume	Slightly decreased	<1 mL/kg/hr	<<1 mL/kg/hr
Urine specific gravity	1.020	1.025	>1.035
BUN	Upper normal	Elevated	High
Blood pH	7.40–7.22	7.30–6.92	7.10–6.8
Thirst	Slightly increased	Moderately increased	Very thirsty or too lethargic to indicate

tions is the mainstay of treatment of fluid and electrolyte losses caused by diarrhea in children with mild to moderate dehydration. ORT can be used regardless of the patient's age, causative pathogen, or initial serum sodium concentration. The basis for the effectiveness of ORT is the phenomenon of glucose-sodium cotransport, where sodium ions given orally are absorbed along with glucose (and other organic molecules) from the lumen of the intestine into the bloodstream.[1] Any of the commercially available oral rehydration solutions can successfully be used to rehydrate otherwise healthy children with mild to moderate dehydration (refer to the table on oral rehydration solutions in textbook Chapter 34 for detailed product information). These products are formulated on physiologic principles and must be distinguished from other nonphysiologic clear liquids that are commonly but inappropriately used to treat dehydration. Clear liquids to be avoided include colas, apple juice, chicken broth, and sports beverages.[3] This patient was inappropriately treated since in addition to an ORT (Pedialyte), her pediatrician recommended a variety of clear liquids including water, Jell-O water, and cola. These liquids have unacceptably low electrolyte concentrations, and cola beverages are hypertonic because of the high glucose concentrations, with osmolalities greater than 700 mOsm.[3]

- *Early feeding of age-appropriate foods.* Although carbohydrate-based ORT is highly effective in replacing fluid and electrolyte losses, it has no effect on stool volume or duration of diarrhea, which can be discouraging to parents. To overcome this limitation, cereal-based ORT has been used investigationally and can reduce stool volume by 20% to 30%. However, there are no commercial products available in the United States. Nevertheless, early feeding of patients as soon as oral rehydration is completed

provides similar reductions in stool volume.[3] Therefore, children with diarrhea requiring rehydration should be fed with age-appropriate diets immediately after completing ORT. Optimal ORT incorporates early feeding of age-appropriate foods. Unrestricted diets generally do not worsen the symptoms of mild diarrhea and decrease the stool output compared with ORT alone.

b. *What feasible pharmacotherapeutic alternatives are available for treatment of this patient's diarrhea?*

- *Antidiarrheal compounds* have been used to treat pediatric gastroenteritis. Their use is intended to shorten the course of diarrhea and to relieve discomfort by reducing stool output and electrolyte losses. However, their usefulness remains to be proven, and antidiarrheal compounds generally should not be used to treat pediatric gastroenteritis. These agents have a variety of proposed mechanisms; their possible benefits and limitations are outlined below.

  ✓ *Antimotility agents* (opiates and opiate/anticholinergic combination products) delay GI transit and increase gut capacity and fluid retention. *Loperamide* with ORT significantly reduces the volume of stool losses, but this reduction is not clinically significant. It also may have an unacceptable rate of side effects (lethargy, respiratory depression, altered mental status, ileus, abdominal distention). Anticholinergic agents (e.g., atropine or mepenzolate bromide) may cause dry mouth that can alter the clinical evaluation of dehydration. Infants and children are especially susceptible to toxic effects of anticholinergics. Antimotility agents can worsen the course of diarrhea in shigellosis, anti-biotic-associated pseudomembranous colitis, and *E. coli* 0157:H7-induced diarrhea. Importantly, reliance on antidiarrheal compounds may shift the focus of treatment away from appropriate ORT and early feeding of the child. They are not recommended by the American Academy of Pediatrics (AAP) to treat acute diarrhea in children because of the modest clinical benefit, limited scientific evidence of efficacy, and concern for toxic effects.

✓ *Antisecretory agents (bismuth subsalicylate)* may have an adjunctive role for acute diarrhea. Bismuth subsalicylate decreases intestinal secretions secondary to cholera and *E. coli* toxins, decreases frequency of unformed stools, decreases total stool output, and reduces the need for ORT. However, the benefit is modest, and it requires dosing every 4 hours. Also, pediatric patients may absorb salicylate (but the effect on Reye's syndrome is unknown). This treatment is also not recommended by the AAP because of modest benefit and concern for toxicity.

✓ *Adsorbent drugs (kaolin & pectin; polycarbophil)* may bind bacterial toxins and water, but their effectiveness remains unproven. There is no conclusive evidence of decreased duration of diarrhea, number of stools, or total stool output. Major toxicity is not a concern with these products, but they may adsorb nutrients, enzymes, and drugs. The FDA recognizes only polycarbophil as an effective adsorbent. These products are not recommended by the AAP because of lack of efficacy.

✓ *Colonic microflora replacement products (Lactobacillus acidophilus, L. bulgaricus)* supposedly replace microflora loss secondary to previous antibiotic therapy. They purportedly suppress growth of pathogenic microorganisms, restoring normal intestinal function. There is no consistent evidence that microflora replacement improves diarrhea, and lactobacillus-containing compounds are not recommended by the AAP because of limited scientific evidence of efficacy.

Optimal Plan

4. *What drug(s), dosage forms, schedule, and duration of therapy are best for this patient?*

• Treatment of a child with dehydration is directed primarily by the degree of dehydration present.[1] This patient had diarrhea with moderate dehydration (6% to 9% loss of body weight). There are four treatment situations[3]:

✓ *Diarrhea without dehydration.* ORT may be given in doses of 10 mL/kg to replace ongoing stool losses. Some children may not take the ORT because of its salty taste. For these few patients, freezer pops are available in a variety of flavors. ORT may not be necessary if fluid consumption and age-appropriate feeding continues. Infants should continue to breastfeed or take regular-strength formula. Older children can usually drink full-strength milk.

✓ *Diarrhea with mild dehydration (3% to 5% weight loss).* Correct dehydration with ORT 50 mL/kg over a 4-hour period. Reassess the status of dehydration and volume of ORT at 2-hour intervals. Concomitantly replace continuing losses from stool or emesis at 10 mL/kg for each stool; estimate emesis loss and replace with fluid. Children with emesis can usually tolerate ORT, but it is necessary to administer ORT in small 5- to 10-mL (1 to

2 teaspoonfuls) aliquots every 1 to 2 minutes. Feeding should start immediately after rehydration is complete, using the feeding guidelines described above.

✓ *Diarrhea with moderate dehydration (6% to 9% weight loss).* Since the patient presented to the ED, this treatment was performed there, but it can usually be accomplished at home. Correct the dehydration with ORT 100 mL/kg plus replacement of ongoing losses (10 mL/kg for each stool, plus estimated losses from emesis as above) during the first 4 hours. Assess rehydration status hourly and adjust the amount of ORT accordingly. Close supervision is required, but this can be continued at home. Rapid restoration of blood volume helps correct acidosis and increase tissue perfusion. Resume feeding of age-appropriate diet as soon as rehydration is completed.

✓ *Diarrhea with severe dehydration (≥10% weight loss).* Severe dehydration and uncompensated shock should be treated aggressively with IV isotonic fluids to restore intravascular volume. Poorly treated pediatric gastroenteritis, especially in infants, can cause life-threatening severe dehydration and should be considered a medical emergency. The patient may be in shock and should be referred to an ED. Administer 20-mL/kg aliquots of normal saline or Ringer's Lactate solution over 15 to 30 minutes (even faster in uncompensated shock). Reassess the patient's status after each completed fluid bolus. Repeat boluses of up to 80 mL/kg total fluid may be used. Isotonic fluid replacement may be discontinued when blood pressure is restored, heart rate is normalized, peripheral pulses are strong, and skin perfusion is restored. Urine output is the best indicator of restored intravascular volume and should be at least 1 mL/kg/hr. If the patient does not respond to rapid IV volume replacement, other underlying disorders should be considered, including septic shock, toxic shock syndrome, myocarditis, cardiomyopathy, pericarditis, and other underlying diseases. ORT may be instituted to complete rehydration when the patient's status is satisfactory. Estimate the degree of remaining dehydration and treat according to the above guidelines. The IV line should be kept in place until it is certain that IV therapy will not be reinstituted. After ORT is complete, resume feeding following the guidelines outlined above.

Outcome Evaluation

5. *What clinical and laboratory parameters should be monitored to evaluate therapy for achievement of the desired therapeutic outcome?*

• Vital signs should normalize with appropriate therapy, but they may be unreliable in patients with fever, agitation, pain, or respiratory illnesses. Tachycardia is usually the first sign of mild dehydration (see Table 29–1). With increasing acidosis and fluid loss, the respiratory rate increases and breathing becomes deeper (hyperpnea). Hypotension is a sign usually of severe dehydration.

• Any existing CNS alterations should be reversed. No CNS changes occur in mild dehydration; some patients may appear listless with moderate dehydration, and severely dehydrated patients appear quite ill with lethargy or irritability.

• Skin changes should be normalized. Mucous membranes should appear moist (previously dry in all degrees of dehydration). Capillary refill is normally <2 seconds and usually is not altered in mild dehydration. Capillary refill in moderately dehydrated patients is 2 to 3 seconds and >3 seconds in severe dehydration. Skin turgor (elasticity) should be normal. There is no change in mild dehydration; but it decreases in moderate dehydration, with "tenting" occurring in patients with severe dehydration. The anterior fontanelle should no longer be sunken, which is seen in moderate to severe dehydration.

- The eyes should appear normal. No change occurs in mild dehydration, but in moderate to severe dehydration, tearing will be absent and the eyes will appear sunken.
- Laboratory tests should be assessed appropriately. Most dehydration occurring with pediatric gastroenteritis is isotonic, and serum electrolyte determinations are unnecessary. However, some patients with moderate dehydration (those whose histories and physical examinations are inconsistent with routine gastroenteritis) and all severely dehydrated patients should have serum electrolytes determined and corrected. Urine volume and specific gravity should be normalized. Progressive decreases in urine volume and increases in specific gravity are expected with increasing severity of dehydration. Urine output will be decreased to <1 mL/kg/hr in moderate dehydration and <<1 mL/kg/hr in severe dehydration (see Table 29–1). Specific gravity will be 1.020 in mild dehydration, 1.025 in moderate dehydration, and maximal in patients with severe dehydration. Adequate rehydration should normalize both urine output and specific gravity.

Patient Counseling

6. *What information should be provided to the child's parents to enhance compliance, ensure successful therapy, and minimize adverse effects?*

- Treatment of diarrhea due to gastroenteritis in your child should begin at home.[1] It is a good idea for you to keep ORT at home at all times (especially in rural areas and poor urban neighborhoods where access to health care may be delayed), and to use it as instructed by your doctor. Sometimes doctors instruct new parents about this treatment at the first newborn visit.
- Early home management will result in fewer complications such as severe dehydration and poor nutrition, as well as fewer office or emergency room visits.
- Any of the commercial oral rehydration products can be used to effectively rehydrate your child. However, rehydration alone does not reduce the duration of diarrhea or the volume of stool output. Early feeding after rehydration can reduce the duration of diarrhea by as much as one-half day.

- Effective oral rehydration always combines early feeding with an age-appropriate diet after rehydration. This will correct dehydration, improve nutritional status, and reduce the volume of stool output.
- Vomiting usually does not preclude the use of oral rehydration. Small amounts (1 to 2 teaspoonfuls) of an oral rehydration product can be given every 1 to 2 minutes, providing as much as 10 ounces/hr of rehydration fluid.
- If the child does not stop vomiting after the appropriate administration of oral rehydration (as above) and appears to be severely dehydrated, contact your doctor, who may refer you to the emergency room for intravenous rehydration therapy.
- Oral rehydration is not sufficient therapy for bloody diarrhea (dysentery). Contact your doctor if this occurs.
- Additional treatments, including antidiarrheal compounds and antimicrobial therapy are almost never necessary in the treatment of pediatric gastroenteritis.
- Proper handwashing technique, diaper changing practices, and personal hygiene can help prevent spread of the disease to other family members.

40 CHRONIC GLOMERULONEPHRITIS

▶ **Annie Brown's Battle With Lupus (Level III)**

Melanie S. Joy, PharmD

A 23-year-old woman with a history of diffuse proliferative glomerulonephritis (DPGN) secondary to systemic lupus erythematosus presents with hematuria and renal biopsy features characteristic of advanced DPGN. In addition to requiring immunosuppressive therapy for DPGN, she also needs treatment for hypertension, dyslipidemia, and corticosteroid-induced osteoporosis. Cyclophosphamide and azathioprine are potent immunosuppressive agents that may be useful as single agents or combined with prednisone for DPGN. Because she received cyclophosphamide on two previous occasions, it should probably be avoided at this time because of the risk of toxicity. Other potential alternatives include cyclosporine or mycophenolate mofetil. This is a complex case because it requires students to develop pharmacotherapeutic plans for all of the patient's medical problems.

▶ **Questions**

Problem Identification

1. a. *Create a list of this patient's drug-related problems.*

- DPGN requiring immunosuppressive drug therapy.
- HTN inadequately treated with present doses of atenolol and clonidine.

- Hypercholesterolemia which is currently untreated.
- Osteoporosis/osteopenia in need of treatment to prevent fractures (*Note:* T score is the SD below or above the expected mean peak BMD obtained).
- Anemia that may be due to renal insufficiency, iron deficiency, or bleeding.

b. *What information obtained from the medical history, physical examination, and laboratory analysis indicates the presence of glomerulonephritis?*

Glomerulonephritis

- Since this patient has had two courses of cyclophosphamide in the past, she should not receive additional courses due to toxicity, unless other options are unavailable. In addition, since she has had renal disease progression while on maintenance prednisone and exhibits long-term adverse effects, try to decrease her exposure if possible.
- Both azathioprine and mycophenolate mofetil would spare her further deterioration in bone disease. Azathioprine doses of up to 4 mg/kg/day orally have been used. Mycophenolate mofetil must be considered an investigational agent until more efficacy trials are completed. Mycophenolate mofetil dosing can begin at 250 mg twice daily and increased at 2-week intervals to a maximum of 1500 mg twice daily. The slow titration upward will help to establish GI tolerance to therapy.
- A lower dose of prednisone (5 to 10 mg daily) may be possible with combination therapy, thereby limiting its adverse effect potential.
- Cyclosporine therapy would be considered later in the treatment options due to its nephrotoxicity and lack of adequate data demonstrating improved outcomes.

Hypertension

- Due to the additional renal protective benefits of ACE inhibitors in glomerular diseases, one of these agents should be used. The choice may depend on the need for enhanced compliance (i.e., a once daily product). Ramipril 2.5 to 5 mg or lisinopril 10 mg po QD could be initiated. Due to the recent data indicating the protective effects of ramipril in nondiabetic renal disease, it may be the preferred agent in this patient.[6] The need to titrate the dosage upward would depend on the BP reduction demonstrated and the response to proteinuria. The serum creatinine should be monitored to detect continued increases, which is common on initiation of therapy.
- Due to the lack of controlled BP reduction and increased risk of adverse acute cardiovascular outcomes with sublingual nifedipine, this agent should be avoided for the acute reduction in blood pressure.
- If an acute reduction is desired due to the high current level (160/115), a 0.1-mg dose of clonidine would be the recommended oral therapy until the ACE inhibitor begins to reduce the pressure. Clonidine is probably not indicated in this patient, since there is no indication of symptoms or end organ damage.
- Atenolol may be able to be discontinued after the efficacy of the ACE inhibitor therapy is determined. Since the data regarding calcium channel blockers and renal disease progression are not as well established as with ACE inhibitors, these agents would not be considered first-line therapy.

Hyperlipidemia

- Since this patient needs at least a 36% decrease in LDL-C to attain a goal of <130 mg/dL, the bile acid sequestrants are not reasonable choices.
- Any of the reductase inhibitors except fluvastatin would be capable of producing a 36% reduction in LDL-C. The most cost-effective therapy should be instituted. Pravastatin may be the preferred agent due to its lack of activity on the cytochrome P450 3A4 enzymes, although this patient is not currently on medications that may interact. Pravastatin 10 to 20 mg at bedtime could be initiated, with the possibility of increasing the dose to 40 mg for increased efficacy, if tolerated.

Osteoporosis

- The patient should begin therapy with a calcium and vitamin D supplement. Oscal 250 mg with D would be a reasonable combination product option. When administered as two tablets BID, the patient will receive 1000 mg elemental calcium and 500 IU vitamin D daily. With the intake of an additional 500 mg of calcium in the diet, the patient will receive the recommended 1500 mg for patients receiving chronic glucocorticoid therapy.
- Since this patient has progressive renal insufficiency with an estimated creatinine clearance of 37 mL/min, alendronate is not a good option, since it is eliminated primarily in the kidneys and is not recommended for patients with clearances of <30 mL/min.
- Although intranasal calcitonin has only demonstrated a 1-year gain in BMD versus the 3-year gain with alendronate in glucocorticoid-treated patients, it would be a reasonable option in this patient with osteoporosis of the spine and a contraindication to alendronate. Calcitonin is administered once daily in the nostril with one spray delivering 200 IU calcitonin.
- The patient should receive some dietary counseling regarding the amount of calcium present in various foods, as well as some physical activity assessment and counseling to enhance weight bearing exercises to prevent worsening osteoporosis.

Outcome Evaluation

5. *Outline a clinical and laboratory monitoring plan for each of the patient's drug-related problems.*

- The patient should return to nephrology clinic in two weeks for assessment of progressive renal insufficiency and safety and efficacy of mycophenolate mofetil and ACE inhibitor therapy.
- Laboratory assessment should include a CBC, liver enzymes, CPK, and electrolytes. Additional follow-up labs and visits should occur at 4- to 6-week intervals to closely follow this patient's rapidly progressive renal disease and ACE inhibitor and lipid-lowering therapy.
- Urinalysis should be performed at each visit and 24-hour urine collections performed at least every six months.
- Blood pressure measurements will be performed at each clinic visit. In addition, the patient should be taught to take her own blood pressure at home.
- Adverse effect questioning at each subsequent clinic visit and appropriate modification in therapy will enhance patient compliance and disease treatment.
- A repeat DEXA scan should be performed in one year from the implementation of osteoporosis therapy to assess efficacy. A 24-hour urine collection to determine the amount of calcium eliminated may be performed to identify whether a thiazide would be indicated to minimize urinary losses.

Patient Counseling

6. *What should the patient be told regarding the drug therapy she is to receive to treat her condition and its complications?*

Mycophenolate Mofetil (CellCept)

- This drug acts to suppress your immune system in order to control your body's response to lupus. Take one tablet (250 mg) twice daily on an empty stomach for best absorption. The dose may be gradually increased every two weeks to minimize gastrointestinal side effects.

- Use appropriate contraception and avoid becoming pregnant while taking this medication, since it may be harmful to a developing fetus.
- You may experience some gastrointestinal side effects such as diarrhea and vomiting; notify your doctor if they become persistent or troublesome.
- The number of white cells in your blood will be monitored monthly because low counts have been reported.

Prednisone

- Prednisone is used to suppress your lupus disease activity. Take your prescribed dose with food to minimize stomach upset.
- Prednisone can cause side effects including increased risk of infection, fluid gain or swelling, increased blood sugar, risk of stomach ulcers, mood swings, and weight gain.

Ramipril (Altace)

- This medication decreases blood pressure, and it may decrease the protein being spilled into your urine.
- Dizziness or lightheadedness may occur if your blood pressure is lowered too much. This will often decrease with chronic therapy. Contact your physician if this persists.
- This drug may increase the concentration of potassium in your bloodstream or cause a nagging cough.
- Contact your physician if you become pregnant because this medication (like mycophenolate mofetil) may harm your unborn child.
- This medication should be taken on an empty stomach for best absorption.

Pravastatin (Pravachol)

- This drug is used to lower cholesterol levels. Take the prescribed 10-mg tablet daily at bedtime. Bedtime is the preferred time to take the drug, since most cholesterol synthesis occurs while you are sleeping.
- Contact your doctor if you experience muscle pain.

Calcium

- Calcium is needed to make the bones strong and to prevent them from breaking. Since you are at high risk of worsening bone disease due to long-term prednisone therapy, you should take 1500 mg of elemental calcium daily. This can be accomplished by taking two Oscal with D tablets twice daily. This will provide you with 1000 mg of your required calcium and 500 I.U. vitamin D. You will need to supplement your diet with high calcium-containing foods such as milk, cheese, beans, yogurt, and ice cream to get the other 500 mg you need. This can be obtained from 2 glasses of milk, 3 to 5 ounces of cheese, 2 cups of yogurt, or 4 cups of ice cream.

- Do not take the calcium with food, since the phosphorus in your diet may reduce its absorption.

Vitamin D

- This vitamin will also prevent your bones from breaking. Since you have been taking prednisone for a long time, you will also require vitamin D. You will receive close to your recommended daily requirement of vitamin D dose of 800 IU by taking the Oscal with D.

Calcitonin (Miacalcin) Nasal Spray

- This medication will prevent continuing bone loss. Administer one spray in one nostril daily. The spray should be alternated between nostrils on a daily basis to prevent irritation.
- Prior to the first dose of medication, the pump should be primed by holding it upright and depressing the two white side arms of the pump until a full spray is produced.
- The opened bottle may be stored at room temperature. Unopened bottles should be stored in the refrigerator.

99   DIABETIC FOOT INFECTION

▶ **Watch Your Step**   (Level II)

Renee-Claude Mercier, PharmD

Accidentally stepping on a piece of metal results in erythema and swelling of the right foot in a 39-year-old homeless woman with poorly controlled type 2 diabetes mellitus. Laboratory evaluation reveals leukocytosis with a left shift. The patient underwent incision and drainage of the lesion with removal of a 2-cm metallic foreign body from the foot. Empiric antimicrobial treatment must be initiated before results of wound culture and sensitivity testing are known. Because of this particular patient's condition, parenteral monotherapy with ampicillin/sulbactam, cefotetan, or cefoxitin would constitute appropriate therapy. Other alternatives include ticarcillin/clavulanate, piperacillin/tazobactam, imipenem/cilastatin, or the combination of clindamycin plus cefazolin. When tissue cultures are reported as positive for methicillin-sensitive *Staphylococcus aureus,* students are asked to change to more specific therapy, which might include parenteral penicillinase-resistant penicillins or first-generation cephalosporins. Although parenteral therapy may be completed as an outpatient, attention must be given to the patient's social situation. Better glycemic control and education on techniques for proper foot care are important components of a comprehensive treatment plan for this patient.

▶ **Questions**

Problem Identification

1. a. Create a list of the patient's drug-related problems.

- Cellulitis and infection of the right foot in a patient with diabetes.

- Poorly controlled type 2 diabetes mellitus, as evidenced by a HbA$_{1c}$ of 11.8% (goal < 7%).
- Non-compliance with medication administration and home glucose monitoring.
- History of depression, which may be inadequately treated (the patient is described as having a "flat affect").
- Poor social conditions; lives in a shelter with minimal family

support. This situation may make it difficult for her to afford medications and glucose monitoring supplies and may contribute to non-adherence with therapy.

- Fungal infection of toenails requiring treatment.

b. What signs, symptoms, or laboratory values indicate the presence of an infection?

- Swollen, sore, and red foot.
- 2+ edema of the foot increasing in amplitude.
- WBC elevated ($20.45 \times 10^3/mm^3$) with increased PMNs and bands.
- X-ray showing the presence of a foreign body in the right foot.

c. What risk factors for infection does the patient have?

- Patient stepped on a foreign object
- She is a poorly controlled diabetic patient.
- Vascular calcifications are present in the foot, indicating a decreased blood supply.
- Poor foot care (presence of fungus and overgrown toenails).

d. What organisms are most likely involved in this infection?

- Aerobic isolates: *Proteus mirabilis,* group D streptococci, *Escherichia coli, Staphylococcus aureus.*[1]
- Anaerobic isolates: *Bacteroides fragilis, Peptococcus, Peptostreptococcus.*

Desired Outcome

2. What are the therapeutic goals for this patient?

- Eradicate the bacteria
- Prevent the development of osteomyelitis and the need for amputation
- Improve control of the diabetes mellitus
- Prevent further recurrence of foot infection
- Improve social conditions and depression by providing her with a secure place to live

Therapeutic Alternatives

3. a. What non-drug therapies might be useful for this patient?

- Deep culture of the wound for both anaerobes and aerobes.
- Appropriate wound care by experienced podiatrists (I & D, debridement of the wound, toenail clipping), nurses (wound care, dressing changes of wound, foot care teaching), and physical therapists (whirlpool treatments, wound debridement, teaching about minimal weight bearing with a walker or crutches).
- Bed rest, minimal weight bearing, leg elevation, and control of edema.
- Proper counseling about wound care and the importance of good diabetes control, glucometer use, and adherence with the medication regimens.

b. What feasible pharmacotherapeutic alternatives are available for the empiric treatment of the foot infection?

- Diabetic foot infections are classified into two categories:
  - ✓ *Non-limb-threatening infections.* Superficial, no systemic toxicity, minimal cellulitis extending less than 2 cm from portal of entry, ulceration not extending fully through skin, no significant ischemia.
  - ✓ *Limb-threatening infections.* More extensive cellulitis, lymphangitis, and ulcers penetrating through skin into subcutaneous tissues, prominent ischemia.
- *An aminoglycoside plus ampicillin IV* has been suggested for limb-threatening infections, but this regimen should not be considered a first empiric choice because it does not have good coverage against the most common anaerobes involved in diabetic foot infection. Use of *IV clindamycin* instead of ampicillin would be more appropriate in this case because it has broader anaerobic coverage. Regimens including an aminoglycoside (which have been associated with the development of nephrotoxicity) should probably be avoided in this patient population because they have an increased risk of developing diabetic nephropathy and renal failure.
- *Cefoxitin* or *cefotetan* (second-generation parenteral cephalosporins) monotherapy is attractive because their spectrum of activity covers the most likely causative organisms. Single-drug therapy is also attractive because of the potential advantages of convenience, cost, and avoidance of toxicities.
- *Ampicillin/sulbactam, piperacillin/tazobactam,* and *ticarcillin/clavulanate* are also appropriate as IV monotherapy but are more costly than second-generation cephalosporins.
- *Imipenem/cilastatin* IV could also be considered, but few studies are available to support its use in this situation. It is also an expensive choice and is a very potent β-lactamase inducer.
- *Clindamycin IV plus either gentamicin or an IV fluoroquinolone* could be used in patients allergic to penicillin.
- *Oral clindamycin* plus an *oral fluoroquinolone* (e.g., ciprofloxacin, ofloxacin) or *cephalexin* could be used in patients in whom osteomyelitis has been ruled out and in those with non-limb-threatening infections.[2] Oral fluoroquinolones have poor activity against *Bacteroides* species and should be used in combination if anaerobes are suspected, such as infections with a foul odor.
- An *oral fluoroquinolone, cloxacillin,* or *clindamycin* alone could be used in patients with non-limb-threatening infection who have not previously received antibiotic therapy because they usually have infections caused by only 1 or 2 species of aerobic organisms, staphylococci and/or streptococci.[3]
- *Becaplermin 0.01% Gel (Regranex)* is FDA approved for the treatment of diabetic ulcers on the lower limbs and feet. Becaplermin is a genetically engineered form of platelet-derived growth factor, a naturally occurring protein in the body that stimulates diabetic ulcer healing. In one clinical trial, becaplermin applied once daily in combination with good wound care significantly increased the incidence of complete healing when compared to placebo gel (50% for becaplermin gel versus 35% for placebo gel). Becaplermin gel also significantly decreased the time to complete healing of diabetic ulcers by 32% (about 6 weeks faster). The incidence of adverse events including infection and cellulitis was similar in patients treated with becaplermin gel, placebo gel, or good diabetic wound care alone. Because becaplermin is a new drug with limited clinical experience, further studies are needed to assess which patients might best benefit from its use.

c. What economic and social considerations are applicable to this patient?

- Simplified drug regimen (less frequent dosing) should be selected due to her history of poor medication adherence.
- In light of the patient's social status, she probably does not have access to health care insurance, which may become an important consideration in selecting her future therapeutic plan.
- In order for this patient to receive appropriate wound care and home IV therapy if judged necessary, she needs to establish secure and comfortable living arrangements for the time of therapy.

Optimal Plan

4. Outline a drug regimen that would provide optimal initial empiric therapy for the infection.

- This diabetic foot infection has significant involvement of the skin and skin structures with deep tissue involvement. Moreover, the area of cellulitis and induration exceeded 2 cm (4 × 5 cm). Even though this is her first foot infection and is more likely to be caused by a single organism, one cannot rule out the presence of a polymicrobial infection because of the extensive skin and skin structure involvement. Initial empiric IV therapy is appropriate in serious cases of diabetic foot infection such as this one.[2–3]
- As discussed, a number of treatment options are appropriate for empiric therapy of diabetic foot infections. The antimicrobial therapy selection may be based on institutional cost and drug availability through the formulary system. Any one of the following regimens is appropriate as monotherapy because each has good coverage of the most commonly involved organisms (including both aerobic and anaerobic bacteria) and a good safety profile.
  - ✓ Ampicillin/sulbactam 1.5 to 3 g IV Q 6 H; the higher dosage should be reserved for serious infections in patients with poor peripheral circulation
  - ✓ Cefotetan 2 g IV Q 12 H
  - ✓ Cefoxitin 1 to 2 g IV Q 8 H
- Other acceptable IV alternatives given as monotherapy include ticarcillin/clavulanate 3.1 g IV Q 6 H, piperacillin/tazobactam 3.375 g IV Q 6 H, or imipenem/cilastatin 500 mg IV Q 6 H. These agents should not be considered first-choice therapy because they are often restricted for more severe/life-threatening nosocomial infections due to their broader spectrum of activity, to prevent the development of resistance, and to reduce treatment costs.
- Clindamycin 900 mg IV Q 8 H in combination with cefazolin 1 to 2 g IV Q 8 H is also appropriate in this case. However, this two-drug regimen is less convenient than monotherapy and is more often associated with *Clostridium difficile* colitis because of clindamycin.

Outcome Evaluation

5. a. What clinical and laboratory parameters are necessary to evaluate your therapy for achievement of the desired therapeutic outcomes and monitoring for adverse effects?

- Regardless of the drug chosen, improvement in the signs and symptoms of infection and healing of the wound with prevention of limb amputation are the primary end points.

- Decreased swelling, induration, and erythema should be observed after 72 to 96 hours of appropriate antimicrobial therapy and surgical debridement. The response to therapy is often patient dependent, and in some cases, improvement may not be seen for up to 7 to 10 days of treatment.
- A decrease in cloudy drainage and formation of new scar tissue are signs of positive response to therapy that may take up to 7 to 14 days to be seen.
- A WBC count and differential should be performed every 48 to 72 hours for the first week or until normalization if less than 1 week, and weekly thereafter until the end of therapy. Monitoring should continue until therapy is completed because neutropenia has been associated with many antibiotics (e.g., ampicillin/sulbactam, cefotetan, cefoxitin).
- BUN and serum creatinine should be monitored weekly while on therapy to detect the development of renal toxicity from certain antibiotics such as nafcillin (acute interstitial nephritis) and aminoglycosides.
- Question the patient to detect any unusual side effects related to the drug or infusion (e.g., rash, nausea, vomiting, diarrhea) daily for the first 3 to 5 days and then weekly thereafter.

▶ ## Follow-up Questions

b. What therapeutic alternatives are available for treating this patient once results of cultures are known to contain MSSA?

- Once the culture results are available and the involved organism(s) is (are) considered pathogenic and responsible for the infectious process, therapy should be targeted at the specific organism(s). Penicillinase-resistant penicillins such as nafcillin, oxacillin, or methicillin are the first-line choices for skin and soft tissue infections caused by MSSA. Methicillin may be more nephrotoxic than the other two agents.
- Other IV therapies that could also be considered include the first-generation cephalosporins (e.g., cefazolin) or ampicillin/sulbactam. Ampicillin/sulbactam is a restricted antibiotic in many institutions and is more expensive than the other alternatives.
- Clindamycin and vancomycin are effective alternatives in penicillin-allergic patients. The use of vancomycin should be limited to patients with severe penicillin allergy in whom the use of cephalosporins or other alternatives should be avoided in order to prevent the development of vancomycin-resistance.

c. Design an optimal drug treatment plan for treating her MSSA infection while she remains hospitalized.

- Because the patient does not have a penicillin allergy, she should be started on either nafcillin 2 g IV Q 4 H or cefazolin 2 g IV Q 8 H. Due to the severity of the infection (i.e., limb-threatening), the possible decrease in blood supply to the area, and the good renal function of the patient, high doses of the antibiotic (>1 g) should be used to assure appropriate drug concentrations at the site of infection.
- The duration of therapy is controversial and based on the patient's personal situation. Therapy should be continued until all signs and symptoms disappear and for at least 2 to 4 weeks total.

Some patients require longer therapy, and wound healing in diabetic patients is often very slow.

- Patients should remain hospitalized until they are afebrile for 24 to 48 hours, have signs of improvement and positive response to therapy (decreased swelling, redness, purulent drainage; normalization of the WBC), and outpatient wound care has been established, either by proper teaching to the patient or through home health care services. This patient will not be able to be discharged until a proper living situation has been found.

d. Design an optimal pharmacotherapeutic plan for completion of her treatment once she has been discharged from the hospital.

- The decision about completion of therapy with IV versus oral therapy is often based on clinical experience, because few clinical trials have been performed on long-term treatment of diabetic foot infections.
- Treatment with oral antibiotics should be considered if the wound is healing well with disappearance of signs and symptoms of infection, there is formation of new scar tissue, and the infection is no longer limb-threatening. Available options are dicloxacillin, cloxacillin, cephalexin, or cephradine, each given in doses of 500 mg po Q 6 H. No studies have demonstrated the superiority of one agent over the others, and the choice is often based on experience, availability, and cost.
- Home IV therapy may be more appropriate in this patient because of the severity of the infection and the very slow improvement observed. Home IV drug therapies suitable for MSSA include nafcillin 2 g IV Q 4 H given via a peristaltic pump, cefazolin 2 g IV Q 8 H, or ceftriaxone 2 g IV Q 24 H. No prospective studies have been performed comparing these 3 agents in this patient population against MSSA. Ampicillin/sulbactam 1.5 to 3 g IV Q 6 H is generally not recommended, because the drug is unstable for the period required with a peristaltic pump and is inconvenient because of the dosing frequency. If the patient was started on nafcillin 2 IV Q 4 H in the hospital, it is more appropriate to continue the same regimen as an outpatient.

Patient Counseling

6. What information should be provided to the patient to enhance compliance, ensure successful therapy, and minimize adverse effects with IV nafcillin?

- Nafcillin, like most antibiotics, may cause diarrhea that could be caused by bacteria known as *Clostridium difficile*. Contact your health care provider immediately if it occurs and before taking any antidiarrheal medicine.
- Contact your doctor or me if any unusual side effects such as rash, shortness of breath, or decreased urine production occur while taking this medicine.
- Contact your home health care provider if pain, redness, or swelling is observed at the IV site.
- The peristaltic pump will deliver the antibiotic every 4 hours for 24 hours, then the bag will need to be changed. Contact your home health care provider if you have any questions or if you notice abnormalities with the pump, such as noise, clogging of the tubing, or air bubbles.

Note: The patient needs to be made aware that osteomyelitis and limb amputation are possible consequences of these infections in diabetic patients. She also needs to be provided with personnel resources (telephone numbers, addresses) to contact if unusual reactions occur while on therapy, if infection worsens, or if she has questions or concerns. Compliance with outpatient clinic follow-up visits is of prime importance for success in this case.